T0212869

Register Now for Online Access to Your Book!

SPRINGER PUBLISHING
CONNECT™

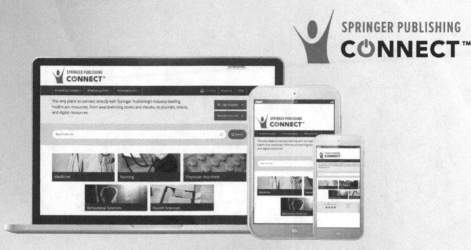

Your print purchase of *Complementary Therapies in Nursing, Ninth Edition*, **includes online access to the contents of your book—**increasing accessibility, portability, and searchability!

Access today at:
http://connect.springerpub.com/content/book/978-0-8261-9499-2
or scan the QR code at the right with your smartphone. Log in or register, then click "Redeem a voucher" and use the code below.

TM7DW0B1

Having trouble redeeming a voucher code?
Go to https://connect.springerpub.com/redeeming-voucher-code

If you are experiencing problems accessing the digital component of this product, please contact our customer service department at cs@springerpub.com

The online access with your print purchase is available at the publisher's discretion and may be removed at any time without notice.

Publisher's Note: New and used products purchased from third-party sellers are not guaranteed for quality, authenticity, or access to any included digital components.

Scan here for quick access.

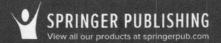

SPRINGER PUBLISHING
View all our products at springerpub.com

Complementary Therapies in Nursing

Ruth Lindquist, PhD, RN, is professor emeritus of nursing and graduate faculty member of the Earl E. Bakken Center for Spirituality and Healing at the University of Minnesota. She is a member of the University of Minnesota Academy of Distinguished Teachers and the Academic Health Center Academy of Excellence in the Scholarship of Teaching and Learning. In her practice and research, Dr. Lindquist uses evidence-based complementary therapies and behavioral strategies to reduce cardiovascular disease risk and promote health-related quality of life. She cofounded an innovative women's only cardiac support group to enhance self-care and transform lifestyles to reduce heart disease risks. As a Densford Scholar in the Katherine J. Densford International Center for Nursing Leadership, she worked with her team to conduct a landmark national survey of critical care nurses' attitudes toward and use of complementary therapies. Complementary therapies have been the core of her care, research, and scholarship for 40 years including co editing this text, now in its 9th edition.

Mary Fran Tracy, PhD, RN, APRN, CCNS, FCNS, FAAN, is an associate professor, University of Minnesota School of Nursing, and an adjunct assistant professor, University of Minnesota Medical School. Dr. Tracy is a fellow of the American Academy of Nursing and a fellow of the Clinical Nurse Specialist Institute, as well as a past president of the American Association of Critical-Care Nurses. Her research focus is on symptom management for acute and critically ill patients. As a Densford Scholar in the Katharine J. Densford International Center for Nursing Leadership, she conducted a national survey of critical care nurses' attitudes toward and use of complementary and alternative therapies, and this survey has been further used by researchers in more than 15 countries.

Mariah Snyder, PhD, is professor emerita, University of Minnesota School of Nursing. Independent nursing interventions and complementary therapies have been the focus of her career. Dr. Snyder studied the effects of complementary therapies in promoting the health and well-being of older adults, particularly those with dementia. She was a founding member of the Earl E. Bakken Center for Spirituality and Healing at the University of Minnesota and instrumental in the establishment of the center's graduate interdisciplinary minor. In retirement, she continues to incorporate complementary therapies in her volunteer activities with women in recovery programs, older adults, and her personal wellness.

Complementary Therapies in Nursing

Promoting Integrative Care

Ninth Edition

Ruth Lindquist, PhD, RN

Mary Fran Tracy, PhD, RN, APRN, CCNS, FCNS, FAAN

Mariah Snyder, PhD

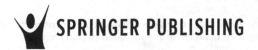

Copyright © 2023 Springer Publishing Company, LLC
All rights reserved.

First Springer Publishing edition 1998 subsequent editions 2001, 2006, 2009, 2013, 2018

No part of this publication may be reproduced, stored in a retrieval system, or transmitted in any form or by any means, electronic, mechanical, photocopying, recording, or otherwise, without the prior permission of Springer Publishing Company, LLC, or authorization through payment of the appropriate fees to the Copyright Clearance Center, Inc., 222 Rosewood Drive, Danvers, MA 01923, 978-750-8400, fax 978-646-8600, info@copyright.com or on the Web at www.copyright.com.

Springer Publishing Company, LLC
11 West 42nd Street, New York, NY 10036
www.springerpub.com
connect.springerpub.com/

Acquisitions Editor: Rachel X. Landes
Compositor: Amnet Systems

ISBN: 978-0-8261-9495-4
ebook ISBN: 978-0-8261-9499-2
DOI: 10.1891/9780826194992

Printed by BnT

The author and the publisher of this Work have made every effort to use sources believed to be reliable to provide information that is accurate and compatible with the standards generally accepted at the time of publication. Because medical science is continually advancing, our knowledge base continues to expand. Therefore, as new information becomes available, changes in procedures become necessary. We recommend that the reader always consult current research and specific institutional policies before performing any clinical procedure or delivering any medication. The author and publisher shall not be liable for any special, consequential, or exemplary damages resulting, in whole or in part, from the readers' use of, or reliance on, the information contained in this book. The publisher has no responsibility for the persistence or accuracy of URLs for external or third-party Internet websites referred to in this publication and does not guarantee that any content on such websites is, or will remain, accurate or appropriate.

Library of Congress Cataloging-in-Publication Data

Names: Lindquist, Ruth (Professor of nursing) editor. | Tracy, Mary Fran, editor. | Snyder, Mariah, editor.
Title: Complementary therapies in nursing : promoting integrative care / [edited by] Ruth Lindquist, Mary Fran Tracy, Mariah Snyder.
Other titles: Complementary & alternative therapies in nursing.
Description: Ninth edition. | New York, NY : Springer Publishing Company, [2023] | Preceded by Complementary and alternative therapies in nursing / Ruth Lindquist, Mary Fran Tracy, Mariah Snyder, editors. Eighth edition. 2018. | Includes bibliographical references and index.
Identifiers: LCCN 2022006702 (print) | LCCN 2022006703 (ebook) | ISBN 9780826194954 (paperback) | ISBN 9780826194992 (ebook)
Subjects: MESH: Holistic Nursing | Complementary Therapies—nursing
Classification: LCC RT42 (print) | LCC RT42 (ebook) | NLM WY 86.5 | DDC 610.73—dc23/eng/20220512
LC record available at https://lccn.loc.gov/2022006702
LC ebook record available at https://lccn.loc.gov/2022006703

Contact sales@springerpub.com to receive discount rates on bulk purchases.

Publisher's Note: New and used products purchased from third-party sellers are not guaranteed for quality, authenticity, or access to any included digital components.

Printed in the United States of America.

We dedicate this book to nurses and other care providers who diligently seek to enhance the healing and well-being of others with the evidence-informed use of complementary therapies. We are continually awed by the ingenuity, love, and kindness flowing at the bedside, in the community, or at a distance with hands, heart and technology. Indeed, the day-to-day courage, commitment, and heart of all healthcare workers truly inspired us as they continued their work of service and caring through the COVID-19 pandemic.

Contents

Contributors

Marilyn P. Bach, MS, RN, CHTP
Independent Practitioner
Eagan, Minnesota

Susan Bee, MS, RN, PMHCNS-BC
Clinical Nurse Specialist
Pain Clinic
Mayo Clinic
Rochester, Minnesota

Frank Bennett, PhD, MDiv, BSc
Senior Fellow, Earl E. Bakken Center for Spirituality and Healing
University of Minnesota
Minneapolis, Minnesota

Kasey R. Boehmer, PhD, MPH, NBC-HWC
Assistant Professor of Health Sciences Research
Knowledge and Evaluation Research (KER) Unit
Division of Health Care Delivery Research
Mayo Clinic
Rochester, Minnesota

Carie A. Braun, PhD, RN, CNE
Professor and Chair
Department of Nursing
College of Saint Benedict/Saint John's University
St. Joseph, Minnesota

Ulf G. Bronäs, PhD, ATC, FSVM, FAHA
Associate Professor and Director of the Laboratory of Vascular
    and Cognitive Health
University of Illinois Chicago
Chicago, Illinois

Miriam Cameron, PhD, MS, MA, RN
Lead Faculty, Yoga and Tibetan Medicine Focus Area and Graduate Faculty
Earl E. Bakken Center for Spiritual and Healing, University of Minnesota
Minneapolis, Minnesota

Kuei-Min Chen, PhD, RN, FAAN
Professor, College of Nursing
Director, Center for Long-Term Care Research
Founding Director, Master Program of Long-Term Care in Aging
Kaohsiung Medical University
Kaohsiung, Taiwan

Corjena K. Cheung, PhD, MS, RN, FGSA
Professor and Associate Dean
Hong Kong Adventist College
Hong Kong, China

Linda L. Chlan, PhD, RN, ATSF, FAAN
Associate Dean for Nursing Research, Division of Nursing Research
Professor of Nursing, Mayo Clinic College of Medicine and
    Science
Mayo Clinic
Rochester, Minnesota

Michael S. Christopher, PhD
Professor and Director of Clinical Training
Clinical Psychology PhD Program
School of Graduate Psychology, Pacific University
Forest Grove, Oregon

Dana Dharmakaya Colgan, PhD, MEd, C-IAYT
Junior Faculty and Licensed Clinical Psychologist
Department of Neurology
Oregon Health and Science University
Portland, Oregon

**Cynthia Lee Dols Finn, DNP, MN, PHN, CNE,
    AHN-BC, CHTP/A**
Associate Professor
Department of Nursing
St. Catherine University
St. Paul, Minnesota

Michele M. Evans, MS, APRN, PMHCNS-BC
Clinical Nurse Specialist, Pain Rehabilitation Center
Assistant Professor of Psychiatry Mayo Clinic
Rochester, Minnesota

Maura Fitzgerald, MS, MA, APRN, CNS
Clinical Nurse Specialist, Retired
Minneapolis, Minnesota

Melissa H. Frisvold, PhD, RN, CNM
Assistant Professor
School of Nursing and Health Sciences, Georgetown University
Washington, D. C.

Thóra Jenný Gunnarsdóttir, PhD, RN
Associate Professor Faculty of Nursing
University of Iceland
Reykjavik, Iceland

Linda L. Halcón, PhD, MPH, RN
Associate Professor Emeritus
School of Nursing, University of Minnesota
Minneapolis, Minnesota

Margo A. Halm, PhD, RN, NEA-BC
Associate Chief Nurse Executive, Nursing Research and Evidence-Based Practice
VA Portland Health Care System
Portland, Oregon

Melodee Harris, PhD, RN, APRN, FAAN
Associate Professor
College of Nursing
University of Arkansas for Medical Sciences
Little Rock, Arkansas

Annie Heiderscheit, PhD, MT-BC, LMFT
Director of Music Therapy
Associate Professor of Music
Augsburg University
Minneapolis, Minnesota

Susan Heitzman, MS, RN, PMHCNS-BC
University of Minnesota Medical Center, Fairview
Minneapolis, Minnesota

Lauren Johnson, MS, RN, CHTP
Independent Practitioner
Richfield, Minnesota

Avis Johnson-Smith, DNP, APRN, CPNP-PC, FNP-BC, CPMHS, CNS, FAANP
Professor, Family Nurse Practitioner Program
Angelo State University
San Angelo, Texas
Healthy Kids and Families Wellness Center, LLC
Albany, Georgia

Mary Jo Kreitzer, PhD, RN, FAAN
Director, Earl E. Bakken Center for Spirituality and Healing
Professor, School of Nursing, University of Minnesota
Minneapolis, Minnesota

Mary Langevin, MSN, RN, FNP-C, CPON
Cancer and Blood Disorders Clinic
Children's Hospitals and Clinics Minnesota
Minneapolis, Minnesota

Angela S. Lillehei, PhD, MPH, RN
Associate Editor and Managing Editor
EXPLORE: The Journal of Science & Healing
Consultant, Health and Healing
Minneapolis, Minnesota

Ruth Lindquist, PhD, RN
Professor Emerita
School of Nursing, University of Minnesota
Minneapolis, Minnesota

Margaret P. Moss, PhD, JD, RN, FAAN
Enrolled Member, Mandan, Hidatsa, and Arikara Nation, North Dakota
Associate Vice President Equity and Inclusion (interim)
Associate Professor, School of Nursing, The University of British Columbia
Director, First Nations House of Learning
Vancouver, British Columbia, Canada

Tenzin Namdul, TMD, PhD
TRACT TL1 Postdoctoral Scholar
Postdoctoral Fellow, Division of Epidemiology and Community Health
School of Public Health, University of Minnesota
Graduate Faculty, Earl E. Bakken Center for Spirituality and Healing
University of Minnesota
Minneapolis, Minnesota

Susan O'Conner-Von, PhD, RN-BC, CNE, FNAP
Professor
School of Nursing, University of Minnesota
Minneapolis, Minnesota

Gregory A. Plotnikoff, MD, MTS, FACP
Minnesota Personalized Medicine
Minneapolis, Minnesota

Barbara Riegel, PhD, RN, FAHA, FAAN
Co-Director, International Center for Self-Care Research
Professor Emerita, School of Nursing, University of Pennsylvania
Philadelphia, Pennsylvania

Debbie Ringdahl, DNP, RN, CNM
Clinical Associate Professor *ad Honorem*
School of Nursing, University of Minnesota
Minneapolis, Minnesota

Dereck L. Salisbury, PhD
Assistant Professor
School of Nursing, University of Minnesota
Minneapolis, Minnesota

Erica Schorr, PhD, RN
Associate Professor
School of Nursing, University of Minnesota
Minneapolis, Minnesota

Akeesha Simmons, MA
PhD Student
School of Graduate Psychology, Pacific University
Forest Grove, Oregon

Mariah Snyder, PhD
Professor Emerita
School of Nursing, University of Minnesota
Minneapolis, Minnesota

Janet Tomaino, DNP, RN
Certified Clinical Aromatherapy Practitioner/
    DNP Integrative Nurse Consultant
Instructor, Earl E. Bakken Center for Spirituality and Healing
University of Minnesota
Minneapolis, Minnesota

Mary Fran Tracy, PhD, RN, APRN, CCNS, FCNS, FAAN
Associate Professor
School of Nursing, University of Minnesota
Minneapolis, Minnesota

Diane Treat-Jacobson, PhD, RN, FAAN
Professor and Associate Dean for Research
Cora Meidl Siehl Chair in Nursing Research for Improved Care
School of Nursing, University of Minnesota
Minneapolis, Minnesota

Alexa W. Umbreit, MS, RN, CHTP, CCP
Independent Practitioner
St. Paul, Minnesota

Shigeaki Watanuki, PhD, RN
Professor
Gerontic Nursing
School of Nursing, National College of Nursing
Tokyo, Japan

Pamela Weiss-Farnan, PhD, MPH, RN, Dip.Ac., L.Ac.
Independent Licensed Acupuncturist
St. Paul, Minnesota

Elizabeth A. Williams, PhD, RN
Assistant Professor
East Carolina University
Greenville, North Carolina

Jaclene A. Zauszniewski, PhD, RN-BC, FAAN
Kate Hanna Harvey Professor in Community Health Nursing
Frances Payne Bolton School of Nursing, Case Western Reserve University
Cleveland, Ohio

Terri Zborowsky PhD, RN, EDAC, CPXP
HGA Design Researcher
St. Paul, Minnesota

INTERNATIONAL CONTRIBUTORS

AUSTRALIA
Trisha Dunning, PhD, RN, CDE, MEd
School of Nursing and Midwifery
Melbourne Burwood Campus
Barwon Health, Deakin University
Victoria, Australia

BRAZIL
Eneida Rejane Rabelo Da Silva, ScD, RN
Professor
School of Nursing, Universidade Federal do Rio Grande do Sul
Researcher, The Brazilian National Council for Scientific
    and Technological Development
Cardiology Division-Heart Failure Clinic and Transplant Group,
    Hospital de Clinicas
Porto Alegre, RS, Brazil

Graziella Badin Aliti, RN, MSc, ScD
Associate Professor
School of Nursing, Universidade Federal do Rio Grande do Sul
Porto Alegre, RS, Brazil

Omar Pereira de Almeida Neto, MSc, ScD, RN
Professor, Department of Heart Failure Research
Universidade Federal de Uberlândia
Minas Gerais, Brazil

Isabel Rossato
Physical Education
Hospital de Clínicas de Porto Alegre
Porto Alegre, RS, Brazil

Paula Eustáquio
Pedagogue
Hospital de Clínicas de Porto Alegre
Porto Alegre, RS, Brazil

Amália de Fátima Lucena, ScD, RN
Professor
Graduate Program in Nursing, Universidade Federal do Rio Grande do Sul
Hospital de Clínicas de Porto Alegre and Grupo de Estudo e Pesquisa em
    Enfermagem no Cuidado ao Adulto e Idoso (GEPECADI)
Porto Alegre, RS, Brazil

Lisiane Pruinelli, PhD, MS, RN
Assistant Professor
School of Nursing, University of Minnesota
Minneapolis, Minnesota

Milena Flória-Santos, PhD, MS, RN
Assistant Professor
Department of Maternal-Infant Nursing and Public Health
Ribeirão Preto College of Nursing, University of São Paulo at Ribeirao
WHO Collaborating Centre for Nursing Research Development
São Paulo, Brazil

CANADA
Margaret P. Moss, PhD, JD, RN, FAAN
Enrolled Member, Mandan, Hidatsa, and Arikara Nation, North Dakota
Director, First Nations House of Learning
Associate Vice President Equity and Inclusion (interim)
Associate Professor, School of Nursing, The University of British Columbia
Faculty of Applied Sciences
Vancouver, British Columbia, Canada

CHINA
Fang Yu, PhD, RN, GNP-BC, FGSA, FAAN
Professor and Edson Chair in Dementia Translational Nursing Science
Edson College of Nursing and Health Innovation, Arizona State University
Phoenix, Arizona

Sarah Walker
ESL Teacher, Abroad
Academy of New York
Warsaw, Poland

DENMARK
Leila Eriksen
Registered Alternative Therapist (RAB)
København, Hovedstaden, Denmark

ECUADOR
Sue Kagel, BSN, RN, HNB-BC, CHTP/I
Healing Touch Practice, Canyon Ranch Health Resort
Andrew Weil Center of Integrative Medicine, University of Arizona
Adjunct Faculty
Past President of Healing Touch International
Tucson, Arizona

FINLAND
Reino Lindqvist, BSc
Agronomist
Marttila, Finland

FRANCE
Chris Lepoutre
Certified in Traditional Chinese Medicine Acupuncture in France
Energy Healing Therapist
North Oaks, Minnesota

GREECE
Ioanna Gryllaki, BSN
School of Nursing, University of Minnesota
Minneapolis, Minnesota

HONG KONG
Corjena K. Cheung, PhD, MS (USA), RN, FGSA (Gerontology)
Associate Academic Dean/Professor
Chair, Deartment of Nursing
Hong Kong Adventist College
Hong Kong

HONG KONG and AUSTRALIA
George Dovas, BCom
Certified Iyengar Yoga Teacher
Director, Iyengar Yoga Centre of Hong Kong
Hong Kong

ICELAND
Thóra Jenný Gunnarsdóttir, PhD, RN
Associate Professor Faculty of Nursing
University of Iceland
Reykjavik, Iceland

INDIA
Sumathy Sundar, PhD
Director, Chennai School of Music Therapy
Director, Center for Music Therapy Education and Research
Mahatma Gandhi Medical College and Research Institute
Sri Balaji Vidyapeeth University
Pondicherry, India
Chair, Education and Training Commission, World Federation of Music Therapy
Founding Member, International Association for Music and Medicine

INDIA and TIBET
Tenzin Namdul, TMD, PhD
TRACT TL1 Postdoctoral Scholar
Postdoctoral Fellow, Division of Epidemiology and Community Health
School of Public Health, University of Minnesota
Graduate Faculty, Earl E. Bakken Center for Spirituality and Healing
Minneapolis, Minnesota

IRAN
Mansour Hadidi, MS (Architecture), MS (Management Information Systems)
Information Technology Specialist
Minnesota Department of Health
St. Paul, Minnesota

JAPAN
Ikuko Ebihara, MBA
Third Degree Reiki Practitioner
NPO Reiki Association, Japanese Reiki Association
St. Paul, Minnesota

Sensei Hyakuten Inamoto
Buddist Monk, Pure Land School
International Reiki Teacher
Kyoto, Japan

Kenji Watanabe, MD, PhD
Keio University Center for Kampo Medicine, Shinjuku-ku
Tokyo, Japan

Shigeaki Watanuki, PhD, RN
Professor of Gerontological Nursing
Faculty of Nursing/Graduate School of Nursing
National College of Nursing
Tokyo, Japan

KENYA
Eunice M. Areba, PhD, RN, PHN
Clinical Assistant Professor
School of Nursing, University of Minnesota
Minneapolis, Minnesota
Mombasa, Kenya

LIBERIA
Maria Tarlue Keita, NP, RN
Allina Health Home Health
St. Paul, Minnesota

MEXICO
Karim Bauza, BSN, RN
Nursing Medical Cardiology ICU
St. Mary's Hospital
Rochester, Minnesota

NEW ZEALAND
Theresa Fleming, PhD
Honorary Academic, Population Health
Medical and Health Sciences
University of Auckland
Auckland, New Zealand
Associate Professor
School of Health, Victoria University of Wellington
Wellington, New Zealand

Matthew Shepherd, DClinPsy, PGHCertHSc, BSW
Associate Professor
School of Psychology
Massey University, University of Auckland
Auckland, New Zealand

NIGERIA
Gladys Igbo, MS, RN
Founder, Synergy Wellness Boutique
Staff Nurse, Abbott Northwestern Hospital
Minneapolis, Minnesota

Onome Henry Osokpo, PhD, MSc, MSN, RN
Provost Postdoctoral Fellow and Postdoctoral Research Fellow
NewCourtland Center for Transitions and Health
School of Nursing, University of Pennsylvania
Philadelphia, Pennsylvania

NORWAY
Ingeborg Pedersen, PhD
Researcher, Department of Public Health Science
Norwegian University of Life Sciences
Ås, Norway

PAKISTAN
Naheed Meghani, PhD, MS, BSN, RN
Medtronic
Minneapolis, Minnesota

PALESTINE and the UNITED ARAB EMIRATES
Jehad Adwan, PhD, RN
Assistant Professor of Nursing
Minnesota State University, Mankato
Mankato, Minnesota

PERU
Miryam Benites Cerna
César Vallejo University
Trujillo, Peru

PHILIPPINES
Marlene Dohm, MS
Retired Clinical Nurse
Minneapolis, Minnesota

Leticia Lantican, PhD
Associate Professor Emerita
School of Nursing, University of Texas at El Paso
El Paso, Texas

SINGAPORE
Siok-Bee Tan, PhD, APN, RN
Deputy Director, Nursing
Singapore General Hospital
Republic of Singapore

SOMALIA
Nasra Giama, DNP, RN, PHN
Clinical Associate Professor
Assistant Director of Inclusivity, Diversity and Equity
School of Nursing, University of Minnesota
Minneapolis, Minnesota
Assistant Professor of Medicine
Mayo Clinic
Rochester, Minnesota

SOUTH AFRICA
Karin Gerber
Nelson Mandela University
Summerstrand, Port Elizabeth, South Africa

SOUTH KOREA
Sohye Lee, PhD, RN
Assistant Professor
Loewenberg College of Nursing, The University of Memphis
Memphis, Tennessee

SWEDEN
Anna Strömberg
Department of Health, Medicine and Caring Sciences (HMV), Division
    of Nursing Sciences and Reproductive Health
Linköping University
Linköping, Sweden

Ulf G. Bronäs, PhD, ATC, FSVM, FAHA
Associate Professor
Department of Biobehavioral Nursing Science
College of Nursing, The University of Illinois at Chicago
Chicago, Illinois

TAIWAN
Jing-Jy Sellin Wang, PhD
Professor and Chair
Department of Nursing
College of Medicine, National Cheng Kung University
Tainan City, Taiwan

Miaofen Yen, PhD, RN, FAAN
Professor and Director of International Studies
Department of Nursing,
College of Medicine, National Cheng Kung University
Tainan City, Taiwan

THAILAND
Kesanee Boonyawatanangkool, APN
Nursing Division
Srinagarind Hospital Faculty of Medicine
Khon Kaen University
Khon Kaen, Thailand

Nutchanart Bunthumporn, PhD, RN
Faculty of Nursing
Thammasat University
Khlong Luang, Pathum Thani, Thailand

Sukjai Charoensuk, PhD, RN
Boromarajonani College of Nursing
Chon Buri, Thailand

Thanchanok Wongvibul, MSN, RN
PhD Student
College of Nursing, The Ohio State University
Columbus, Ohio

TIBET
Tashi Llamo, DTMS, BSN, RN
Tibetan Medicine Practitioner
Mercy Hospital, Unity Campus
Fridley, Minnesota

UGANDA
Faith R. K. Sebuliba, PhD, RN/M, DHT
Lecturer, Nursing and Midwifery Department
Uganda Christian University
Mukono, Uganda

UNITED KINGDOM
Graeme D. Smith, PhD, BA, FEANS, RGN
Professor
School of Health Sciences, Caritas Institute of Higher Education
Edinburgh, United Kingdom

Jacqui Stringer
Clinical and Research Lead, Complementary Health and Wellbeing Services
The Christie NHS Foundation Trust
Manchester, United Kingdom

UNITED STATES
Nicole Englebert, PhD, LP
Psychologist
Children's Hospital and Clinics of Minnesota
Minneapolis, Minnesota

Michelle McGrorey, BSN, RN, HNB-BC, HTCP, NCCA, OCN, HMIP
Integrative Therapies Nurse
University Medical Center of Southern Nevada
Las Vegas, Nevada

Deborah McKinney, BSN, RN, HMIP
Integrative Therapies Nurse
University Medical Center of Southern Nevada
Las Vegas, Nevada

Foreword

Complementary therapies unmask the self-healing wisdom of the body. Complementary therapies blend well with self-awareness: an awareness of one's human evolution toward natural healing and environmental health. Ideally, we have within us an evolutionary inclination to restore our health spontaneously, enhance the health of those around us, and instinctively protect the world in which we live. Neglect of these naturally evolving, self-healing abilities may cause us to experience various diseases for which chosen remedies often contradict natural processes. Often labeled "natural," some complementary therapies may be ineffective and possibly harmful when combined with some allopathic medicines if deep self-awareness is not involved. Such deep awareness can be achieved through mindfulness and meditation or at least an ability to ponder on what is invited into our bodies, minds, and souls.

Perhaps the original, foundational element of complementary therapy is intentionality, essentially an inclination toward seeking and intending that an intervention is of benefit to self, others, or both. Within the past several decades, an evolving understanding of the power of intentionality, especially in terms of interpersonal human reciprocity with the natural environment, has been achieved through research within the discipline of caring science, and it portends to have an ever-greater influence over universal human activity in the future. Intentionality is, perhaps, the only means of human survival. Much of modern medicine originates from natural resources. However, a respect for, awareness of, and communion with those same natural resources appear to have been overshadowed by commercial interests. Such interests not only obscure access to natural remedies but also cloud interpersonal human caring relationships, so essential to healing.

Born and raised in Bath, United Kingdom, I was exposed to complementary therapy at an early age. My dad once obtained from an herbalist a plant-derived anxiolytic for me to take prior to a piano recital. He sometimes used herbals to supplement the typical medical remedies my mother would obtain from our family physician. My own willingness to combine valid complementary therapies with Western medical interventions persists to this day. For example, my current physician endorsed my use of tart cherry juice as an effective therapy for gouty arthritis and referred to his own coauthorship of research findings that tart cherry juice can be as effective as ibuprofen in relieving this type of pain.

There appears to be no doubt that a complementary relationship between natural and artificial medicines is essential and necessary. Natural evolution is perhaps a process of refinement, a process no less important than the evolution of modern medicine. However, nature does not appear to ignore and neglect its origins, since without direct access to its past, there would be no ability to return to a natural beginning from which alternative paths can be taken. In essence, complementary and alternative therapies provide a time-transcendent portal to return to the original gifts of nature and self-healing in a never-ending process of discovery and rediscovery. An ongoing evolution of complementary therapies with modern medicines is full of promise for the future, especially in a greater potential synergy of subjective patient self-awareness pertaining to what is suggested by the wisdom of nature and its skilled interpreters, as well as in research that evolves from objective assessments of group responses to large-scale organized medicine. The practice-relevant and evidence-based information related to complementary therapies contained in *Complementary Therapies in Nursing: Promoting Integrative Care, Ninth Edition,* will assist more nurses and healthcare professionals to integrate these therapies into the provision of care to their clients.

Patrick J Dean, RN, EDD, OSTJ
Clinical Associate Professor *ad Honorem*
School of Nursing, University of Minnesota
Past-President, International Association for Human Caring

Preface

EQUIPPING NURSES AND NURSING STUDENTS FOR GLOBALLY AWARE, CULTURALLY SENSITIVE CARE

The ninth edition of this award-winning book continues to offer fresh, new, readily accessible, and timely information regarding important and most commonly used complementary therapies. These can be introduced to graduate and undergraduate nursing students in educational programs and used by entry-level, more experienced, and advanced practice nurses for professional practice and self-care. Credible information is needed to provide the safe and effective use of complementary therapies, both for consumers and for practitioners (Lin et al., 2021; World Health Organization, 2019). This book is a valuable resource as a handbook for nursing students, working nurses, and advanced practice nurses who desire to increase the use of complementary therapies in their practice. Using these therapies can enhance health, well-being, and the quality of life of patients; improve the quality of care; and improve satisfaction outcomes. Complementary therapies and integrative health approaches can be used by nurses to address the needs of the whole person, including their body, mind, emotion, and spirit (American Holistic Nurses Association, 2016; American Holistic Nurses Association/American Nurses Association, 2019).

We are excited to share what's new in complementary therapies and their application to the care of patients. The ninth edition significantly expands on the content of previous editions and brings the most current research and practice advances together within the cover of one book. Outdated information has been removed while fresh new topics and content have been added. The book highlights many recent advances in technology, including digital apps that can help nurses stay informed to effectively apply the therapies to patient populations. There is carefully considered safety and precaution content, with helpful tips for selecting practitioners for therapy delivery or referral. Expanded content is included related to technology and digital resources fostering safe, informed, effective, and efficient delivery of therapies.

What is unique about this book is that it is written with a specific focus on therapy delivery by nurses and nursing students. There are countless therapies or derivations of therapies existent in the world—too many to be included in one text! The therapies selected for inclusion in this text were those that are generally associated with the term complementary therapies, commonly used by nurses, and most are included in the National Center for Complementary and Integrative Health (NCCIH, 2021) A to Z index. Those most familiar and commonly used by nurses were selected because they were also deemed to have the most promise for nurses to readily apply in their practice. Thus, all the therapies in this text were selected because they are within the scope of nursing practice. The therapy chapters follow a standard format for ease of comprehension and quick reference for the practicing nurse. Along with definitions and descriptions of the selected therapies, the book provides a background for each therapy, as well as the scientific basis and current evidence for the use of therapies for a variety of patient populations. The therapies expand what nurses can offer in the scope of their practice to meet the diverse needs of their patients for a broad range of health conditions. Each chapter contains a practice protocol that describes the basic steps of an intervention along with a section on measurement of outcomes. There is updated information regarding regulation, legal concerns, and credentialing. Useful information from credible national and international web and text-based sources is included throughout each chapter along with the inclusion of websites at the end of the chapters for readers who want more information.

The chapters are written by prominent experts in their field. In this edition, the Foreword is written by Patrick Dean, a national leader in human caring. His thoughtful reflections in the Foreword reflect his keen vision and leadership roles in the national organization of the International Association of Human Caring, where he models the philosophy of culturally sensitive humanistic patient-centered care. Many of the therapies included in this text can also be self-administered by nurses, students, patients, and families as part of their self-care regimen. To that end, there is new and enhanced content on using complementary therapies for nurses' and patients' self-care included in the chapter written by Dr. Barbara Riegel, a prominent nurse scientist and international leader in the field. Likewise, the authors of each chapter have considered the relevance of their topic to self-care. Importantly, the chapter on integrating therapies into practice has been significantly revised, including numerous examples of institution-wide or organization-wide complementary therapy programs. This chapter (Chapter 28), written by Dr. Cynthia Lee Dols Finn, provides useful strategies and models that can serve as readily modifiable blueprints for their integration in other practice settings.

There is literally a *world of therapies!* Indeed, in this text, an amazing group of more than 80 contributing professionals share perspectives on complementary therapies from more than 30 countries and 6 continents, spanning the globe (Figure 1).

The ninth edition features new and expanded international content and content highlighting Indigenous culture-based therapies. The global perspectives provided in each chapter are uniquely needed in today's world in which immigration, refugees, and travel create a necessity to know the health practices of other cultures. Indeed, complementary therapies are used by nurses around the globe. The international sidebars included in each chapter insert rich global perspectives on the therapies and enrich our appreciation for cultural derivations and applications of the therapies. The sharing of stories and perspectives of their use by nurses and individuals in numerous other countries and cultures in the section on cultural uses within the chapters and the international sidebars included deepens our understanding of our diverse patients and fosters the delivery of more culturally sensitive care.

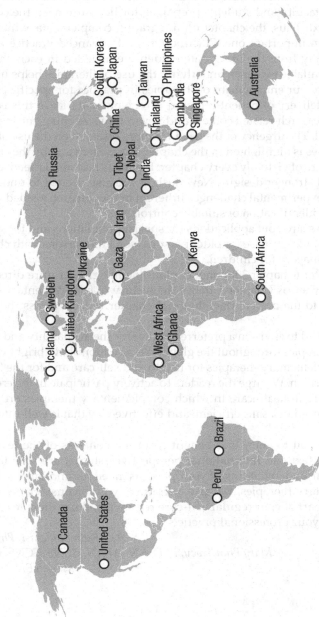

Figure 1 Contributors from around the world. A sampling of the wide-ranging geographic locations depicted here.

This edition satisfies the requirement of the American Association of Colleges of Nursing for knowledge of complementary therapies as essential content for BSN and post-BSN programs and will assist students in their study for the NCLEX-RN® exam (National Council of State Boards of Nursing [NCSBN®], 2018). With complementary therapies integrated into the NCLEX-RN® exam, now more than ever nursing faculty and students preparing for licensure need the content provided by the text. Thus, the chapter on integrating complementary therapies into education is an important one. Practitioners and advanced practice nurses can benefit especially from the up-to-date evidence embedded in each chapter. The inclusion of available evidence underlying the use of therapies helps us consider the wisdom of our employment of therapies in practice for specific patient conditions in the delivery of patient-centered care. New material in this edition includes updated research-related content and new references citing cutting-edge research in the field. The urgency of the need for more research on the use of complementary therapies is highlighted in the chapter on research and by the chapter authors in the closure of virtually every chapter. Rigorous research is needed with larger samples and stronger designs. New designs are also needed to undergird and overcome the experimental challenges inherent in the research needed in this area, including the identification of suitable controls.

We continue to search out applications for special populations and for special conditions, for example, exercise for older persons, yoga for persons with chronic pain, and guided imagery for children.

The final chapter (Chapter 30) ponders plausible imagined future directions of the field. And, whereas Chapter 1 traces the history of complementary therapies through time to the present day, the final chapter reflects across therapies and future trends.

Readers are asked to envision a preferred future for the availability and use of complementary therapies throughout the globe. We, as editors, have bright visions for the use of complementary therapies for health and self-care and for the "new" therapies on the horizon. We urge the readers to actively participate in the creation of a preferred future in healthcare in which complementary therapies are available, selected, and used in a safe, efficient, and effective way that is well-informed by the evidence.

We encourage you to enjoy and benefit from the contents of the text. The information in the text and international perspectives shared are sure to help you to grow in your understanding of your patients' need for and interest in the use of complementary therapies. We also encourage you to consider the use of these therapies as part of your regular self-care regimen and use them to expand the dimensions of your professional practice.

Ruth Lindquist, PhD, RN
Mary Fran Tracy, PhD, RN, APRN, CCNS, FCNS, FAAN
Mariah Snyder, PhD

REFERENCES

American Holistic Nurses Association. (2016). *Position on the role of nurses in the practice of complementary and integrative health approaches* (CIHA). http://www.ahna.org/LinkClick.aspx?fileticket=Gdt_dxWvaqk%3Dportalid=66

American Holistic Nurses Association/American Nurses Association. (2019). *Holistic nursing scope and standards of practice* (3rd ed.). AHNA/ANA. ISBN # 978-1-947800-39-7

National Center for Complementary and Integrative Health. (2021). *Health topics A to Z.* https://www.nccih.nih.gov/health/atoz

National Council of State Boards of Nursing. (2018). *NCLEX-RN® examination: Test plan for the National Council Licensure Examination for Registered Nurses. NCSBN®.* https://www.ncsbn.org/2019_RN_TestPlan-English.pdf

Lin, L. W., Ananthakrishnan, A., Teerawattananon, Y. (2021). Evaluating traditional and complementary medicines: Where do we go from here? *International Journal of Technology Assessment in Health Care, 37,* e45, 1–6. https://doi.org/10.1017/S0266462321000179

World Health Organization. (2019). *WHO global report on traditional and complementary medicine 2019.* https://apps.who.int/iris/bitstream/handle/10665/312342/9789241515436-eng.pdf?sequence=1isAllowed=y. ISBN 978-92-4-151543-6

Foundations for Practice

KUEI-MIN CHEN

Complementary therapies have become widely known and used in Western healthcare, particularly in nursing. According to the National Center for Complementary and Integrative Health (NCCIH, 2017), a national survey in the United States documented that 62% of American adults use complementary therapies. The use of these therapies also occurs on a global scale. Throughout the text, perspectives from individuals worldwide provide a view of the use of complementary therapies in their respective countries. Not only are complementary therapies used within conventional healthcare, but other systems of care and the healing practices initiated a millennium ago are also receiving increasing attention. Expanding the perspectives on therapies used in other health systems will provide nurses with knowledge about therapies that are practiced by people in multiple cultures across the globe and will lead to more personalized quality care.

Chapter 1 provides an overview of the long tradition of using complementary therapies in nursing and the growing acceptance of their place in healthcare. In accordance with this growing acceptance and integration into healthcare, the National Center for Complementary and Alternative Medicine changed its title to the NCCIH. The term *integrative health* reflects the blending of complementary therapies and conventional health practices into a healthcare delivery system. Globally, as people migrate for economic reasons, wars, drought, or political factors, it is paramount that healthcare providers be more aware of the great diversity in health practices that exist and secure from patients a thorough assessment of the practices used as some, particularly natural, products may interact with medications being prescribed.

Two therapies—presence (Chapter 2) and therapeutic listening and communication (Chapter 3)—are critical elements in the implementation of any complementary therapies. Many patients and families voice appreciation for a nurse who was "really present when providing care." *Presence* is difficult to define. An adage goes "You know it when you see it." The multiple facets of therapeutic listening and communication (Chapter 3), both verbal and nonverbal, are likewise important keys to providing holistic care. Nonverbal communication, including really listening and observing, can assume even greater importance when interacting with people from other cultures in the context of a therapeutic relationship. The knowledge of customs—as basic as whether it is acceptable to shake the hands of the patient and family or touch someone of another gender—is foundational in establishing the kind of therapeutic relationship integral to the success of complementary therapies.

Chapter 4 focuses on creating an optimal healing environment. A base of evidence about the creation of optimal healing environments is emerging from many disciplines, including nursing, interior design, architecture, neuroscience, psychoneuroimmunology, and environmental psychology. More health facilities are devoting attention to light, color, and other aspects of the environment. In the post-COVID-19 pandemic world, nurses need to be informed about the ways in which the physical environment affects health outcomes so that they can contribute to the design of patient care units and other healthcare facilities that will optimize the health and well-being of patients, their families, and the staff. Research is beginning to substantiate the impact that the environment has on outcomes of care.

Systems of care (Chapter 5), well illustrated by the example of Tibetan medicine, is a chapter describing systems and practices that differ significantly from the conventional system of care with which readers are most familiar. Having a basic understanding of other systems will assist nurses in providing care to the growing diversity of cultures found in patient populations. Although it is unlikely that nurses will ever embrace an entire system of nonconventional healthcare, they may identify a practice or therapy from a system that would be useful for them to use for their patients or for self-care.

Self-care (Chapter 6) was the primary form of healthcare long before the medical establishment as we now know it came into existence. It is performed in both healthy and ill states, although self-care for the healthy general population differs from that prescribed for individuals with a chronic illness. Establishing healthy habits and lifestyle routines early in life can make self-care easier later in life when chronic illness is most likely to mandate some level of self-care. The evidence is convincing that self-care is associated with positive health outcomes. However, for a variety of reasons, people routinely defer self-care, and the formal healthcare system fails to emphasize it. The focus of this chapter is on self-care for nurses and nursing students and the role they play in educating communities, patients, caregivers, and families about the importance of self-care.

REFERENCE

National Center for Complementary and Integrative Health. (2017). *The use of complementary and alternative medicine in the United States.* https://nccih.nih.gov/research/statistics/2007/camsurvey_fs1.htm

1

Evolution and Use of Complementary Therapies and Integrative Health Approaches

MARIAH SNYDER, RUTH LINDQUIST, MARY FRAN TRACY,
AND KUEI-MIN CHEN

Complementary and alternative therapies, or, as occasionally labeled, *unconventional* therapies, have become an integral part of healthcare in the United States and other countries around the world. The word *complementary* conveys that a procedure is used as an adjunct to Western or conventional therapies. The term *alternative*, which had also been in the title of previous editions of this text, is used when a therapy is utilized *in place of* a Western approach to healthcare. This text focuses on selected complementary therapies commonly used by nurses in practice. A term receiving increasing use is *integrative health approaches*, which conveys that both biomedical and complementary therapies or other systems of care are offered by a provider or part of the offerings at a healthcare facility.

The National Institutes of Health (NIH) has changed the title for the unique center that had been created to focus on complementary therapies. Whereas the founding title of the center was the National Center for Complementary and Alternative Medicine (NCCAM), it was more recently changed to the National Center for Complementary and Integrative Health (NCCIH). What is important to note is that in addition to dropping the word *alternative*, the new title also uses a more inclusive and positively stated phrase "integrative health" and eliminates the more professionally restrictive medicine-centric word *medicine*. The history, goals, and mission of NCCIH are further elaborated later in this chapter.

DEFINITION AND CLASSIFICATION

Numerous definitions of *complementary therapies* exist. The broad scope of the therapies and the many health professionals and therapists who are involved in delivering them create challenges for finding a definition that captures the breadth of this field. The NCCIH describes *complementary health approaches* as the use of nonmainstream practices and products together with conventional medicine, whereas *integrative health* is the term used when complementary therapies/practices and conventional healthcare approaches are used together in a coordinated way (NCCIH, 2021a). These definitions convey the inclusion of different therapies in countries in which Western biomedicine predominates, as opposed to countries in which another health system is dominant, such as traditional Chinese medicine (TCM). According to the World Health Organization (WHO, 2019a), a large number of healing practices in developing countries comprise Indigenous traditional health practices rather than Western biomedical approaches.

The lack of precision in the definition of *complementary therapies* poses challenges when comparing findings across surveys that have been conducted on the use of complementary procedures. Some surveys have included a large number of complementary practices, whereas others have been limited in scope. For example, in the NCCAM/National Center for Health Statistics Survey, adding prayer for health purposes to the analyses increased the percentage of use of complementary therapies from 36% to 62% (Barnes et al., 2004).

The NCCIH classifies complementary health approaches into two categories: natural products and mind and body practices. Exhibit 1.1 identifies common therapies in each category. In addition, some of the other systems of care are noted. A number of these common therapies have been a part of nursing for many years. The NCCIH lists do not include a number of the complementary therapies

---

Exhibit 1.1 *NCCIH Classification for Complementary Approaches with Examples*

Nutritional
These include such things as probiotics, prebiotics, phytochemicals, dietary plants, herbs and spices, dietary supplements, vitamins, and minerals.

Psychological
This category includes a diverse group of therapies: Mindfulness and spiritual practices, psychotherapy, meditation, breathing and relaxation techniques, art, music, dance, movement education, yoga, and tai chi.

Physical
This category includes manual therapies and heat and cold therapies.

Other Complementary Health Approaches
Some therapies do not fit neatly into other categories such as traditional healers, Ayurvedic medicine, traditional Chinese medicine, homeopathy, naturopathy, and functional medicine.

Source: National Center for Complementary and Integrative Health. (2021a). *Complementary, alternative, or integrative health: What's in a name?* https://nccih.nih.gov/research/statistics/2007/camsurvey_fs1.htm

included in this text, such as presence, active listening, and biofeedback. However, these are therapies often used by nurses.

According to findings from two sequential National Health Interview Surveys (NHIS), yoga was the most commonly used complementary health approach among adults in the United States in 2012 and 2017 (Clarke et al., 2018). Natural products are also widely available and widely used. Nearly 18% of American adults used a dietary supplement other than vitamins and minerals despite the fact that there is little regulation in this area.

The class of mind and body practices encompasses a wide spectrum of practices and ranges from massage and yoga to energy therapies such as healing touch and acupuncture. As can also be observed in the most recent (2021) NCCIH complementary therapies classification, chiropractic and osteopathic manipulation are included in the mind and body practice category. Some view chiropractic and osteopathy as specific systems of care. A significant number of the therapies found in the mind and body practices class have been used by nurses for years, whereas others have recently become therapies that a number of nurses incorporate into their nursing care.

The NCCIH has over the years developed a number of classifications for complementary therapies and integrative approaches. To the most recent classification, we would add *systems of care* (Chapter 5), which covers a broad array of systems of care, including Tibetan medicine. The field of complementary therapies is constantly changing as new therapies are identified; a number of these are from other systems of care or used in Indigenous cultures. Indeed, many systems of care have been used for millennia by Indigenous people around the globe. Many Indigenous systems of care have very sophisticated ideas of health and well-being that more closely approximate the health definition proposed by the WHO, in which health is more than the absence of disease; indeed, health is a fundamental right and "resource for living" (WHO, 2019b).

Other methods for classifying complementary therapies exist. One of these is provider-based versus non-provider-based administration. Therapies that are provider-based require a health professional or therapist to administer them, whereas therapies that are non-provider-based do not require the presence of a professional. For example, a therapist is required for acupuncture, but one is not necessarily required for acupressure. Herbal preparations and food supplements—the most used groups of complementary therapies—are self-administered. For a number of therapies, once the technique has been taught, a therapist is not needed. Meditation is an example of this type of self-administered therapy. Non-provider administered therapies are less costly than provider-administered therapies.

Globally, as people migrate for economic reasons, wars, drought, or political factors, health professionals are becoming increasingly aware of culture-specific health practices used in other countries. These practices may be carried out by shamans, healers, family members, or the patient. Knowledge about common practices in various ethnic groups assists nurses in providing culturally sensitive and safe care to promote health. A danger that health professionals face is assuming all people from a country or an area of the world engage in the same health practices. For example, Africa is a vast continent, and cultural practices vary significantly across the continent, as do practices across the tribes within a nation. This is also true for Native American tribes, with practices depending on the plants available for healing within given geographical areas.

USE OF COMPLEMENTARY THERAPIES

Interest in, and use of, complementary/alternative therapies has remained fairly constant in the United States, with slightly more than 30% of adults reporting use of complementary therapies (NCCIH, 2016). Prior to the emergence of health professionals' interest in complementary therapies, many individuals used these therapies (e.g., massage, meditation, herbal preparations); however, they did not refer to them as being complementary therapies. Surveys have addressed use by adults in the United States (Clarke et al., 2015; Laiyemo et al., 2015). Clarke et al. (2015), using data from the NHIS for 2012, found a slight decrease in reported adult use of complementary therapies from the NHIS 2007 survey: 35% in 2007 to 33.2% in 2012. Findings from the 2012 NHIS revealed a lower use of complementary therapies by Hispanic adults (22%) and non-Hispanic Black adults (19.3%) compared with non-Hispanic White adults (37.9%; Clarke et al., 2015). Interestingly, the percentage of children 4 to 17 years who reported using yoga and meditation increased from the 2012 to the 2017 survey (Black et al., 2018).

Interest in the use of complementary therapies is a phenomenon found not only in the United States but also in many other countries across the globe. In a recent survey of member states, the WHO reported that 88% of the members indicated using Traditional and Complementary Therapies (WHO, 2019a). Research on the use of these therapies has been conducted in various countries, including Canada (Qureshi et al., 2018), Germany (Linde et al., 2014), Japan (Motoo et al., 2019), Hong Kong (Lam et al., 2021), Iran (Balouchi et al., 2016), and Taiwan (Huang et al., 2019). The number of people using complementary therapies varied in these survey reports, but it was 50% or higher, indicating a wide use of these therapies. In a large cross-sectional online survey of a representative sample of Australians 18 years of age and older ($N = 2,019$), the prevalence and characteristics of the use of complementary medicine practices and products were assessed (Steel et al., 2018). The prevalence of any complementary medicine use was 63.1%; vitamin/mineral supplements were used by nearly half of survey respondents. Users of complementary medicine in this sample were more likely to be female with higher education levels and a chronic disease diagnosis (Steel et al., 2018).

Numerous studies have explored the use of complementary therapies in specific health conditions, including cancer (Lee et al., 2019), asthma (George & Topaz, 2013), neck pain (Brosseau et al., 2012), and COVID-19 (Paudyal, 2021). Since complementary therapies have been used in the prevention and treatment of stress, it would be expected that they would be widely used during the COVID-19 pandemic. Across the world, during the global COVID-19 pandemic, many nations experienced pressure to consider traditional medicines for preventing and treating COVID symptoms (Lin et al., 2021). The Cochrane Database of Systematic Reviews (2021) contains reviews of the efficacy of numerous complementary therapies in the treatment of specific conditions. In addition to their use for health conditions, complementary therapies are often used to promote a healthy lifestyle. An example would be the use of tai chi to promote flexibility and prevent falls in older adults. A search of the Cochrane database of the term "complementary therapies" generated 171 unique published Cochrane reviews for a wide range of health conditions and complementary therapy interventions.

Researchers have attempted to identify characteristics of users of complementary therapies. Nguyen et al. (2011) found that more women than men use these therapies. They also noted that a higher percentage of individuals using complementary therapies have academic degrees compared with a nonuser group. This may relate to economics and the ability to pay out of pocket for complementary therapies. These findings were further validated in the 2007 NHIS conducted by the National Center for Health Statistics of the Centers for Disease Control and Prevention (CDC) (Barnes et al., 2008). Goetz et al. (2013) compared the use of complementary therapies by people in active military service with the use by civilians. Their findings revealed a much higher use by active military personnel (44.5%) compared with civilians (36%).

In the large landmark national survey conducted in 2012, natural products were the most commonly used complementary therapy by both adults and children (Clarke et al., 2015). Exhibit 1.2 displays the 10 most commonly used therapies by adults identified by the 2012 NHIS.

The growing interest in and use of complementary therapies has prompted groups to explore why people elect to use a complementary therapy or integrative health approach. In a report from an international panel looking at the economic factors related to the use of complementary therapies, Coulter et al. (2013) noted that complementary and integrative health therapies often target the whole person rather than a specific symptom or disease. This holistic philosophy underlying many of the complementary therapies differs significantly from the dualistic or Cartesian philosophy that for several centuries has permeated Western medicine. Although use for a specific symptom or condition may be the focus of the

Exhibit 1.2 *10 Most Commonly Used Complementary Health Approaches Among Adults in 2012*

Natural products	17.7%*
Deep breathing	10.9%
Yoga, tai chi, qi gong	10.1%
Chiropractic or osteopathic manipulation	8.4%
Meditation	8.0%
Massage	6.9%
Special diets	3.0%
Homeopathy	2.2%
Progressive relaxation	2.1%
Guided imagery	1.7%

*This listing does not compute to 100% because there were other therapies on the survey that were used by less than 1.7% of those surveyed.
Source: Clarke, T., Black, L., Stussman, B., Barnes, P., & Nahin, R. (2015). Trends in the use of complementary health approaches among adults: United States, 2002–2012. *National Health Statistics Reports, 79,* 1–15.

therapy, often the person who is treated reports a greater sense of harmony or balance. People often seek care from complementary therapists or care at facilities that offer complementary therapies because they want to be treated as a whole person—and not treated as "a heart attack" or "a fractured hip." Indeed, the whole person is a central focus of the 2021–2025 strategic plan of NCCIH (2021b).

The integration of complementary therapies with biomedical therapies is a growing trend in healthcare as the scientific basis for the use of numerous complementary therapies increases. With the growing number of older adults and the increase in chronic health conditions, complementary therapies and practices that may be used to manage symptoms and increase quality of life have great appeal.

The personal qualities of a complementary practitioner (whether a nurse, physician, or other therapist) are key in the healing process. Having a practitioner who is caring, which has been integral to the nursing profession through the years, is also a key component in administering complementary therapies. Two aspects central to the effective administration of complementary therapies—presence and active listening—are covered in subsequent chapters; both convey caring. Remen (2000), a physician who is involved in cancer care, has stated:

> I know that if I listen attentively to someone, to their essential self, their soul, as it were, I often find that at the deepest, most unconscious level, they can sense the direction of their own healing and wholeness. If I can remain open to that, without expectations of what the someone is supposed to do, how they are supposed to change in order to be better, or even what their wholeness looks like, what can happen is magical. By that I mean that it has a certain coherency or integrity about it, far beyond any way of fixing their situation or easing their pain that I can devise on my own. (p. 90)

Historically, the high public interest in complementary therapies prompted the NIH to establish the Office of Alternative Medicine in 1992, which was elevated to the NCCAM in 1998. The name was changed to the NCCIH in 2014. What was significant about the establishment of the center in 1992 was that consumers, rather than health professionals, led the lobbying for its creation. As stated in the NCCIH's 2021–2025 strategic plan:

> The mission of NCCIH is to determine, through rigorous scientific investigation, the fundamental science, usefulness, and safety of complementary and integrative health approaches and their roles in improving health and health care. (NCCIH, 2021b, p. 1)

A new emphasis of the research agenda is whole-person health. The new strategic plan for 2021 to 2025 includes five major objectives (NCCIH, 2021b):

- advance fundamental science and methods development
- advance research on the whole person and on the integration of complementary and conventional care
- foster research on health promotion and restoration, resilience, disease prevention, and symptom management

- enhance the complementary and integrative health research workforce
- provide objective evidence-based information on complementary and integrative health interventions

The NCCIH's website, www.nccih.nih.gov, contains information about complementary therapies, research opportunities, and outcomes of recent surveys.

REIMBURSEMENT AND REGULATION

The costs and cost-effectiveness of complementary therapies are difficult to determine. Thus, scientifically sound investigations of the outcomes of specific interventions are needed. Many of the current studies have used a small sample size and/or have design flaws. Because people may use a complementary therapy to accomplish several outcomes, it becomes a challenge to measure all of these outcomes and to find tools that capture these seemingly diverse goals.

Are complementary therapies cost-effective in terms of outcomes of care? Lind et al. (2010) examined differences in costs of healthcare for patients with back pain, fibromyalgia, and menopause symptoms who used complementary therapies and for those who did not. They found that those using complementary therapies had overall lower healthcare costs—$1,420 less on average—than those who did not use these therapies. Other researchers reported that individuals with chronic illnesses who used complementary therapies were more likely to report feeling healthier (Nguyen et al., 2011).

With the continuing emphasis on controlling healthcare costs in the United States, studies examining the costs of complementary therapies and integrative health approaches will receive increasing attention. The impact that a therapy has on producing positive health outcomes is highly important, but also outcomes such as quality of life, satisfaction with care, and adherence are good inclusions in investigations. This is especially true in those with multiple chronic illnesses, such as in the aging population.

Some of the challenges relate to the holistic focus of many of the complementary therapies. Does massage relieve knee pain? Does a reduction in pain result in fewer days missed from work? Does the reduction in pain result in a better mood state that has an effect on social interactions? These are only a small number of outcomes that may result from massage reducing knee or other pain. The multitude of possible outcomes poses many challenges for researchers in terms of determining the cost-effectiveness of a specific therapy.

Third-party payers such as insurance companies pay for a limited number of complementary therapies. The therapies most frequently covered are chiropractic medicine, acupuncture, and biofeedback. In some instances, a physician referral is required for reimbursement. Patients should consult with their insurer to see if and what complementary therapies may be covered. According to the NHIS 2012 survey, Americans spend $30.2 billion out of pocket each year on complementary therapies. This money was divided among health practitioners ($14.7 billion), natural products ($12.8 billion), and other complementary therapy approaches ($2.7 billion; NCCIH, 2016). Obviously, people must believe that complementary techniques produce positive results if they continue to personally pay for these aids. Although the amount spent on complementary therapies seems large, it is less than 10% of out-of-pocket payments made by Americans for healthcare (NCCIH, 2016).

Some states (e.g., Washington) have long included complementary therapists in private, commercial insurance offerings. Other states have instituted legislation that provides protection for persons using complementary procedures. The NCCIH (2016) has information on its website to help consumers gather information from their health insurance provider to determine out-of-pocket costs versus insurance coverage for specific complementary therapies and services. Consumers are also encouraged to ask practitioners about costs for the initial and follow-up visits and the length or number of treatments proposed.

Practitioners administering complementary therapies may or may not be licensed health professionals. Concern has been voiced about the preparation of all who administer complementary therapies but particularly about non-healthcare professionals. Regulation of both healthcare and nonhealthcare professionals is done by states and in some instances at the city level. A number of professional organizations, such as the National Board of Chiropractic Examiners, the Healing Touch Program, and the National Holistic Nurses, establish standards and administer certification examinations for practitioners in these therapies. Many healthcare facilities have requirements for complementary therapists working in their facility. For example, they may require that practitioners administering healing touch be certified.

Because of the diversity in educational preparation and the lack of state requirements for some complementary therapy practitioners, it is important that the individual seeking a therapist inquire about practitioner/provider experience and background. Also, if concerns exist, the person should contact the specific state's Department of Health for further information.

CULTURE-RELATED ASPECTS OF COMPLEMENTARY THERAPIES

Human cultures pervade the globe. One's culture lends structure to a shared way of life in health and illness. All cultures have either systems of healthcare or numerous healthcare practices/therapies used by the members of that culture.

Entire systems of healthcare have survived for thousands of years in various regions of the world. With the increasing movement of people either for short periods of time such as for study, business, or vacation or for permanent immigration, aspects of diverse systems of care will be encountered both by those in transit and by healthcare providers in their home country. The impact of Western medicine in most areas of the world is growing. However, individuals will continue to use all or portions of their familiar traditional systems of healthcare. These different ways of healing can work well together; however, it is imperative for Western care providers to assess for therapies or practices being used so that the patient receives safe care. Because minimal information is known about the outcomes of many of these therapies, close observations are needed to ensure that they are enhancing, not interfering with, biomedical treatment. For example, Quinlan (2011) stated that 85% of traditional remedies are herbal, and more than 70% of the world's population depends on common herbal medicine for their primary care. Beliefs about the cause of a number of chronic conditions point to the type of therapies selected to treat or "cure" that condition. Sidebar 1.1 details the therapeutic use of plant medicines that have been used over the centuries in Peru as part of the traditional system of healthcare.

Although some healthcare practices of other cultures, such as yoga, have become part of the compendium of complementary therapies, many of these remedies remain unknown to Western healthcare providers. Because of the largest refugee

Sidebar 1.1 *The Use of Medicinal Plants in Peru*

Miryam Benites Cerna

I am a nurse and have been working for more than 25 years in rural and urban areas of northern Peru. During this time, I have been able to observe and guide the use of herbs or plants used for medicinal purposes.

There is evidence that ancient Peruvians used plants for therapeutic purposes 6,000 years before Christ. The inhabitants of pre-Inca cultures were keen observers of the environment that surrounded them and, therefore, of the plants that grew in their environment. For thousands of years, the inhabitants of Peru, especially those living in rural areas, have used various plants for medicinal purposes; some were grown in the wild, and others were cultivated especially for this purpose. This cultural practice has not been lost because it has been transmitted orally from one generation to the next. Families and communities are the depositories and practitioners of this ancient wisdom.

In some cases, the whole plant or part of it is used to cure or alleviate pain, and in other cases, infusions are administered to the patient. Some of the disorders that are treated with medicinal plants are trauma to the skeletal system; bacterial, fungal, or viral infections; parasites; and respiratory, digestive, and urinary disorders. They are also used as regulators of the hormonal, reproductive, and even psychic systems.

Here are some examples of well-known and commonly used plants:

- *Cola de caballo* is used as a diuretic to improve kidney function and heal wounds.
- *Manzanilla* is an infusion of stems, leaves, and flowers used to relieve stomach pains. It is also used as a tranquilizer and for diarrhea in children.
- *Altamisa* involves heating branches and then rubbing them on limb areas affected by rheumatism. Fresh branches are placed under a bed to expel fleas.
- *Cerraja* is a concoction of leaves used to relieve digestive disorders and hepatitis.
- *Supiquegua* or *pedorrera* is an infusion used for indigestion and stomach gases.
- *Toronjil* is an aromatic plant used as an antispasmodic or as a relaxant and sedative of the nervous system.
- *Panisara* is used to relieve symptoms of a light cold and cough and strengthen the respiratory system.
- *Matico* is an infusion of leaves taken for flu and coughs. Dried and crushed leaves are used to heal wounds.
- *Llantén* is a concoction prepared from leaves and used to heal wounds. An infusion of the leaves serves as an anti-inflammatory agent.
- *Pie de perro* is an infusion used as an anti-inflammatory for the kidneys.
- *Cedron* is used as an infusion for digestive problems and intestinal gases.

population since World War II, large numbers of immigrants, migrations of people due to climate changes, and an increase in global travel, knowledge of the health-care practices of other cultures has become paramount in providing healthcare.

The migration of people brings not only their diseases but also their health-care practices. Traditional healers traveling in populations of refugees include midwives, herbalists, shamans, priests or priestesses, bonesetters, and surgeons. There is a great need for healers because 47% of global morbidity is attributable to chronic conditions, with 60% mortality arising from such conditions (Manderson & Smith-Morris, 2010). Some individuals may seek care from a sorcerer. Humoral balance is a focus in some cultural systems of care such as TCM (yin/yang) and Latin American medicine (hot/cold). Therapies to promote this balance such as chi in TCM and other systems in Latin American medicine may be used by immigrants from these areas.

One area in which knowledge is particularly needed is the use of herbal preparations. The use of herbs as medicines has been common throughout the world since ancient times. In many cultures, it is not one herb but a combination of multiple herbal preparations that is used. Thus, information on the entirety of all herbs in any mixtures being taken is needed so that its potential health-related effects or interactions with Western therapeutics may be established. Traditional healing practices, herbs, and certain health-giving foods may be highly valued and closely linked to one's worldview and cultural identity as illustrated in the account of traditional practices shared in Sidebar 1.2 by a nurse from Palestine.

Sidebar 1.2 *International Perspective—Palestine*

Jehad Adwan

Wedged in the southwestern gate between Asia and Africa, Palestine sits at the crossroads of ancient civilizations. Almost 1 million Palestinians—my family included—became refugees during the 1948 war that led to the establishment of the state of Israel in Palestine. Although my father's village was only a half-hour drive from where he lived until he died in 2018, he never saw it again since he was forced out of it 70 years earlier. I was born and grew up in a refugee camp in the Gaza Strip—a small strip of land in the southwest corner of Palestine on the border with Egypt. I was brought up dreaming about and living the stories of a stolen homeland and a distorted culture. I had heard from my grandparents and parents so many of the stories and methods my ancestors used to treat a variety of ailments. They used combinations of spirituality, herbs, oils, and inherited skills passing from father to son and mother to daughter. It is believed that using warm extra virgin olive oil for massages along with reciting verses from the Quran and drinking herbal teas would cure the toughest of colds and other respiratory and gastrointestinal illnesses.

To a Palestinian, Palestine's comfort foods have healing superpowers. They comfort us when we are upset or sad and give us a sense of returning to our deeply held roots to the land and its holiness. Any Palestinian would tell you that sitting with family and friends around a woodfire toasting pita bread and dipping it in olive oil and *Zaater* (rubbed thyme leaves mixed in with other herbs, seasoning,

Sidebar 1.2 *International Perspective—Palestine (continued)*

sumac, and sesame seeds) along with eating pickled olives, is the best meal that heals the soul. When I feel sad or lonely—being away from home for more than 23 years—I toast pita bread and dip it in olive oil and *Zaater*. That lifts my spirit and takes me back to my roots.

My paternal grandfather was a *Darwish* or a man of God. I was told that he could predict evil things before they happened. He used that gift to help others. His wife inherited the skill of massage from her mother and grandmother. My maternal grandfather was a genius farmer whose hobbies included playing the flute, poetry, and tree grafting. When I was young, he told me he had left behind, in his village in Palestine, an almond tree he had grafted using buds from sweet peach, apricot, and plum trees—altogether. He lived the rest of his days in a refugee camp.

I had always looked up to my father for his strength and admired his personality and hard work to raise his three daughters and six sons. When I broke my arm in gym class when I was 13, he took me to a traditional healer in a nearby town. He watched as the healer tried to rectify my broken bones with no analgesia, of course. My father kept cheering me up. "Be strong! Don't cry!" He cheered. I saw his tearful eyes looking away from me. I saw that and could not hold back anymore. We both burst into tears. The healer wrapped my arm up with long white cloth bandage after spreading parts of it with a special blend of herbs and olive oil. I will never forget the aroma that emanated from my rudimentary cast whenever it came close to my nose.

My oldest brother, Mohammed, who has a unique taste for herbal teas, had a pleasant surprise in the mail earlier this year when he received a package from me containing a variety of herbal teas I sent to him from the United States. He enjoyed the teas sent from across the globe. My brother, Ra'ed, is 6 years older than I am. He has always been my go-to person for advice. He always had a recipe of teas, herbs, and oils ready for everything. When I grew up and became a nurse, I tried to sway him away from traditional medicines to no avail. I get some recipes from him through social media every now and then. I smile and click "like" on his messages.

I believe that social media is ruining our traditional healing methods and practices. With the convergence of social media and the COVID-19 pandemic, I see a lot of misuse and abuse of authentic Palestinian traditional methods of healing being thrown around in friends' and relatives' social media posts. It saddens me to see such deterioration and makes me fear that this long-held tradition is on its way to extinction someday. I remain hopeful, however, because Palestine—the holy land—is the essence of this culture and as long as Palestine exists, tradition is nothing but a living, growing, and evolving being that will sustain itself despite aberrations of modern-day tools of division and destruction.

The importance of knowledge about cultural health practices can be illustrated by examining Native American traditional healthcare practices. As noted previously, the health professional must not make broad generalizations about the health practices of Native Americans because great variations exist among the more than 500 Native American nations. Traditional healing practices of Native American cultures were often embedded in stories, legends, symbolism, ceremonies, and spiritual treatments; these healing traditions have played an important role in the well-being of traditional Native American people (Vemireddy, 2020). Purifying the body is a foundational healing component of health rituals in a number of Native American nations. The basis for cleansing is to rid the person of bad feelings, negative energy, or bad spirits. The individual is cleansed both physically and spiritually (Borden & Coyote, 2012). Cleansing can take a variety of forms, such as smudging or sweat lodges. Sage and sweetgrass are commonly used by Great Plains Native Americans for their smudging ceremonies. Native American families may wish to use smudging for family members who are hospitalized. It requires creativity on the part of nurses, safety officers, administrators, and others to make this possible.

The rights of Indigenous peoples to their cultural beliefs and healthcare practices are receiving increasing attention. In 2007, the United Nations adopted and disseminated the Declaration on the Rights of Indigenous Peoples (Carrie et al., 2015; United Nations, n.d.). Although the declaration is not binding for member nations, it behooves healthcare practitioners to become more aware of the practices of peoples coming to biomedical facilities for healthcare. It is important for healthcare workers to inquire about the use of healthcare practices and not show repugnance at seemingly "strange" practices.

The inclusion of immigrants and indigenous persons in research on complementary therapies and other biomedical research is sorely needed, as is the exploration of the effectiveness of the health practices of Indigenous cultures. One area in which research on the practices of Indigenous people has been done is in the use of sweat lodges in the treatment of addiction in Native Americans. These practices were found to be effective both with the addiction and in the spiritual well-being of persons (Rowan et al., 2014).

Chapters in Section I include concepts foundational to the health-promoting structural or relational context of complementary therapies or environment. Therapeutic presence and listening are foundational to the delivery of complementary therapies. Healing environments can also be established to promote the goals of therapy. Light, a common element of a healing environment, is universally present and utilized throughout the world for its aesthetic, health, and mood-enhancing potential. In early times, it had been considered a sacred element by some cultures. Recognition of its beauty, its importance for life, and its energy-giving nature evident in the built environments and structures in Persia is illustrated in Sidebar 1.3.

Sidebar 1.3 *Use of Light as an Architectural Asset in Iran*

Mansour Hadidi

Light (fire) was one of the four sacred elements in ancient Persia; the other three were Water, Earth (soil), and Air (wind). Zoroastrians (followers of the Persian prophet Zoroaster) believed that fire must never be extinguished in the temple. Zoroaster is thought to have lived in eastern Persia (today's Iran) in 600 BCE. Zoroastrians (Persians) probably were the first to introduce the idea of binary powers (as opposed to the Greeks who believed in multiple gods and goddesses). Ahura Mazda was the god of light and goodness; Angra Mainyu was the god

Sidebar 1.3 *Use of Light as an Architectural Asset in Iran (continued)*

of darkness and "evil spirit," who, at the end, was believed to be defeated by goodness. The words *ahura* and *mazda* mean "light" and "wisdom," respectively.

Iran is a light-rich country, located between 25° north at its southernmost and 39° north at its northernmost latitude. There is a broad range of temperatures, climate and elevations, and water and desert areas, with some regions seeing no rain for half the year. Due to the country's global position, sunlight is a beautiful asset of it. The elevation in the mountainous regions also contributes to the intensity and effects of sunlight. The climate is temperate, and there is plentiful sunshine on most days, especially in the arid desert areas.

Architects in Iran, even from early times, have understood the importance of light in the design and construction of buildings. Natural light, plentiful in Iran, plays an important role in the illumination of buildings. The beauty of natural light can be observed in homes, workspaces, hotels, hospitals, schools, mosques, and other buildings. Exposure to light can be uplifting and energizing. It can improve mood and vitality with potential effects on human productivity. Early-morning exposure has wakening effects and can be more effective.

Stained glass was used to soften the light where the heat from light was excessive. Architects used a balance between light and heat. Another approach was using indirect light. For example, in areas close to the desert, small patios were designed to bring in light while preventing direct sunshine and heat as a result. An important consideration is the direction of windows in buildings. Although southern exposures are the most popular for daytime living areas (such as the living and family rooms) because they receive the highest amount of natural light during the day, northern windows are best for bedrooms and spaces that are used at night.

With the advent of electricity, air-conditioning, and heating appliances, architects had more freedom to design buildings with other factors in mind. For example, although architects were aware that light could add to the beauty and illumination of a building, the view of the vista's surroundings became a higher priority. In old structures, reticular stone panels were often used to prevent excessive heat from sunshine. However, in modern buildings, large glass windows mostly cover the facade.

The individual complementary therapy chapters that follow in subsequent sections of this text include descriptions of how these specific therapies are implemented in many different cultures and countries other than the United States. Although similarities across nations and cultures in administering therapies are noted, cultural differences are recognized in the handling of therapies globally. International sidebars that highlight both cross-cultural similarities and differences are included in most chapters.

IMPLICATIONS FOR NURSING

Although the term *complementary therapies* was not used until relatively recently, numerous therapies and their underlying philosophies have been a part of the nursing profession since its beginnings. In *Notes on Nursing* (1859/1992), Florence

Nightingale stressed the importance of creating an environment in which healing could occur and the significance of therapies such as music in the healing process. Complementary therapies today simply provide yet another opportunity for nurses to demonstrate caring for patients.

As noted in the chapters on self-care, education, practice, and research, nursing has embraced complementary practices. Although it is indeed gratifying to see that medicine and other health professions are recognizing the importance of listening and presence in the healing process, nurses need to assert that many of these therapies have been taught in nursing programs and have been practiced by nurses for centuries. Complementary practices, including meditation, imagery, music intervention, journaling, massage, healing touch, therapeutic listening, and presence, have been valued and employed by nurses throughout time.

In a survey of the Nursing Practice Acts in all states, the American Holistic Nurses Association (AHNA) found that 18 states referred to or had specific position statements regarding holistic nursing and/or complementary therapies (AHNA, 2020). This inclusion acknowledges that nursing is becoming more aware of the use of complementary therapies as an important aspect of nursing care. The New York State Nurses Association (2021) has developed a position statement on the use of complementary therapies in nursing that includes 10 recommendations to guide nurses in using complementary therapies in practice. In the last section of this text, specific attention is given to complementary therapies and integrative health in education and practice.

Complementary therapies are receiving increasing attention within nursing. Journals such as the *Journal of Holistic Nursing* and *Complementary Therapies for Clinical Practice* are devoted almost exclusively to complementary solutions. Many professional journals have devoted entire issues to exploring the use of complementary remedies. Articles inform nurses about complementary therapies and ways that specific procedures can be used with various conditions, including use for promoting health.

Because of the increasing use of complementary therapies by patients, it is critical that nurses possess basic knowledge about these therapies. Chang and Chang (2015) reviewed studies done on nurses' knowledge and attitudes about complementary therapies. Although 66.4% of the participating nurses reported positive attitudes about these therapies, 77.4% did not possess a good understanding of the risks and benefits of complementary therapies, and many nurses felt uncomfortable about discussing using these therapies with their patients.

It is not feasible for nurses to know about *all* the vast number of therapies, but the following are some skills and knowledge nurses should possess:

- skills in obtaining a comprehensive health history to accurately ascertain patients' use of a broad range of complementary therapies
- ability to assess the appropriateness and safety of therapies used
- ability to answer basic questions about the use of complementary techniques
- knowledge to refer patients to reliable sources of information
- knowledge to suggest therapies having evidence of benefit for specific conditions
- knowledge to provide guidelines for identifying competent therapists
- ability to assist in determining whether insurance will reimburse for a specific therapy
- knowledge and skills to administer a select number of complementary remedies

Obtaining a complete health history requires that questions about the use of complementary and alternative therapies be an integral part of the health history. Many patients may not volunteer information about using complementary and/or alternative therapies unless they are specifically asked; others may be reluctant to share this information unless the practitioner overtly displays an acceptance of these therapies. Although facts are needed about all complementary therapies, getting feedback about using herbal preparations is critical because interactions between certain prescription drugs and certain herbal preparations may pose a threat to health.

The vast number of complementary therapies makes it impossible for nurses to be knowledgeable about all of them, but familiarity with the more common therapies will assist health providers in answering basic questions. Many organizations, professional associations, individuals, and groups have excellent websites that provide information about specific therapies. Caution is needed, however, in accepting information from any website. These are some questions to consider when accessing a website for unbiased and honest information about a complementary therapy:

- What is the purpose of the site?
- What group/organization operates and/or funds the site?
- Who, such as an editorial board, selects the data contained on the site?
- How often is the content updated?
- Is there a way for the user to contact someone if questions arise about site content?

Each complementary therapy chapter in this book lists websites from reputable sources that can provide the reader with additional credible information. Some authors also list other resources related to that therapy for the interested reader.

CONCLUSION

More and more people not only know about complementary therapies but are using them or considering using them as well. Thus, it is essential for nurses to increase their knowledge about these therapies, which are often used in conjunction with Western biomedical treatments. Patients may desire an emphasis on holistic care (or whole-person care) that underlies many complementary techniques. Holistic practice has permeated nursing for centuries, and incorporating complementary procedures into nursing care carries on this tradition.

REFERENCES

American Holistic Nurses Association. (2020). *State nurse practice acts*. https://www.ahna.org/Home/Resources?State-Practice-Acts

Balouchi, A., Rahanama, M., Hastings-Tolsma, M., Shoja, M., & Bolaydehyi, E. (2016). Knowledge, attitude and use of complementary and integrative health strategies: A preliminary survey of Iranian nurses. *Journal of Integrative Medicine, 14*, 121–127. https://doi.org/10.1016/S2095-4964(16)60245-5

Barnes, P. M., Bloom, B., & Nahin, R. L. 2008 *Complementary and alternative medicine use among adults and children: United States, 2007*. (National Health Statistics Report No. 12). National Center for Health Statistics. https://www.cdc.gov/nchs/data/nhsr/nhsr012.pdf

Barnes, P. M., Powell-Griner, E., McFann, K., & Nahin, R. L. (2004). Complementary and alternative medicine use among adults: United States, 2002. *Seminars in Integrative Medicine, 2*(2), 54–71. https://doi.org/10.1016/j.sigm.2004.07.003

Black, L. I., Barnes, P. M., Clarke, T. C., Studdman, B. J., & Nahin, R. L. (2018). *Use of yoga, meditation, and chiropractors among U. S., children aged 4–17 years* (NCHS data brief, 324). National Center for Health Statistics. https://www.cdc.gov/nchs/data/databriefs/db324-h.pdf

Borden, A., & Coyote, S. (2012). *The smudging ceremony.* http://www.asunam.com/smudge_ceremony.html

Brosseau, L., Wells, G., Tugwell, P., Casimiro, L., Novikov, M., Loew, L., Sredic, D., Clement, S., Gravelle, A., Hua, K., Kresic, D., Lakic, A., Menard, G., Cote, P., Leblanc, G., Sonier, M., Cloutier, A., McEwan, J., Poitras, S., & Cohoon, C. (2012). Ottawa panel evidence-based clinical practice guidelines on therapeutic massage for neck pain. *Journal of Bodywork and Movement Therapies, 16*(3), 300–325. https://doi.org/10.1016/j.jbmt.2012.04.001

Carrie, H., Mackey, T., & Laird, S. (2015). Integrating traditional indigenous medicine into Western biomedical health systems: A review of Nicaraguan health policies and Miskitu health services. *International Journal for Equity in Health, 1,* 129. https://doi.org/10.1186/s12939-015-0260-1

Chang, H., & Chang, H. (2015). A review of nurses' knowledge, attitudes, and ability to communicate the risks and benefits of complementary and alternative medicine. *Journal of Clinical Nursing, 24,* 1466–1478. https://doi.org/10.1111/jocn.12790

Clarke, T. C., Barnes, P. M., Black, L. I., Stussman, B. J., & Nahin, R. L. (2018). *Use of yoga, meditation, and chiropractors among U. S. Adults aged 18 and over* (NCHS Data Brief No. 325). National Center for Health Statistics. https://www.cdc.gov/nchs/data/databriefs/db325-h.pdf

Clarke, T. C., Black, L. I., Stussman, B. J., Barnes, P. M., & Nahin, R. L. (2015). Trends in the use of complementary health approaches among adults: United States, 2002–2012. *National Health Statistics Reports, 79,* 1–15.

Cochrane Database of Systematic Reviews. (2021). *Cochrane database of systematic reviews.* https://www.cochranelibrary.com/cdsr/about-cdsr

Coulter, I. D., Herman, P. M., & Nataraj, S. (2013). Economic analysis of complementary, alternative, and integrative medicine: Considerations raised by an expert panel. *BMC Complementary and Alternative Medicine, 13,* 191. https://doi.org/10.1186/1472-6882-13-191

George, M., & Topaz, M. (2013). A systematic review of complementary and alternative medicine for asthma self-management. *Nursing Clinics of North America, 48,* 53–149. https://doi.org/10.1016/j.cnur.2012.11.002

Goetz, C., Marriott, B. P., Finch, M. D., Bray, R. M., Williams, T. V., Hourani, L. L., Hadden, L. S., Colleran, H. L., & Jonas, W. B. (2013). Military report more complementary and alternative medicine use than civilians. *Journal of Alternative and Complementary Medicine, 19*(6), 509–517. https://doi.org/10.1089/acm.2012.0108.

Huang, C. W., Tran, D. N. H., Li, T. F., Sasaki, Y., Lee, J. A., Lee, M. S., Arai, I., Motoo, Y., Yukawa, K., Tsutani, K., Ko, S. G., Hwang, S. J., & Chen, F. P. (2019). The utilization of complementary and alternative medicine in Taiwan: An internet survey using an adapted version of the international questionnaire (I-CAM-Q). *Journal of the Chinese Medical Association, 82*(8), 665–671. https://doi.org/10.1097/JCMA.0000000000000131

Laiyemo, M. A., Nunlee-Bland, G., Adams, G., Laiyemo, A. O., & Lombardo, F. A. (2015). Characteristics and health perceptions of complementary and alternative medicine users in the United States. *Clinical Investigation, 349*(2), 140–144. https://doi.org/10.1097/MAJ.0000000000000363

Lam, C. S., Koon, H. K., Chung, V. C., & Cheung, Y. T. (2021). A public survey of traditional, complementary and integrative medicine use during COVID-19 outbreak in Hong Kong. *PLoS ONE, 16*(7), e0253890. https://doi.org/10.1371/journal.pone.0253890

Lee, S. M., Choi, H. C., & Hyun, M. K. (2019). An overview of systematic reviews: Complementary therapies for cancer patients. *Integrative Cancer Therapies, 18,* 1534735419890029. https://doi.org/10.1177/1534735419890029

Lin, L. W., Ananthakrishnan, A., & Teerawattananon, Y. (2021). Evaluating traditional and complementary medicines: Where do we go from here? *International Journal of Technology Assessment in Health Care, 37*, e45, 1–6. https://doi.org/10.1017/ S0266462321000179

Lind, B. K., Lafferty, W. E., Tyree, P. T., & Diehr, P. K. (2010). Comparison of health care expenditures among insured users and nonusers of complementary and alternative medicine in Washington state: A cost minimization analysis. *Journal of Alternative and Complementary Medicine, 16*, 411–417. https://doi.org/10.1089/acm.2009.0261

Linde, K., Alscher, A., Friedrichs, C., Joos, S., & Schneider, A. (2014). The use of complementary and alternative therapies in Germany: A systematic review of nationwide surveys. *Forschende Komplementarmedizin, 21*, 111–118. https://doi.org/10.1159/000360917

Manderson, L., & Smith-Morris, C. (2010). *Chronic conditions, fluid states: Chronicity and the anthropology of illness*. Rutgers University Press.

Motoo, Y., Yukawa, K., Arai, I., Hisamura, K., & Tsutani, K. (2019). Use of complementary and alternative medicine in Japan: A cross-sectional internet survey using the Japanese version of the International Complementary and Alternative Medicine Questionnaire. *JMA Journal, 2*(1), 35–46. https://doi.org/10.31662/jmaj.2018-0044

National Center for Complementary and Integrative Health. (2016). *Paying for complementary and integrative health approaches*. https://www.nccih.nih.gov/health/paying-for-complementary -and-integrative-health-approaches#:~:text=%20Paying%20for%20Complementary%20 and%20Integrative%20Health%20Approaches,If%20you%E2%80%99re%20 planning%20to%20see%20a...%20More%20

National Center for Complementary and Integrative Health. (2021a). *Complementary, alternative, or integrative health: What's in a name?* https://nccih.nih.gov/research/statistics/2007/ camsurvey_fs1.htm

National Center for Complementary and Integrative Health. (2021b). *Strategic plan: FY 2021–2025. Mapping a pathway to research on whole person health*. https://files.nccih.nih.gov/nccih-strategic -plan-2021-2025.pdf

New York State Nurses Association. (2021). *Position statement on the use of complementary and alternative therapies in the practice of nursing*. https:www.nysna.org/position-statement -use-complementary-and-alternative-therapies-practice-nursing#.YV7wmdpKUI

Nguyen, L. T., Davis, R. B., Kaptchuk, T. J., & Phillips, R. S. (2011). Use of complementary and alternative medicine and self-rated health status: Results from a national survey. *Journal of General Internal Medicine, 26*(4), 399–404. https://doi.org/10.1007/s11606-010-1542-3

Nightingale, F. (1992). *Notes on nursing*. Lippincott. (Original work published 1859)

Paudyal, V., Sun, S., Hussain, R., Abulaleb, M. H., & Hedima, W. (2021). Complementary and alternative uses in COVID-19: A global perspective on practice, policy, and research. *Research in Social and Administrative Pharmacy, 18*, 2524. https://doi.org/10.1016/j.sapharm,2021.05.004.

Quinlan, M. (2011). Ethnomedicine. In M. Singer & P. Erickson (Eds.), *A companion to medical anthropology* (pp. 381–404). Wiley-Blackwell.

Qureshi, M., Zelinski, E., & Carlson, L. E. (2018). Cancer and complementary therapies: Current trends in survivors' interest and use. *Integrative Cancer Therapies, 17*, 844–853. https://doi .org/10.1177/1534735418762496

Remen, R. N. (2000). *My grandfather's blessings*. Riverhead Books.

Rowan, M., Poole, N., Shea, B., Gone, J. P., Mykota, D., Farag, M., Hopkins, C., Hall, L., Mushquash, C., & Dell, C. (2014). Cultural interventions to treat addictions in Indigenous populations: Findings from a scoping study. *Substance Abuse Treatment, Prevention, and Policy, 9*, 34. https:// doi.org/10.1186/1747-597X-9-34

Steel, A., McIntyre, E., Harnett, J., Foley, H., Adams, J., Sibbritt, D., Wardle, J., & Frawley, J. (2018). Complementary medicine use in the Australian population: Results of a nationally-representative cross-sectional survey. *Scientific Reports, 8*, 17325. https://doi.org/10.1038/ s41598-018-35508-y

United Nations. (n.d.). *United Nations declaration on the rights of Indigenous peoples.* https://www
.un.org/development/desa/indigenouspeoples/declaration-on-the-rights-of-indigenous
-peoples.html
Vemireddy, R. (2020). The role of Native American healing traditions within allopathic
medicine. *Inquiries Journal, 12*(12), 1. http://www.inquiriesjournal.com/articles/1849/
the-role-of-native-american-healing-traditions-within-allopathic-medicine
World Health Organization. (2019a). *WHO global report on traditional and complementary medicine
2019.* https://www.who.int/publications/i/item/978924151536
World Health Organization. (2019b). *World Health Organization (WHO) definition of health.* https://
www.publichealth.com.ng/world-health-organizationwho-definition-of-health

2

Presence

FRANK B. BENNETT

> It does not mean to be in a place where there is no noise, trouble or hard work.
> It means to be in the midst of those things and still be calm in your heart.
> —*Unknown*

Presence can be hard to describe in words but easy to recognize in ourselves or others. We know presence when we experience it. When we make eye contact with another person, pay close attention to their verbal and nonverbal communication, engage in active listening, and demonstrate we are focused on being with them in that moment, then we could say we're truly present. By contrast, we've all experienced moments when either we or the person we're with is not present and we feel a sense of separation. In Mitch Albom's (1997) book *Tuesdays with Morrie*, Morrie, a mentor and colleague of Albom's who is living with advanced amyotrophic lateral sclerosis, describes the essence of presence:

> I believe in being fully present. That means you should be with the person you're with. When I'm talking with you now, Mitch, I try to keep focused only on what is going on between us. I am not thinking about something we said last week. I am not thinking about what's coming up this Friday. I am not thinking about doing another Koppel show, or about medications I'm taking. I am talking to you; I am thinking about you. (pp. 135–136)

Presence is the awareness and actions a nurse intentionally brings to an authentic patient relationship to support patients in the present moment, empowering patient-centered care and decision-making. Presence describes the awareness and actions a nurse intentionally brings to this relationship to improve the patient's health, support them in becoming more authentic and empower them to take responsibility for defining and shaping their present and future life (Covington, 2003). It transcends cultures and modes of communication. Nursing presence is a model for understanding the nature of the relationship between nurse and patient and the effects of presence, or its absence, on patients' experiences.

Presence is an important element in complementary therapies that supports therapeutic nurse–patient relationships (Ellison & Meyer, 2020). Health professionals use presence in their daily interactions with patients and families as an integral part of complementary therapies during diagnostic assessments and therapeutic interventions. Being fully present adds to the effectiveness of therapies administered by the nurse. The context for nursing presence lies within the nurse–patient relationship. Nursing presence occurs in all care settings: acute, postacute, long term, and home care. Even if a nurse and patient are unable to communicate verbally, the patient can perceive the presence of a caring nurse.

DEFINITION AND ATTRIBUTES

The origins of nursing presence can be found in existential philosophy with Sartre's (1943/1984) description of "awareness of the other" as a means toward knowing a person and a way of presence. The connection between the concept of presence and nursing began to emerge in the 1960s. Vaillot (1962) used the phenomenon of presence to describe therapeutic relationships that are crucial to nurses' patient care. In their theory of humanistic nursing, Paterson and Zderad (1976) defined *presence* as an integral component of both nursing care interventions that establish patient relationships and as a process in which the nurse is available with their whole selves to the patient's experience through reciprocal interpersonal encounters.

Multiple perspectives on nursing presence have evolved over time, each contributing to a broader understanding of the concept. Benner (1984) coined the verb *presencing* to denote the existential practice of being with a patient, identifying it as one of the eight competencies in the helping role of the nurse. Parse (1992) defined *presence* as an interrelationship that honors the ever-changing reality of the other, requiring an attentiveness to the moment, a centering of self, and a focus on the other. Nelms (1996) believed presence was the heart of nursing practice. Doona and colleagues (1997) defined *presence* "as an intersubjective encounter between a nurse and a patient in which the nurse encounters the patient as a unique human being in a unique situation and chooses to spend her/himself on the patient's behalf. . . . As a consequence . . . both the nurse and patient are changed" (p. 12). Smith (2001) defined presence in nursing as "synonymous with both 'being there' and 'being with'" (p. 309). Jonsdöttir and colleagues (2004) documented the universal association between nursing presence and caring. McMahon and Christopher (2011) built on Benner's work to develop their midrange theory of nursing presence which identified five variables that characterize presence: individual client characteristics, characteristics of the nurse, shared characteristics within the nurse–patient dyad, the environment, and the intentional decisions of the nurse related to practice. Stockman and colleagues (2018) found that nursing presence is multidimensional, integrating therapeutic listening with nurses' intention to improve patient outcomes.

Although many nursing situations require close proximity of the nurse and another person, proximity does not constitute presence. Presence encompasses much more than being physically present in proximity of another. To be truly present, a nurse conveys openness to a "person-with-needs" with an "availability-in-a-helping way" (Paterson & Zderad, 1976). Presence implies nurses' openness, receptivity, readiness, and availability to an interpersonal relationship with the patient. Presence changes nurses' experience too, moving them beyond a role as an instrument of care to that of a cocreator of care, bearing witnesses to the mystery of healing contained within the nurse–patient relationship (Clemence, 1996). Reciprocity often emerges through this type of interaction. Melnechenko (2003) noted, "To be invited to share in another's unfolding health, to be asked to journey with another through the process of moving and choosing, is, without a doubt, an honor and privilege" (p. 24).

Nursing presence has five prerequisites: awareness, time, openness, trust, and initiative. It also has four attributes:

1. **It is intentional:** Nurses choose to be present in service of aims and purpose instead of agendas and scripts.
2. **It is based on attunement:** The nurse must bring multiple aspects of awareness to being present.
3. **It is relational:** It happens within the experience of a relationship between nurse and patient.
4. **It is dynamic:** It is always evolving and changing from moment to moment, elusive, and fragile.

Kostovich (2012) described presence through qualities nurses incorporate into their actions and approach to patient encounters: teaching, surveillance, concern, empathy, companionship, educated skillfulness, availability, responsive listening, spiritual enhancement, reassurance, personalization, and coordination of care. Anderson (2007) identified an extensive list of 22 attributes to describe nursing presence.

SCIENTIFIC BASIS

Conducting research on presence poses many challenges due to its subjective nature. Nurse scientists have described presence as a subconstruct of the broad concept of caring (Nelms, 1996; Watson, 1985). Caring requires the nurse to be keenly attentive to the needs of the patient, the meaning the patient attaches to the illness or problem, and the way that the patient wishes to proceed. Although the use of presence helps the patient heal, discover others, and find meaning in life, it is difficult to measure.

Research on the expert practice of critical care nurses has demonstrated the importance of presence. Minick (1995) found that connectedness with the patient was important not only as a caring behavior but also because it assisted the nurse in the early identification of postoperative problems. Therapeutic presence may help nurses be more attentive and detect subtle changes that may not be evident without it. Nurses lacking connectedness were perceived by their patients as detached. Wilkin and Slevin (2004) further validated the importance of the critical care nurse being present to the patient as essential, as were the skills needed to reach unresponsive and intubated patients.

When presence is used as a complementary therapy, it has effects on the patient, family, and nurse. Easter (2000) reported a decrease in pain for the patient, an increase in satisfaction for the nurse, and improved mental well-being for the nurse through presence. According to Drick (2003), presence creates healing and changes the atmosphere in the nurse–patient relationship. Jonas and Crawford (2004) reported lower, more stable heart rates as a result of healing presence within minutes to hours of the intervention. Tavernier (2006) identified relationship, healing, and reward as consequences of presence. Nursing presence has been shown to improve patient outcomes by decreasing their stress and anxiety and recovery time while increasing their feelings of safety and satisfaction with their care (Ellison & Meyer, 2020). Stuck and Rogers (2019) found that nursing presence promoted trust between nurses and home healthcare patients. Further investigation on why and how presence plays a positive and vital role in health outcomes needs to be encouraged.

INTERVENTION

Nursing presence interventions are recognized and valued as integral to the nurse–patient relationship and to patient care. In McMahon and Christopher's (2011) midrange theory of nursing presence, it is used as an intervention by nurses in all settings, but it requires constant intention by the nurse due to increased workflow and compressed time for patient care. With practice, nurses learn to become available to the patient with the wholeness of their individual being. Although nursing presence can be evidenced by behaviors and characteristics (see Exhibit 2.1), it is essentially about a nurse's perspective and attitude toward the patient relationship, "a being with rather than doing to" (McGivergn, 2009, p. 722). Edvardsson and colleagues (2017) used the term *patient-centeredness* to capture the focus of presence on the patient. Hessel's (2009) concept analysis of presence noted the spiritual connection that was felt when a nurse and patient share an experience of being together. Hessel observed that nurses need to completely focus their attention on their patients, free of other thoughts and responsibilities, to allow for a true connectedness through sharing the human experience (p. 278).

Exhibit 2.1 *Anderson's Attributes of Nursing Presence*

Listening	Authenticity
Understanding	Commitment
Reassurance	Openness
Touch	Confidence
Silence	Humor
Compassion	Vigilance
Sharing	Nonabandonment
Competence	Self-awareness
Trust	Respect
Affirming	Coaching
Continuity	Conscience

Nursing presence can be learned through practice and reflection (Kostovich et al., 2017). Indeed, every healthcare professional needs to learn how to become present, because "the gift of presence is something every caregiver can cultivate" (Chapman, 2003, p. 94). Nurses may increase their use of true presence by being with a patient through mindfulness or centering practices. These activities enable a person to experience presence and evoke it as an intervention.

MINDFULNESS

Jon Kabat-Zinn, a pioneer in mindfulness practice, teaching, and research, defines mindfulness as "awareness that arises through paying attention, on purpose, in the present moment, non-judgmentally . . . as if your life depended on it" (Kabat-Zinn, 2012, p. 17). He added the last phrase based on the results of his research, which showed that mindfulness practice has beneficial effects on both the perception of stress and the capacity to cope with it. Kabat-Zinn describes a mindful person as one who is attentive, aware, and fully present in the moment without judgment of the persons involved or the circumstances (Kabat-Zinn, 1990). Ziemann's (2019) meta-analysis of 61 studies found that mindfulness training was associated with lowered posttraumatic stress symptoms. Mindfulness practice can be conceived as a nurse's intention to nonjudgmental attention, focusing thoughts on the patient and the context of the present moment. It incorporates both a nurse's intentional awareness of the patient and a commitment, or motivation, to provide that patient with support and care. Jones and colleagues (2016) found that mindfulness was a significant factor in regulating a person's thoughts and feelings when they were engaged in supportive communication with another. A mindfulness-based intervention demonstrated an increase in nurses' compassion, satisfaction, well-being, and nursing presence (Kostovich et al., 2021). Given the significant stress that nurses have recently experienced while caring for patients during a global pandemic, mindfulness training may present an opportunity to increase their presence and improve resiliency and the capacity for coping with stress.

CENTERING

Presence entails a nurse's conscious attention before an upcoming interaction with the patient, whether in person or remotely through telehealth technology. Through centering, a nurse can be available with their whole self, open to the patient and their care needs. As a practice, centering is a process that helps a nurse refocus to truly be with the patient they are caring for at the moment. One centering technique is to take a short pause for 10 to 20 seconds to eliminate other thoughts or distractions and become present with the patient. This pause may entail closing the eyes prior to engaging with the patient or taking a few deep breaths while donning protective equipment or handwashing. Centering may also be as simple as pausing before contact with the patient, repeating the patient's name, and remembering their care needs to focus attention on that person. Bartels (2014) discusses the use of "The Pause" for being with a person who has died. The nurse or team would take 45 to 60 seconds to pause and focus on the life of the patient who had died. This practice could also be implemented with cognitively impaired or unresponsive patients.

Exhibit 2.2 *Skills for Implementing Presence*	
Key Component	**Skills**
Holistic attention to patient	Centering Active listening Openness to others Sensitivity Verbal communication at the patient's eye level Use of touch when culturally appropriate Nonverbal demonstration of acceptance

Exhibit 2.2 lists some key components of presence and the skills that support cultivating presence. Sensitivity to others requires the nurse to be an excellent listener and observer. (Therapeutic listening is addressed in Chapter 3.) Good observation skills assist the nurse in identifying nonverbal communication and nuances in expression that may reveal unexpressed patient concerns, issues, and questions. Presence can often entail periods of silence in which subtle, nonverbal interchanges occur between the nurse and patient. The nurse's continuing attentiveness is a critical aspect of therapeutic presence. Both the nurse and the patient experience a sense of union or joining for a moment in time. Mindfully focusing on the moment—not the past or the future—is inherent in being present.

It is important to note that presence is episodic and not continuous, occurring over minutes of a nurse–patient encounter. Because of the intense nature of these focused interactions, trying to extend presence for long periods can be mentally and emotionally exhausting for both the nurse and the patient (Koloroutis & Trout, 2014). Little is known about the optimal length of a presence session or the times when therapeutic presence should be used. Often, the nurse identifies it intuitively: "It just seems like this patient truly needs me now." Although presence can be used with another therapy or treatment, identifying when patients need someone to just be present for a few minutes may be the most effective technique in helping the patient feel cared for.

MEASUREMENT OF OUTCOMES

Employing validated measurement tools in research is crucial to reliably measure nursing presence. Measuring outcomes of presence interventions involves both the patient and the nurse because of their reciprocal interaction. Comments from the patient about feeling cared for, being able to express concerns, and perceiving understanding are some outcome measures derived from patient satisfaction tools. McMahon and Christopher (2011) reviewed the literature on presence and identified potential patient outcomes, including increased motivation, comfort, support, care satisfaction, self-worth, and sense of peace and hope, as well as decreased pain, anxiety, stress, and loneliness.

Kostovich (2012) used her elements of nursing presence as the foundation for her development of the Presence of Nursing Scale, which measured patients' perceptions of nurses' presence. Subsequently, she modified this scale to develop the Presence of Nursing-RN Scale, which measured nurses' perceptions of their own presence with patients (Kostovich et al., 2016). This scale has been used to measure nursing students' increased perception of presence through high-fidelity simulations (Kostovich et al., 2017), correlations between patient satisfaction and person-centered care (Edvardsson et al., 2017), and patient satisfaction in acute care (Hansbrough & Georges, 2019).

Two other validated instruments, Bodie's (2011) Active-Empathic Listening Scale and Baer and colleagues' (2006) Five-Facet Mindfulness Questionnaire, could also be employed to measure nurses' attention to their thoughts, behaviors, and emotions in the present moment. Incorporating the effects of presence in patient surveys should be considered among the important outcomes that indicate a patient's positive health experience and healing. Because of the intangibles that often occur with the use of presence, finding words or indices to measure presence can be challenging, and further development of, and research on, tools to measure presence is needed.

PRECAUTIONS

The major precaution in the use of presence is that nurses should take their cue, or invitation from, patients' verbal and nonverbal communication. It is important for nurses not to force a presence encounter. A true presence encounter considers the wants and needs of the patient, it is not for the nurse's primary benefit. If the nurse is truly centered on the patient and their needs, then the nurse will act in accordance with the wishes and needs of the patient (Paterson & Zderad, 1976).

A negative consequence of presence is that colleagues may be critical of nurses who spend time "just being" with patients and/or families. Certainly, this should not be a deterrent to the use of presence but an opportunity for interprofessional discussion and education through sharing evidence regarding the positive effects of presence on patient outcomes and resolution regarding the application of presence as a therapeutic intervention. Finfgeld-Connett (2006) stated that a supportive work environment that starts with the facility's highest administrative level helps promote the use of presence.

USES

Nursing presence has clinical applications across the healthcare spectrum, from birth (MacKinnon et al., 2005) to hospice (Trout, 2013) and in community (DeLashmutt, 2007), acute (Kostovich et al., 2021), and long-term care settings (An & Jo, 2009; O'Conner-Von & Bennett, 2020). It can be used in all nursing situations but may have particular usefulness when caring for patients in critical care, those struggling with a new diagnosis, exacerbation of a condition, or isolation and loss. Patients and their families in high-tech acute or critical care settings often feel lost. The use of presence helps prevent critical care nurses from being viewed by their patients as emotionally distant and focusing only on tasks and technology (Wilkin & Slevin, 2004; Wiman & Wikblad, 2004). Presence has also been shown to be significant in caring for women with postpartum psychosis (Engqvist et al., 2010), in midwifery practice (Hunter, 2009), and with cancer patients (Karlou et al., 2015). Rushton and colleagues (2009) employed mindfulness practices to train hospice nurses to use their presence while caring for dying patients. Although the dying person may not give any acknowledgment of presence during these "being with" encounters, the act of holding a hand or touching conveys that they are not alone.

Educators using distance teaching have been investigating the impact of instructors' emotional presence on students and their learning outcomes. Sandelowski (2002) noted that nurses and people involved in designing technology are interested in creating environments for patients and nurses to produce feelings of interaction that are immediate, intimate, and real. The rapidly increasing use of home monitoring and other forms of telehealth challenge nurses to convey their presence and attentive care. Researchers have begun exploring the application of virtual presence in online or telehealth contexts (Barrett, 2017; Grumme et al., 2016). Nurses providing care in telehealth or online settings might ask themselves, "Am I truly listening to and present with this patient?"

CULTURAL APPLICATIONS

Cultural elements, including nationality, race/ethnicity, social norms, boundaries, definitions of health and disease, traditions and religion, language, and diet and food are all important considerations when determining the use and meaning of presence for the nurse, the patient, and their family. Past experience or family influences may also impact an individual's interpretation of presence. It is important to explore and acknowledge the meaning of presence for the patient and those members of their community with whom they have a close relationship. Mitchell (2006) examined the concepts of presence and intentional attention among young, middle-aged, and older adults, finding that cultural perspectives about the role of presence in healing and bringing meaning to life experiences vary across generations.

Patients, family members, and nurses all have communication style preferences, which may be influenced by respective cultural influences. In some cultures, indicating respect and taking time to get to know a person are important in establishing trust-based relationships that may lead to presence. In other cultures, too much eye contact may be seen as offensive. Conversational silence is necessary in some cultures to become present with another person or the environment. Communication and trust are shown to be the largest factors that create a connection among Hispanic families (Evans et al., 2007). Buddhists are comfortable with long periods of silence as a respectful technique to cultivate being present.

A nurse in an unfamiliar situation, such as interacting with patients and families from a different culture than their own may need more time to become accustomed to using presence. Patience, as a form of presence, may be required for comprehension, responses, or decisions within certain cultures. Nurses may have to rely on their presence through close attention to patients' and families' nonverbal communication when verbal communication is reduced or inadequate. A warm smile and just standing by the bed for a moment convey a nurse's presence, attentive care, and intention and improve patient outcomes.

In Sidebar 2.1, a nurse from Pakistan relates the use of presence while caring for a patient in her country. It conveys the universality of the use of presence by nurses across the world.

Sidebar 2.1 *Use of "Presence in Nursing" in Pakistan*

Naheed Meghani

Pakistan, being a developing country, has fewer resources than many countries. There is a nursing shortage, and hence, cultural and socioeconomic realities intersect. In Pakistan, when possible, nurses rely on family members or volunteers to be with the patient. In Pakistani culture, there is a family value system, and a family member's illness is regarded as a family matter. The nurses work collaboratively with the family member or members who stay with the patient, and their presence is comforting and healing to the patient. Nurses' presence is also reassuring to the patients to allay fear and anxiety. Having the familiar face of a family member helps in achieving the goal of promoting comfort and healing. In the event when nurses have too many patients assigned and are pressed for time, they prioritize which patients would benefit most from their presence.

One of the examples I remember vividly from my nursing experience was of a patient (a truck driver) who was brought into the hospital after an accident. I found in the patient's chart that some roadside witnesses of the accident brought him to the hospital. He was unconscious and did not have any family members with him. When he regained consciousness and was stable, he was transferred to our unit. This patient was always quiet, disinterested, and staring at the ceiling. He would not finish his meals and sometimes skip them, saying he wasn't hungry. He started refusing his medications, too. I had 30 patients assigned to me, but I prioritized that this particular patient needed my presence. I sat on the chair beside his bed and asked him, while making appropriate eye contact, what he would like to share. He started crying and revealed that he missed his family, who lived in a rural area quite distant and probably were unable to visit. He wasn't sure if they even knew that he had been in an accident. He worried that he would never see them again.

I told him it was all right to cry about not being with his family and offered him some water. I sat by him and told him that as his nurse, I was concerned about his health and well-being and that although it was not possible for his family to visit, perhaps there was a way he could talk to them over the phone or write them. He told me that they did not have a telephone and that although he knew how to read and write, no one at his home knew how to do so. I felt very sad and quite helpless. I asked him if there was anything he would like changed in his surroundings to make him feel better. He asked if we could move his bed by the window so that he can see the tree that reminded him of a tree in the front of his house. I asked permission from another patient, and we switched the bed assignments so the trucker had the bed closer to the window. He was very grateful. I gave him paper and a pen so that he could draw a picture of the tree for his family. I sent that to his family. I also connected him with other patients on the unit and their family members. I reassured him that we were figuring out a way to connect with his family and coordinating the next steps of care. The patient started to connect with other patients and their families. The patient became stable and was discharged home. When he was leaving the unit, he gave me a paper (a thank-you note), on which he had drawn a tree and a sun rising. He said, "That tree gave me hope and reminded me of my home. Then I wanted to get better so I could see my family. You helped me see that there was hope."

This was emotionally and spiritually uplifting for me, knowing that my attentiveness and presence made a difference in this patient's life. I believe that it is essential to assess, understand, and respond to what is a meaningful presence for a patient from a cultural perspective. Presence is meaningful when the nurse is open to the reciprocal interaction; however, with sensitivity to the knowledge of the culture, any related previous experiences or cues from the patient or family will assist the nurse in these interactions.

FUTURE RESEARCH

Nurses document assessments performed and treatments administered but rarely document the use of presence as an integral part of patient care as a complementary therapy. Despite the challenges in measuring the outcomes of presence, current interest and a growing body of evidence about the effectiveness of presence as a therapeutic intervention provides nurses with opportunities for nurses to report outcomes from the use of presence. Areas in which research is needed include the following:

- Although every patient could benefit from presence, which assessments could help identify patients who want or might benefit the most from the therapeutic application of presence?
- What strategies can be used to teach nursing students and other health professionals ways to implement presence? Several articles cited in this chapter (DeLashmutt, 2007; Kostovich et al., 2017; Rushton et al., 2009) suggest educational strategies that may be useful in developing nurses' capacity for and discernment about applying presence as an intervention.
- With telehealth applications growing rapidly, how can presence be introduced into these contexts with patients? Is physical presence essential for patients to feel caring and personal interest by nurses?
- As diversity in patient populations increases, in what ways can nurses learn about cultural factors that influence the practice of presence in an appropriate manner?

REFERENCES

Albom, M. (1997). *Tuesdays with Morrie*. Doubleday.

An, G., & Jo, K. (2009). The effect of a nursing presence program on reducing stress in older adults in two Korean nursing homes. *Australian Journal of Advanced Nursing, 26,* 79–85. https://doi .org/10.3316/informit.248943163813707

Anderson, J. (2007). Nursing presence in a community heart failure program. *Nurse Practitioner, 32,* 14–21. https://doi.org/10.1097/01.NPR.0000294223.14054.04

Baer, R., Smith, G., Hopkins, J., Krietemeyer, J., & Toney, L. (2006). Using self-report assessment methods to explore facets of mindfulness. *Assessment, 13*(1), 27–45. https://doi.org/10.1177/1073191105283504

Barrett, D. (2017). Rethinking presence: A grounded theory of nurses and teleconsultation. *Journal of Clinical Nursing, 26*(19–20), 3088–3098. https://doi.org/10.1111/jocn.13656

Bartels, J. (2014). The pause. *Critical Care Nurse, 34,* 74–75. https://doi.org/10.4037/ccn2014962

Benner, P. (1984). *From novice to expert: Excellence and power in clinical nursing practice*. Addison-Wesley.

Bodie, G. D. (2011). The Active-Emphatic Listening Scale (AELS): Conceptualization and evidence of validity within the interpersonal domain. *Communication Quarterly, 59,* 277–295. https://doi.org/10.1080/01463373.2011.583495/

Chapman, E. (2003). *Radical loving care: Building the healing hospital in America*. Baptist Healing Hospital Trust.

Clemence, M. (1966). Existentialism: A philosophy of commitment. *The American Journal of Nursing, 66*(3), 500–505. https://doi.org/10.2307/3419729

Covington, H. (2003). Caring presence. Delineation of a concept for holistic nursing. *Journal of Holistic Nursing, 21*(3), 301–317. https://doi.org/10.1177/0898010103254915

DeLashmutt, M. (2007). Students' experience of nursing presence with poor mothers. *Journal of Obstetric, Gynecologic & Neonatal Nursing, 36*(2), 183–189. https://doi.org/10.1111/j.1552-6909.2007.00135.x

Doona, M., Haggerty, L., & Chase, S. (1997). Nursing presence: An existential exploration of the concept. *Scholarly Inquiry for Nursing Practice, 11*(1), 3–16. https://doi.org/10.1891/0889-7182.11.1.3

Drick, C. A. (2003). Back to basics: The power of presence in nursing care. *Journal of Gynecologic Oncology Nursing, 13*(3), 13–18.

Easter, A. (2000). Construct analysis of four modes of being present. *Journal of Holistic Nursing, 18,* 362–377. https://doi.org/10.1177/089801010001800407

Edvardsson, D., Watt, E., & Pearce, F. (2017). Patient experiences of caring and person-centeredness are associated with perceived nursing care quality. *Journal of Advanced Nursing, 73,* 217–227. https://doi.org/10.1111/jan.13105

Ellison, D., & Meyer, C. (2020). Presence and therapeutic listening. *Nursing Clinics of North America, 55*(4), 457–465. https://doi.org/10.1016/j.cnur.2020.06.012

Engqvist, I., Ferszt, G., & Nilsson, K. (2010). Swedish registered nurses' description of presence when caring for women with post-partum psychosis: An interview study. *International Journal of Mental Health Nursing, 19,* 193–196. https://doi.org/10.1111/j.1447-0349.2010.00691.x

Evans, B., Coon, D., & Crogan, N. (2007). *Personalismo* and breaking barriers: Accessing Hispanic populations for clinical services and research. *Geriatric Nursing, 28*(5), 289–296. https://doi.org/10.1016/j.gerinurse.2007.08.008

Finfgeld-Connett, D. (2006). Meta-synthesis of presence in nursing. *Journal of Advanced Nursing, 55,* 708–714. https://doi.org/10.1111/j.1365-2648.2006.03961.x

Grumme, V., Barry, C., Gordon, S., & Ray, M. (2016). On virtual presence. *Advances in Nursing Science, 39*(1), 48–59. https://doi.org/10.1097/ANS.0000000000000103

Hansbrough, W., & Georges, J. (2019). Validation of the presence of nursing scale using data triangulation. *Nursing Research, 68*(6), 439–444. https://doi.org/10.1097/NNR.0000000000000381

Hessel, J. (2009). Presence in nursing practice: A concept analysis. *Holistic Nursing Practice, 23,* 276–281. https://doi.org/10.1097/HNP.0b013e3181b66cb5

Hunter, L. (2009). A descriptive study of "being with women" during labor and birth. *Journal of Midwifery & Women's Health, 54,* 111–118. https://doi.org/10.1016/j.jmwh.2008.10.006

Jonas, W., & Crawford, C. (2004). The healing presence: Can it be reliably measured? *Journal of Alternative and Complementary Medicine, 10,* 751–756. https://doi.org/10.1089/acm.2004.10.751

Jones, S., Bodie, G., & Hughes, S. (2016). The impact of mindfulness on empathy, active listening, and perceived provisions of emotional support. *Communication Research, 46*(6), 838–865. https://doi.org/10.1177/0093650215626983

Jonsdóttir, H., Litchfield, M., & Pharris, M. D. (2004). The relational core of nursing practice in partnership. *Journal of Advanced Nursing, 47,* 241–248. https://doi.org/10.1111/j.1365-2648.2004.03088_1.x

Kabat-Zinn, J. (1990). *Full catastrophe living.* Delacorte.

Kabat-Zinn, J. (2012). *Mindfulness for beginners: Reclaiming the present moment—And your life.* Sounds True.

Karlou, C., Papathanassoglou, E., & Patiraki, E. (2015). Caring behaviors in cancer care in Greece: Comparison of patients', their caregivers', and nurses' perceptions. *European Journal of Oncology Nursing, 19,* 244–250. https://doi.org/10.1016/j.ejon.2014.11.005

Koloroutis, M., & Trout, M. (2014). See me as a person: A therapeutic framework for mindful care of hospice patients and their loved ones (P14). *Journal of Pain and Symptom Management, 47*(2), 379. https://doi.org/10.1016/j.jpainsymman.2013.12.015

Kostovich, C. (2012). Development and psychometric assessment of the Presence of Nursing Scale. *Nursing Science Quarterly, 25,* 167–175. https://doi.org/10.1177/0894318412437945

Kostovich, C., Bormann, J., Gonzalez, B., Hansbrough, W., Kelly, B., & Collins, E. (2021). Being present: Examining the efficacy of an internet mantram program on RN-delivered patient-centered care. *Nursing Outlook, 69,* 136–146. https://doi.org/10.1016/j.outlook.2021.01.001

Kostovich, C., Dunya, B., Schmidt, L., & Collins, E. (2016). A Rasch rating scale analysis of the presence of nursing scale-RN. *Journal of Applied Measurement, 17*(4), 476–488.

Kostovich, C., Van Denack, J., & Bachmeier, P. (2017). *"I Will Be Here for You:" Nursing Students' perceptions of being present for their patients.* Sigma Theta Tau International 44th Biennial Convention.

MacKinnon, K., McIntyre, M., & Quance, M. (2005). The meaning of the nurse's presence during childbirth. *Journal of Obstetric, Gynecologic, & Neonatal Nursing, 34*(1), 28–36. https://doi .org/10.1177/0884217504272808

McMahon, M., & Christopher, K. (2011). Toward a mid-range theory of nursing presence. *Nursing Forum, 46*(2), 71–82. https://doi.org/10.1111/j.1744-6198.2011.00215.x

Melnechenko, K. (2003). To make a difference: Nursing presence. *Nursing Forum, 38*, 18–24. https://doi.org/10.1111/j.1744-6198.2003.tb01207.x

Minick, P. (1995). The power of human caring: Early recognition of patient problems. *Scholarly Inquiry for Nursing Practice: An International Journal, 9*, 303–317. https://doi.org/10.1891/0889 -7182.9.4.303

Mitchell, M. (2006). Understanding true presence with elders: A story of joy and sorrow. *Perspectives, 30*(3), 17–19.

Nelms, T. P. (1996). Living a caring presence in nursing: A Heideggerian hermeneutical analysis. *Journal of Advanced Nursing, 24*, 368–374. https://doi.org/10.1046/j.1365-2648.1996.20020.x

O'Conner-Von, S., & Bennett, F., (2020). Long-term care nurses and their experiences with patients' and families' end-of-life preferences: A focus group study *Journal of Gerontological Nursing, 46*(12), 23–29. https://doi.org/10.3928/00989134-20201106-05

Parse, R. (1992). Human becoming: Parse's theory of nursing. *Nursing Science Quarterly, 5*(1), 35–42. https://doi.org/10.1177/089431849200500109

Paterson, J., & Zderad, L. (1976). *Humanistic nursing.* Wiley.

Rushton, C., Sellers, D., Heller, K., Spring, B., Dossey, B., & Halifax, J. (2009). Impact of a contemplative end-of-life training program: Being with dying. *Palliative & Supportive Care, 7*(4), 405–414. https://doi.org/10.1017/S1478951509990411

Sandelowski, M. (2002). Visible humans, vanishing bodies, and virtual nursing: Complications of life, presence, place, and identity. *Advances in Nursing Science, 24*, 58–70. https://doi .org/10.1097/00012272-200203000-00007

Sartre, J. (1943/1984). *Being and nothingness.* Washington Square Press.

Smith, T. (2001). The concept of nursing presence: State of the science. *Scholarly Inquiry for Nursing Practice, 15*(4), 299–322. https://doi.org/10.1891/oo89-7182.15.4.299

Stuck, R., & Rogers, W. (2019). Supporting trust in home healthcare providers: Insights into the care recipients' perspective. *Home Health Care Services Quarterly, 38*(2), 61–79. https://doi.org/ 10.1080/01621424.2019.1604462

Tavernier, S. (2006). An evidence-based conceptual analysis of presence. *Holistic Nursing Practice, 20*, 152–156.

Trout, L. (2013). *Nursing presence from the perspective of hospice nurses* [Doctoral dissertation]. Widener University.

Vaillot, S. M. C. (1962). *Commitment to nursing: A philosophical investigation.* Lippincott.

Watson, J. (1985). *Nursing: Human science and human care: A theory of nursing.* Appleton-Century-Crofts.

Wilkin, K., & Slevin, E. (2004). The meaning of caring to nurses: An investigation into the nature of caring work in an intensive care unit. *Journal of Clinical Nursing, 13*, 50–59. https://doi .org/10.1111/j.1365-2702.2004.00814.x

Wiman, E., & Wikblad, K. (2004). Caring and uncaring encounters in nursing in an emergency department. *Journal of Clinical Nursing, 13*, 422–429. https://doi.org/10.1111/j.1365-2702.2004.00902.x

Ziemann, K. (2019). *A meta-analysis of research examining the relationship between mindfulness and posttraumatic stress symptoms* [Doctoral dissertation]. University of Minnesota.

Therapeutic Listening

MARY FRAN TRACY, SHIGEAKI WATANUKI, AND RUTH LINDQUIST

Listening is an active and dynamic process of interaction that requires intentional effort to attend to a client's verbal and nonverbal cues. Listening is an integral part and foundation of nurse–client relationships and one of the most effective therapeutic techniques available to nurses. The theoretical underpinnings of listening can be traced back to counseling psychology and psychotherapy. Rogers (1957) used counseling and listening to foster independence and promote the growth and development of clients. Rogers also emphasized that empathy, warmth, and genuineness with clients were necessary and sufficient for therapeutic changes to occur. Listening is a significant component of therapeutic communication with patients and foundational to the building of an effective therapeutic nurse–patient relationship. Listening is also a key to improving patient safety in complex clinical settings (Berzins et al., 2018; Loos, 2021; Villar et al., 2020). Listening is foundational in the administration of complementary therapies. Listening is a process that is important in human interactions. Therapeutic listening is particularly important in the context of the nurse–patient relationship and is a foundational skill taught in nursing schools and honed throughout one's professional career.

DEFINITION

Many modifiers are used with the word *listening—active, attentive, empathic, therapeutic,* and *holistic.* Unless active listening was explicitly used by researchers in the articles reviewed in this chapter, the term *therapeutic listening* is used here to focus on the formal, deliberate actions of listening for therapeutic purposes (Lekander et al., 1993). *Therapeutic listening* is defined as "an interpersonal, confirmation process involving all the senses in which the therapist attends with empathy to the client's verbal and nonverbal messages to facilitate the understanding, synthesis, and interpretation of the client's situation" (Kemper, 1992, p. 22). Beyond the therapist, this empathetic attending pertains to nurses and to other care providers.

SCIENTIFIC BASIS

Therapeutic listening is a topic of interest and concern to a variety of disciplines. A number of qualitative and quantitative studies provide a scientific basis of intervention effects in relation to process—behavioral changes of providers that foster communication—and outcomes, including improved client satisfaction and other clinical indicators. The process of therapeutic listening may also lead to greater provider job satisfaction and retention. Listening conveys caring and is central to a nurse's role.

Evidence from a neuropsychological experiment using functional brain imaging demonstrates the powerful interpersonal impact of listening (Kawamichi et al., 2015). When the study participants perceived the experience of "being actively listened to" or had a positive emotional appraisal of such an interaction and the listener, their brains showed an activated "reward system," as evidenced by neural activation in the ventral striatum and the right anterior insula (Kawamichi et al., 2015). When the participants believed they were being actively listened to, they also expressed increased willingness to cooperate with the listener.

Garcia and colleagues (2018) conducted a randomized controlled trial, assigning 25 surgical patients to receive therapeutic listening and 25 surgical patients to a control group. Patients were assessed for changes in physiological (e.g., salivary cortisol, heart rate, blood pressure) and psychological indicators for anxiety and surgical fear. While there were no significant differences between the two groups on any of the variables, the authors postulated that contact with the researchers may have resulted in changes in the control group or that perhaps only one therapeutic listening session was inadequate to demonstrate differences.

Qualitative studies provide a rich understanding of the nature of therapeutic listening and explore the meaning and experience of being listened to in the context of real-world settings. Thirty patients who had been seen in an emergency department participated in a semistructured interview to elicit perceptions of their communication with nurses and providers (Hermann et al., 2019). Patients expressed recognition of verbal and nonverbal behaviors that conveyed respect, dignity, and feeling valued: "really listening, sitting at eye level, and smiling. They expressed satisfaction when they believed nurses were being attentive to them by providing undivided attention.

An integrative review of therapeutic interpersonal relationships in the acute care setting included 10 studies from Australia, the United Kingdom, Canada, the United States, Denmark, and the Netherlands (Kornhaber et al., 2016). Participants included patients, nurses, and providers, and the methodologies were qualitative and mixed methods in nature. The researchers found that patients saw therapeutic listening as promoting healing and recovery and helped strengthen provider relationships. They also reported patient-perceived improved quality of care after staff attended communication skills training. Therapeutic listening is key to improving therapeutic relationships.

Researchers explored the perceptions of adults aged 50 years and older of nurse listening posthospital admission (Loos, 2021). Thirty-three adults in Southern California participated in semistructured interviews, describing verbal and nonverbal behaviors where they "knew" they were being listened to. These behaviors included eye contact, attentiveness, body language, asking appropriate questions, speaking to the patient rather than facing the computer, and appearing caring. Patients stated these interactions only needed to occur once per shift in light of how busy they perceived nurses were. These listening interactions made them feel connected, put them at ease, and gave a sense of safe care. When these patients perceived listening did not occur, they felt vulnerable, discounted, distrustful, and angry (Loos, 2021).

The utility of active listening training has been shown in an experiment with undergraduate students (Bodie et al., 2015). The undergraduate students were randomly assigned to disclose their upsetting problem to either trained listeners or untrained listeners. The study results showed that active listening behavior promoted a greater emotional improvement in the students; however, active listening did not affect perceived improvement in relational assurance and problem-solvingof the students (Bodie et al., 2015).

A combination of learning sessions (cognitive interventions), administrative support, and coaching activities (affective and behavioral interventions) enables long-term improvement in the communication styles of nurses. A quasi-experimental study was undertaken to test the effectiveness of an integrated communication skills training program for 129 oncology nurses at a hospital in China. Continued significant improvements in overall basic communication skills, self-efficacy, outcome expectancy beliefs, and perceived support in the training group were observed after 1 and 6 months of training intervention. No significant improvements were found in the control group (Liu et al., 2007).

These studies attempted to identify complex relationships among multiple phenomena and variables, including the immediate and long-term effects of training interventions, clinical supervision and support, and cognitive and behavioral changes on the part of nurses. Further systematic studies are needed to enhance knowledge related to intervention effectiveness, especially the link between client characteristics, client satisfaction, and type of interventions. This is particularly important in light of today's healthcare emphasis and reimbursement aligned with patient satisfaction, patient engagement, and symptom management such as alleviating pain. The Centers for Medicare & Medicaid Services (CMS) views RN–patient communication as one of several critical aspects of patients' hospital experiences (CMS, 2014, 2015). That is why a question regarding RN–patient communication is on the *Hospital Consumer Assessment of Healthcare Providers and Systems (HCAHPS) Survey*, a patient satisfaction survey that all hospitals are required to conduct and publicly report and on which a portion of their reimbursement is based (CMS, 2014, 2015).

INTERVENTION

Therapeutic listening enables clients to better understand their feelings and to experience being understood by another caring person. It has been said that there may be no more fundamental behavior for supporting others in the process of disclosing stress than through active listening (Bodie et al., 2015), and it is thought to be a crucial skill for nurses and healthcare providers (Halpern, 2012). Effective engagement in therapeutic listening requires nurses to be aware of verbal and nonverbal communication that conveys explicit and implicit messages. Nonverbal behaviors tend to convey more than verbal messaging. It has been estimated that verbal communication impacts only 7% of the total communication interaction, whereas 55% of the impact comes from facial expressions, and 39% of the impact from vocal tones (Mehrabian & Ferris, 1967). Nonverbal communication is inextricably linked to verbal communication; differences in cultural norms also impact the interpretation of the interaction (Ellison & Meyer, 2020).

DEVELOPING THERAPEUTIC LISTENING SKILLS

Listening is a skill that needs to be practiced and refined as a nursing student and in one's professional nursing role, just like other more tangible nursing skills. In today's healthcare environment with ever-present time pressures, it may be easy to become a "provider" of listening using visible behaviors, such as nodding, eye contact, and not monitoring the time, rather than being an empathetic listener who truly engages and actively participates with the discloser (Halpern, 2012). Nurses may view others or be viewed themselves as not being productive when taking the time to act as a listener rather than performing other more visible, tangible nursing interventions. It is important to recognize that it requires practice and education to transform "ordinary" listening skills into "therapeutic" listening. In the process of learning therapeutic listening, the listener may actually learn to do less than more, undoing habitual reactions and interactions (Lee & Prior, 2013), since there can be a tendency for nurses to talk more and offer advice rather than to stay in the listening mode.

One must learn to be aware of what is occurring when listening: Am I filtering content through my personal lens? What am I doing with my body? Am I having an emotional reaction to what is being said? Am I formulating a response rather than staying engaged in listening? (Lee & Prior, 2013).

There are multiple ways to practice and refine therapeutic listening skills, both in education programs and in clinical practice. In education, using traditional and contemporary methods, such as role-playing and simulations, may be helpful; both of those scenarios developed specifically around therapeutic-listening situations or were embedded within scenarios that are emotionally charged, such as end-of-life conversations after acute physiological events. Scenarios can occur with colleagues, instructors, or actors playing the part of clients. They can also be videotaped or audiotaped and reviewed for learning opportunities. It is also important for instructors and preceptors to both role model in the clinical setting and provide feedback after observations of the student. The Calgary–Cambridge Referenced Observation Guide may be a helpful tool for instructors to use when educating nursing students in this skill (Bagacean et al., 2020; Taylor et al., 2018).

In clinical practice, more experienced colleagues and leaders can also role-model, mentor, and provide feedback in daily interactions, as well as in more formal conversations with patients and families such as care conferences. Mentors can offer phrases and techniques to improve listening skills as a vital component of building therapeutic relationships.

GUIDELINES

Listening is an active process, incorporating explicit behaviors, as well as attention to the choice of words, quality of voice (pitch, timing, and volume), and full engagement in the process (Burnard, 1997). Therapeutic listening requires a listener to tune in to the client and to use all the senses in analyzing, inferring, and evaluating the stated and underlying meaning of the client's message. As providers feel increasing time pressures, it can be easy to attempt to guide or limit the conversation rather than allowing the patient to fully express concerns. However, to be fully heard without interruption and using appropriate nonverbal behaviors can be viewed by the patient as providing a sense of security, well-being, and safety (Loos, 2021); can strengthen the individual's sense of self (Delaney et al., 2017); and may ultimately strengthen the therapeutic relationship. Therapeutic listening requires concentration and an ability to differentiate between what is actually being said and what one wants or expects to hear. It may be difficult to listen accurately and interpret messages that one finds difficult to relate to or to listen to information that one may not want to hear. When not fully engaged, it can be easy to become distracted or to start formulating a response rather than to stay focused on the message.

Therapeutic listening is both a cognitive and an emotional process. Jones and Cutcliffe (2009) state that therapeutic listening requires a critical competency of self-management and resilience in the midst of emotional situations. Furthermore, it involves the need to be comfortable with ambiguity and emotional discomfort. Nurses should be prepared with statements to use in response to expressions of negative emotions to encourage the speaker to further discuss their feelings (Adams et al., 2012). Several components have been identified as being foundational to therapeutic listening:

1. Rephrasing the patient's words and thoughts to ensure clarity and accuracy
2. Reflecting feeling
3. Conveying an understanding of the speaker's perceptions
4. Assumption checking
5. Asking questions and prompting to clarify (Bodie et al., 2015; De Vito, 2006)

These and other techniques for therapeutic listening intervention are presented in Exhibit 3.1.

Therapeutic listening with children can be even more complex because it frequently involves the presence or participation of more parties: nurse, child, parents, and/or other family members. This may take particular skill on the part of the nurse, who attends to both the spoken messages and the nonverbal communication/reactions of two or more people simultaneously. In addition, the nurse must be sensitive to the information and cues of either the child or the caregiver, depending on the child's age and developmental stage.

Adolescents especially may be willing to talk openly with an adult who is not a family member. However, they may respond quickly, abruptly, or defensively to any perceived indications of judgment, indifference, or disrespect on the part of the listener. With adolescents, it is extremely important to be fully attentive, allow for complete expression of thoughts, and avoid statements or facial expressions that imply disapproval or that can be misinterpreted.

Barriers are ever-present in today's healthcare settings to challenge the full use of therapeutic listening. These barriers can include the time required to fully engage; the pressure to focus on completing tasks such as patient care, paperwork, and charting; and a lack of opportunity (Ellison & Meyer, 2020). However, through initiatives such as "Commit to Sit," nurses may find more opportunities to embed therapeutic listening as a routine part of their day. Nurses on a medical telemetry unit made a commitment to sit with each patient at least once during the shift (at eye level, with eye contact, and undistracted). The unit saw improvements in their patient satisfaction scores for nursing (Lidgett, 2016).

Exhibit 3.1 *Therapeutic Listening Techniques*

Active presence: Active presence involves focusing on clients to interpret the message that they are trying to convey, on recognizing themes, and on hearing what is left unsaid. Short responses such as "yes" or "uh-huh" with appropriate timing and frequency may promote clients' willingness to talk.

Accepting attitude: Conveying an accepting attitude is assuring and can help clients feel more comfortable about expressing themselves. This can be demonstrated by short affirmative responses or gestures.

Clarifying statements: Clarifying statements and summarizing can help the listener verify message interpretation and create clarity, as well as encourage specificity rather than vague statements to facilitate communication. Rephrasing and reflection can assist the client in self-understanding. Using phrases such as "Tell me more about that," and "What was that like?" may be helpful rather than asking, "Why?" which may elicit a defensive response. Typically statements such as these are used with an introductory phrase that conveys speculation and an attempt to clarify (e.g., it seems that, it appears that, etc.)

Paraphrasing: The listener repeats what speakers said using their own words to the best of how the listener understood it.

Reflecting feelings: The listener references the speaker's statements in an attempt to accurately convey and mirror the feelings underlying the statements, which is different from paraphrasing.

Assumption checking: The listener uses short questions to verify accuracy in understanding the speaker's disclosure.

Use of silence: The use of silence can encourage the client to talk, facilitate the nurse's focus on listening rather than the formulation of responses, and reduce the use of leading questions. Sensitivity toward cultural and individual variations in the seconds of silence may be developed by paying detailed attention to the patterns of client communication.

Tone: Tone of voice can express more than words through empathy, judgment, or acceptance. The intensity of the tone should be matched to the message received to avoid minimizing or overemphasizing.

Nonverbal behaviors: Clients relaying sensitive information may be very aware of the listener's body language, which will be viewed as either accepting of the message or closed to it, judgmental, and/or disinterested. Eye contact or nodding is essential to conveying the listener's true interest and attention. Maintaining a conversational spatial distance and judicious use of touch may increase the client's comfort. Cultural and social awareness is important so as to avoid undesired touch as well as misinterpretation of gestures or expressions.

Environment: Distractions should be eliminated to encourage therapeutic interchange. Therapeutic listening may require careful planning to provide time for undivided attention or may occur spontaneously. Some clients may feel very comfortable having family present; others may feel inhibited when others are present.

A listening technique referred to as *change-oriented reflective listening* targets behavioral change in healthcare providers (Strang et al., 2004) and has a strong potential for incorporating the repertoire of nursing interventions. This technique has been adapted from the core principles of motivational interviewing

(Rollnick et al., 2002). Change-oriented reflective listening is a brief motivational enhancement intervention that encourages providers' consideration of the quality of primary care and then stimulates their intent to change behavior in the direction desired. This method takes the form of a brief telephone conversation (15–20 minutes), in which reflective listening statements are interspersed with open questions about the issue at hand. A menu of questions with a range of possible areas for discussion is constructed in advance. The technique has been successfully piloted with general practitioners to motivate them to intervene with opiate users and as part of alcohol intervention (McCambridge et al., 2004; Strang et al., 2004).

Communicating with a patient and family in difficult situations necessitates careful and considerate listening skills. Basic communication skills, such as the "ask–tell–ask" and "tell me more" principles, have been introduced to oncology settings (Back et al., 2005) and end-of-life care in critical care settings (Hollyday & Buonocore, 2015). The first "ask" is used for the provider to assess the perceptions and understanding of a patient or family regarding the current situation or issue at hand. This step would help the provider to obtain a basic idea about the patient's or family's level of knowledge or emotional state. The "tell" portion is used for the provider to convey the most pressing needed or desired information to the patient/family. The information should be provided in understandable, brief chunks, kept to no more than three pieces of information at a time. Then the second "ask" is used to check the understanding of the patient/family and to answer their additional questions. The "ask–tell–ask" cycle would be repeated until a final "ask" is a summary of agreed-on decisions or plans. "Tell me more" can be used to get back on track when the conversation appears diverted. It also can be used to allow the patient/family to share more of their emotions while letting the health provider get past initial reactions and respond in a less defensive or emotional mode (Back et al., 2005; Shannon et al., 2011).

MEASUREMENT OF OUTCOMES

Including multiple measurements, such as self-report, behavioral observation, physiological indicators, and qualitative accounts, provides rich data for the study of therapeutic listening. For example, the Active Listening Observation Scale (ALOS-global) is a validated seven-item behavioral observational scale that measures the general practitioner's attentiveness and acknowledgment of suffering among patients presenting minor ailments (Fassaert et al., 2007).

Challenges for outcome measurement may include the isolation of therapeutic listening as an independent variable from other confounding variables. Other challenges may be related to the complexity of the multifaceted phenomenon of therapeutic listening that may necessitate different study designs. Antecedents to interventions, such as clients' characteristics, have to be taken into consideration; likewise, the process-related components of interventions, such as short- and long-term improvements in nurses' knowledge, skills, and attitudes after training and client outcomes, need to be evaluated (Harrington et al., 2004; Kruijver et al., 2000).

Positive changes in psychological variables such as anxiety, depression, hostility, nurse–patient communication, or nursing care satisfaction are potential client outcomes of therapeutic listening. It may also be useful to examine physiological measures (e.g., heart rate, blood pressure, respiratory rate, immunological measures, electroencephalography results) as outcomes of therapeutic interchange. Outcomes may include clinical variables such as patients' response to illness, mood, treatment adherence, disease control, morbidity, and healthcare cost. Boudreau et al. (2009) believe that therapeutic listening can result in multiple outcomes: Listening gives patients opportunities to articulate concerns that provide insight into their "personhood"; it can generate data for providers to use in the provision of optimal care, and it may actually assist in healing.

PRECAUTIONS

Therapeutic listening has at its heart the intent to be helpful; however, a few precautions are warranted. Questions that start with the word *why* may take clients out of the context of their experience or feelings and direct them into an intellectual thinking mode or cause defensive responses. Rather, phrases such as "Tell me more about that," or "What was that like?" (Shattell & Hogan, 2005, p. 31) may be helpful.

The provider needs to be engaged fully when using therapeutic listening. If the provider is only half-listening, is using selective listening, or is distracted, patients may sense that their concerns are being minimized, or the provider may reach an inaccurate diagnosis. This weakens the therapeutic relationship between patient and provider (Boudreau et al., 2009).

The provider also needs to be aware of the potential negative self-consequences if the caregiver is involved in emotionally charged situations. Clinical supervision may be helpful for the provider in addressing such difficulties (Jones & Cutcliffe, 2009).

Practitioners and clinicians are encouraged to raise positive expectations and cautioned to selectively use active listening skills, especially with patients with minor ailments. When patients were in a good mood state before the consultation, the active listening behavior of general practitioners was observed to correlate with nonadherence to medication regimens. Rather, general practitioners' sensitivity to the emotional state of a patient and provision of clear explanations of the condition and preferable prognosis were observed to correlate with patients' reduced anxiety and better overall health (Fassaert et al., 2008).

Maintaining professional boundaries during therapeutic listening is important; empathy should be demonstrated but within the professional relationship with clients. Referrals for professional counseling may be indicated in cases such as psychiatric crises. Ethical dilemmas may result if the principle of respecting clients' autonomy and confidentiality conflicts with the principle of maintaining professional responsibility and integrity, such as taking action based on sensitive information shared in the therapeutic exchange. Open discussion and negotiating the use of such sensitive information, within the context of the nurse–client relationship, relies on the trust relationship that has been established such that the trust is retained or even deepened.

USES

Therapeutic listening is an intervention applicable to a virtually unlimited number of care situations. Selected patient population–based examples in which the use of listening is described are included in Exhibit 3.2. The Websites section that follows presents websites of national and international professional organizations where online resources for therapeutic listening can be found.

Exhibit 3.2 *Selected Uses of Listening With Patient Populations or in Care Settings*
• Emergency care for pediatric patients (Grahn et al., 2016) • Emergency care for adults (Hermann et al., 2019) • End-of-life care in critical care settings (Myers & Hyrkas, 2021) • Family-centered care in neonatal intensive care (Naef et al., 2020) • Heart failure: to improve self-care (Riegel et al., 2017) • Major depressive disorder (Davidson et al., 2015) • Neonatal intensive care unit (NICU): mothers' depression management (Segre et al., 2016) • Preschoolers with developmental disabilities (Bazyk et al., 2010) • Spiritual care for patients with life-threatening cancer (Kang & Kim, 2020) • Spiritual interventions in diabetes prevention (Long, 2020) • Teen mothers (SmithBattle & Freed, 2016) • Women with breast cancer (Cohen et al., 2012) • Young people in foster care (Murphy & Jenkinson, 2012)

MENTAL HEALTH SETTINGS

Therapeutic listening can be particularly impactful in mental health settings and situations. Patient mentions of hints and expressions of concerns are more prevalent in mental health nursing interactions compared to patients in medical settings (Griep et al., 2016). Psychiatric mental health nurses use short responses to these cues and expressions rather than long responses or providing advice, allowing the patient to have space to talk more about their emotions. While this is positive, Griep and colleagues also saw opportunities for the nurses to continue developing their active listening skills.

A case example by Faccio et al. (2021) relays a patient perspective on the frustration of not feeling heard, which can lead to aggression and potential violence in this population. The authors provide recommendations for using listening techniques to engage in therapeutic relationships with patients. Expert psychiatric nurses viewed active listening as a means to be attentive to the patient's message and to facilitate finding meaning behind the messages (Thomson et al., 2019).

TECHNOLOGY

With the increased use of technology in everyday healthcare environments (e.g., telehealth, telemedicine, charting at the bedside through electronic health records), it is imperative to consider how the use of technology can either impede or enhance the use of therapeutic listening skills.

Technology is ever-advancing and becoming increasingly important in ensuring that patients have effective means to communicate and ways to be fully heard and understood. Devices such as Passy–Muir tracheal valves that can allow mechanically ventilated patients to speak, computer programs that can "speak" the patient's electronic input, and laryngeal devices are now more frequently available and expected to promote communication. When alternative methods are being used, nonverbal communication is even more important to observe and monitor.

Telehealth and telephone visits were being implemented prior to the COVID-19 pandemic, but their use exponentially increased with the onset of the pandemic. While telehealth provides opportunities to provide care to individuals who are not able to meet in person, it is too early to definitively state the effectiveness of therapeutic listening via telehealth. Itamura and colleagues (2021) identified communication shortcomings with this interactive methodology when used with otolaryngologic patients when comparing surveys from 1,284 in-person visits pre-pandemic to 221 virtual visits post-pandemic onset. They noted a significant reduction in patient satisfaction with careful listening with virtual visits compared to in-person visits ($p = 0.003$). This reduction in perceived careful listening was similar to the overall satisfaction with the virtual visit compared to in person. While this may be a unique population in which communication can be challenging, it is important to continue to study this area in light of the likelihood that virtual visits will remain well after the pandemic is resolved. Regardless, focused training of providers will be needed on how to convey therapeutic listening via telehealth.

LISTENING FOR NURSES

In light of the rise in burnout and fatigue for all healthcare providers (National Academies of Science, Engineering, and Medicine, 2019), but especially nurses, it is worthwhile to consider how therapeutic listening can be used to support the well-being of nurses, and thus their ability to optimally care for patients. Active-empathic listening on the part of supervisors in Iceland was shown to have a significant positive relationship with employee work engagement ($p < 0.001$; Jonsdottir & Kristensson, 2020). The authors recommend further research and support of supervisor training to improve active-empathic listening skills.

Supporting resilience and mitigating burnout have been particularly compelling issues for healthcare workers during the COVID pandemic. One healthcare system implemented a multipronged program to address resilience and burnout during the pandemic. A component of this program included an adaptation of the U.S. Army's "Battle Buddy" system (Abbott et al., 2020), in which buddies assist each other in and out of combat with the goal to make sure no one is "left behind." Healthcare workers were paired with buddies based on like areas such as clinical practice and responsibility, experience and role, and life situations outside work. One of the goals of the program was to encourage daily conversations between buddies to promote a sense of being connected, provide mutual support, and develop a sense of trust (Abbott et al., 2020)—in other words, feeling that there was someone there to listen and provide insights. Resources for more formal mental health consultation were available if a buddy noticed escalating anxiety or other concerning behaviors. The overarching purpose was to offer a safe place at work to discuss the unique challenges experienced during the pandemic with coworkers who understood so that time outside work could truly be focused on relaxation and rest (Abbott et al., 2020). While the authors have not yet published the results of the program at the time of this writing, this intervention certainly aligns with using therapeutic listening as a complementary therapy to decrease anxiety and support resilience.

CULTURAL APPLICATIONS

Sensitivity and awareness of cultural variations in communication styles are vital to intervention effectiveness. Cultural differences in meanings of certain words, styles, and approaches or in certain nonverbal behaviors such as silence, touch, eye contact, or smile, may adversely affect the effectiveness of therapeutic communication. For example, there may be tendencies for clients from certain cultures to talk loudly, to be direct in conversation, and to come to the point quickly. Clients from other cultures may tend to talk softly, be indirect in their communication, or "talk around" points while emphasizing attitudes and feelings. In some cultures, it is believed that open expression of emotions is unacceptable. Whether in the dominant culture or in nondominant cultures, however, people may simply smile when they do not comprehend. The skills of therapeutic listening are particularly useful in ensuring that communication in such cases is effective.

The need is urgent for nursing to reduce health inequities in healthcare (NASEM, 2019). One of the beginning steps to accomplishing this is to utilize therapeutic listening with patient populations that are particularly vulnerable, marginalized, or disadvantaged. Through listening, nurses can minimize the gaps between human interactions where each person can have a different interpretation based on culture, ethnicity, language, and experiences (Alicea-Planas, 2016). Listening can contribute to the formation of meaning and outcomes in a therapeutic provider–patient relationship and reduce barriers these populations encounter (Alicea-Planas, 2016).

It is important that nurses explore and understand clients' cultural values and assumptions, as well as their patterns of behavior related to communication, while avoiding stereotyping (Seidel et al., 2011). Awareness of cultural differences is key to therapeutic communication. Sidebars 3.1 through 3.3 illustrate the importance of therapeutic listening in very diverse cultural contexts. Sidebar 3.1 provides an exemplar of the use of therapeutic listening in the context of a healthcare setting in Japan. It underscores the challenge of working within an Asian culture wherein older adults may hesitate to express concerns and when they may perceive questioning medical providers to be improper or socially unacceptable. Sidebar 3.2 presents the challenge of overcoming barriers of cultural differences in healthcare and the need for establishing trust in the therapeutic relationship through careful listening to achieve mutually desired healthcare outcomes. A final cultural example is provided in Sidebar 3.3, which emphasizes the centrality of family and proposes their inclusion in therapeutic listening surrounding the patients' care.

Sidebar 3.1 *Nurses' Therapeutic Listening Skills Used for Older Postesophagectomy Patients in Tokyo, Japan*

Shigeaki Watanuki

Many esophageal cancer patients in Japan undergo thoracoabdominal esophageal surgery. Such patients frequently experience multiple signs and symptoms after surgery for months and sometimes even years due to gastrointestinal (GI) conditions. These conditions may include vocal cord paralysis, esophageal stenosis, or reflux, which may result in coughing, dysphagia, difficulty swallowing, vomiting, weight loss, or reduced physical activity.

Surgeons, due to their limited time and the large number of patients, have only a few minutes to listen to postsurgical patients in outpatient departments. Older Japanese patients usually hesitate to ask their primary doctors (surgeons) about their signs and symptoms, changes in daily life, or biopsychosocial concerns. It is as though these older adults think they have problems that are "too small" to ask their doctors. Such problems, however, are often very important and may actually be an indication of major complications or GI conditions; reporting them may aid in diagnosis.

(continued)

Sidebar 3.1 *Nurses' Therapeutic Listening Skills Used for Older Postesophagectomy Patients in Tokyo, Japan (continued)*

Nurses' therapeutic listening skills play a key role in detecting patients' problems. Nurses at this hospital are trained in the "ask–tell–ask" and "tell me more" educational programs. Designated nurses are assigned to the GI surgical outpatient department to see postsurgical patients and to listen to their stories. In addition, nurses are specifically trained to use systematic questions and assessment skills that enhance identifying the patients' GI problems and symptoms. Such questions include general (e.g., fatigue, insomnia), GI-related (e.g., nausea and vomiting, constipation, diarrhea, constipation), and esophagectomy-related symptoms (e.g., dysphagia, reflux, difficulty swallowing, choking, coughing). If the nurses "sense" patients' problems through a therapeutic exchange, they continue to explore the type and degree of the patients' problems and the way that the problems affect their daily lives. The nurses listen to the patients' entire experiences of living after esophagectomy while paying attention to any potential signs of hesitation or emotional distress that the patients may not show or state clearly. The nurses are aware that older Japanese patients usually do not want to admit they "have problems or difficulties"; however, they do have problems or difficulties. With nurse reassurance and encouragement, patients may go on: "Actually, I am concerned this symptom may be . . . ," or "Yeah, I was going to say I have been bothered by this symptom for weeks. . . ."

One day, a nurse saw a patient who complained of nothing special but had eaten sushi the previous evening as a celebration of his 80th birthday—3 months after his esophagectomy. The nurse kept exploring the patient's story and found that he had continuously experienced a decline in food intake because of an increased difficulty in passing food through his esophagus. The nurse assessed that such a condition might be associated with esophageal stenosis, an indication of a need for balloon or bougie dilation by his surgeon. The nurse immediately reported this to the surgeon. The surgeon examined the patient and, as expected, diagnosed severe esophageal stenosis. This patient's condition might otherwise have been overlooked by nurses and surgeons if this nurse had not had an outstanding "sense" and effective therapeutic listening skills.

The nurses also provide assurance and positive feedback if the patients are on the right track and are trying to adhere to the expected "healthy behavior." Such behavior includes eating small amounts of food slowly, engaging in regular physical activity, and keeping the upper body elevated while asleep. If patients would benefit from behavioral changes in their daily lives, nurses work with them to find acceptable common ground.

After seeing patients, the nurses convey the clients' critical information or questions to the surgeon if indicated and desired. Otherwise, nurses encourage the patients to relay their concerns to the surgeons or may ask surgeons questions on behalf of patients. The patients and surgeons of this department have reported that the nurses are sensitive to the patients' needs and have noted how helpful nurses are in working together on behalf of the patients. The nurses' outstanding therapeutic listening skills truly enhance the quality of care in the outpatient department of this hospital.

Sidebar 3.2 *The Role of Complementary and Alternative Therapies in Caring for Somali Patients*

Nasra Giama

Therapeutic listening as part of therapeutic communication with Somali patients may not only build trust but also help provide culturally sensitive care. It can help avoid adverse interactions between traditional therapies and those used in Western medicine.

Numerous types of complementary and alternative therapies are used by Somalis, including massage, prayer and spiritual healing, plant-based treatments, and herbs. The most popular herbs are fenugreek and black seed (oil or seed form), and specialized diets are used to treat certain diseases. For example, natural products may be used to induce diarrhea to cleanse the colon and digestive system (*qaras bixin*); the purpose is to expel sickness-causing pathogens. Traditional healers and spiritual leaders may be called on to use the Qur'an, as well as the teachings from the Prophet, to provide tailored treatment remedies and prayers for sick individuals. Listening to recitations of the Qur'an is calming, healing, and humbling; through the recitations, one may come to appreciate God's (Allah's) blessings and may ask for the higher being to send healing (Ahmed, 1988).

Trained traditional healers in Somalia may use cutting (bloodletting to remove spoiled blood), burning/cauterization (consistent with the Somali saying, "Disease and fire cannot stay together in the same place"), and cupping (Ahmed, 1988). Traditional healers typically find it difficult to practice in the Western world because of laws prohibiting certain practices. However, Somalis may seek traditional care because it is what they know and how they perceive their illness. They seek it from healers and spiritual leaders whom they trust. Often, these are sought before entry into the more foreign Western healthcare system.

To provide patient-centered, culturally sensitive care to Somali patients, therapeutic listening is important (Guerin et al., 2004). There are important questions to be asked related to complementary and alternative therapies and healing practices, and the nurse should listen carefully and respectfully to the answers. Tips for nurses:

1. Ask patients for their understanding or explanations of the illnesses they are experiencing. What do they think is the cause?
2. Ask what patients have done at home for self-care or ask about other remedies or healing practices they may have sought and used. Identify through conversation with patients and caregivers what things they do (or have done), in addition to the treatment plan recommended by the healthcare team?

(continued)

Sidebar 3.2 *The Role of Complementary and Alternative Therapies in Caring for Somali Patients (continued)*

3. Provide a "showing," or demonstration, of any complementary or alternative therapy if offered to a Somali patient in the context of the Western healthcare system. Clearly explain its purpose. A Somali patient may know and have used certain therapies but be unfamiliar with the English terms for them. The nurse can listen carefully to the patient to determine whether the therapy is understood and, if so, whether it is desired.

References

Ahmed, A. (1988). Somali traditional healers, role and status. *Medicine and Traditional Medicine*, 240–247.   http://dspace-roma3.caspur.it/bitstream/2307/1050/5/33_A.%20M.%20AHMED%20-%20Somali%20traditional%20healers,%20role%20and%20status.pdf;jsessionid=E66E51EF5CAA227F7FA8BC1C378E8DA0

Guerin, B., Guerin, P., Diiriye, R., Omar, R., & Yates, S. (2004). Somali conceptions and expectations concerning mental health: Some guidelines for mental health professionals. *New Zealand Journal of Psychology*, 33(2), 59–67.

Sidebar 3.3 *Therapeutic Communication With Mexican Patients Includes Listening to Families*

Karim Bauza

First, in providing care to Mexican patients, one must understand the absolute importance of family. Culturally, in Mexico and other Latin American countries, family holds things together. From the perspective of my culture and Mexican/Latina heritage, I know that if something happens to me, I have a strong family support system to rely on. The importance of family extends to medical care contexts. Some nurses would like to care for patients without the family present; working with family members in difficult healthcare contexts can be frustrating. Having family in the room or answering their questions may be difficult, but family have expectations and responsibilities to be on top of the care and to help in making decisions for their family member. If I were injured and hospitalized, my whole family would be in the room. Someone would be with me (or desire to be) 100% of the time.

Listening to the family in the hospital is important. If a family member were to be intubated, you would be able to get significant information from family (e.g., patient allergies and personal preferences). In Latina cultures, family is a resource. It would be unusual for family not to be present or not to visit regularly when a family member is hospitalized. Coming from this family-centered culture, it is shocking when I care for non-Latino patients and sometimes family may

(continued)

Sidebar 3.3 *Therapeutic Communication With Mexican Patients Includes Listening to Families (continued)*

not be there or visit for days at a time. Family is a great resource that is often underutilized. If I had a family member who was hospitalized, I would want the nurse to make me feel included. I would be listening to how my family member will get better. How could my loved one be more comfortable? How are their holistic needs being met?

The difference in knowledge and practice between the large urban tertiary care centers and what is available in small towns or locations in Mexico is significant. There are "medical deserts" in Mexico. There are cultural differences that should be considered. For example, in the Mexican culture, someone with sniffles may take penicillin—penicillin for everything. It is available without a prescription. If a patient arrives in the United States from Mexico requiring healthcare, they would have many questions, which may go unasked and unanswered if a therapeutic relationship is not developed through mutual listening. In this process, nurses should try their best to include the family. We learned this in our basic education, but its importance cannot be overemphasized.

So, what would I recommend a nurse do? Listen. Many Mexican or Latina patients may not know why they are taking their prescribed medications; listen to what they think is the purpose of the treatment or medication. Use therapeutic listening skills to build the bridge to get closer to them in a therapeutic relationship to close the gap between what they are thinking about their care and health and what they may need to know to ensure desired therapeutic outcomes. Use listening skills to gather important information about Latina patients' medical and cultural backgrounds and understanding of their health or illness. As a nurse, a priority is to understand their expectations of treatment outcomes. To achieve positive healthcare outcomes, it is important to reach common understandings with the patient and family members who may support the patients or provide care. Otherwise, problems with medical adherence to the prescribed drugs, medical treatments, or therapies are likely. Without careful listening for understanding and reaching mutual expectations and goals for care, medical therapies may be doomed to fail. For example, in the case of wound care, it is important that the patient and family have the supplies and understanding of the timing and techniques of dressing changes—otherwise, the wound won't be properly dressed and the patient is likely to return with infection.

Listening needs to occur on both sides of a relationship. It should not only be the nurse or provider saying, "This is my expectation for your treatment and outcome." The nurse may also need to be the one who listens first; nurses can model listening and respect. Two-sided listening has an important role in the caregiving relationship. Nurses can listen to hear what the patient and family understand and what they are seeking from care. Only through listening and truly hearing can the nurse know and understand patient and family preferences and demonstrate caring. In this manner, trust is developed, and patients and families can be confident that the nurse and providers have their best interest at heart.

LANGUAGE CHALLENGES

Interpreter-mediated healthcare encounters can be a challenge for therapeutic interchange. Using appropriately trained and experienced interpreters is a necessity for clients who have language barriers.

Roter and colleagues (2020) studied the outcomes of professional interpreter use for patients speaking Spanish, Cantonese, and Mandarin for primary care visits in a large, urban academic practice. A total of 55 patient visits with 31 clinicians (physicians, nurse practitioners, residents) were recorded. Conversations were coded using the Roter Interactions Analysis System (RIAS) looking for patient-centered statements related to psychosocial, lifestyle, and socioemotional talk. The researchers found that there were significantly fewer RIAS-coded statements between clinicians and interpreters-as-clinicians. Findings were similar for RIAS-coded statements between patients and interpreters-as-patients. Differences were higher for Spanish translations than for Cantonese or Mandarin translations. In other words, patients and clinicians made substantially more RAIS-coded statements than were conveyed by the translators (Roter et al., 2020). This has the potential to substantially alter the perception of therapeutic listening and the promotion of patient-centered care.

Another study showed that non-English-speaking family members are at an increased risk of receiving less information about the patient's condition, as evidenced by less family conference time, shorter duration, and less proportion of clinician speech during a conference (Thornton et al., 2009). This study also showed that non-English-speaking families receive less reported emotional support from their healthcare providers, including valuing families' input, easing emotional burdens, and actively listening (Thornton et al., 2009). Healthcare professionals' cultural sensitivity and considerations are vital to promoting quality of care for patients/families with language barriers.

FUTURE RESEARCH

Many research questions have the potential for exploration in the area of therapeutic listening. Systematic studies are needed to develop a body of knowledge. The study designs will require new paradigms beyond traditional randomized controlled trials for, among other things, ethical and feasibility reasons. Qualitative studies, case reports, or mixed-method designs may be better options for understanding the nature and effects of therapeutic listening. Some potential questions for future research include the following:

- Can caring, through therapeutic listening via telephone or virtual telehealth visits, be effectively conveyed?
- What are the effects of listening by healthcare providers on patient satisfaction and other outcomes of care?
- Are interventions to enhance listening on the part of healthcare providers cost-effective and legitimate areas on which to focus continuous quality improvement to increase patient safety and quality of care?
- How do multicultural differences manifest in the processes and effectiveness of therapeutic listening?

WEBSITES

- International Listening Association (www.listen.org)
- EACH: International Association for Communication in Health Care (www .each.eu)
- AACH: Academy on Communication in Healthcare (www.achonline.org)

REFERENCES

Abbott, C. S., Wozniak, J. R., McGlinch, B. P., Wall, M. H., Gold, B. S., & Vinogradov, S. (2020). Battle buddies: Rapid deployment of a psychological resilience intervention for health care workers during the COVID-19 pandemic. *Anesthesia & Analgesia, 131*(1), 43–54. https://doi .org/10.1213/ANE.0000000000004912

Adams, K., Cimino, J. E. W., Arnold, R. M., & Anderson, W. G. (2012). Why should I talk about emotion? Communication patterns associated with physician discussion of patient expressions of negative emotion in hospital admission encounters. *Patient Education and Counseling, 89*(1), 44–50. https://doi.org/10.1016/j.pec.2012.04.005

Alicea-Planas, J. (2016). Listening to the narratives of our patients as part of holistic nursing care. *Journal of Holistic Nursing, 34*(2), 162–166. https://doi.org/10.1177/0898010115591396

Back, A. L., Arnold, R. M., Baile, W. F., Tulsky, J. A., & Fryer-Edwards, K. (2005). Approaching difficult communication tasks in oncology. *CA: A Cancer Journal for Clinicians, 55*(3), 164–177. https://doi.org/10.3322/canjclin.55.3.164

Bagacean, C., Cousin, I., Ubertini, A-H., El Idrissi, M. E. Y., Bordron, A., Mercadie, L., Garci a, L. C., Ianotto, J-C., DeVries, P., & Berthou, C. (2020). Simulated patient and role play methodologies for communication skills and empathy training of undergraduate medical students. *BMC Medical Education, 20*(1), 491. https://doi.org/10.1186/s12909-020-02401-0

Bazyk, S., Cimino, J., Hayes, K., Goodman, G., & Farrell, P. (2010). The use of therapeutic listening with preschoolers with developmental disabilities: A look at the outcomes. *Journal of Occupational Therapy, Schools, and Early Intervention, 3*(2), 124–138. https://doi.org/10.1080/19411243.210.49103

Berzins, K., Baker, J., Brown, M., & Lawton, R. (2018). A cross-sectional survey of mental health service users', carers' and professionals' priorities for patient safety in the United Kingdom. *Health Expectations, 21*(6), 1085–1094. https://doi.org/10.1111/hex.12805

Bodie, G. D., Vickery, A. J., Cannava, K. E., & Jones, S. (2015). The role of "active listening" in informal helping conversations: Impact on perceptions of listener helpfulness, sensitivity, and supportiveness and discloser emotional improvement. *Western Journal of Communication, 79*(2), 151–173. https://doi.org/10.1080/10570314.2014.943429

Boudreau, J. D., Cassell, E., & Fuks, A. (2009). Preparing medical students to become attentive listeners. *Medical Teacher, 31*, 22–29. https://doi.org/10.1080/01421590802350776

Burnard, P. (1997). *Effective communication skills for health professionals* (2nd ed.). Nelson Thornes.

Centers for Medicare and Medicaid Services. (2014). *HCAHPS: Patients' perspectives of care survey*. https://www.cms.gov/Medicare/Quality-Initiatives-Patient-Assessment-Instruments/HospitalQualityInits/HospitalHCAHPS.html

Centers for Medicare and Medicaid Services. (2015). *HCAHPS fact sheet*. http://hospitalcoremeasures.com/pdf/hcahps/HCAHPS_Fact_Sheet_June_2015.pdf

Cohen, M., Anderson, R. C., Jensik, K., Xiang, Q., Pruszynski, J., & Walker, A. P. (2012). Communication between breast cancer patients and their physicians about breast-related body image issues. *Plastic Surgical Nursing, 32*(3), 101–105. https://doi.org/10.1097/PSN.0b013e3182650994

Davidson, S. K., Harris, M. G., Dowrick, C. F., Wachtler, C. A., Pirkis, J., & Gunn, J. M. (2015). Mental health interventions and future major depression among primary care patients with subthreshold depression. *Journal of Affective Disorders, 177*, 65–73. https://doi.org/10.1016/j.jad.2015.02.014

Delaney, K. R., Shattell, M., & Johnson, M. E. (2017). Capturing the interpersonal process of psychiatric nurses: A model for engagement. *Archives of Psychiatric Nursing, 31*, 634–640. https://doi.org/10.1016/j.apnu.2017.08.003

De Vito, J. A. (2006). *The interpersonal communication book* (11th ed.). Allyn & Bacon.

Ellison, D. L., & Meyer, C. K. (2020). Presence and therapeutic listening. *Nursing Clinics of North America, 55*(4), 457–465. https://doi.org/10.1016/j.cnur.2020.06.012

Faccio, E., Anonymous Author, & Rocelli, M. (2021). It's the way you treat me that makes me angry, it's not a question of madness: Good and bad practice in dealing with violence in the mental health services. *Mental Health Nursing, 28*, 481–487. https://doi.org/10.1111/jpm.12690

Fassaert, T., van Dulmen, S., Schellevis, F., & Bensing, J. (2007). Active listening in medical consultations: Development of the Active Listening Observation Scale (ALOS-global). *Patient Education and Counseling, 68*(3), 258–264. https://doi.org/10.1016/j.pec.2007.06.011

Fassaert, T., van Dulmen, S., Schellevis, F., van der Jagt, L., & Bensing, J. (2008). Raising positive expectations helps patients with minor ailments: A cross-sectional study. *BMC Family Practice, 9*, 38. https://doi.org/10.1186/1471-2296-9-38

Garcia, A. C. M., Simão-Miranda, T. P., Carvalho, A. M. P., Elias, P. C. L., Pereira, M. D. G., & Carvalho, E. C. (2018). The effect of therapeutic listening on anxiety and fear among surgical patients: Randomized controlled trial. *Revista Latino-Americana de Enfermagem, 9*(26), e3027. https://doi.org/10.1590/1518-8345.2438.3027

Grahn, M., Olsson, E., & Mansson, M. E. (2016). Interactions between children and pediatric nurses at the emergency department: A Swedish interview study. *Journal of Pediatric Nursing, 31*, 284–292. https://doi.org/10.1016/j.pedn.2015.11.016

Griep, E. C., Noordman, J., & van Dulmen, S. (2016). Practice nurses mental health provide space to patients to discuss unpleasant emotions. *Journal of Psychiatric and Mental Health Nursing, 23*(2), 77–85. https://doi.org/10.1111/jpm.12279

Halpern, J. (2012, Spring). Attending to clinical wisdom. *Journal of Clinical Ethics, 23*(1), 41–46. https://doi.org/10.1111/j.1467-8519.2010.01817.x

Harrington, J., Noble, L. M., & Newman, S. P. (2004). Improving patients' communication with doctors: A systematic review of intervention studies. *Patient Education and Counseling, 52*(1), 7–16. https://doi.org/10.1016/s0738-3991(03)00017-x

Hermann, R. M., Long, E., & Trotta, R. L. (2019). Improving patients' experiences communicating with nurses and providers in the emergency department. *Journal of Emergency Nursing, 45*(5), 523–530. https://doi.org/10.1016/j.jen.2018.12.001

Hollyday, S. L., & Buonocore, D. (2015). Breaking bad news and discussing goals of care in the intensive care unit. *AACN Advanced Critical Care, 26*(2), 131–141. https://doi.org/10.1097/NCI.0000000000000082

Itamura, K., Tang, D. M., Higgins, T. S., Rimell, F. L., Illing, E. A., Ting, J. Y., Lee, M. K., & Wu, A. (2021). Comparison of patient satisfaction between virtual visits during the COVID-19 pandemic and in-person visits during the COVID-19 visits pre-pandemic. *Annals of Otology, Rhinology, & Laryngology, 130*(7), 810–817. https://doi.org/10.1177/0003489420977766

Jones, A. C., & Cutcliffe, J. R. (2009). Listening as a method of addressing psychological distress. *Journal of Nursing Management, 17*(3), 352–358. https://doi.org/10.1111/j.1365-2834.2009.00998.x

Jonsdottir, I. J., & Kristinsson, K. (2020). Supervisors' active-empathetic listening as an important antecedent of work engagement. *International Journal of Environmental Research and Public Health, 17*(21), 7976. https://doi.org/10.3390/ijerph17217976

Kang, K. A., & Kim, S. J. (2020). Comparison of perceptions of spiritual care among patients with life-threatening cancer, primary family caregivers, and hospice/palliative care nurses in South Korea. *Journal of Hospice and Palliative Nursing, 22*(6), 532–551. https://doi.org/10.1097/NJH.0000000000000697

Kawamichi, H., Yoshihara, K., Sasaki, A. T., Sugawara, S. K., Tanabe, H. C., Shinohara, R., Sugisawa, Y., Tokutake, K., Mochizuki, Y., Amme, T., & Sadato, N. (2015). Perceiving active listening activates the reward system and improves the impression of relevant experiences. *Social Neuroscience, 10*(1), 16–26. https://doi.org/10.1080/17470919.2014.954732

Kemper, B. J. (1992). Therapeutic listening: Developing the concept. *Journal of Psychosocial Nursing and Mental Health Services, 30*(7), 21–23. https://doi.org/10.3928/0279-3695-19920701-07

Kornhaber, R., Walsh, K., Duff, J., & Walker, K. (2016). Enhancing adult therapeutic interpersonal relationships in the acute health care setting: An integrative review. *Journal of Multidisciplinary Healthcare, 14*(9), 537–546. https://doi.org/10.2147/JMDH.S116957

Kruijver, I. P., Kerkstra, A., Francke, A. L., Bensing, J. M., & van de Wiel, H. B. (2000). Evaluation of communication training programs in nursing care: A review of the literature. *Patient Education and Counseling, 39*, 129–145. https://doi.org/10.1016/s0738-3991(99)00096-8

Lee, B., & Prior, S. (2013). Developing therapeutic listening. *British Journal of Guidance & Counseling, 41*(2), 91–104. https://doi.org/10.1080/03069885.2012.705816

Lekander, B. J., Lehmann, S., & Lindquist, R. (1993). Therapeutic listening: Key nursing interventions for several nursing diagnoses. *Dimensions of Critical Care Nursing, 12*, 24–30. https://doi.org/10.1097/00003465-199301000-00012

Lidgett, C. D. (2016). Improving the patient experience through a commit to sit service excellence initiative. *Patient Experience Journal, 3*(2), 67–72. https://doi.org/10.35680/2372-0247.1148

Liu, J. E., Mok, E., Wong, T., Xue, L., & Xu, B. (2007). Evaluation of an integrated communication skills training program for nurses in cancer care in Beijing, China. *Nursing Research, 56*, 202–209. https://doi.org/10.1097/01.NNR.0000270030.82736.8c

Long, S. E. P. (2020). Faith community nursing: Using spiritual interventions in diabetes prevention. *Journal of Christian Nursing, 37*(4), 243–249. https://doi.org/10.1097/CNJ.0000000000000752

Loos, N. M. (2021). Nurse listening as perceived by patients: How to improve the patient experience, keep patients safe, and raise HCAHPS Scores. *Journal of Nursing Administration, 51*(6), 324–328. https://doi.org/10.1097/NNA.0000000000001021

McCambridge, J., Platts, S., Whooley, D., & Strang, J. (2004). Encouraging GP alcohol intervention: Pilot study of change-oriented reflective listening (CORL). *Alcohol & Alcoholism, 39*(2), 146–149. https://doi.org/10.1093/alcalc/agh027

Mehrabian, A., & Ferris, S. R. (1967). Inference of attitudes from nonverbal communication in two channels. *Journal of Consulting and Clinical Psychology, 31*(3), 248–252. https://doi.org/10.1037/h0024648

Murphy, D., & Jenkinson, H. (2012). The mutual benefits of listening to young people in care, with a particular focus on grief and loss: An Irish foster carer's perspective. *Child Care in Practice, 18*(3), 243–253. https://doi.org/10.1080/13575279.2012.683772

Myers, J. C., & Hyrkas, K. (2021). End-of-life care: Improving communication and reducing stress. *Critical Care Nursing Quarterly, 44*(2), 235–247. https://doi.org/10.1097/CNQ.0000000000000357

Naef, R., Kläuser-Troxler, M., Ernst, J., Huber, S., Dinten-Schmid, B., Karen, T., & Petry, H. (2020). Translating family systems care into neonatal practice: A mixed method study of practitioners' attitudes, practice skills and implementation experience. *International Journal of Nursing Studies, 102*, 103448. https://doi.org/10.1016/j.ijnurstu.2019.103448

National Academies of Science, Engineering, and Medicine. (2019). *Taking action against clinician burnout: A systems approach to professional well-being.* The National Academies Press. https://doi.org/10.17226/25521

Riegel, B., Dickson, V. V., Garcia, L. E., Masterson Creber, R., & Streur, M. (2017). Mechanisms of change in self-care in adults with heart failure receiving a tailored, motivational interviewing intervention. *Patient Education and Counseling, 100*, 283–288. https://doi.org/10.1016/j.pec.2016.08.030

Rogers, C. R. (1957). The necessary and sufficient conditions of therapeutic personality change. *Journal of Consulting Psychology, 21*, 95–103. https://doi.org/10.1037/0033-3204.44.3.240

Rollnick, S., Allison, J., Ballasiotes, S., Barth, T., Butler, C. C., Rose, G. S., & Rosengren, D. B. (2002). Variations on a theme: Motivational interviewing and its adaptations. In W. R. Miller & S. Rollnick (Eds.), *Motivational interviewing: Preparing people for change* (2nd ed., pp. 270–283). Guilford Press.

Roter, D. L., Gregorich, S. E., Diamond, L., Livaudais-Toman, J., Kaplan, C., Pathak, S., & Karliner, L. (2020). Loss of patient centeredness in interpreter-mediated primary care visits. *Patient Education and Counseling, 103*(11), 2244–2251. https://doi.org/10.1016/j.pec.2020.07.028

Seidel, H. E., Ball, J. W., Dains, J. E., Flynn, J. A., Solomon, B. S., & Stewart, R. W. (Eds.). (2011). Cultural awareness. In *Mosby's guide to physical examination* (7th ed., pp. 32–45). Mosby.

Segre, L. S., Orengo-Aguayo, R. E., & Siewert, R. C. (2016). Depression management by NICU nurses: Mothers' views. *Clinical Nursing Research, 25*, 273–290. https://doi.org/10.1177/1054773815592596

Shannon, S. E., Long-Sutehall, T., & Coombs, M. (2011). Conversations in end-of-life care: Communication tools for critical care practitioners. *Nursing in Critical Care, 16*(3), 124–130. https://doi.org/10.1111/j.1478-5153.2011.00456.x

Shattell, M., & Hogan, B. (2005). Facilitating communication: How to truly understand what patients mean. *Journal of Psychosocial Nursing and Mental Health Service, 43*(10), 29–32. https://doi.org/10.3928/02793695-20051001-04

SmithBattle, L., & Freed, P. (2016). Teen mothers' mental health. *MCN: American Journal of Maternal Child Nursing, 41*(1), 31–36. https://doi.org/10.1097/NMC.0000000000000198

Strang, J., McCambridge, J., Platts, S., & Groves, P. (2004). Engaging the reluctant GP in care of the opiate users. *Family Practice, 21*(2), 150–154. https://doi.org/10.1093/fampra/cmh208

Taylor, S., Bobba, S., Roome, S., Ahmadzai, M., Tran, D., Vickers, D., Bhatti, M., De Silva, D., Dunstan, L., Falconer, R., Kaur, H., Kitson, J., Patel, J., & Shulruf, B. (2018). Simulated patient and role play methodologies for communication skills training in an undergraduate medical program: Randomized, crossover trial. *Education for Health (Abingdon), 31*(1), 10–16. https://doi.org/10.4103/1357-6283.239040

Thomson, A. E., Racher, F., & Clements, K. (2019). Person-centered psychiatric nursing interventions in acute care settings. *Issues in Mental Health Nursing, 4*(8), 682–689. https://doi.org/10.1080/01612840.2019.1585495

Thornton, J. D., Pham, K., Engelberg, R. A., Jackson, J. C., & Curtis, J. R. (2009). Families with limited English proficiency receive less information and support in interpreted intensive care unit family conferences. *Critical Care Medicine, 37*(1), 89–95. https://doi.org/10.1097/CCM.0b013e3181926430

Villar, V. C. F. L., Duarte, S. D. C. M., & Martins, M. (2020). Patient safety in hospital care: A review of the patient's perspective. *Cadernos de Saude Publica, 36*(12), e00223019. https://doi.org/10.1590/0102311X00223019

Creating Optimal Healing Environments

THERESA ZBOROWSKY AND MARY JO KREITZER

Nurses have long been leaders in creating optimal healing environments (OHEs). Florence Nightingale, the founder of modern nursing, described the role of the nurse as helping the patient attain the best possible condition so that nature can act and self-healing occur (Dossey, 2000). Nightingale recognized the nurse's role in both caring for the patient and managing the physical environment. She wrote about the importance of natural light, fresh air, noise reduction, and infection control, as well as spirituality, presence, and caring. Her philosophy embodied the notion that people have the innate capacity to heal, and as nurses, we create the conditions that support healing within a person. Increasingly, a base of evidence about the creation of OHEs is emerging from many disciplines, including nursing, interior design, architecture, neuroscience, psychoneuroimmunology, and environmental psychology, among others. Just as evidence-based practice informs clinical decision-making, evidence-based design impacts the planning and construction of healthcare facilities. Nurses need to be informed about the ways in which the physical environment affects health outcomes so that they can contribute to the design of patient care units and other healthcare facilities that will optimize the health and well-being of patients, their families, and the staff. Nurses are also in a unique position to carry out needed research on the impact of specific design interventions on intended outcomes. This need is heightened now. In the post-COVID-19 pandemic world, the idea of a staff healing environment is critical. As images of nurses sleeping in hallways flooded our screens, it quickly became apparent that aspects of the environment are critical to staff wellbeing.

DEFINITION

The word *healing* comes from the Anglo-Saxon word *haelen*, which means "to make whole." Healing environments are designed to promote harmony or balance of mind, body, and spirit; to reduce anxiety and stress; and to be restorative. An OHE model developed by Zborowsky and Kreitzer (2009) and depicted in Figure 4.1 illustrates that an OHE is created through a deep and dynamic interplay among people, place, and process. In this model, "people" includes the caregivers and

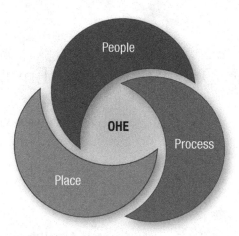

Figure 4.1 People, place, and process: The role of place in creating OHEs.
OHEs, optimal healing environments.
Source: Reprinted from Zborowsky, T., & Kreitzer, M. J. (2009). People, place, and process:
The role of place in creating optimal healing environments. *Creative Nursing, 15*(4), 186–190.
https://doi.org/10.1891/1078-4535.15.4.186

support team who surround the patient. The characteristics and competencies of the staff and the knowledge, skills, and attitudes that they embody are some of the most critical elements of an OHE. The "place" element focuses on the physical space where care is provided and the geography that surrounds the patient, family, and caregiver. "Place" elements include meeting functional requirements or program needs, access to nature, positive distractions, design elements that help create aesthetics, ambient environment, and ecosystem sustainability (see Exhibit 4.1 for definitions). The "process" element refers to the care processes as well as the leadership processes that support a culture aligned with creating an OHE. Care processes include conventional, integrative, and behavioral interventions.

This model of OHE illustrates that optimally, there is coherence and alignment between the "people—nurses, patients and families," the "processes—caregiving in the context of patient-centered care," and in a "place—physical environment" that is designed to maximize positive outcomes for patients, their family, and staff. The reality is that much of care occurs in old, dysfunctional facilities. Even healthcare facilities built 20 years ago lack the available space and mechanical systems to function well today due to changes in building codes, guidelines, and best practices in care models. An inadequate space makes it more difficult to attain a truly healing environment, although the elements of the caregiver and the care provided are even more critical than the physical place or space.

Today, there is a deeper understanding of and rigorous research describing the ways to choose elements of "place" that support and enable an OHE. The primary emphasis of this research is on the evidence and clinical applications of complementary and alternative therapies that nurses can use to enhance their practice. This chapter focuses on the physical environment in which care is provided and the ways in which evidence can be used to create environments that contribute to positive health outcomes.

> ### Exhibit 4.1 *OHE "Place" Element Definitions*
>
> **Meets Functional Requirements:** functional requirements are identified during the programming phase of the design process (see the Facility Guidelines Institute's guidelines for more information: https://fgiguidelines.org/guidelines/2018-fgi-guidelines). Guideline requirements include patient and staff safety, space for social support, and staff work areas, among others.
>
>   **Access to Nature:** includes actual or visual access to natural settings or designed nature settings. Access to daylight.
>
>   **Positive Distractions:** includes elements of the design environment that are of a two- or three-dimensional nature (e.g., artwork, water features, fireplaces).
>
>   **Design Elements:** includes the design elements—color, texture, shape, form, and volume—that contribute to the creation of furniture, fabric, and room layout, among other design artifacts.
>
>   **Ambient Environment:** includes the design elements of artificial light, sound, odor, and heating, ventilation, and air conditioning (HVAC).
>
>   **Supports a Sustainable Ecosystem:** includes the economic, social, and ecological impact of the design elements of the building and impact of any construction.
>
> OHEs = optimal healing environments.

SCIENTIFIC BASIS

A growing body of evidence links the physical environment to health outcomes. According to a review of the research literature on evidence-based healthcare design (Ulrich et al., 2008), more than 1,000 rigorous empirical studies link the design of a hospital's physical environment with healthcare outcomes. The studies cover a broad scope, with evidence linking

- *single-bed rooms* with reduced hospital-acquired infections, reduced medical errors, reduced patient falls, improved patient sleep, and increased patient satisfaction;
- *decentralized supplies* with increased staff effectiveness;
- *appropriate lighting* with decreased medical errors and decreased staff stress; and
- *ceiling lifts* with decreased staff injuries.

Since 2008 a number of systematic literature reviews have focused on specific aspects of the physical environment linked to health outcomes. The following are examples of these studies:

- Gharaveis et al. (2018) found that environmental design, which involves nurses, support staff, and physicians, is one of the critical factors that promotes the efficiency of teamwork and collaborative communication. Layout design, visibility, and accessibility levels are the most cited aspects of design that can affect the level of communication and teamwork in healthcare facilities.

- Bosch and Laurosso (2019) found that a modest amount of evidence indicates that the physical environment may affect patient- and family-engaged care. Designs that are comfortable and foster control of one's physical and social environment, that access social support, and that provide positive distractions may enhance the patient and family experience and promote engagement in care delivery.
- Shahheidari and Homer (2012) found that there were two main designs of NICUs: open bay and single-family room. The open-bay environment develops communication and interaction with medical staff and nurses and has the ability to monitor multiple infants simultaneously. The single-family rooms were deemed superior for patient care and parent satisfaction. Key factors associated with improved outcomes included increased privacy, increased parental involvement in patient care, assistance with infection control, noise control, improved sleep, decreased length of hospital stay, and reduced rehospitalization.

Although many of the studies focus on topics such as infection control, patient falls, staff productivity, and staff injuries, a growing number of studies focus on other aspects of the environment that contribute to healing.

As described by Malkin (2008), design strategies that focus on creating healing environments have in common the goal of stress reduction and include:

- connections to nature (e.g., artwork with a nature theme, views to the outside, interior gardens, plants);
- options that give patients choices and control (e.g., room service menu, choice of music and art, ability to control lighting and temperature);
- spaces that provide access to social support (e.g., family zones within patient rooms that offer sleeping space, storage, and adequate seating);
- positive distractions (e.g., music, water features, aviaries, videos of nature, aquariums, sculpture); and
- reductions of environmental stressors such as noise and glare from direct light sources (e.g., carpet, indirect lighting, elimination of overhead paging).

DESIGN THEORIES AND BEST PRACTICES RELATED TO HEALING ENVIRONMENTS AND CLINICAL APPLICATIONS

ACCESS TO NATURE

OHE "place" elements include theories that support creating healing spaces in healthcare. For example, biophilia is a theory that supports the concept of access to nature. Biophilia is the inherent human inclination to "affiliate" with natural systems and processes. The concept, originally proposed by eminent biologist Edward O. Wilson (1984), has grown into a broader framework that increasingly is shaping the design of the man-made environment, including hospitals and other healthcare facilities. Biophilic design emphasizes the necessity of maintaining, enhancing, and restoring the beneficial experience of nature and describes attempts to do so through the use of environmental features that embody characteristics of the natural world, such as color, water, sunlight, plants, natural materials, and exterior views and vistas (Kellert, 2008).

The theory of biophilia has been empirically tested in clinical settings. Outcomes measured most often include stress and pain reduction. The following are examples:

- A study of older adult residents in an urban long-term care facility revealed that residents attach considerable importance to having access to window views of outdoor spaces with prominent features such as plants, gardens, and birds (Kearney & Winterbottom, 2005).
- Patients in a dental clinic reported less stress on days when a large nature mural was hung in the waiting room compared with days when there was no nature scene (Heerwagen, 1990).
- In a prospective randomized trial of blood donors, it was found that donors who viewed a wall-mounted television playing a nature videotape had lower blood pressure and pulse rates than subjects who were viewing a television playing either a videotape of urban scenes or game or talk shows (Ulrich et al., 2003).
- Ulrich et al. (1993) found that following heart surgery, patients who viewed photos of trees and water required fewer doses of strong pain medication and reported less anxiety than patients who viewed abstract images or were assigned to a control group with no picture.

There is some evidence that the more engrossing a nature distraction, the greater the potential for pain alleviation. Miller et al. (1992), in a study of burn patients, found that distracting patients during burn dressings by having them view nature scenes on a bedside TV accompanied by music lessened both pain and anxiety. In a randomized prospective trial of patients undergoing bronchoscopy, patients who viewed a ceiling-mounted nature scene and listened to nature sounds reported less pain than patients in the control group who looked at a blank ceiling. Following a review of the literature on the use of virtual reality as an adjunct analgesic technique, Wismeijer and Vingerhoets (2005) concluded that "nature exposures" may tend to be more diverting, and hence pain-reducing, if they involve sound as well as visual stimulation and maximize realism and immersion.

Roe and Aspinall (2011) reported on two quasi-experiments that compared the restorative benefits of walking in urban and rural settings in two groups of adults with good and poor mental health. The authors examined two aspects of restoration, mood, and personal project techniques to capture an underexplored aspect of cognitive restoration through reflection on everyday life tasks. Results were consistent with a restorative effect of landscape. The rural walk was advantageous to affective and cognitive restoration in both health groups when compared with an urban walk. However, a beneficial change took place to a greater extent in the poor health group. Differential outcomes between health groups were found in the urban setting, which was most advantageous to restoration in the poor mental health group. This study extends restorative environments research by showing that the amount of change and context for restoration can differ among adults with variable mental health.

Emerging research uses a multimethod approach to understand the effect nature has on patients. In a case study of 19 subjects living in an assisted living facility, Goto et al. (2013) found that exposure to organized gardens can affect both the mood and the cardiac physiology of older adults. Among other findings, they revealed that the subjects' heart rates were significantly lower in the

Japanese garden than in the other environments studied; measures of subjects' sympathetic function were also significantly lower.

In a study relevant to our current crisis, the COVID pandemic, Nejati et al. (2016) investigated the main restorative components of staff break areas in healthcare facilities. Statistical analysis revealed that ratings increased significantly based on higher levels of nature content, from no added amenities to indoor plants to nature artwork to window views and, finally, to direct access to the outdoors through a balcony. This study supports the proposition that access to nature, daylight, and outdoor environments are perceived to have significantly more restorative potential in healthcare workplaces.

POSITIVE DISTRACTIONS

Art falls under another of the "place" elements of positive distractions. A number of studies have examined patient preferences for art and the effect of art on stress, recovery, and pain, among other outcomes. Studies have consistently documented that patients prefer nature over other subject matter and that they overwhelmingly prefer realistic art and strongly dislike abstract images (Winston & Cupchik, 1992). Findings such as these, consistent with the theory of biophilia, have led to the use of evidence-based design guidelines in healthcare facilities to guide the selection of art. According to Ulrich and Gilpin (2003), visual art should be unambiguously positive. Recommended subject matter includes waterscapes with calm or nonturbulent water, landscapes with visual depth or openness, nature settings depicted during warmer seasons when vegetation is verdant and flowers are visible, garden scenes, and outdoor scenes in sunny conditions while avoiding overcast or foreboding weather. Pati and Nanda (2011) used a quasi-experimental design to examine pediatric patients' behavior during five distraction conditions ranging from a slideshow to video with music. All distraction conditions were created on one flatscreen plasma TV monitor mounted on a stand in the waiting areas. Data analysis showed that the introduction of distraction conditions was associated with more calm behavior and less fine and gross movement, suggesting significant calming effects associated with the distraction conditions. Data also suggest that positive distraction conditions are significant attention grabbers and could be an important contributor to enhancing the waiting experience for children in hospitals by improving environmental attractiveness. Nanda et al. (2012) conducted a systematic review of neuroscience articles on the emotional states of fear, anxiety, and pain to understand how emotional response is linked to the visual characteristics of an image at the level of brain behavior. Findings indicate that there is a paucity of research in this area and a compelling area for future research on the direct impact the imagery of artwork can have on emotional processing centers in the brain.

Nanda et al. (2010) investigated the impact of different visual art conditions on agitation and anxiety levels of patients by measuring the rate of pro re nata (PRN; as needed) incidents and collecting nurse feedback. Results showed that PRN medication dispensed by nurses for anxiety and agitation was significantly lower on days when a realistic nature image of a landscape was displayed as compared with days when abstract or no art was displayed. The authors concluded that positive distractions, such as visual art depicting restorative nature scenes, could help reduce mental health patients' anxiety and agitation in healthcare settings. It also makes a case that the environment can have a powerful impact on healing in mental health settings. The emergence of simulated nature products has raised the question regarding the effectiveness of these approaches. Pati et al. (2016) conducted a between-subject experimental design, in which outcomes from five inpatient rooms with sky-composition ceiling fixtures were compared with corresponding outcomes in five identical rooms without the intervention. The experimental group of subjects exhibited shorter times spent in the room, lower diastolic blood pressure, lower acute stress, lower anxiety, less pain, better sleep quality, and higher environmental satisfaction. The authors concluded that the salutogenic benefits of photographic sky compositions render them better than traditional ceiling tiles and offer an alternative to other nature interventions.

To evaluate how a positive environmental distraction intervention impacted pediatric radiography patient behavioral stress responses, mood states, and parental satisfaction, Quan et al. (2016) conducted a multimethod study. Researchers added a wall-projected image that was age-appropriate to one imaging room, while the control room had none. A technician rotated between rooms while researchers conducted behavioral observations and parents filled out a questionnaire. This study found that under interventional conditions, patients exhibited less low-stress coping behaviors ($p = .001–.007$) and more verbal behaviors indicating positive affect ($p = .003$); parents more favorably rated environmental pleasantness ($p < .001$), sense of environmental control ($p = .002$), and willingness to return and recommend the facility ($p = .001–.005$). More studies are needed, but these initial results are promising.

AMBIENT ENVIRONMENT

Light is an aspect of the "place" element, the ambient environment. Chronobiology is an interdisciplinary field of inquiry that focuses on biological rhythms. Discoveries in "chronotherapeutics" have documented that time patterning of medications in synchrony with body rhythms can enhance effectiveness and safety. Other studies have focused on the impact of environmental factors such as light and temperature on body rhythms. A significant body of literature has focused on the impact of light on depression. In a study of psychiatric patients, Beauchemin and Hays (1996) found that patients in sunnier rooms stayed an average of 2.6 fewer days than those in sunless rooms. A meta-analysis of 20 randomized controlled trials by Golden et al. (2005) on the impact of light treatment on nonseasonal and seasonal depression quantified the effect of light treatment as equivalent to that of antidepressant pharmacotherapy trials. Light has also been found to be related to patients' perception of pain. In a study (Walch et al., 2005) of post–spinal surgery experiences, patients who were admitted to rooms with greater sunlight intensity reported less pain and stress and took 22% fewer analgesic medications. Results such as these support careful site planning to ensure adequate access to daylight and provide justification for larger windows in patient rooms or the use of bright (but diffused) artificial light in areas where sufficient daylight is inaccessible. Using a pretest/posttest quasi-experimental study in two ICUs, Shepley et al. (2012) studied the impact of daylight and window views on patient pain levels, length of stay, staff errors, absenteeism, and vacancy rates. Researchers concluded that high levels of natural light and window views may positively affect staff absenteeism and staff vacancy, whereas factors such as medical errors, patient pain, and length of stay still require additional research. In summary, there is growing evidence that nature views and light are beneficial for patients as well as staff.

Interestingly, evolving research explores the impact of lighting, both daylight and electrical lighting, on the circadian entrainment of older adults who live with neurocognitive disorders. In a systematic literature review, Joseph et al. (2015) found one multidimensional intervention, which included a daily sunlight exposure of 30 minutes or more, resulted in a significant decrease in daytime sleeping in intervention participants with no change in controls. In addition, there was a modest decrease in the mean duration of nighttime awakenings in intervention participants versus an increase in controls. They noted that although there is inconsistent support for the impact of bright light on direct sleep measures, findings do consistently suggest that bright-light treatment may be effective in improving rest–activity rhythms (which results in better sleep at night and greater wakefulness in the daytime) for residents with dementia (Ancoli-Israel et al., 2003; Dowling et al., 2005). Figueiro et al. (2008) conducted a study that incorporated a 24-hour lighting design intervention to meet the physiological needs of older adults in residential care environments (see Exhibit 4.2). Although this study did not find a significant difference in sleep quality, nighttime sleep, or daytime awake hours in the small sample of seven assisted living residents, residents overwhelmingly preferred the new lighting conditions and felt they could read better under this condition compared with the old lighting condition. In the discussion section of the review, Joseph et al. (2015) noted that this study is significant because it offered concrete lighting design solutions that can be incorporated within new or existing environments.

Recent studies on the impact of work lighting on staff hold promise for positive environmental changes. McCunn and Safranek (2020) found that nurses and patients desire greater control over the lighting in patient rooms. In this qualitative analysis of interviews, a general theme of environmental control over both overhead and task lighting in patient rooms emerged from the data. Daylighting was also considered to be among the best lighting-related design attributes in patient rooms. Control over the light level in patient rooms by providing additional

---

Exhibit 4.2 *Applied Lighting Interventions*

Figueiro et al. (2008) applied the following architectural lighting scheme to improve the circadian entrainment and increase the architectural legibility for older adults with dementia:

1. high circadian stimulation during the day and low circadian stimulation during the night
2. good visual conditions during waking hours
3. nightlights that provide perceptual cues for navigation and that improve postural stability and control for transitioning from a sitting into a standing position
4. high contrasts between daytime and nighttime light levels
5. glare-free lighting
6. shadow-free visual environments

These lighting interventions appear to be applicable to many other settings of care, including home environments.

dimming capabilities for patients, as well as additional light sources, came forward as prominent points in nurses' narratives across the four hospitals in the United States. Despite differences in the level of technology and sophistication in lighting frameworks among the four facilities, lighting control continues to be a primary concern for medical-surgical nurses. The use of color light to affect night staff was explored by Figueiro and Pedler (2020). To examine the use of red-light exposures at night to promote alertness and improve performance while not negatively affecting melatonin secretion, they conducted a crossover, mixed (within- and between-subjects) design field study. Preliminary results indicated that response times were improved by the red and blue interventions but not accuracy and hit rates. Blue light was associated with improvements in self-reported sleep disturbances compared to dim light. The authors conclude that red light may be used to improve response times in shift workers but that continued research will elucidate the lighting interventions' effects on melatonin and objective sleep measures (actigraphy).

This area of study—the impact of place on creating OHEs—is growing rapidly. In a 2014 study, Zborowsky analyzed a sample of 67 healthcare design–related research articles from 25 nursing journals to validate the extent to which current topics align with Nightingale's environmental theory. She found that sound and noise ranked high among the dependent variables and sleep among the independent variables (the result of sound and noise). As stated by Nightingale, "Unnecessary noise is the most cruel absence of care which can be inflicted either on sick or well" (Nightingale, 1860, p. 27). Like Nightingale, nurses today are in a strategic position to study and design healing environments that optimize health outcomes for patients, families, and staff.

INTERVENTION

CASE STUDY APPLICATIONS OF OHE

The following case studies represent three important healthcare settings along the continuum of care: a large academic medical center, a regional outpatient cancer center, and a behavioral health treatment facility. Each healthcare setting promotes the creation of optimal healing environments for their patients, staff, and community members.

University of Kentucky Children's Hospital Neonatal Intensive Care Unit (NICU)

The University of Kentucky Children's Hospital is a hospital within a hospital. The new 72-bed NICU department incorporates all private patient rooms in neighborhoods of 12 rooms. Within the neighborhoods, there are decentralized nursing and staff spaces, along with a staff huddle space that allows for a collaborative environment. As it is part of an academic medical center, there are resident rooms, conference spaces, educational areas, and simulation rooms to enable students to learn and complete research. Private respite spaces were included for staff to encourage huddles, support, and learning for the academic institution. The staff breakroom has an outdoor balcony for their use.

Environmental graphics were utilized to create a sense of place for the hospital and the neighborhoods within the department. Four Kentucky-related natural themes provide visual ownership of the 12-bed communities to promote ease of wayfinding for parents under stress. Themes are seen through large tile mosaics at the entrance and smaller artwork throughout the neighborhoods. Attention was paid to driving as much natural light into the space as possible, through skylights and large-scale windows. Inside the patient rooms, architectural cycled lighting was incorporated to provide visual cues for day to night.

Additionally, family-centered care was important to the success of the project. There are areas for the family to sleep, lounges for respite and connection with others, and "Care by Parent" rooms, which provide space for parents to care solely for an infant to make the transition home easier.

ThedaCare Regional Cancer Center

ThedaCare's regional cancer center in Wisconsin reflects its philosophy of delivering convenient, compassionate, patient-centered care, practiced in a highly integrated and collaborative way. The center provides a full spectrum of care, including advanced medical and radiation oncology treatments and procedures in addition to wellness programs, such as art and music therapy, cooking classes, yoga, and cosmetology services.

Memorable First Impression: Upon entry, patients and family members enjoy an environment that feels as though they are entering a high-end hotel lobby rather than a cancer treatment center. Inspired by the surrounding meadows, wetlands, and dense forest, the palette is familiar to the community and rooted in nature. Custom pendants above a variety of seating groupings reduce the scale of the impressive two-story atrium, while built-in planters create privacy.

Design solutions within patient treatment areas were selected to reduce stress, provide a greater sense of control, and create positive distractions for patients. Understanding the length and frequency of treatments, along with input gathered from past patients and families, informed the design helping enhance patient experiences. With chemo treatments lasting up to six hours, access to daylight and views, as well as options for privacy during infusion and comfortable furnishings, were top priorities. Conversely, radiation treatments, typically quick and frequent, required a different approach. Radiation vaults, windowless by design, are wrapped in panoramic nature scenes and lit with colored LED lights, allowing patients to change the colors to suit their preferences. Designed to improve outcomes, enhance collaboration and provide patients with an excellent experience, the new Cancer Center brings advanced cancer care to the regional and the surrounding community.

Hazelden Betty Ford Foundation Campus in St. Paul, Minnesota

In April 2016, the Hazelden Betty Ford Foundation addiction treatment center in St. Paul, Minnesota, expanded significantly by adding a new building on remediated land and connecting it to the center's historic existing structure, built 130 years earlier. The facility provides outpatient mental health and addiction care, sober living residences, and a hub for community Twelve Step and other mutual-aid recovery-support meetings. Design elements support healing through safety for staff and patients, areas of pause and reflection, access to nature, and community engagement.

Overlooking the Mississippi River, a redbrick mansion with a mansard roof, built in the 1880s, had long served as Hazelden Betty Ford's Fellowship Club.

The new building, which is now connected to the mansion, was built to accommodate a growing population seeking outpatient treatment for substance use and mental health disorders. The addition doubled the number of people the facility serves, with 55 new beds in the low-slung brick volume as well as outpatient treatment rooms and offices on the upper level. To create a sense of hospitality upon entry, the foyer opens into a light-filled lobby with a stone fireplace, wood reception and admission desks, a coffee bar, and a staircase.

Panels of colored glass were incorporated into windows throughout the addition, a nod to the mansion's stained-glass windows. Patterns in the mansion's stained glass and ornate wood banisters were abstracted and incorporated into the addition's open staircase and wood privacy screens. The addition was given a 15-degree turn on the site to take advantage of a bluff and views while creating a visual link back to the mansion. A glass-and-brick-clad walkway connects the addition to the mansion, where there's a newly renovated mental health clinic.

To promote healing and a sense of well-being throughout the addition, large windows, including a full-glass wall in the lecture auditorium, bring in abundant daylight and views of gardens, a Twelve Step path and labyrinth, and the river outside. Cherry and walnut (woods also used in the mansion) introduce warmth, as does the limestone (similar to that of the river bluffs) used for the fireplace.

CULTURAL APPLICATIONS AND PRECAUTIONS

The increased diversity of the U.S. population has added a level of complexity to the design of healthcare environments. As noted by Kopec and Han (2008), entering a healthcare environment can be frightening and disempowering, particularly when a patient's traditional and spiritual beliefs differ from that of the dominant culture. Thus, it is becoming increasingly important to carefully weigh all design decisions that impact the physical environment, including the use of color and cultural symbols, as well as other visual, auditory, and tactile design elements.

To Asians, for example, the color red symbolizes good luck whereas the color white is associated with mourning and death. The color green has positive associations within the Islamic tradition because it is associated with vegetation and life and is believed to have been the Prophet Muhammad's favorite color. Kopec and Han (2008) have identified a number of ways in which the needs of Muslim patients might be accommodated. A curtain inside the door, for instance, could help patients maintain visual privacy and modesty while allowing healthcare providers on rounds to announce their presence, giving patients time to prepare themselves to be seen. Understanding that followers of Islam face the northeast when they pray could be taken into consideration when orienting the bed and furnishings in the room. Given the diversity of spiritual, religious, and cultural beliefs and practices, however, it would be nearly impossible—from a design perspective, as well as practically and financially—to accommodate all the specifics and nuances of every tradition in the design of healthcare settings. Thus, the goal of design can only be to strive to express core, universal values while seeking to devise design elements that can be flexible. Sidebar 4.1, written by a nurse from Liberia, reminds us that it is not only the physical environment that can enhance healing. It is also important to understand diverse cultural perspectives of healing and healing environments so that nurses can work to overcome the challenges that these present in the provision of culturally sensitive, patient-centered care.

Another cultural perspective is presented in Sidebar 4.2. This sidebar emphasizes the healing potential of natural and builds environments and the ancient understanding of their potential effects on healing.

Sidebar 4.1 *Healing Environments in Liberia, West Africa*

Maria Tarlue Keita

I am from the Krahn tribe, a small tribe in Liberia, West Africa, which is one of 16 tribes in Liberia. However, I am confident in saying that the healing environment I describe reflects the culture of the Liberian people in general.

When I think of the healing environment in the United States, what comes to mind are the beautiful, well-designed rooms, readily available medications, and high-tech medical devices. The healing environment in my culture consists of four major parts: family presence, food, spirituality, and complementary therapies.

Presence

When people from Liberia are in the hospital, it is important for staff to understand the importance of presence. Family and friends come in dozens to visit. However, there are always one or two people who stay in the room at all times to support the sick person. The role of the assigned person(s) is to coordinate the care of the patient between the hospital caregiver and the family and to provide direct support, such as encouragement and reassurance, to the patient. The presence of friends and family reduces anxiety and builds trust with hospital staff. A healing environment is incomplete without the presence of a family member or a friend with the sick.

It is an expectation in my culture that people stay with one who is ill. The role of the family is to help in the care of the sick with activities of daily living, even when in a formal hospital setting.

Food

Food is another very important part of the healing environment in my culture. Special foods, such as a pepper soup made with hot spices, are offered to sick people. If solid food is prepared, it is usually anything that can be easily swallowed. *Depa* and *fufu* are like mashed potatoes made from fresh or dried cassava, yams, or plantains. So-called slippery soups are also easy to swallow. Sick people, it is believed, obtain cleansing and nasal decongestion from various soups.

Spirituality

Providing regular prayers and the presence of religious symbols is an essential part of the healing environment; however, these may come with different levels of spirituality. Many families may believe that without intervention from above, conventional medicine will not bring about healing.

Sidebar 4.1 *Healing Environments in Liberia, West Africa (continued)*

Complementary Therapies

A warm bath with or without herbs is considered to be very therapeutic in my culture and is therefore offered to sick people. A routine daily bath is an expectation. Herbs are often boiled with the bathwater, and the hot bath is given to the patient.

The combination of conventional medicine and a healing environment in the Liberian culture is sometimes a challenge to healthcare providers in the United States. Family involvement in conventional medicine is limited based on how a healing environment is perceived by Liberians. Hospital staff are usually overwhelmed by the presence of many family members in rooms of patients from Liberia or most African cultures.

Sidebar 4.2 *Ancient Healing Environments of Greece*

Ioanna Gryllaki

I have given the topic of the environment's role in healing much consideration. After reflecting on my own most recent experience in the public hospitals of Greece and consulting my resident family members about their experiences, I have come to the conclusion that unfortunately, modern Greece does not have the resources or motivation to use its beautiful landscape to induce healing. The reality of the economic depression in Greece has taken a hit not only on its natural and financial resources but also on the spirit of the Greek people. In ancient Greece, the most famous healing temples were the 2,400-year-old Asclepions, which were dedicated to the god of healing, Asclepius (Holloway, 2015). The estimated 320 beautiful healing temples acted as hospitals in ancient Greece, with the most famous temples located in Epidaurus, Cos, and Pergamum (Holloway, 2015). In ancient days, the priests and physicians who oversaw the care provided at the Asclepions embraced a holistic approach to healing that included treatments such as massage and herbal medicines—treatments embedded in the context of soul-uplifting healing environments to optimize the body's power for health and healing. The healers of the day held a view that one's soul needed mending as well as one's body (Holloway, 2015). However, these ancient temples are no longer being funded or used by Greeks. Although this is the stark reality of Greece today, the dormant power of the healing environments within these treasures awaits future reawakening to benefit its people and visitors to this historic land.

Reference

Holloway, A. (2015, October 25). 2,400-year-old healing temple dedicated to Asclepius, god of healing, excavated in Greece. *Ancient Origins.* http://www.ancient-origins.net/news-history -archaeology/2400-year-old-healing-temple-dedicated-asclepius-god-healing-excavated-020587

Exhibit 4.3 *Creating Healing Environments and Enhancing Well-Being: Tips for the Home*

- *Open a window.* Allowing fresh air to circulate through your home lets you breathe easier. This also rids the air of pollutants, including harmful chemicals that may accumulate from products, equipment such as air conditioners, and furniture.
- *Bring the outside in.* Studies have demonstrated that exposure to nature can reduce stress levels and improve well-being. Viewing nature from a window or looking at nature-related images can give a sense of retreat throughout the day.
- *Create a quiet, comfortable space* that allows you to escape and reflect. Meditation is an important part of overall well-being and has been shown to increase (hard-to-access) alpha-wave patterns in the brain that have been associated with less stress and anxiety.
- *Use calming colors.* Color can have a wide range of effects on human mood and emotions. Colors with blue undertones have the ability to calm the mind and create a greater sense of relaxation. Light waves corresponding to the color blue are found to have the greatest effect on regulating the circadian rhythms that are directly related to moods.
- *Avoid clutter in the home;* it can create unnecessary stress! Because our brains are constantly categorizing what we see, it is important to keep the space around us organized and free of clutter.
- *Personalize your space* with items, furnishings, and finishes that bring you joy and that have meaning. Personalizing one's space gives one a sense of control and a deeper connection to a space.
- *Have a sense of control* in your home environment. This can include temperature controls, space allocation and organization, noise levels, security, and safety. Most important, your home should function according to the way you live.

Source: Adapted from Angelita Scott, personal communication, April 1, 2013.

Nurses can promote health and well-being by providing simple tips for modifying and enhancing the environment of patients' homes. These simple, yet effective tips are presented in Exhibit 4.3.

FUTURE RESEARCH

More research is needed to understand the impact of design interventions on the environment of care. Future studies need to rigorously examine the many factors that contribute to healing environments and should focus on staff, as well as patient outcomes. Healthcare outcomes for patients may include the reduction of stress, reduced length of stay, decreased incidence of nosocomial infections, reduced pain, improved sleep, increased satisfaction, and reduced number of falls. Outcomes for nursing staff may include decreased injuries, decreased stress, reduced number of sick days taken, and increased effectiveness, productivity, and satisfaction. The OHE framework provides one way to help establish study parameters. As U.S. healthcare facility construction spending continues to be robust, nurses need to be actively engaged in contributing to the design and evaluation of healing environments that will optimize the health and well-being of patients, family members, and staff.

WEBSITES

The following websites contain additional information on healing environments:

- The Center for Health Design (www.healthdesign.org)
- Earl E. Bakken Center for Spirituality & Healing, University of Minnesota (www.takingcharge.csh.umn.edu/what-is-a-healing-environment)
  (www.takingcharge.csh.umn.edu/explore-healing-practices/healing-environment)
  (www.takingcharge.csh.umn.edu/explore-healing-practices/healing-environment/what-impact-does-environment-have-us)

REFERENCES

Ancoli-Israel, S., Gehrman, P., Martin, J. L., Shochat, T., Marler, M., Corey-Bloom, J., & Levi, L. (2003). Increased light exposure consolidates sleep and strengthens circadian rhythms in severe Alzheimer's disease patients. *Behavioral Sleep Medicine, 1,* 22–36. https://doi.org/10.1207/S15402010BSM0101_4

Beauchemin, K. M., & Hays, P. (1996). Sunny hospital rooms expedite recovery from severe and refractory depressions. *Journal of Affective Disorders, 40*(1–2), 49–51. https://doi.org/10.1016/0165-0327(96)00040-7

Bosch, S. J., & Lorusso, L. N. (2019). Promoting patient and family engagement through health-care facility design: A systematic literature review. *Journal of Environmental Psychology, 62,* 74–83. https://doi.org/10.1016/j.jenvp.2019.02.002

Dossey, B. M. (2000). *Florence Nightingale: Mystic, visionary, healer.* Springhouse.

Dowling, G. A., Mastick, J., Hubbard, E. M., Luxenberg, J. S., & Burr, R. L. (2005). Effect of timed bright light treatment for rest-activity disruption in institutionalized patients with Alzheimer's disease. *International Journal of Geriatric Psychiatry, 20,* 738–743. https://doi.org/10.1002/gps.1352

Figueiro, M. G., & Pedler, D. (2020). Red light: A novel, non-pharmacological intervention to promote alertness in shift workers. *Journal of Safety Research, 74,* 169–177. https://doi.org/10.1016/j.jsr.2020.06.003

Figueiro, M. G., Saldo, E., Rea, M. S., Kubarek, K., Cunningham, J., & Rea, M. S. (2008). Developing architectural lighting designs to improve sleep in older adults. *The Open Sleep Journal, 1,* 40–51. https://doi.org/10.2174/1874620900801010040

Gharaveis, A., Hamilton, D. K., & Pati, D. (2018). The impact of environmental design on teamwork and communication in healthcare facilities: A systematic literature review. *HERD: Health Environments Research & Design Journal, 11*(1), 119–137. https://doi.org/10.1177/1937586717730333

Golden, R. N., Gaynes, B. N., Ekstrom, R. D., Hamer, R. M., Jacobsen, F. M., Suppes, T., Wisner, K. L., & Nemeroff, C. B. (2005). The efficacy of light therapy in the treatment of mood disorders: A review and meta-analysis of the evidence. *American Journal of Psychiatry, 162*(4), 656–662. https://doi.org/10.1176/appi.ajp.162.4.656

Goto, S., Park, B. J., Tsunetsugu, Y., Herrup, K., & Miyazaki, Y. (2013). The effect of garden designs on mood and heart output in older adults residing in an assisted living facility. *Health Environments Research & Design Journal, 6*(2), 27–42. https://doi.org/10.1177/193758671300600204

Heerwagen, J. H. (1990). The psychological aspects of windows and window design. In K. H. Anthony, J. Choi, & B. Orland (Eds.), *Proceedings of 21st Annual Conference of the Environmental Design Research Association* (pp. 269–280). Environmental Design Research Association.

Joseph, A., Choi, Y., & Quan, X. (2015). Impact of the physical environment of residential health, care, and support facilities (RHCSF) on staff and residents: A systematic review of the literature. *Environment & Behavior, 48*(10), 1203–1241. https://doi.org/10.1177/0013916515597027

Kearney, A. R., & Winterbottom, D. (2005). Nearby nature and long-term care facility residents: Benefits and design recommendations. *Journal of Housing for the Elderly, 1*(3/4), 7–28. https://doi.org/10.1300/J081v19n03_02

Kellert, S. R. (2008). Dimensions, elements and attributes of biophilic design. In S. R. Kellert, J. H. Heerwagen, & M. L. Mador (Eds.), *Biophilic design* (pp. 3–20). John Wiley.

Kopec, D., & Han, L. (2008). Islam and the healthcare environment: Designing patient rooms. *Health Environments Research and Design Journal, 1*(4), 111–121. https://doi.org/10.1177/193758670800100412

Malkin, J. (2008). *A visual reference for evidence-based design.* The Center for Health Design.

McCunn, L. J., Safranek, S., Wilkerson, A., & Davis, R. G. (2020). Lighting control in patient rooms: Understanding nurses' perceptions of hospital lighting using qualitative methods. *HERD: Health Environments Research & Design Journal.* Advanced online publication. https://doi.org/10.1177/1937586720946669

Miller, A. C., Hickman, L. C., & Lemasters, G. K. (1992). A distraction technique for control of burn pain. *Journal of Burn Care and Rehabilitation, 13*(5), 576–580. https://doi.org/10.1097/00004630-199209000-00012

Nanda, U., Eisen, S., Zadeh, R., & Owen, D. (2010). Effect of visual art on patient anxiety and agitation in a mental health facility and implications for the business case. *Journal of Psychiatric and Mental Health Nursing, 18,* 386–393. https://doi.org/10.1111/j.1365-2850.2010.01682.x

Nanda, U., Zhu, X., & Jansen, B. H. (2012). Image and emotion: From outcomes to brain behavior. *Health Environments Research & Design Journal, 5*(4), 40–59. https://doi.org/10.1177/193758671200500404

Nejati, A., Rodiek, S., & Shepley, M. (2016). Using visual simulation to evaluate restorative qualities of access to nature in hospital staff break areas. *Landscape and Urban Planning, 148,* 132–138.

Nightingale, F. (1860). *Notes on nursing: What it is, what it is not.* Harrison and Sons. https://doi.org/10.1177/2165079915612097

Pati, D., Freier, P., O'Boyle, M., Amor, C., & Valipoor, S. (2016). The impact of simulated nature on patient outcomes: A study of photographic sky compositions. *Health Environments Research & Design Journal, 9*(2), 36–51. https://doi.org/10.1177/1937586715595505

Pati, D., & Nanda, U. (2011). Influence of positive distractions on children in two clinic waiting areas. *Health Environments Research & Design Journal, 4,* 124–140. https://doi.org/10.1177/193758671100400310

Quan, X., Joseph, A., Nanda, U., Moyano-Smith, O., Kanakri, S., Ancheta, C., & Loveless, E. A. (2016) Improving pediatric radiography patient stress, mood, and parental satisfaction through positive environmental distractions: A randomized control trial. *Journal of Pediatric Nursing, 31,* e11–e22. https://doi.org/10.1016/j.pedn.2015.08.004

Roe, J., & Aspinall, P. (2011). The restorative benefits of walking in urban and rural settings in adults with good and poor mental health. *Health & Place, 17,* 103–113. https://doi.org/10.1016/j.healthplace.2010.09.003

Shahheidari, M., & Homer, C. (2012). Impact of the design of neonatal intensive care units on neonates, staff, and families. *Journal of Perinatal & Neonatal Nursing, 26*(3), 260–266. https://doi.org/10.1097/JPN.0b013e318261ca1d

Shepley, M. M., Gerbi, R. P., Watson, A. E., Imgrund, S., & Sagha-Zadeh, R. (2012). The impact of daylight and views on ICU patients and staff. *Health Environments Research & Design Journal, 5*(2), 46–60. https://doi.org/10.1177/193758671200500205

Ulrich, R. S., & Gilpin, L. (2003). Healing arts. In S. B. Frampton, L. Gilpin, & P. Charmel (Eds.), *Putting patients first: Designing and practicing patient-centered care* (pp. 117–146). Jossey-Bass.

Ulrich, R. S., Lunden, O. L., & Eltinge, J. L. (1993). Effects of exposure to nature and abstract pictures on patients recovering from heart surgery. [Paper presented at the 33rd Meeting of the Society for Psychophysiological Research.] *Psychophysiology, 30*(Suppl. 1), 7.

Ulrich, R. S., Simons, R. F., & Miles, M. A. (2003). Effects of environmental simulations and television on blood donor stress. *Journal of Architectural & Planning Research, 20*(1), 38–47. https://www.jstor.org/stable/43030641

Ulrich, R. S., Zimring, C., Zhu, X., DuBose, J., Seo, H-B., Choi, Y-S., Quan, X., & Joseph, A. (2008). A review of the research literature on evidence-based healthcare design. *Health Environments Research & Design Journal, 1*(3), 61–125. https://doi.org/10.1177/193758670800100306

Walch, J. M., Rabin, B. S., Day, R., Williams, J. N., Choi, K., & Kang, J. D. (2005). The effect of sunlight on post-operative analgesic medication usage: A prospective study of patients undergoing spinal surgery. *Psychosomatic Medicine, 67*, 156–163. https://doi.org/10.1097/01.psy.0000149258.42508.70

Wilson, E. O. (1984). *Biophilia: The human bond with other species*. Harvard University Press.

Winston, A. S., & Cupchik, G. C. (1992). The evaluation of high art and popular art by naive and experienced viewers. *Visual Arts Research, 18*, 1–14. https://jstor.org/stable/20715763

Wismeijer, A. J., & Vingerhoets, J. J. (2005). The use of virtual reality and audiovisual eyeglass systems as adjunct analgesic techniques: A review of the literature. *Annals of Behavioral Medicine, 30*(3), 268–278. https://doi.org/10.1207/s15324796abm3003_11

Zborowsky, T., & Kreitzer, M. J. (2009). People, place, and process: The role of place in creating optimal healing environments. *Creative Nursing, 15*(4), 186–190. https://doi.org/10.1891/1078-4535.15.4.186

Systems of Care: Tibetan Medicine

MIRIAM E. CAMERON AND TENZIN NAMDUL

Conventional healthcare is burdened by caring for individuals whose health problems result in part from unhealthy choices. As people become more health-conscious, they are looking outside of conventional healthcare for answers to well-being. Often, they turn to diverse systems of care, such as the myriad of Native American and Asian healing systems, that support the power of the mind and body to establish, maintain, and restore health. These traditions may lack scientific evidence. The scientific method doesn't easily adapt to investigating holistic systems. Their profound therapies may affect the mind and body in ways that are not measurable. People may engage in these practices without understanding their context, meaning, and safety (National Center for Complementary and Integrative Health [NCCIH], 2021b).

The goal of integrative nursing is to advance health and wellbeing through person-centered, evidence-based care that incorporates complementary therapies and conventional healthcare (Earl E. Bakken Center for Spirituality & Healing, University of Minnesota, 2021b). To practice quality care, nurses need to learn about diverse care systems. For example, homeopathy and naturopathy are recent care systems that may be effective but currently lack high-quality scientific evidence (Natural Medicines, 2021b, 2021c). Education and licensing differ for the various types of homeopathic (American Institute of Homeopathy, 2021) and naturopathic practitioners (American Association of Naturopathic Physicians, 2021).

Homeopathy developed in Germany at the end of the 18th century. The central tenets are that (a) like cures like, which means a disease can be cured by a substance that produces similar symptoms in healthy people, and (b) the law of minimum dose, meaning that the *lower* the dose of medication, the *greater* its effectiveness (NCCIH, 2021d). Naturopathy as a care system evolved from a combination of traditional practices and healthcare approaches popular in Europe during the 19th century. Naturopaths practice according to these principles: (a) Treat the individual, (b) stimulate and support the body's inherent ability to heal, (c) identify the root cause of dysfunction, (d) address the cause naturally and gently, and (e) teach clients how to create wellness and prevent illness (NCCIH, 2021e).

In contrast, Tibetan medicine from Tibet and Ayurveda from India are ancient, yet timely, systems of care (NCCIH, 2021a). Publications are exploding with studies about the benefits of their therapies (Lindquist et al., 2018; Natural Medicines, 2021a). Both traditions use natural, holistic approaches to physical, mental, and spiritual health, often in combination with yoga (NCCIH, 2021c). They teach that health is balance and disease (lack of ease) is imbalance. Each person is born with a unique combination of three vital energies that link body and mind: (a) movement energy (*loong* in Tibetan; *vata* in Ayurveda), (b) hot energy (*tripa* in Tibetan; *pitta* in Ayurveda), and (c) cold energy (*baekan* in Tibetan; *kapha* in Ayurveda). To create physical, mental, and spiritual health, the person needs to make informed, mindful choices that keep the current levels of these energies about the same as their levels in the individual's inborn constitution (Cameron & Namdul, 2020; Earl E. Bakken Center for Spirituality & Healing, University of Minnesota, 2020; Gonpo, 2015a, 2015b).

This chapter explores Tibetan medicine as an example of a care system that fits well with integrative nursing. Tibetan medicine, called *Sowa Rigpa* in Tibetan, teaches that the purpose of life is to be happy! Nursing and Tibetan medicine aim to address an individual's unique, interrelated mental, physical, and spiritual needs. Both disciplines share these principles: (a) Treat the whole individual; (b) Support the person's innate healing capacity; (c) Behave in harmony with nature; (d) Practice relationship-based care; (e) Start with mild treatments, rather than strong ones; and (f) Engage in self-care. Nurses will benefit by using Tibetan medicine for integrative care and for their own and clients' self-care. Including Tibetan medicine in integrative nursing expands healing options and promotes individualized quality care.

DEFINITION

HISTORY, PHILOSOPHY, AND PSYCHOLOGY OF TIBETAN MEDICINE

The earliest inhabitants of Tibet learned to thrive in the Himalayas, the tallest mountains on earth. Observing wildlife, Tibetans relied on natural resources to heal and sustain them. They practiced *Bon*, Tibet's Indigenous shamanism that teaches the interrelatedness of mind, body, and the natural world. When Buddhism came to Tibet, Tibetan medicine practitioners blended *Bon* and Buddhism with influences from Ayurveda, yoga, and Chinese, Persian, and Greek traditions. In the 8th century, Yuthok Yonten Gonpo, a famous Tibetan doctor, compiled these teachings into the *Gyueshi*, the fundamental text of Tibetan medicine (Gonpo, 2015a, 2015b; Tsona & Dakpa, 2017).

Today Tibetan medical colleges base their educational programs on the *Gyueshi*, commentaries, other texts, traditional and Western scientific research, and theories of health and disease. A graduate of Men-Tsee-Khang Tibetan Medical Colleges in Dharamsala and Bengaluru, India, is called a Tibetan Medicine Doctor. Tso-Ngon (Qinghai) University Tibetan Medical College in Amdo, Tibet (Xining, China), offers master's degrees and a PhD in Tibetan medicine, as well as a bachelor's degree in Tibetan medicine nursing.

Tibetan medicine is based on four profound concepts: *karma, suffering, healing,* and *happiness*. *Karma* is the universal law of cause and effect: "As one sows, so does one reap." To be healthy and happy, one needs to make choices that create health and happiness. Ethical behavior is essential to avoid the turmoil resulting from unethical actions. Sometimes choices have immediate, obvious effects, but other times, the results may not be clear right away. For example, eating unhealthy food or telling lies may not reap poor consequences immediately but eventually will cause suffering and even disease. One needs to develop an awareness of both immediate and long-term effects of one's choices (Tsona & Dakpa, 2017).

Suffering results from interpreting life from a negative perspective and making things worse. The Sanskrit term for suffering is *dukkha*, meaning "dissatisfaction" (lack of satisfaction). Most of human life is spent trying to avoid suffering and increase pleasure, too often in ways that inadvertently cause suffering. Pain and suffering are not the same (Gonpo, 2015a, 2015b). For example, one feels pain from a sprained ankle. One also will suffer by angrily asking, "Why do bad things always happen to me?" Anger and other negativity adversely affect the mind and body. One can avoid suffering by seeing the situation from a neutral or positive view, such as saying, "I'm glad that I didn't break my ankle."

Healing means to reestablish balance and create optimal health. One needs to purify negativity, reverse what's wrong, behave ethically, and create a healthy mind. A more neutral, compassionate mindset empowers one to interpret life accurately and make choices that create balance. Even on one's deathbed, healing the mind is advisable and possible, although the body is deteriorating (Cameron & Namdul, 2020).

Happiness is the very purpose of life! Happiness means joy, peace of mind, and well-being resulting from a healthy mind and balanced living. One creates meaning by seeing one's life as part of a bigger, purposeful picture and behaving with integrity according to one's best ethical values. Like a lotus flower growing in mud, one transforms life's "mud" into nourishment to rise and bloom (Cameron & Namdul, 2020, p.1).

FIVE ELEMENTS, THREE ENERGIES, AND SEVEN CONSTITUTIONS

Tibetan medicine teaches that energy (life force or *prana* in Sanskrit) is the very source of existence. Because all phenomena, including human beings, consist of energy, everyone is interconnected with everyone else and the natural world. Energy has five major characteristics, called elements. The five elements explain functions that work synergistically to maintain physical, mental, and spiritual health in mind and body. Tibetans used everyday terms to name and illustrate the five elements' universal, energetic qualities, as described in Exhibit 5.1 (Gonpo, 2015a, 2015b; Tsona & Dakpa, 2017).

Exhibit 5.1 *The Five Elements of Tibetan Medicine*

- *Earth* is the aspect of energy that produces stability and structure.
- *Water* is the aspect of energy that provides moisture, lubrication, and smoothness.
- *Fire* is the aspect of energy that drives growth, development, metabolism, and digestion.
- *Air* is the aspect of energy that governs movement, including blood and lymph circulation.
- *Space* is the aspect of energy that allows the other four elements to interact and coexist.

Source: Adapted from Gonpo, Y. Y. (2015a). *Root tantra and explanatory tantra (Gyueshi)* (T. Paljor, P. Wangdu, & S. Dolma, Trans.). Men-Tsee-Khang.

The five elements interact to form three primary energies: loong, tripa, and baekan. Each of the three vital energies has divisions, subdivisions, and defining characteristics. Everyone is born with a constitution consisting of a unique combination of loong, tripa, and baekan. The dominant energy or energies gives the name to the individual's constitution (Gonpo, 2015a). Exhibit 5.2 lists the three primary energies, the Romanized phonetic and transliterated Tibetan terms, and the element(s) composing each vital energy. Exhibit 5.3 lists the seven general constitutions.

Ordinarily, one's inborn constitution does not change. However, the three primary energies can rise, fall, or become disturbed due to multiple variables, such as thoughts, diet, stress, weather, environment, other people, lifestyle, season, time of day, and stage in life. To be healthy and happy, one must make choices that keep the current levels of loong, tripa, and baekan consistent with their levels in one's constitution. Understanding one's constitution will help to maintain balance, enhance strengths, and transform weaknesses into assets, or at least keep them from becoming obstacles (Gonpo, 2015a).

Exhibit 5.2 *The Three Primary Energies, the Romanized Phonetic and Transliterated Tibetan Terms, and the Five Elements*

Primary Energy	Tibetan Term	Element
Movement	*Loong* or *rLoong* (pronounced LOONG)	*Air*
Heat	*Tripa* or *mKhrispa* (pronounced TEE-pa)	*Fire*
Cold	*Baekan* or *Bad kan* (pronounced BA-kan)	*Earth, Water*

Source: Adapted from Gonpo, Y. Y. (2015a). *Root tantra and explanatory tantra (Gyueshi)* (T. Paljor, P. Wangdu, & S. Dolma, Trans.). Men-Tsee-Khang.

Exhibit 5.3 *The Seven Constitutions of Tibetan Medicine*

- *loong* constitution: *Loong* dominates *tripa* and *baekan.*
- *tripa* constitution: *Tripa* dominates *loong* and *baekan.*
- *baekan* constitution: *Baekan* dominates *loong* and *tripa.*
- *loong/tripa* or *tripa/loong* constitution: *Loong* and *tripa* dominate *baekan.*
- *tripa/baekan* or *baekan/tripa* constitution: *Tripa* and *baekan* dominate *loong.*
- *loong/baekan* or *baekan/loong* constitution: *Loong* and *baekan* dominate *tripa.*
- *loong/tripa/baekan* constitution: All three energies are equal, a rare, highly evolved constitution.

Source: Adapted from Gonpo, Y. Y. (2015a). *Root tantra and explanatory tantra (Gyueshi)* (T. Paljor, P. Wangdu, & S. Dolma, Trans.). Men-Tsee-Khang.

For example, one may be born with about 45% tripa, 40% baekan, and 15% loong (tripa/baekan constitution, as illustrated in Figure 5.1). To be healthy and happy, one must keep the current percentages of the three primary energies at about these inborn levels. Change in one energy affects the other two energies. Increasing tripa (hot energy) can decrease baekan (cold energy) and vice versa. Imbalance occurs well before physical symptoms of disease appear (Tsona & Dakpa, 2017).

Regardless of one's inborn constitution, baekan rises in the first stage of life to help children grow and develop. Tripa is high during the second and third stages of life when adults need enough hot energy to set and meet goals, establish a career, go back to school, create partnerships, raise a family, and do other adult tasks. In the fourth (final) stage, loong rises so elders become less grounded and more spiritual as they prepare to let go and die (Cameron & Namdul, 2020).

RELATIONSHIP BETWEEN THE THREE PRIMARY ENERGIES AND THREE MENTAL POISONS

Suffering begins in the mind. Thoughts impact the three primary energies, health, and happiness. Happy, compassionate thoughts calm mind and body. In contrast, anger raises the heart rate and blood pressure; causes shallow, irregular breathing; and depresses the immune system. When engaging in any of three mental poisons, one is likely to make unhealthy choices that result in suffering and illness, rather than happiness and health, as listed in Exhibit 5.4 (Cameron & Namdul, 2020, pp. 22–23).

Greed causes and results from loong imbalance; anger causes and results from tripa imbalance; delusion causes and results from baekan imbalance. When one vital energy goes out of balance, the other two energies are likely to go out of balance, too. Often, anxiety and insomnia begin the process, and then loong rises, which affects tripa and baekan. Chronic imbalance in all three energies is challenging to unravel and can produce complex health problems, such as cancer, cardiovascular disease, and autoimmune disorders. Creating a healthy mind and making good choices is the first step to healing and health (Gonpo, 2015a; Tsona & Dakpa, 2017).

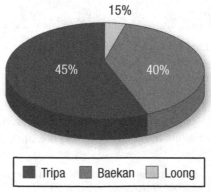

Figure 5.1 Example of a *Tripa/Baekan* constitution.

Exhibit 5.4 *Three Mental Poisons Promote Imbalance in the Three Primary Energies; How to Heal Resulting Health Problems*		
Mental Poison	**Promotes Imbalance in Primary Energy**	**How to Heal Resulting Health Problems**
Greed, attachments, desire	*Loong* (Movement Energy)	**Health Problems:** Anxiety, insomnia, lack of focus, headaches, heart and blood pressure issues, irritable digestion/bowel, movement disorders, addictions, mental illness **Heal:** Do what is warm, grounded, peaceful; meditate on impermanence; behave with generosity and acceptance
Anger, hostility, aggression	*Tripa* (Heat energy)	**Health Problems:** Inflammations, infections, headaches, autoimmune disorders, rashes, metabolic/hormonal issues, sensitive small intestine, cardiovascular disease **Heal:** Do what is dry and cool; meditate on compassion; engage in actions that relieve suffering for others and benefit the earth
Delusion, confusion, close-mindedness	*Baekan* (Cold energy)	**Health Problems:** Respiratory disorders, weak metabolism/digestion, poor blood circulation, kidney and bladder dysfunction, obesity, diabetes, tendency to dementia **Heal:** Do what is dry and warm; meditate on wisdom; reach out to help others and work to create a more compassionate, just world

Source: Adapted from Cameron, M. E., & Namdul, T. (2020). *Tibetan medicine and you: A path to wellbeing, better health, and joy (Blessing by His Holiness the Dalai Lama)*. Rowman & Littlefield (pp. 22–23, 100–108, 255).

SCIENTIFIC BASIS

Scientific research on Tibetan medicine is lacking. Investigating this ancient, holistic system is challenging because the physical, mental, and spiritual components work synergistically. Studying only one isolated component is inadequate to understand the power of Tibetan medicine. Qualitative methodologies may be needed to conduct such research. Even so, research results are promising for nursing.

THERAPIES

Since ancient times, Tibetan medicine doctors have conducted traditional, evidence-based research. They document the outcomes of therapies and prescribe what is most effective. Now numerous Western scientific studies are affirming the benefits of practices essential to Tibetan medicine. Researchers are finding positive results for meditation, mindfulness, yoga, art, chanting, breathing techniques, therapeutic listening, massage, imagery, aromatherapy, acupressure, music, biofeedback, nutrition, healing touch, reflexology, presence, relaxation, exercise, and Reiki (Lindquist et al., 2018; NCCIH, 2021c).

Western scientific researchers are starting to validate Tibetan medicine's teaching about seeing the whole person, not just separate organs, body systems, and specific diseases. Whole-person health focuses on restoring health, promoting resilience, and preventing diseases across the lifespan. Multiple interconnected factors promote health and disease: genes, nurturing, culture, environment, thoughts, diet, behavior, weather, climate, toxins, work, and others. Whole-person health empowers individuals, families, communities, and populations to create biological, behavioral, social, and environmental health (NCCIH, 2021g).

NATURE

Tibetan medicine teaches that human beings are part of nature, not separate from nature. Living in harmony with nature and spending time in nature promote healing and rejuvenation, as reported by researchers worldwide (Izenstark et al., 2021; Javelle et al., 2021; Kang & Chae, 2021; Kuhn et al., 2021; Peterfalvi et al., 2021; Tomasso et al., 2021). A synthesis of studies showed the positive effects of nature on immunological health (Andersen et al., 2021), the cardiovascular system, and mental health (Stier-Jarmer et al., 2021). A brief work break in nature regenerated hospital staff during stressful health emergencies (Gola et al., 2021). Tibetan medicine and researchers, Robinson et al. (2021), advocate conserving, restoring, and designing nature-centric environments that promote resilient societies and planetary health.

COMPASSION

Compassion, the essence of Tibetan medicine, is a philosophical stance of kindness toward all beings based on an understanding that all phenomena consist of the same five elements. Tibetan medicine teaches that the way to be happy is to practice compassion. Compassion cultivates conflict-proof well-being (Ho et al., 2020). So-called compassion fatigue does not result from too much compassion but from codependency, which is reliance on others for approval and identity (Cameron, 2018).

Tibetan medicine teaches a positive relationship among self-compassion, compassion, healing, and health, which numerous studies have confirmed (Alquwez et al., 2021; Andel et al., 2021; Arli, 2021; Beato et al., 2021; Fagan et al., 2021; Garcia et al., 2021; Hansen et al., 2021; Mesquita Garcia et al., 2021; O'Loghlen & Galligan, 2021; Roca et al., 2021; Siwik et al., 2021; Wakelin et al., 2021). Mindful self-compassion was an appropriate therapeutic approach for patients with chronic pain (Torrijos-Zarcero et al., 2021). Self-compassion predicted lower levels of daily physical symptoms and was associated with fewer increases in chronic illness in advanced old age (Herriot & Wrosch, 2021). Durkin et al. (2021) found that patients described receiving compassion through the use of touch that made them feel safe; nurses used touch to create an authentic connection with patients and were aware of the different meanings of touch; and avoiding touch, being wary of touch, or considering touch taboo robbed patients of compassion moments.

Compassion can be taught (Watts et al., 2021). Nursing students reported higher ratings of well-being when given compassion-based feedback (Bond et al., 2021). Self-compassion was positively related to resilience, engagement, motivation, and mental well-being, prompting Kotera et al. (2021) to recommend including a self-compassion component in nursing education. Ortega-Galan et al. (2021) found that nurses confuse the concepts of empathy and compassion as if they were synonymous, which necessitates clarifying compassion through educational interventions. Tibetan medicine offers an in-depth understanding of compassion that will benefit nursing education and integrative nursing (Cameron, 2018; Cameron & Namdul, 2020).

TIBETAN MEDICINES

Most published studies of Tibetan medicine focus on particular Tibetan medicines. This research is challenging to conduct because recipes for making Tibetan medicines are not readily available to Western scientific researchers. Tibetan medicines often are composites of 100 or more plants picked in the mountains of Tibet, China, India, and Nepal. Some herbs treat symptoms, others reverse imbalance, and still others promote healing. Unlike pharmaceuticals, the potency of plants varies because of weather, pollution, when and how they are picked, and other factors. Often, Tibetan medicinal preparations consist of easily available ingredients. For example, boiled water cooled enough to sip can relieve indigestion. Tibetan medicine doctors conduct evidence-based research on these medicinal preparations (Kalsang, 2016).

Western scientific researchers are validating Tibetan medicine doctors' claims about Tibetan medicines. Recent studies found that Tibetan medicines were helpful for persons with rheumatoid arthritis (Dong et al., 2021; Huang et al., 2021; Liu et al., 2021), antihypoxia capability and inflammation (Hua et al., 2021), cardioprotection in atherosclerosis (Wang et al., 2021), liver disease, COVID-19, and other dysfunctions (Y. Zhang et al., 2021). Researchers study rats to investigate whether Tibetan medicines can benefit human beings. The most recent studies showed alleviation of type 2 diabetes by regulating gut microbiota composition (Xu et al., 2021) and a positive effect on pneumonia (C. Zhang et al., 2021). More research is needed to learn if Tibetan medicines can be helpful for persons with cancer, autoimmune disorders, regeneration, and other health issues.

INTERVENTION

Tibetan medicine has numerous, research-tested, easy-to-use therapies, including breathing techniques, nutrition, meditation, mindfulness, relaxation, yoga, music, art, massage, imagery, aromatherapy, and acupressure. Besides these practices, nurses can do and teach their clients other Tibetan medicine interventions.

TECHNIQUES AND GUIDELINES
Complete a Constitutional Assessment

The gold standard is to have a consultation with a qualified, experienced Tibetan medicine doctor, called a Tibetan medicine practitioner in the United States. The practitioner asks questions, reads the radial pulses, analyzes the urine, and inspects the tongue. This information helps the practitioner identify the person's inborn constitution, energy imbalance, and the best treatment. The practitioner chooses natural remedies from mild to strong in this order: diet, behavior, Tibetan medicines, and accessory therapies (Tsona & Dakpa, 2017).

Because few people have access to a Tibetan medicine practitioner, nurses can do and encourage clients to do the Constitutional Self-Assessment Tool (CSAT) and the Lifestyle Guidelines Tool (LGT), the first published, research-based self-assessment tools based on Tibetan medicine. In a mixed-methods study, Cameron and Namdul (2020) created, tested, and refined the CSAT and LGT. The purpose was to provide valid, research-based self-assessment tools for individuals who don't have access to a Tibetan medicine doctor. Both tools had high content validity. The CSAT had moderate criterion validity. When participants followed instructions in Exhibit 5.5, the CSAT's assessment accuracy (criterion validity) increased.

Create a Healthy Body

An accurate CSAT assessment identifies one's current dominant energy, which may not be the same as the dominant energy in one's inborn constitution. Using the CSAT result, follow the LGT to calm loong, cool tripa, or warm baekan. If, for example, one's CSAT result is tripa, do what is listed in the LGT tripa column to cool tripa. For a dual constitution, such as loong/tripa, follow both the loong and tripa LGT columns.

When an energy rises too high or falls too low, engage in the opposite behavior to reverse the imbalance. For example, sit quietly and listen to calming music and/or eat warm, nutritious soup when stressed out and loong is high. On a hot day when tripa is elevated, transform anger into compassion, avoid the sun, and eat cooling foods like salads. During a cold winter when baekan rises, eat warm, spicy foods, and exercise vigorously to increase metabolism. Doing the CSAT and LGT regularly helps to create balance and reverse imbalance, as described in Exhibit 5.4 (Cameron & Namdul, 2020, pp. 35–50).

Exhibit 5.5 *Instructions for Completing the Constitutional Self-Assessment Tool (CSAT)*

- Before completing the CSAT, learn the basic teachings of Tibetan medicine explained in this chapter.
- Complete the CSAT in a quiet, reflective environment, without time pressure.
- Do an accurate, honest assessment of who you *really* are, not the person you wish to be.
- Consult with someone who knows you well to help you assess yourself accurately.
- Base your answers on your overall life, not just your current situation.
- Use the CSAT result to complete the LGT and calm *loong*, cool *tripa*, and/or warm *baekan*.

Source: Adapted from Cameron, M. E., & Namdul, T. (2020). *Tibetan medicine and you: A path to wellbeing, better health, and joy (Blessing by His Holiness the Dalai Lama)*. Rowman & Littlefield (pp. 37–46).

Create a Healthy Mind

Creating a healthy mind is essential for making mindful, informed choices leading to happiness. Tibetan medicine integrates ethics, spirituality, and healing. A healthy mind results from an ethical, spiritual life. Meditation is a powerful tool to create optimal health. As researchers have found, meditation opens the heart, promotes compassion, and enhances the immune system (Lindquist et al., 2018). The mind may feel like a jumping monkey. Tibetan meditation tames the monkey mind. Bring unconscious/subconscious thoughts into consciousness and heal what is negative. Transform the three mental poisons into qualities of happiness: love, compassion, gratitude, wisdom, kindness, honesty, integrity, meaning, joy, forgiveness, peace, tolerance, altruism, humility, equanimity, responsibility, and patience (Cameron & Namdul, 2020. p. 98).

Many options exist. Meditate while sitting, walking, lying down, dancing, or listening to calming music. Try meditating while walking safely in a forest, along the beach, around a lake, or in another beautiful area. Sitting comfortably can reduce distractions and enhance deep meditation. Exercising first may promote quiet during sitting meditation. For example, do yoga postures before sitting down to meditate. The ideal is to cultivate a meditative mindset all the time (Cameron & Namdul, 2020).

Nurses can meditate and teach clients to meditate before and after treatments and surgery to calm the mind and body. Start with a 2-minute meditation on the breath (Exhibit 5.6). Do Tonglen Meditation to fill the heart with compassion and purify the mind and body (Exhibit 5.7). Do Loving-Kindness Meditation to enhance the immune system (Exhibit 5.8). Engaging in circular breathing all the time, not just during meditation, brings in life force (*prana* in Sanskrit), oxygenates cells, and releases toxins (Cameron & Namdul, 2020).

Create a Good Death

Tibetan medicine teaches that death is part of life, not separate from life. One dies as one lives. To die well, one must live well. Now is the time to create a good life and a good death, the kind of life and death that one wants and is feasible. Identify and heal all negativity, or disturbing thoughts and feelings likely will cause suffering during life and the dying process. Develop beliefs about death

---

Exhibit 5.6 *Two-Minute Meditation on Your Breath*

- Make yourself comfortable sitting, standing, walking, or lying down.
- Straighten your back, relax your body, breathe deeply, and focus on your breath.
- Engage in circular breathing: Breathe slowly, deeply, and evenly through your nose, from your abdomen, with your in-breath the same length as your out-breath, and no break between.
- When your attention moves away from your breath, bring it back to your breath.

Source: Adapted from Cameron, M. E., & Namdul, T. (2020). *Tibetan medicine and you: A path to wellbeing, better health, and joy (Blessing by His Holiness the Dalai Lama).* Rowman & Littlefield (p. 256).

Exhibit 5.7 *Tonglen Meditation: "Breathe in suffering and breathe out compassion"*

- Make yourself comfortable sitting, standing, walking, or lying down.
- Straighten your back, relax your body, breathe deeply, and focus on your breath.
- Engage in circular breathing: Breathe slowly, deeply, and evenly through your nose, from your abdomen, with your in-breath the same length as your out-breath, and no break between.
- *Do Tonglen for yourself*: As you breathe in, let all negativity in your mind and body come to the surface. On your out-breath, breathe out these toxins completely and fill yourself with compassion.
- *Do Tonglen for someone you love*: Breathe in your loved one's suffering and breathe out compassion to the person. Open your heart to your loved one.
- *Do Tonglen for someone about whom you feel neutral (clerk in a store, etc.)*: Breathe in the person's suffering, and breath out compassion to the person. Open your heart to this individual.
- *Do Tonglen for someone you dislike*: Breathe in the person's suffering and breathe out compassion for this individual. Open your heart to the person and let go of any negativity.
- *Do Tonglen for the world*: Breathe in the suffering of the world and breathe out compassion to the world. Open your heart to everyone's suffering and let go of any negativity.
- *Purification*: Visualize the suffering you breathed in as black smoke in your heart's center and breathe it out completely. Fill your heart with compassion for yourself, everyone, and everything.

Source: Adapted from Cameron, M. E., & Namdul, T. (2020). *Tibetan medicine and you: A path to wellbeing, better health, and joy (Blessing by His Holiness the Dalai Lama)*. Rowman & Littlefield (pp. 63–65, 166–167).

Exhibit 5.8 *Loving-Kindness Meditation*

- Make yourself comfortable sitting, standing, walking, or lying down.
- Straighten your back, relax your body, breathe deeply, and focus on your breath.
- Engage in circular breathing: Breathe slowly, deeply, and evenly through your nose, from your abdomen, with your in-breath the same length as your out-breath, and no break between.
- When you are deeply relaxed and focused, say these words with an altruistic intention:
  - May I be well; may all beings be well.
  - May I be happy; may all beings be happy.
  - May I be peaceful; may all beings be peaceful.
  - May I be loved; may all beings be loved.

Source: Adapted from Cameron, M. E., & Namdul, T. (2020). *Tibetan medicine and you: A path to wellbeing, better health, and joy (Blessing by His Holiness the Dalai Lama)*. Rowman & Littlefield (pp. 183–184).

that make sense, provide comfort, and alleviate fears involving one's own death and the death of one's loved ones. By creating a healthy mind, one will be able to face death with acceptance, peace, and even joy (Cameron & Namdul, 2020, pp. 149–167; Namdul, 2021).

MEASUREMENT OF OUTCOMES

To determine the effectiveness of these interventions, nurses can ask themselves and clients if they feel better after the interventions. Conventional care can be excellent when Western pharmaceuticals, technology, and surgery are needed. Tibetan medicine can be effective to create a healthy mind and body, heal or manage disease, and die peacefully. The two approaches complement each other. For example, someone with cancer can use Tibetan medicine to prepare for and recover from chemotherapy and radiation (Cameron & Namdul, 2020).

Even beginners can use Tibetan medicine to decrease stress, anxiety, and headaches, and to improve digestion and sleep. However, most health problems develop over time; Tibetan medicine may not alleviate them right away. A serious imbalance may require careful, long-term rebalancing. Tibetan medicine advocates gradual change. Optimal benefits occur from systematic use (Earl E. Bakken Center for Spirituality & Healing, University of Minnesota, 2020; Gonpo, 2015a).

PRECAUTIONS

Exhibit 5.9 lists precautions to ensure coordinated, safe care. Because Tibetan medicine is not yet widespread in the United States, standardization, accreditation, and licensure have not yet been established. Some people lacking credentials claim to be Tibetan medicine practitioners. Only consult with experienced practitioners who graduated from a legitimate Tibetan medical college (Cameron, 2018; Earl E. Bakken Center for Spirituality & Healing, University of Minnesota, 2020).

Exhibit 5.9 *Precautions When Using Tibetan Medicine*

- *Do not use* Tibetan medicine to replace effective conventional healthcare or as a reason to postpone seeing conventional health professionals about health problems.
- Learn as much as you can about your inborn constitution and your health problems.
- Carefully select qualified professionals you trust while listening to your internal wisdom.
- Advocate for yourself, rather than just accepting what health professionals tell you.
- Explain to your health professionals how you manage your health and any medications you take.

Source: Adapted from Cameron, M. E., & Namdul, T. (2020). *Tibetan medicine and you: A path to wellbeing, better health, and joy (Blessing by His Holiness the Dalai Lama)*. Rowman & Littlefield (pp. 258–260).

In the United States, Tibetan medicine practitioners must follow state laws regulating unlicensed practitioners of complementary and alternative healthcare. For example, Chapter 146A of the Minnesota Statutes (2020) states that unlicensed practitioners cannot call themselves a doctor, refer to clients as patients, or use treatments such as acupuncture covered by other licensing boards. They must give each client a detailed bill of rights about their qualifications and the client's rights and responsibilities. The Minnesota Statute lists the detailed information required in the client's bill of rights.

Precautions are needed if Tibetan medicine practitioners prescribe Tibetan medicines. Tibetan herbal preparations generally work slowly and have few, if any, side effects. In the United States, Tibetan medicines are categorized as dietary supplements regulated by the U.S. Food and Drug Administration. In general, U.S. government regulations involving dietary supplements are less stringent than for Western pharmaceuticals.

A few Tibetan medicines contain minute amounts of detoxified minerals and poisonous plants to stimulate healing. In two studies, Tibetan medicines containing detoxified mercury did not lead to mercury in the participants' blood (Sallon et al., 2017). However, L. Zhang et al. (2021) investigated a Tibetan medicine used by Tibetans for over a thousand years to treat advanced gastroenteropathy diseases. The researchers concluded that precautions should be taken to monitor the medicine's toxicity if given over a long period.

Until more testing is done, one probably is best off avoiding Tibetan medicines containing minerals and poisonous plants. Many other Tibetan medicines are available. Do not take a Tibetan medicine at the same time as a Western pharmaceutical because they may interact and be unsafe. Or maintain a gap of at least 1 hour between taking a Tibetan medicine and a Western pharmaceutical. Pregnant or nursing women and parents who want to use Tibetan medicines for their children first need to consult with qualified health professionals.

USES

Nurses will benefit by using Tibetan medicine as self-care and integrative care for themselves. Moreover, they can teach Tibetan medicine to their clients and use Tibetan medicine as part of integrative nursing.

CULTURAL APPLICATION

Millions of people around the world use Tibetan medicine instead of or as a complement to conventional healthcare. Tibetan medicine doctors hold clinics in North and South America, Europe, Asia, Australia, and Africa. Tibetan medicine can be adapted to any individual, culture, and values. In Sidebar 5.1, Tashi Lhamo, a registered nurse and Tibetan medicine doctor, explains how she integrates nursing and Tibetan medicine.

FUTURE RESEARCH

Published studies about Tibetan medicine report positive results. However, much more scientific research is needed. Tibetan medicine's holistic philosophy and psychology pose challenges for conducting scientific research. The profound

Sidebar 5.1 *A Tibetan Nurse Integrates Nursing and Tibetan Medicine*

Tashi Lhamo

My parents grew up in Tibet and moved to India, where I was born. Because I wanted to help others, I entered the Tibetan medicine program at Men-Tsee-Khang Tibetan Medical College in Dharamsala, India. I graduated as a Tibetan Medicine Doctor and worked with senior doctors. After immigrating to the United States in 2002, I went to college and studied nursing. Now I am a staff nurse on a busy medical–surgical unit of a large metropolitan hospital and a student in a Doctor of Nursing Practice program. Tibetan medicine is essential to my nursing practice.

Tibetan medicine teaches that the purpose of life is to be happy. Everyone is born with a unique combination of three principal energies: loong (movement energy), tripa (hot energy), and baekan (cold energy). What we think, eat, drink, and do can cause them to rise, fall, or become disturbed. Health is balance, and disease is imbalance. To be happy and healthy, we need to make lifestyle choices that keep the current percentages of these energies consistent with our inborn constitution. By using Tibetan medicine as self-care, we become aware of how our thoughts and behaviors affect our body, mind, health, and happiness.

Tibetan medicine helps me give quality nursing care by understanding my clients on the level of their three principal energies. I view each client as unique and encourage the person to make healthy choices, let go of negativity, and create optimal health. Tibetan medicine teaches me to be mindful of my surroundings and treat each client with compassion, loving-kindness, empathetic joy, and equanimity. Also, Tibetan medicine reminds me to practice self-compassion and nurture myself to be healthy physically, mentally, and spiritually. Medical–surgical nursing is challenging. Stressed-out nurses will benefit by using Tibetan medicine for self-care and integrative nursing.

---

therapies affect the mind and body in ways that may not be reproducible and quantifiable. The multiple components of Tibetan medicine work together synergistically to promote healing and health. Testing only one small component, as in reductionist, quantitative research, won't yield accurate results about Tibetan medicine. New qualitative methods may be needed.

Well-designed studies can test these and other research questions:

- How accurate are theories about the five elements, three primary energies, and seven constitutions?
- What is the relationship between energy imbalance and specific health problems?
- Are an individual's health, illness, and negative or positive emotions related?
- How does Tibetan medicine affect happiness, mental health, immunity, longevity, and dying?
- What are the relationships between each of the seven constitutions and measurements of compassion, anxiety, insomnia, anger, depression, addictions, biological markers, and specific illnesses?

■ Which Tibetan medicines are helpful for which individuals?
■ How can nurses and their clients be taught to use Tibetan medicine for self-care?
■ What are effective ways for nurses to integrate Tibetan medicine and nursing?
■ How can nurses be taught to practice self-compassion and become true healers?

In summary, integrative nurses bring together the best of ancient and modern wisdom about health and healing. Tibetan medicine complements nursing. Both integrative nursing and Tibetan medicine promote mindfulness, self-understanding, and healthy choices, and they are based on scientific evidence. Nurses who use Tibetan medicine for self-care and integrative nursing enhance health and healing. People who make informed, healthy choices benefit themselves, conventional healthcare, society, and the planet.

WEBSITES

■ Book: *Tibetan Medicine and You: A Path to Wellbeing, Better Health, and Joy,* with a Blessing by His Holiness the Dalai Lama: https://rowman.com/ISBN/9781538135013/Tibetan-Medicine-and-You-A-Path-to-Wellbeing-Better -Health-and-Joy
■ Example of Graduate Courses: www.csh.umn.edu/education/credit-courses/csph-5315-traditional-tibetan-medicine-ethics-spirituality-and-healing
■ Online Tools: Constitutional Self-Assessment Tool and Lifestyle Guidelines Tool: www.csh.umn.edu/education/focus-areas/tibetan-medicine/assessment -and-guidelines-tools
■ Online Overview of Tibetan Medicine: www.takingcharge.csh.umn.edu/tibetan-medicine

REFERENCES

Alquwez, N., Cruz, J. P., Al Thobaity, A., Almazan, J., Alabdulaziz, H., Alshammari, F., Albloushi, M., Tumala, R., & Albougami, A. (2021). Self-compassion influences the caring behaviour and compassion competence among Saudi nursing students: A multi-university study. *Nursing Open, 8,* 2732. https://doi.org/10.1002/nop2.848

American Association of Naturopathic Physicians. (2021). *About us.* https://naturopathic.org/page/AboutUs

American Institute of Homeopathy. (2021). *About the American Institute of Homeopathy.* https://homeopathyusa.org/about-aih-2.html

Andel, S. A., Shen, W., & Arvan, M. L. (2021). Depending on your own kindness: The moderating role of self-compassion on the within-person consequences of work loneliness during the covid-19 pandemic. *Journal of Occupational Health Psychology, 26,* 276. https://doi.org/10.1037/ocp0000271

Andersen, L., Corazon, S. S. S., & Stigsdotter, U. K. K. (2021). Nature exposure and its effects on immune system functioning: A systematic review. *International Journal of Environmental Research & Public Health, 18,* 1416. https://doi.org/10.3390/ijerph18041416

Arli, S. K. (2021). An investigation of the relationship between attitudes towards caring for dying patients and compassion. *Omega: Journal of Death & Dying,* 302228211004805. https://doi.org/10.1177/00302228211004805

Beato, A. F., da Costa, L. P., & Nogueira, R. (2021). "Everything is gonna be alright with me": The role of self-compassion, affect, and coping in negative emotional symptoms during coronavirus quarantine. *International Journal of Environmental Research & Public Health, 18,* 2017. https://doi.org/10.3390/ijerph18042017

Bond, C. A. E., Tsikandilakis, M., Stacey, G., Hui, A., & Timmons, S. (2021). The effects of compassion-based feedback on wellbeing ratings during a professional assessment healthcare task. *Nurse Education Today, 99*, 104788. https://doi.org/10.1016/j.nedt.2021.104788

Cameron, M. E. (2018). Systems of care: Sowa Rigpa—The Tibetan knowledge of healing. In Lindquist, R., Tracy, M. S., & Snyder, M. (Eds.), *Complementary & alternative therapies in nursing* (8th ed., pp. 63–80). Springer Publishing Company.

Cameron, M. E., & Namdul, T. (2020). *Tibetan medicine and you: A path to wellbeing, better health, and joy (Blessing by His Holiness the Dalai Lama).* Rowman & Littlefield.

Dong, Z. Y., Wei, L., Lu, H. Q., Zeng, Q. H., Meng, F. C., Wang, G. W., Lan, X. Z., Liao, Z. H., & Chen, M. (2021). Ptehoosines a and b: Two new sesamin-type sesquilignans with antiangiogenic activity from *Pterocephalus hookeri* (C.B. Clarke) Hoëck. *Fitoterapia, 151*, 104886. https://doi.org/10.1016/j.fitote.2021.104886

Durkin, J., Jackson, D., & Usher, K. (2021). The expression and receipt of compassion through touch in a health setting: A qualitative study. *Journal of Advanced Nursing, 77*, 1980–1991. https://doi.org/10.1111/jan.14766

Earl E. Bakken Center for Spirituality & Healing, University of Minnesota. (2020). *Tibetan medicine.* https://www.takingcharge.csh.umn.edu/tibetan-medicine

Earl E. Bakken Center for Spirituality & Healing, University of Minnesota. (2021b). *Integrative nursing.* https://www.csh.umn.edu/education/focus-areas/integrative-nursing

Fagan, S., Hodge, S., & Morris, C. (2021). Experiences of compassion in adults with a diagnosis of borderline personality disorder: An interpretative phenomenological analysis. *Psychological Reports, 332941211000661*. https://doi.org/10.1177/00332941211000661

Garcia, A. C. M., Camargos Junior, J. B., Sarto, K. K., Silva Marcelo, C. A. D., Paiva, E. M. D. C., Nogueira, D. A., & Mills, J. (2021). Quality of life, self-compassion and mindfulness in cancer patients undergoing chemotherapy: A cross-sectional study. *European Journal of Oncology Nursing, 51*, 101924. https://doi.org/10.1016/j.ejon.2021.101924

Gola, M., Botta, M., D'Aniello, A. L., & Capolongo, S. (2021). Influence of nature at the time of the pandemic. *HERD: Health Environments Research & Design Journal, 14*(2), 49–65. https://doi.org/10.1177/1937586721991113

Gonpo, Y. Y. (2015a). *Root Tantra and Explanatory Tantra (Gyueshi)* (T. Paljor, P. Wangdu, & S. Dolma, Trans.). Men-Tsee-Khang.

Gonpo, Y. Y. (2015b). *Subsequent Tantra (Gyueshi)* (T. Paljor, Trans.). Men-Tsee-Khang.

Hansen, N. H., Juul, L., Pallesen, K. J., & Fjorback, L. O. (2021). Effect of a compassion cultivation training program for caregivers of people with mental illness in Denmark: A randomized clinical trial. *JAMA Network Open, 4*, e211020. https://doi.org/10.1001/jamanetworkopen.2021.1020

Herriot, H., & Wrosch, C. (2021). Self-compassion as predictor of daily physical symptoms and chronic illness across older adulthood. *Journal of Health Psychology, 13591053211002326*. https://doi.org/10.1177/13591053211002326

Ho, S. S., Nakamura, Y., & Swain, J. E. (2020). Compassion as an intervention to attune to universal suffering of self and others in conflicts: A translational framework. *Frontiers in Psychology, 11*, 603385. https://doi.org/10.3389/fpsyg.2020.603385

Hua, H., Zhu, H., Liu, C., Zhang, W., Li, J., Hu, B., Guo, Y., Cheng, Y., Pi, F., Xie, Y., Yao, W., & Qian, H. (2021). Bioactive compound from the Tibetan turnip (*Brassica rapa* L.) elicited anti-hypoxia effects in OGD/R-injured HT22 cells by activating the PI3K/AKT pathway. *Food & Function, 12*, 2901. https://doi.org/10.1039/d0fo03190a

Huang, X. J., Wang, J., Muhammad, A., Tong, H. Y., Wang, D. G., Li, J., Ihsan, A., & Yang, G. Z. (2021). Systems pharmacology-based dissection of mechanisms of Tibetan medicinal compound ruteng as an effective treatment for collagen-induced arthritis rats. *Journal of Ethnopharmacology, 272*, 113953. https://doi.org/10.1016/j.jep.2021.113953

Izenstark, D., Ravindran, N., Rodriguez, S., & Devine, N. (2021). The affective and conversational benefits of a walk in nature among mother-daughter dyads. *Applied Psychology, Health and Well-being, 13*, 299. https://doi.org/10.1111/aphw.12250

Javelle, F., Laborde, S., Hosang, T. J., Metcalfe, A. J., & Zimmer, P. (2021). The importance of nature exposure and physical activity for psychological health and stress perception. *Frontiers in Psychology, 12*, 623946. https://doi.org/10.3389/fpsyg.2021.623946

Kalsang, T. (2016). *Cultivation and conservation of endangered medicinal plants: Tibetan medicinal plants for health.* Men-Tsee-Khang.

Kang, H., & Chae, Y. (2021). Effects of integrated indirect forest experience on emotion, fatigue, stress, and immune function in hemodialysis patients. *International Journal of Environmental Research & Public Health, 18*, 1701. https://doi.org/10.3390/ijerph18041701

Kotera, Y., Cockerill, V., Chircop, J., Kaluzeviciute, G., & Dyson, S. (2021). Predicting self-compassion in UK nursing students. *Nurse Education in Practice, 51*, 102989. https://doi.org/10.1016/j.nepr.2021.102989

Kuhn, S., Forlim, C. G., Lender, A., Wirtz, J., & Gallinat, J. (2021). Brain functional connectivity differs when viewing pictures from natural and built environments using FMRI resting state analysis. *Scientific Reports, 11*, 4110. https://doi.org/10.1038/s41598-021-83246-5

Lindquist, R., Tracy, M. F., & Snyder, M. (Eds.). (2018). *Complementary & alternative therapies in nursing* (8th ed.). Springer Publishing Company.

Liu, C., Zhao, Q., Zhong, L., Li, Q., Li, R., Li, S., Li, Y., Li, N., Su, J., Dhondrup, W., Meng, X., Zhang, Y., Tu, Y., & Wang, X. (2021). Tibetan medicine Ershiwuwei Lvxue pill attenuates collagen-induced arthritis via inhibition of JAK2/STAT3 signaling pathway. *Journal of Ethnopharmacology, 270*, 113820. https://doi.org/10.1016/j.jep.2021.113820

Mesquita Garcia, A. C., Domingues Silva, B., Oliveira da Silva, L. C., & Mills, J. (2021). Self-compassion in hospice and palliative care: A systematic integrative review. *Journal of Hospice & Palliative Nursing, 23*, 145–154. https://doi.org/10.1097/njh.0000000000000727

Minnesota Statutes. (2020). *Chapter 146A. Complementary and alternative health care practices.* https://www.revisor.mn.gov/statutes/cite/146A#stat.146A.001

Namdul, T. (2021). Re-examining death: Doors to resilience and wellbeing in Tibetan Buddhist practice. *Religions, 12*, 522. https://doi.org/10.3390/rel12070522

National Center for Complementary and Integrative Health. (2021a). *Ayurvedic medicine: In depth.* https://www.nccih.nih.gov/health/ayurvedic-medicine-in-depth

National Center for Complementary and Integrative Health. (2021b). *Complementary, alternative, or integrative health.* https://www.nccih.nih.gov/health/complementary-alternative-or-integrative-health-whats-in-a-name

National Center for Complementary and Integrative Health. (2021c). *Health topics A-Z.* https://www.nccih.nih.gov/health/atoz#linkA

National Center for Complementary and Integrative Health. (2021d). *Homeopathy: What you need to know.* https://www.nccih.nih.gov/health/homeopathy

National Center for Complementary and Integrative Health. (2021e). *Naturopathy.* https://www.nccih.nih.gov/health/naturopathy

National Center for Complementary and Integrative Health. (2021g). *Whole person health: What you need to know.* https://www.nccih.nih.gov/health/whole-person-health-what-you-need-to-know?nav=govd

Natural Medicines. (2021a). *Ayurveda.* Therapeutic Research Center. https://naturalmedicines-therapeuticresearch-com.ezp3.lib.umn.edu/databases/health-wellness/professional.aspx?productid=1201

Natural Medicines. (2021b). *Homeopathy.* Therapeutic Research Center. https://naturalmedicines-therapeuticresearch-com.ezp3.lib.umn.edu/databases/health-wellness/professional.aspx?productid=1154

Natural Medicines. (2021c). *Naturopathy.* Therapeutic Research Center. https://naturalmedicines-therapeuticresearch-com.ezp3.lib.umn.edu/databases/health-wellness/professional.aspx?productid=1198

O'Loghlen, E., & Galligan, R. (2021). Disordered eating in the postpartum period: Role of psychological distress, body dissatisfaction, dysfunctional maternal beliefs, and self-compassion. *Journal of Health Psychology*, 1359105321995940. https://doi.org/10.1177/135910532 1995940

Ortega-Galan, A. M., Perez-Garcia, E., Brito-Pons, G., Ramos-Pichardo, J. D., Carmona-Rega, M. I., & Ruiz-Fernandez, M. D. (2021). Understanding the concept of compassion from the perspectives of nurses. *Nursing Ethics*, 969733020983401. https://doi.org/10.1177/0969733020 983401

Peterfalvi, A., Meggyes, M., Makszin, L., Farkas, N., Miko, E., Miseta, A., & Szereday, L. (2021). Forest bathing always makes sense. *International Journal of Environmental Research & Public Health*, 18. https://doi.org/10.3390/ijerph18042067

Robinson, J. M., Brindley, P., Cameron, R., MacCarthy, D., & Jorgensen, A. (2021). Nature's role in supporting health during the covid-19 pandemic. *International Journal of Environmental Research & Public Health*, 18, 2227. https://doi.org/10.3390/ijerph18052227

Roca, P., Vazquez, C., Diez, G., Brito-Pons, G., & McNally, R. J. (2021). Not all types of meditation are the same: Mediators of change in mindfulness and compassion meditation interventions. *Journal of Affective Disorders*, 283, 354–362. https://doi.org/10.1016/j.jad.2021.01.070

Sallon, S., Dory, Y., Barghouthy, Y., Tamdin, T., Sangmo, R., Tashi, J., Yangdon, S., Yeshi, T., Sadutshang, T., Rotenberg, M., Cohen, E., Harlavan, Y., Sharabi, G., & Bdolah-Abram, T. (2017). Is mercury in Tibetan medicine toxic? Clinical, neurocognitive, and biochemical results of an initial cross-sectional study. *Experimental Biology & Medicine*, 242, 316–332. https://doi .org/10.1177/1535370216672748

Siwik, C. J., Phillips, K., Zimmaro, L., Salmon, P., & Sephton, S. E. (2021). Depressive symptoms among patients with lung cancer: Elucidating the roles of shame, guilt, and self-compassion. *Journal of Health Psychology*, 1359105320988331. https://doi.org/10.1177/1359105320988331

Stier-Jarmer, M., Throner, V., Kirschneck, M., Immich, G., Frisch, D., & Schuh, A. (2021). The psychological and physical effects of forests on human health. *International Journal of Environmental Research & Public Health*, 18. https://doi.org/10.3390/ijerph18041770

Tomasso, L. P., Yin, J., Cedeno Laurent, J. G., Chen, J. T., Catalano, P. J., & Spengler, J. D. (2021). The relationship between nature deprivation and individual wellbeing across urban gradients under Covid-19. *International Journal of Environmental Research & Public Health*, 18, 1511. https://doi.org/10.3390/ijerph18041511

Torrijos-Zarcero, M., Mediavilla, R., Rodriguez-Vega, B., Del Rio-Dieguez, M., Lopez-Alvarez, I., Rocamora-Gonzalez, C., & Palao-Tarrero, A. (2021). Mindful self-compassion program for chronic pain patients. *European Journal of Pain*, 25, 930–944. https://doi.org/10.1002/ejp.1734

Tsona, L. T. T., & Dakpa, T. (2017). *Fundamentals of Tibetan medicine*. Men-Tsee-Khang.

Wakelin, K. E., Perman, G., & Simonds, L. M. (2021). Effectiveness of self-compassion-related interventions for reducing self-criticism. *Clinical Psychology & Psychotherapy*, 29. https://doi .org/10.1002/cpp.2586

Wang, C., Nan, X., Pei, S., Zhao, Y., Wang, X., Ma, S., & Ma, G. (2021). Salidroside and isorhamne-tin attenuate urotensin II-induced inflammatory response *in vivo* and *in vitro*: Involvement in regulating the RhoA/ROCK II pathway. *Oncology Letters*, 21, 292. https://doi.org/10.3892/ ol.2021.12553

Watts, K. J., O'Connor, M., Johnson, C. E., Breen, L. J., Kane, R. T., Choules, K., Doyle, C., Buchanan, G., & Yuen, K. (2021). Mindfulness-based compassion training for health professionals providing end-of-life care: Impact, feasibility, and acceptability. *Journal of Palliative Medicine*, 24, 1364. https://doi.org/10.1089/jpm.2020.0358

Xu, T., Ge, Y., Du, H., Li, Q., Xu, X., Yi, H., Wu, X., Kuang, T., Fan, G., & Zhang, Y. (2021). Berberis kansuensis extract alleviates type 2 diabetes in rats by regulating gut microbiota composition. *Journal of Ethnopharmacology*, 273, 113995. https://doi.org/10.1016/j.jep.2021.113995

Zhang, C., Liu, C., Qu, Y., Cao, Y., Liu, R., Sun, Y., Nyima, T., Zhang, S., & Sun, Y. (2021). Lc-MS-based qualitative analysis and pharmacokinetic integration network pharmacology strategy reveals the mechanism of *Phlomis brevidentata* H. W. Li treatment of pneumonia. *ACS Omega, 6*, 4495–4505. https://doi.org/10.1021/acsomega.0c06201

Zhang, L., Rezeng, C., Wang, Y., & Li, Z. (2021). Changes in copper, zinc, arsenic, mercury, and lead concentrations in rat biofluids and tissues induced by the "Renqing Changjue" pill, a traditional Tibetan medicine. *Biological Trace Element Research, 199*, 4646. https://doi.org/10.1007/s12011-021-02586-5

Zhang, Y., Zhou, Q., Ding, X., Ma, J., & Tan, G. (2021). Chemical profile of *Swertia mussotii* franch and its potential targets against liver fibrosis revealed by cross-platform metabolomics. *Journal of Ethnopharmacology, 274*, 114051. https://doi.org/10.1016/j.jep.2021.114051

6

Self-Care and Use of Complementary Therapies

BARBARA RIEGEL AND RUTH LINDQUIST

Self-care is essential for health and everyone engages in some form of self-care daily with food choices, tooth brushing, sleeping, controlling stress, and so on. Self-care was the primary form of healthcare long before the medical establishment as we now know it came into existence. By necessity, people have been managing their own health and that of their loved ones since the beginning of humankind. Taylor (2019) argues that Socrates was the founder of the self-care movement, when he promoted care, the Greek word was understood to include meditation, regular fasting, prayer, education, music, and exercise. These behaviors were intended to train the body and the mind to prepare to comprehend the truth. Modern medicine emerged in the 19th century, during the Industrial Revolution in America, with scientific and medical discoveries, technological advances, and the development of the healthcare professions (International Self Care Foundation, 2021).

Broadly speaking, self-care can also be understood to embrace choices and wisdom related to environmental exposures (e.g., elements of heat and cold, air quality, light and sun), stress management, recreation, recreational drugs, and dietary supplements. Environmental factors such as air pollution the quality of drinking water, the availability of fresh produce, and environmental toxins affect the health of individuals and virtually any geographic setting in the world. Despite even the potentially worst adverse environmental conditions, individuals can act defensively to sustain their health or promote health. That is, for example, one may limit sun exposure, filter the air or avoid outdoor exposure when toxins are airborne or air quality is poor, boil or treat contaminated water, and avoid, test for, and effectively mitigate environmental conditions—for example, radon.

Partnership in care with healthcare providers, particularly a primary care provider, is important. Today we are enculturated to seek medical care early in the course of an illness and to expect a pharmaceutical solution to whatever ails us, although the majority of care is still self-care. Indeed, time spent with a provider (an estimated 15 minutes annually) is minuscule compared to the time individuals may spend outside the provider's office engaged in self-care (60 min/hour × 24 hr/day × 365 days/year = 525,600 minutes). Persons may visit a primary care provider or health clinic for an annual or periodic visit to be screened or examined for adverse conditions or given a clean bill of health. The amount of time in observation and presence of a primary healthcare provider, and the exchange of information—although relevant and important—pales in comparison to the time spent by an individual apart from the primary provider's office whether at home or in the context of the many other living environments and routines familiar to the individual. It is during these times that routines are forged and health habits formed that, as they are repeated and "practiced" day after day, impact health. It is thus outside the provider's office that significant time is spent that could influence health, good or bad. The sustained and conscious efforts of individuals to attend to their own health needs (self-care) can go far to maintain and promote their health, well-being, as well as the length and health-related quality of life.

Self-care is performed in both healthy and ill states, although self-care for the healthy general population differs from that prescribed for individuals with a chronic illness. Chronic illness requires behaviors intended to control the illness, decrease symptoms, and improve survival. Once chronic illness occurs, providers partner in self-care, often expecting that the patient will adhere to the medication regimen and share responsibility for monitoring and report back when changes occur. However, the person with a chronic illness still needs to engage in general self-care behaviors. For this reason, establishing healthy habits and lifestyle routines early in life can make self-care easier later in life when chronic illness is most likely to mandate some level of self-care.

As described in some detail below, the evidence is convincing that self-care is associated with positive health outcomes. However, for a variety of reasons, people routinely defer self-care and the formal healthcare system fails to emphasize it. Surprisingly, although the SARS-CoV-2 (COVID) pandemic has encouraged and sometimes mandated self-care with routine handwashing, masking in public, and vaccinations, even this shared event has not convinced everyone regarding the importance of self-care to patients, families, communities, and providers. Historical documents from the 1918 influenza epidemic illustrate that self-care was emphasized then as it is now (Figure 6.1). For a variety of reasons, these basic self-care messages are not uniformly endorsed during this pandemic.

Self-care is also important to nonprofessional and professional caregivers. Indeed, a nonprofessional caregiver is unable to provide care if too fatigued or worn down to do so. Likewise, self-care is important to nurses, nursing students, and other healthcare providers. In fact, the Code of Ethics for Nurses of the American Nurses Association identifies self-care as a duty to self beyond their duty to their patients (American Nurses Association, 2015; Linton & Koonmen, 2020). Thus, the focus of this chapter is on self-care for nurses and nursing students and the role they play in educating communities, patients, caregivers, and families about the importance of self-care.

DEFINITION

Riegel and colleagues defined *self-care* as a process of maintaining health through health promoting practices and managing illness when it occurs (Riegel et al., 2012). Unfortunately, multiple terms are used as synonyms for self-care. In 2011, Godfrey and colleagues identified 139 different definitions of self-care (Godfrey

Do's and Don't's for Influenza Prevention.

(Douglas Island News.)

Wear a mask.

Live a clean, healthy life.

Keep the pores open—that is bathe frequently.

Wash your hands before each meal.

Live in an abundance of fresh air, day and night.

Keep warm.

Get plenty of sleep.

Gargle frequently (and always after having been out) with a solution of salt in water. (Half teaspoon of salt to one glass—eight ounces—of water).

Report early symptoms to the doctor at once.

Respect the quarantine regulations.

Avoid crowds. You can get the influenza only by being near some one who is infected.

Avoid persons who sneeze or cough.

Do not neglect your mask.

Do not disregard the advice of a specialist just because you do not understand.

Do not disregard the rights of a community—obey cheerfully the rules issued by the authorities.

Do not think you are entitled to special privileges.

Do not go near other people if you have a cold or fever—you may expose them to the influenza and death. See the doctor.

Do not think it is impossible for you to get or transmit influenza.

Keep your hands out of your mouth.

Do not cough or sneeze in the open.

Do not use a public towel or drinking cup.

Do not visit the sick or handle articles from the sick room.

DON'T WORRY.

Figure 6.1 *Do's and Don'ts for Influenza Prevention* from the Douglas Island News, published in 1918 during the most severe pandemic in recent history, prior to the COVID pandemic.

et al., 2011). The term most used is *self-management*, advocated by the National Institute for Nursing Research (NINR). The NINR definition of *self-management* is the strategies used by individuals with chronic conditions and their caregivers to better understand and manage their illness and improve their health behaviors (NINR, 2021). Jonkman and colleagues proposed a new operational definition of self-management interventions as interventions that "aim to equip patients with skills to actively participate and take responsibility in the management of their chronic condition in order to function optimally through at least knowledge acquisition and a combination of at least two of the following: stimulation of independent sign/symptom monitoring, medication management, enhancing problem-solving and decision-making skills for medical treatment management, and changing their physical activity, dietary, and/or smoking behavior" (Jonkman et al., 2016a, p. 862). This definition captures many of the elements of our definition of self-care.

Health professional definitions of self-care differ significantly from self-care as used in other disciplines and the lay press. A recent article from the humanities identified five possible dimensions of self-care: mindfulness, self-compassion, habits, time, and agency (Lemon, 2021). These dimensions are not too different from definitions of self-care in popular magazines where lay press authors talk about self-care as self-soothing, self-coddling, self-compassion, and self-love. This focus has been effective: In 2014, the self-care industry had an estimated value of $10 billion, which increased in 2021 to $450 billion. Nearly nine out of 10 Americans report actively practicing self-care. In just 1 year (2019 to 2020), Google Search Trends documented a 250% increase in Internet searches related to self-care. For these reasons, Riegel argued that the marketing industry has usurped the science of self-care (Riegel, 2021).

SCIENTIFIC BASIS

Nurses will want to use a precise definition of self-care that is relevant to both healthy and ill populations. Riegel and colleagues developed both a middle-range theory of self-care of chronic illness (Riegel et al., 2012) and a situation-specific theory of heart failure self-care that may be useful in fully understanding self-care (Riegel et al., 2016). In defining self-care for people with a chronic illness, three concepts were specified: self-care maintenance, self-care monitoring, and self-care management. Self-care maintenance refers to the behaviors used to maintain physical and emotional stability. These behaviors may be self-determined (e.g., choosing to eat a vegan diet) or reflect recommendations of the healthcare provider such as routine medication adherence.

Self-care monitoring is defined as the process of actively observing oneself for changes in symptoms and checking for the presence of bodily changes. Although self-care monitoring is emphasized for people with a chronic illness, everyone engages in monitoring. *Did I get enough sleep? Should I worry about this sore throat?* Self-care monitoring begins with symptom detection. Once detected, perception involves becoming consciously aware of a symptom. For example, imagine that you are busy studying or working. Then you realize that you have a headache. This realization is detection while perception involves categorizing and interpreting what is sensed. Once detected and fully perceived, symptom recognition occurs, which involves evaluation, interpretation, and the assignment of meaning. That is, recognition adds reasoning, which stimulates a judgment, a decision, and a behavioral response. The noticing of typical bodily changes promotes symptom monitoring, which creates a feedback loop between symptom monitoring and perception (Lee et al., under review).

The third concept, self-care management, is defined as the response to signs and symptoms when they occur. This concept of self-care management is particularly relevant for people with a chronic illness. Once someone goes through the process of detection, perception, and recognition of a symptom, self-care management can be used to respond. Ideally, a response to a symptom will be judged as effective or ineffective so that effective responses can be repeated in the future. See Figure 6.2 for an illustration of the specific behaviors captured by the concepts of self-care maintenance, self-care monitoring, and self-care management.

The middle-range and situation-specific theories are very similar; the major difference is in self-care monitoring, which is operationalized as symptom perception in the situation-specific theory of heart failure self-care because heart failure patients have difficulty perceiving symptoms. Prior research has demonstrated that patients with heart failure and other conditions have damage to the insular cortex, an area of the brain associated with symptom perception (Critchley et al., 2004; Mehling et al., 2018). This damage may be responsible for poor symptom perception in patients with heart failure, but further research is needed to test this hypothesis.

Since publication, these theories have been used widely. The situation-specific theory, published originally in 2008 (Riegel & Dickson, 2008) and updated in 2016 (Riegel et al., 2016), has been tested 13 times and referenced 413 times as of July 2021. The middle-range theory was published in 2012 (Riegel et al., 2012), and updated in 2019 (Riegel et al., 2019b). Since the original publication, this theory has been tested 26 times and referenced 361 times. A variety of self-report instruments reflecting the theoretical concepts are freely available to users through this website: www.selfcaremeasures.com. These instruments measure the self-care behaviors of people with heart failure (Riegel et al., 2019a), diabetes (Ausili et al., 2017), chronic obstructive lung disease (Matarese et al., 2020), hypertension (Dickson et al., 2017), coronary heart disease (Vaughan Dickson et al., 2017), and chronic illness in general (Riegel et al., 2018). Another instrument was designed to assess the self-care behaviors of essentially healthy individuals (Luciani et al., under review), and other measures self-care self-efficacy (Luciani, 2022; Yu et al., 2021). Another set of instruments is available to assess the contribution of caregivers to

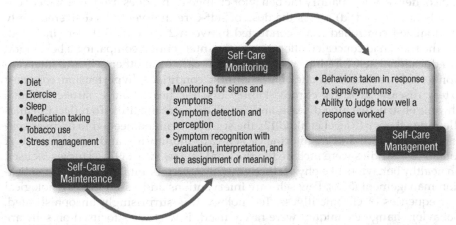

Figure 6.2 Examples of self-care maintenance, self-care monitoring, and self-care management behaviors.

the self-care of patients (Vellone et al., 2020a, 2020b). With the availability of valid, reliable, free, and locally translated instruments, self-care research has blossomed worldwide.

A large body of research exists describing the effectiveness of self-care. These studies can be classified as studies of specific individual self-care behaviors (e.g., diet, exercise) and studies of general self-care behaviors (e.g., management of diabetes). Many of the studies testing general self-care behaviors address the behaviors of individuals with a chronic illness because these patients need to engage in numerous self-care behaviors simultaneously (e.g., medication adherence, monitoring of signs and symptoms, response to changes in symptoms; Riegel et al., 2017).

There has been so much self-care research over the past two decades that it is easy to find systematic reviews and meta-analyses of general self-care interventions. In patients with heart failure, self-care decreases readmission rates (Jovicic et al., 2006; McAlister et al., 2004), and improves quality of life (Grady, 2008). In patients with chronic obstructive lung disease, using a focused self-care exacerbation action plan reduces in-hospital healthcare use (Howcroft et al., 2016; Jonkman et al., 2016c). In patients who suffered a stroke, there is evidence across multiple trials and several systematic reviews that self-care improves activities of daily living and quality of life, and decreases premature death (Fryer et al., 2016; Parke et al., 2015). In patients with chronic kidney disease, self-care interventions control interdialytic weight gain (Cho & Kang, 2021). Self-care maximizes independence in patients with a spinal cord injury (Conti et al., 2020). In patients with diabetes, self-care decreases complications (da Rocha et al., 2020). This is just a brief summary of a large body of evidence supporting self-care interventions for chronic illness as a way to improve outcomes; however, interventions vary immensely, and it is difficult to identify the most effective elements (Jonkman et al., 2016b).

In a recent scoping review, Riegel et al. (2021b) examined interventions designed to improve *specific* self-care behaviors of adults with various chronic conditions to (a) identify what self-care concepts and behaviors had been evaluated in self-care interventions, (b) classify and quantify heterogeneity in mode and type of delivery, (c) quantify the behavior change techniques used to enhance self-care behavior, and (d) assess the dose of self-care interventions delivered. Only randomized controlled trials conducted between 2008 and 2019 were included. All the trials had concealed allocation to the intervention comparing a behavioral or educational self-care intervention to usual care or another self-care intervention tested in adults with one of nine chronic conditions: hypertension, coronary artery disease, arthritis, chronic kidney disease, heart failure, stroke, asthma, chronic obstructive lung disease, and Type 2 diabetes mellitus. To reflect the middle-range theory (Riegel et al., 2012), the studies included needed to address self-care maintenance and monitoring or self-care monitoring and management. A total of 233 studies were included in the final review. Most (97%) studies focused on healthy behaviors like physical activity (70%), dietary intake (59%), and medication management (52%). Few self-care interventions addressed the psychological consequences of chronic illness. Technology was surprisingly unsophisticated. Behavior change techniques were rarely used. Few studies focused on self-care management, and the interventions tested were rarely innovative. Research reporting was generally poor.

After conducting this scoping review, Lee and colleagues used 145 of the 233 trials involving participants with asthma, coronary artery disease, chronic obstructive pulmonary disease, Type 2 diabetes mellitus, heart failure, or hypertension to compare the efficacy of specific self-care interventions on relevant outcomes compared with controls (Lee et al., under review). Data were pooled using random-effects meta-analyses. Meta-regression was used to test the effect of potential moderators on trial efficacy. The trial reports were generally poor with multiple areas of high risk of bias. Overall, the effect size of self-care interventions on improving outcomes was small (Hedges' g = 0.29, 95% CI [0.25–0.33], $p <$ 0.001), with significant heterogeneity across trials (Q = 514.85, $p <$ 0.001, I2 = 72.0%). There was no significant difference in trial efficacy regarding the use of theory, specific components of self-care, the number of modes of delivery, the number of behavioral change techniques, modes of delivery, or specific behavioral change techniques. Overall, the conclusion was that the individual self-care interventions tested were modestly efficacious in improving outcomes. However, poor trial quality compromised the ability to make definitive conclusions.

A theme identified from all these studies was poor quality. That is, the studies were often poor in quality as was the reporting of published studies. Poor quality makes it difficult to find significant intervention effects. Without significant intervention effect sizes, it will be challenging to convince decision-makers in charge of allocating healthcare resources to fund self-care programs in the future.

INTERVENTION

Directors of the International Center for Self-Care Research (www.selfcareresearch.org/) argue that self-care should be the first-line approach in all healthcare encounters. Giving self-care this level of priority and significance would change the emphasis from the prescription of medications to the prescription of behavior such as exercise, sleep, and a healthy diet. Imagine a healthcare system in which a well-child visit involved discussion of diet, exercise, and sleep patterns. The annual adult visit to a provider might focus less on the "chief complaint" and more on the anticipated benefits of self-care. Such an approach would help establish healthy goals, practices, habits, and lifestyle routines and promote health and disease prevention. Spending time educating about self-care during visits with a provider would produce informed consumers and support self-care as a fundamental philosophy in the population.

In a recent article summarizing work in the International Center for Self-Care Research, Riegel and colleagues articulated a focused research agenda intended to provide guidance to investigators studying self-care (Riegel et al., 2021a). Major reasons why self-care is challenging were identified. Many of these reasons reflect known difficulties with behavioral change: attachment to unhealthy behaviors (e.g., cigarette smoking, high fat diet), a lack of motivation to change, difficulty deciding when in the life span to adopt a healthy lifestyle, and difficulty in maintaining healthy behavior over time. For example, maintaining weight loss is known to be difficult over time (Spreckley et al., 2021).

Illness-related factors also make self-care difficult. People who have multiple illnesses find it difficult to perform self-care because they may have difficulty determining which condition is causing symptoms. Furthermore, different conditions typically require different self-care behaviors. For example, if someone with lung disease and heart failure develops shortness of breath, it may be difficult to discern the cause of the symptom. Without knowledge of the cause, choosing a self-care management behavior is difficult: *Should I take an extra diuretic or use my inhaler?* Another common issue is a poor response to symptoms. Many ill individuals "wait and see" when they have symptoms because they are unsure of the right time to seek help. Another issue is that life events may interfere with healthy behavior. In a qualitative study, a patient deferred seeking acute care for heart failure because he was responsible for caring for his young child (Riegel et al., 2013). These illness-related factors are reflected in naturalistic decision-making, which focuses on how people use experiences to make decisions and how contextual factors influence this process (Zsambok & Klein, 1997). According to naturalistic decision-making, the decision-maker may experience uncertainty when the situation is ambiguous, the environment is changing, or necessary information is missing. Decisions are often influenced by time stress, the perception that there is much at stake, and conflicting input and influence from multiple individuals (Zsambok & Klein, 1997).

To address these behavioral and illness-related challenges, six specific areas for future research are suggested. First, habit formation has a strong influence on behavior change. Once habits form, they provide a default response that can help to overcome the need to repeatedly choose healthy behaviors (Wood et al., 2014). Many unhealthy behaviors, such as food choices, are learned early in life and habits are hard to change (Miller et al., 2018). Other important areas thought to influence self-care are resilience in the face of stressful life events that interfere with self-care, the influence of culture on self-care behavioral choices, the difficulty performing self-care with multiple chronic conditions, self-care in persons with severe mental illness, and the influence of others (caregivers, family, peer supporters, healthcare professionals) on self-care.

A factor with a strong positive influence on behavior change is self-care confidence or self-efficacy. Numerous investigators have found that confidence in the ability to perform self-care, or self-care self-efficacy, is extremely important in predicting someone's ability to perform self-care (Fivecoat et al., 2018; Vellone et al., 2015, 2016). Interestingly, people with multiple chronic conditions often have a decrease in self-efficacy (Buck et al., 2015; Dickson et al., 2013), which may help to explain why multiple chronic conditions interfere with self-care.

A major challenge that behavioral scientists face is trying to change the behavior of individuals who are nested within families, communities, and societies. The Self-Care Matrix (SCM; Figure 6.3) illustrates a synthesis of 32 existing models and frameworks, which makes it possible to consider self-care in its wider context (El-Osta et al., 2019). This unifying framework portrays the relationships between the various dimensions of self-care—systems, social networks, individuals, and person-centered capabilities. According to the SCM, self-care is influenced by macrolevel environmental determinants such as culture, fiscal policy, health policy, and the built environment. This self-care context (meso-level) influences daily choices, lifestyle, and the management of acute and chronic conditions. At the micro level, individual capacities and capabilities influence specific self-care activities such as physical activity, healthy eating, risk avoidance, good hygiene, and rational use of

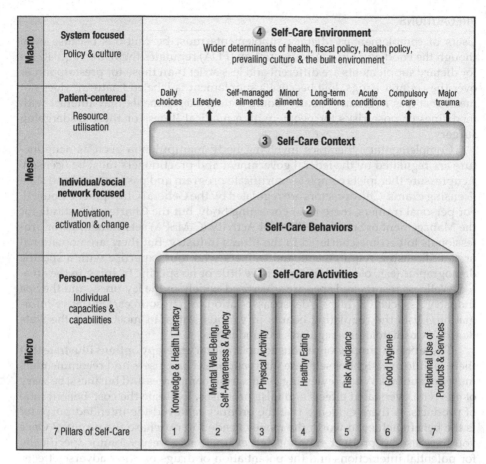

Figure 6.3 The Self-Care Matrix. This figure illustrates the relationships between four core dimensions of self-care—systems, patients, individuals, and individual capabilities. This Self-Care Matrix (SCM) is a synthesis of 32 existing models and frameworks which makes it possible to consider self-care in its totality (El-Osta et al., 2019). These micro, meso, and macro elements describe the level of focus and the perspective relevant to each dimension of self-care. The schema also shows how self-care activities, behaviors, and resources are connected. The self-care environment exerts its influence on all other three dimensions of self-care, illustrating the importance of addressing policy and culture to promote self-care.
Source: Courtesy of Austen El-Osta. Reprinted from El-Osta, A., Webber, D., Gnani, S., Banarsee, R., Mummery, D., Majeed, A., & Smith, P. (2019). The self-care matrix: A unifying framework for self-care. *Self Care, 10*(3), 38–56. https://doi.org/10.6084/m9.figshare.12578741.

products and services. Choices about these self-care activities are influenced by knowledge, health literacy, mental well-being, self-awareness, and agency.

General self-care interventions are best selected from the professional literature. But there are many complementary therapies available for self-care that could be personally useful or beneficial to patients. A process for selecting and evaluating therapies, providers, products and evaluating their effectiveness is described later.

PRECAUTIONS

Users of complementary dietary supplements must be cautious because even though the Food and Drug Administration (FDA) regulates them, the regulations for dietary supplements are different and less strict than those for prescription or over-the-counter drugs. Just because a supplement is labeled "natural" does not mean that it is necessarily "safe." Some dietary supplements may interact with medicines or pose risks for people with a medical illness or those undergoing surgery.

Complementary therapies involving body manipulation such as acupuncture are regulated by the federal government and practitioners must be licensed. Acupressure therapists complete a certificate program and pass national and state licensing exams. Chiropractors are regulated by the General Chiropractic Council. For personal trainers, there is no governing body, but the Chartered Institute for the Management of Sport and Physical Activity (CIMSPA) sets standards for professionals to become chartered in the fitness industry. But there are no national or state licensing requirements and trainers who tout expertise with a specific demographic (e.g., older adults) may have little or no specific training in the area.

Wellness resorts and spas are advertised widely in the lay press, and the Spa Industry Association (https://dayspaassociation.com/resources/legislative-information/) lists the regulating boards in various states. In most states, the State Board of Cosmetologists regulates this industry.

These brief examples of various complementary therapy options illustrate that there is little oversight of self-care interventions. Thus, users and recommenders must be cautious. When reviewing claims from companies and business, be wary of ads with overstated effects and false promises. Evaluate the cost–benefit ratio of products. Is there evidence that the product achieved the intended purpose? Is the benefit achieved worth the money needed to purchase the product? Once you have used a product, monitor and evaluate its safety. Monitor specifically for potential interactions and the potentiation of drugs or other adverse effects. Always report your use of complementary therapies in discussion with a health-care provider.

USES

Complementary therapies are useful for specific self-care needs, especially those related to self-care maintenance behaviors of sleep, weight loss, exercise, and stress reduction. See Chapter 18 for a review of exercise. Several of the chapters in this book address complementary therapies that are particularly useful for stress management including Chapters 7 (imagery) and Chapter 11 (meditation). Therapies described in other chapters are useful for relaxation and/or sleep including Chapter 10 (biofeedback), Chapter 15 (Massage), and Chapter 17 (relaxation therapies). Some brief research exemplars follow.

EXEMPLARS

- **Research exemplar: sleep in children:** A mindfulness program was tied to more sleep in children: Researchers found that children who received a school-based program in mindfulness training, which included yoga movements, deep breathing, and being present in the moment, during their physical education period twice a week for about 2 years gained 74 minutes of sleep per night and 24 minutes of REM sleep compared with controls, who lost about 63 minutes of sleep per night (Chick et al., 2021).

▨ **Research exemplar: sleep in adults:** Tang and colleagues demonstrated that 2 weeks of 30 min of bedtime active open-loop audiovisual stimulation (AVS) can improve sleep onset but not sleep maintenance in older adults with insomnia and osteoarthritic pain (Tang et al., 2021). A subsequent study provided a mechanistic foundation for future AVS research in sleep promotion by examining quantitative electroencephalogram (QEEG) responses to AVS. A significant elevation of mean baseline gamma (35–45 Hz) power supported cortical hyperarousal. Findings demonstrate that delta induction, which can promote sleep, is achievable using a 30-minute open-loop AVS program (Tang et al., 2019).

▨ **Research exemplar: weight loss:** Tai chi improved body mass index (BMI) in persons with type 2 diabetes mellitus (T2DM). A systematic review and meta-analysis of 18 intervention studies found a decrease in BMI (MD = −1.53 [95% CI = −2.71 to −0.36] $p < 0.001$) compared with control group (wait list; no intervention; usual care; sham exercise; Qin et al., 2020).

▨ **Research exemplar: smoking cessation:** Neurofeedback (NF) is thought to facilitate smoking cessation by teaching self-regulation of craving and stress. Studies are underway to determine if self-regulation, once learned, transfers to behavioral outcomes (Pandria et al., 2020).

▨ **Research exemplar: meditation:** When 6 weeks of high-resistance inspiratory muscle strength training (IMST, 30 breaths/day, 6 days/week) was compared to sham training (15% maximal inspiratory pressure), IMST improved blood pressure, endothelial function, and arterial stiffness in midlife/older adults with systolic blood pressure ≥120 mm Hg. (Craighead et al., 2021). Casual systolic blood pressure decreased from 135±2 mm Hg to 126±3 mm Hg (P<0.01) with IMST, which was about 75% sustained 6 weeks after IMST ($p < 0.01$); blood pressure was unaffected by sham training (all $p > 0.05$).

CULTURAL APPLICATIONS

As noted earlier, we know relatively little about the influence of culture on self-care behavioral choices, and Riegel and colleagues have called for more work in the area (Riegel et al., 2021a). A recent integrative review revealed that the influence of culture may be predominantly in self-care maintenance behaviors (Osokpo & Riegel, 2021). Findings from that review focused on traditional cultural beliefs such as collectivism, family and kinship ties, fatalism, cultural norms, normative thinking, and traditional gender roles. These cultural beliefs were found to influence dietary adherence in African American and South Asian populations.

Another area influenced by cultural beliefs is decision-making about medication adherence and using complementary medicine. Cultural beliefs and social norms also influence the interpretation and response to symptoms. When African immigrants were studied, Osokpo and colleagues found that acculturation was not associated with self-care practices among these immigrants (Osokpo et al., 2021). Instead, self-care self-efficacy was a strong determinant of self-care maintenance ($p < 0.0001$), self-care monitoring ($p < 0.0001$), and self-care management ($p < 0.0001$). In that study, the perception of inadequate income was a significant determinant of poor self-care management ($p = 0.03$) while self-care self-efficacy and perceived income adequacy were better determinants of self-care than acculturation.

Sidebars 6.1, 6.2, and 6.3 describe the self-care practices and approaches of geographically and culturally disparate peoples. These illustrate similarities and differences among persons and societies across the globe.

Sidebar 6.1 *Self-Care in Nigeria*

Onome Henry Osokpo

Nigeria is a multiethnic country with different subcultures. In Nigeria, there are two major approaches to self-care. Nigerians often use Western approaches; in the event of an illness or symptoms of a chronic medical condition, people go to a local pharmacy store often called a "chemist" and request that either a pharmacy technician or a pharmacist prescribe a medication to treat their condition (e.g., high blood pressure) or symptoms. Typically, a physician's prescription is not required to purchase medicines from a chemist. Almost all drugs are considered "over the counter." People may also visit a local government clinic or go to a private hospital to see a physician with their complaints and be prescribed medicines that can be purchased from the chemist or from the clinic's pharmacy. Once medicines are prescribed, people may or may not continue to take the medicine or follow up with the provider. Some adjust the prescribed regimen based on recommendations from family, friends, and sometimes from the chemist.

Herbal remedies are widely used for the management and treatment of acute and chronic conditions. People in rural areas and also those in urban cities in Nigeria use herbal remedies, irrespective of ethnic background, educational level, occupation, or social class. Nigerians use a variety of soups, concoctions (multi-herbal preparations), and other traditional approaches for general health maintenance or to manage illnesses. There are traders and retailers with Indigenous knowledge about medicines derived from trees, leaves, herbs, fruits, and so on that has been passed down from generation to generation before Western medicines came to Nigeria. These traders will recommend specific concoctions depending on the illness or health situation described. Indigenous knowledge about natural remedies may be common knowledge within a family, passed down from prior generations, or people may ask neighbors and friends if they have had specific symptoms and what worked for them. There is a perception in Nigeria that westerners only repackaged these formations into tablets and capsules after learning about these leaves from Indigenous people.

Herbal preparations might range from a mixture of vegetables like garlic and ginger to bark on trees and grass. They may include fruits like lemon and lime or their extracts. The mixture of these items, usually with no specific proportion, is washed with clean water and added to a pot with water. A popular concoction is "Agbo" (e.g., "Agbo iba," "Agbo jedi- jedi")—a liquid mixture of the bark of fruit paw paw, "Dongoyaro" leaves, scent leaves or basil, lemongrass, fruits (lemon), vegetables (ginger), and other items depending on the specific illness or health issue. These items are put into clean water and boiled for a few minutes. The liquid preparation is cooled and then drunk a couple of times during the day. These herbal preparations

(continued)

Sidebar 6.1 *Self-Care in Nigeria (continued)*

may also be used in a bath or inhaled under the covering of a blanket. In certain instances, the mixture is not boiled at all. In some parts of the country, like Delta State, alcohol is sometimes added to the liquid preparation to make the mixture more potent. "Agbo" drink or bath is believed to have anti-infective properties against a wide range of bacteria, fungi, and protozoans. It is used for malaria or typhoid fever treatment and other conditions (e.g., nausea, high blood pressure, intestinal worms, measles). These concoctions can also be used to supplement Western medicine.

For high blood pressure, a liquid blend of garlic and ginger is often used to lower blood pressure. The garlic and ginger can be also soaked in water or boiled in water and the liquid is drunk. A mixture of garlic, ginger, bitter leaf, and sometimes aloe vera is also used for the management of diabetes. Lemongrass is often used for the treatment of fevers and joint pains. The peels of grapefruits, pineapple, and other citrus fruits are boiled and used to treat different conditions, for example, fever. Certain soups are often used to manage a common cold and fevers: pepper soup with special condiments, herbs, and spices. The soups are thought to clear the system of toxins and symptoms of a cold and runny nose. The milky sap of papaya is taken to treat roundworms and other stomach disorders.

Spiritual healing and prayer can be used alone or with traditional or western medicine. Massage is another approach used in managing body and muscle aches. Certain oils (e.g., "Ori" [shea butter]) are often used for massage.

In rich neighborhoods, people may engage in physical activities like running, cycling, and going to the gym. However, the typical Nigerian does not set aside special time for physical activity since they walk long distances to get to the bus stop or go to the market to buy food and other household items. It is challenging for people to make changes to their diet if advised to do so by a physician or nurse because cooking is done for the entire family and done with limited resources. Families may consider making separate foods for a family member if someone they know reports that changing their diet improved their health or resolved their symptoms. These approaches cannot be generalized due to the multiethnic context of Nigeria, but a variation of these approaches may be observed in the various regions of the country.

Sidebar 6.2 *Self-Care of Heart Failure in Southern Brazil*

Eneida Rejane Rabelo da Silva, Graziella Badin Aliti, and Omar Pereira de Almeida Neto

Brazil is a culturally heterogeneous country. The southern region in particular is influenced not only by its early Indigenous inhabitants but also by African, Portuguese, German, Italian, Polish and Japanese immigrants, as well as people from neighboring countries (Uruguay and Argentina). The "gaucho" diet (as the people of Rio Grande do Sul are called) is rich in animal protein, saturated

(continued)

Sidebar 6.2 *Self-Care of Heart Failure in Southern Brazil (continued)*

fat, simple carbohydrates, and salt; major foods include barbecue, sausages, pasta, and polenta with little fruit or vegetable intake. Overweight, obesity, and sedentary lifestyle are prevalent. Other important issues affecting self-care are beliefs and values. The Brazilian population as a whole, as well as the gaucho, is remarkably spiritual and religious. Higher spirituality is associated with better treatment adherence.

In Brazil, a common belief of the population is that lifestyle habits (i.e., a diet high in salt/fat/sugar, alcohol intake, sedentary lifestyle) are not related to illness. Thus, Brazilians, particularly older adults, typically ignore health promotion and disease prevention messages. People turn their attention to self-care only when disease occurs, and even then, only if they experience signs and symptoms that compromise their activities of daily living or their livelihood. These deep-rooted cultural beliefs make it very difficult to convince people to adopt positive self-care behaviors. Teaching daily self-care behaviors, influencing patient attitudes, and helping patients to correlate their improvement over time with what we teach them is our biggest challenge. These multicultural habits are ultimately a financial burden on the public health system, as they directly impact clinical outcomes.

Self-care of heart failure (HF) has become a cornerstone of treatment worldwide—as important an element of therapy as the drugs shown to reduce mortality and improve symptoms. People with decompensated HF in Brazil exhibit the classic signs of lower limb edema and pulmonary congestion. A plausible explanation goes back to the food culture in the country; on average, Brazilians consume 12 g of table salt (sodium chloride) per day. Brazilians typically salt food after preparation, even salads, and always have a salt-shaker at the table. Additionally, Brazil has a high output and intake of processed and ultra-processed foods, which increases sodium consumption. Ensuring adherence to a low-sodium diet is a major challenge, compounded by the loss in taste observed in older adults as a result of advancing age. Although we have a range of spices that can be used to season food, salt is still the condiment of choice for Brazilians. For these reasons and others, pharmacological management of HF emphasizing an increased dose of diuretics may be ineffective.

Physical exercise rates are low in the Brazilian population. Cold, wet weather (especially in the southern region of the country) and a lack of public safety are some of the barriers to regular physical activity. Furthermore, public cardiovascular rehabilitation programs for patients with HF are lacking. Some clinical trials have included physical activity, but there is a pressing need for further progress in this respect.

Unfortunately, complementary and alternative medicine measures such as homeopathy are not usually explored by patients with HF, although a wide variety of medicinal plants are available in Brazil. Clinical trials of such alternative treatments are lacking. However, especially in the central areas of the country, herbal teas and infusions with diuretic and hypoglycemic effects are widely used to treat comorbidities commonly associated with HF. It is noteworthy that, in Brazilian

(continued)

Sidebar 6.2 *Self-Care of Heart Failure in Southern Brazil (continued)*

culture, this use of herbal medicines does not replace conventional medicine; patients concomitantly take the medications prescribed by their cardiologist.

Another interesting issue is the difference between age groups in the understanding of HF self-care behavior. Younger patients find it easier to understand the importance of self-care as an adjunct to pharmacologic therapy. Whether this is due to higher educational attainment or because they have younger partners or spouses to help them is unclear. Older patients experience additional barriers to implementing healthy habits, hindering HF control and management, mainly because they remain alone during the day, or because their partners or spouses are also older and perhaps experiencing cognitive decline and cannot help them. Although younger patients may ascribe greater value to self-care, they face challenges of their own, such as increased sodium intake (eating at restaurants more often), increased consumption of alcohol and other drugs, and working long days. These issues make it challenging for younger patients to attend follow-up appointments at the HF clinic. Once lost to outpatient clinical follow-up, these patients are at higher odds of HF decompensation and hospital readmission.

Another challenge in Brazil is that physicians are more valued than nurses although in recent years nurses have gained respect. In Brazil, patients have come to trust nurses with their concerns and challenges in adhering to recommended treatment, especially nonpharmacological management measures, which include self-care behaviors. Nurses prescribe nonpharmacological management measures that improve clinical outcomes, resolve psychosocial barriers, link patients with the health service, and promote self-care. These skills have created trust, especially in nurse specialists who are highly valued as a link between the medical and multidisciplinary teams. Nurse-led clinical trials in HF contribute to the increase in trust. Brazilian patients are very fond of participating in clinical trials; they understand that trial results have the potential to aid in the treatment of HF and improve their quality of life and constantly ask their care team about new guidelines and developments in the treatment of HF. However, personal beliefs and attitudes vary among individuals. So, a critical challenge remains in helping patients to attribute their clinical improvements to self-care behaviors and not just to the medications they take or to other treatments.

Sidebar 6.3 *Self-Care in Sweden*

Anna Strömberg and Tiny Jaarsma

In Sweden, peoples' attitudes toward self-care are in general very positive. If a person is diagnosed with an acute or chronic illness, most of them will immediately ask their healthcare provider what they can do themselves to feel better and to have a better prognosis. It is also natural, as well as mandatory, for doctors,

(continued)

Sidebar 6.3 *Self-Care in Sweden (continued)*

nurses, and other healthcare professionals to always provide self-care advice when interacting with patients. This mandatory advice is discussed further later.

Sweden is a multicultural community, and there are a number of ethnic differences regarding attitudes to self-care. It is therefore impossible to define a uniform attitude toward self-care for all Swedes, but most in the population have a very positive attitude and feel responsible to do self-care. Some even prefer self-care over care from a healthcare provider. As in many other countries worldwide, there are also socioeconomic aspects influencing attitudes and skills of self-care in Sweden. Individuals with higher levels of education, better income, and more social support perform self-care to a higher extent.

There is easy access to self-care support through the national hub for information and services within healthcare in Sweden. This hub, called *1177* after the telephone number 1177, offers an open line where registered nurses are available to respond to nonurgent health issues. The line is accessible 24 hours a day, 7 days a week. 1177 is hosted and operated by the healthcare regions and municipalities in Sweden, working collectively for better national public health. Each of the 21 healthcare regions in Sweden operates its own healthcare consulting center, but collectively, these centers are part of the Swedish national healthcare network and comply with common self-care guidelines. Nurses responding to the calls give self-care advice, consult on the potential need for further care, and provide guidance regarding the need for further services. The nurses respond to about 5 million calls every year.

The Swedish healthcare guide 1177 can also be found on the web at www.1177.se where a variety of healthcare topics are addressed. The objectives of the national healthcare guide are to promote health, increase public knowledge, and strengthen the position of patients and family caregivers. The website offers comprehensive information concerning diseases, treatments, and self-care, as well as rules and rights. Patients and their caregivers can find extensive information about where to find various healthcare services, including e-health services. The website offers both quality-assured and user-friendly information as well as services that facilitate self-care. Healthcare and pharmacy workers, schools, media, and libraries also benefit from the website as a resource in their day-to-day work. When visiting www.1177.se, the website automatically provides local news, information, and links to e-services relevant in a specific region. This joint initiative for all citizens is possible since Sweden has a tax-paid healthcare system.

It is the Swedish Medical Products Agency that decides whether a medicine can be bought over-the-counter or if a prescription is needed. This agency also decides which medicines may be sold in places other than pharmacies (e.g., grocery stores and supermarkets). Factors influencing these decisions are what it contains and what it is to be used for. In order for a drug to be over the counter, it

(continued)

Sidebar 6.3 *Self-Care in Sweden (continued)*

must be possible to use it for self-care. This means that it should be used for minor ailments that can be diagnosed and treated by laypeople.

An increasing number of medications are over the counter in small amounts, but when the same medication needs to be taken on a regular basis, a prescription is required. The smaller amounts are suitable for temporary self-care, but if the medication is needed for longer treatment, consultation with a doctor and a prescription are needed. With consultation, the costs of medication are subsidized. Medicines that have complicated dosages or the potential for serious side effects, even at the recommended dose, are prescription-only.

Being informed about treatment, participating in shared decision-making, and being educated and supported to perform self-care are legal rights in Sweden according to Swedish healthcare legislation (Health and Medical Services Act). In Sweden, the National Board of Health and Welfare, a government agency under the Ministry of Health and Social Affairs, has ruled that healthcare professionals are responsible for assessing patients' abilities and the availability of support before prescribing self-care (SOSFS 2009:6). This statute is implemented collaboratively between primary, secondary, and community care providers. The goal of the statue is to safely transfer the burden of care from healthcare professionals to laypersons.

According to this Swedish self-care legislation (SOSFS 2009:6), a self-care assessment is done by registered healthcare providers who assess patients to determine if a self-care task can be performed safely and if support is needed to perform the self-care task. There are two levels of assessment: (a) general assessment regarding if a task should be performed as self-care or healthcare and (b) Individual assessment to determine if the patient can perform self-care alone. This assessment is followed by implementation and documentation of the assessment, the final decision, and plans for follow-up. The Swedish National Agency for Education has a specific regulation for children with a chronic disease (e.g., diabetes). These children have the right to be assisted with self-care while at school.

In summary, self-care is a well-established, highly accepted, and important concept, and even a legal right in Sweden.

FUTURE RESEARCH

There are many areas in which additional knowledge will help people develop a personal self-care plan that includes complementary therapies. A few of these areas include the following:

1. What complementary and integrative health approaches do nurses recommend and what is the evidence behind those recommendations?
2. Where do individuals obtain information about the complementary therapies that they incorporate into their personal self-care health regimen?

3. What are the most effective strategies to teach patients, families, and communities about the selection and use of complementary therapies and integrative approaches as part of their self-care?
4. What evidence-based strategies can be used to initiate and sustain the effective use of complementary therapies as part of self-care regimens for patients, nurses, and nursing students?
5. What are ways to measure and monitor the effects of self-care strategies employed?
6. What are measurable outcomes of selected complementary therapies when used alone or in combination as self-care practices?
7. How often and how long do selected complementary therapies need to be sustained to realize a benefit of their use as part of self-care?

In addition, to address knowledge gaps in how habit formation, resilience, culture, multimorbidity, severe mental illness, and other people influence self-care, future research on motivation through human contact and empathy (e.g., presence, Chapter 2, or therapeutic listening and communication, Chapter 3) and the use of tailored interventions using technology such as biofeedback (Chapter 10) is recommended (Riegel et al., 2021a). Further research is needed into the influences of culture, support from others (e.g., animal-assisted therapy, Chapter 14), and use of decision algorithms, handheld technologies of measuring and monitoring, and tools (e.g., online meditation programs, Chapter 11) designed to promote informed self-care. Finally, policy changes are needed in areas that influence self-care because major societal changes influence habit formation and a context of a healthy environment. For example, a city with bike lanes encourages bicycle riding while an unsafe environment may discourage exercise (Halali et al., 2016), and restrictions on indoor smoking have encouraged tobacco users to quit (Abdullah et al., 2015).

WEBSITES

Knowledge is essential but not sufficient for self-care (Tinoco et al, 2021). Thus, lifelong learning about one's body and the avenues and behaviors that may sustain and improve health through informed self-care can promote healthy habits that promote self-care. These habits are beneficial to one's patients and for the nurse's or nursing student's own self-care. Good sources of information may be found on these selected websites:

- National Center for Complementary and Integrated Health: nccih.nih.gov
- PubMed: www.ncbi/nih/gov/pubmed
- Cochrane Database of Systematic Reviews: www.cochranelibrary.com/cochrane-database-of-systematic-reviews
- International Center for Self-Care Research: www.selfcareresearch.org/
- International Self-Care Foundation: https://isfglobal.org/
- Mayo Clinic. (2021). Integrative medicine: Find out what works. www.mayoclinic.org/tests-procedures/complementary-alternative-medicine/in-depth/alternative-medicine/art-20046087
- Self-Care Measures: http://self-care-measures.com/

REFERENCES

Abdullah, A. S., Driezen, P., Quah, A. C., Nargis, N., & Fong, G. T. (2015). Predictors of smoking cessation behavior among Bangladeshi adults: Findings from ITC Bangladesh survey. *Tobacco Induced Diseases, 13*(1), 23. https://doi.org/10.1186/s12971-015-0050-y

American Nurses Association. (2015). *Code of ethics for nurses with interpretive statements* (p. 9).

Ausili, D., Barbaranelli, C., Rossi, E., Rebora, P., Fabrizi, D., Coghi, C., Luciani, M., Vellone, E., Di Mauro, S., & Riegel, B. (2017). Development and psychometric testing of a theory-based tool to measure self-care in diabetes patients: The self-care of diabetes inventory. *BMC Endocrine Disorders, 17*(1), 66. https://doi.org/10.1186/s12902-017-0218-y

Buck, H. G., Dickson, V. V., Fida, R., Riegel, B., D'Agostino, F., Alvaro, R., & Vellone, E. (2015). Predictors of hospitalization and quality of life in heart failure: A model of comorbidity, self-efficacy and self-care. *International Journal of Nursing Studies, 52*(11), 1714–1722. https://doi.org/10.1016/j.ijnurstu.2015.06.018

Chick, C. F., Singh, A., Anker, L. A., Buck, C., Kawai, M., Gould, C., Cotto, I., Schneider, L., Linkovski, O., Karna, R., Pirog, S., Parker-Fong, K., Nolan, C. R., Shinsky, D. N., Hiteshi, P. N., Leyva, O., Flores, B., Matlow, R., Bradley, T., . . . O'Hara, R. (2021). A school-based health and mindfulness curriculum improves children's objectively measured sleep: a prospective observational cohort study. *Journal of Clinical Sleep Medicine.* Advanced online publication. https://doi.org/10.5664/jcsm.9508

Cho, M. K., & Kang, Y. (2021). Effect of self-care intervention for controlling interdialytic weight gain among patients on haemodialysis: A systematic review and meta-analysis. *Journal of Clinical Nursing, 30*(15–16), 2348–2365. https://doi.org/10.1111/jocn.15773

Conti, A., Clari, M., Kangasniemi, M., Martin, B., Borraccino, A., & Campagna, S. (2020). What self-care behaviours are essential for people with spinal cord injury? A systematic review and meta-synthesis. *Disability and Rehabilitation,* 1–16. https://doi.org/10.1080/09638288.2020.1783703

Craighead, D. H., Heinbockel, T. C., Freeberg, K. A., Rossman, M. J., Jackman, R. A., Jankowski, L. R., Hamilton, M. N., Ziemba, B. P., Reisz, J. A., D'Alessandro, A., Brewster, L. M., DeSouza, C. A., You, Z., Chonchol, M., Bailey, E. F., & Seals, D. R. (2021). Time-efficient inspiratory muscle strength training lowers blood pressure and improves endothelial function, NO bioavailability, and oxidative stress in midlife/older adults with above-normal blood pressure. *Journal of the American Heart Association, 10*(13), e020980. https://doi.org/10.1161/jaha.121.020980

Critchley, H. D., Wiens, S., Rotshtein, P., Ohman, A., & Dolan, R. J. (2004). Neural systems supporting interoceptive awareness. *Nature Neuroscience, 7*(2), 189–195. https://doi.org/10.1038/nn1176

da Rocha, R. B., Silva, C. S., & Cardoso, V. S. (2020). Self-care in adults with type 2 diabetes mellitus: A systematic review. *Current Diabetes Reviews, 16*(6), 598–607. https://doi.org/10.2174/1573399815666190702161849

Dickson, V. V., Buck, H., & Riegel, B. (2013). Multiple comorbid conditions challenge heart failure self-care by decreasing self-efficacy. *Nursing Research, 62*(1), 2–9. https://doi.org/10.1097/NNR.0b013e31827337b3

Dickson, V. V., Lee, C., Yehle, K. S., Abel, W. M., & Riegel, B. (2017). Psychometric testing of the self-care of hypertension inventory. *Journal of Cardiovascular Nursing, 32*(5), 431–438. https://doi.org/10.1097/jcn.0000000000000364

El-Osta, A., Webber, D., Gnani, S., Banarsee, R., Mummery, D., Majeed, A., & Smith, P. (2019). The self-care matrix: A unifying framework for self-care. *Self Care, 10*(3), 38–56. https://doi.org/10.6084/m9.figshare.12578741

Fivecoat, H. C., Sayers, S. L., & Riegel, B. (2018). Social support predicts self-care confidence in patients with heart failure. *European Journal of Cardiovascular Nursing, 17*(7), 598–604. https://doi.org/10.1177/1474515118762800

Fryer, C. E., Luker, J. A., McDonnell, M. N., & Hillier, S. L. (2016). Self management programmes for quality of life in people with stroke. *Cochrane Database of Systematic Reviews, 2016*(8), CD010442. https://doi.org/10.1002/14651858.CD010442.pub2

Godfrey, C. M., Harrison, M. B., Lysaght, R., Lamb, M., Graham, I. D., & Oakley, P. (2011). Care of self-care by other – care of other: The meaning of self-care from research, practice, policy and industry perspectives. *International Journal of Evidence-Based Healthcare, 9*(1), 3–24. https://doi .org/10.1111/j.1744-1609.2010.00196.x

Grady, K. L. (2008). Self-care and quality of life outcomes in heart failure patients. *Journal of Cardiovascular Nursing, 23*(3), 285–292. https://doi.org/10.1097/01.JCN.0000305092.42882.ad

Halali, F., Mahdavi, R., Asghari Jafarabadi, M., Mobasseri, M., & Namazi, N. (2016). A cross-sectional study of barriers to physical activity among overweight and obese patients with Type 2 diabetes in Iran. *Health and Social Care in the Community, 24*(5), e92–e100. https://doi .org/10.1111/hsc.12263

Howcroft, M., Walters, E. H., Wood-Baker, R., & Walters, J. A. (2016). Action plans with brief patient education for exacerbations in chronic obstructive pulmonary disease. *Cochrane Database of Systematic Reviews, 12*(12), Cd005074. https://doi.org/10.1002/14651858.CD005074.pub4

International Center for Self-Care Research. (2019). *Our mission.* http://www.selfcareresearch.org/

International Self Care Foundation. (2021). *A brief history of self-care.* https://isfglobal.org/ what-is-self-care/a-brief-history-of-self-care/

Jonkman, N. H., Schuurmans, M. J., Groenwold, R. H. H., Hoes, A. W., & Trappenburg, J. C. A. (2016a). Identifying components of self-management interventions that improve health-related quality of life in chronically ill patients: Systematic review and meta-regression analysis. *Patient Education and Counseling, 99*(7), 1087–1098. https://doi.org/10.1016/j.pec.2016.01.022

Jonkman, N. H., Schuurmans, M. J., Jaarsma, T., Shortridge-Baggett, L. M., Hoes, A. W., & Trappenburg, J. C. (2016b). Self-management interventions: Proposal and validation of a new operational definition. *Journal of Clinical Epidemiology, 80,* 34–42. https://doi.org/10.1016/j .jclinepi.2016.08.001

Jonkman, N. H., Westland, H., Trappenburg, J. C., Groenwold, R. H., Bischoff, E. W., Bourbeau, J., Bucknail, C. E., Coultas, D., Effing, T. W., Epton, M. J., Gallefoss, F., Garcia-Aymerich, J., Lloyd, S. M., Monninkof, E. M., Nguyen, H. Q., van der Palen, J., Rice, K. L., Sedeno, M., Taylor, S. J. C., . . . Schuurmans, M. J. (2016c). Do self-management interventions in COPD patients work and which patients benefit most? An individual patient data meta-analysis. *International Journal of Chronic Obstructive Pulmonary Disorders, 11,* 2063–2074. https://doi .org/10.2147/COPD.S107884

Jovicic, A., Holroyd-Leduc, J. M., & Straus, S. E. (2006). Effects of self-management intervention on health outcomes of patients with heart failure: A systematic review of randomized controlled trials. *BMC Cardiovascular Disorders, 6,* 43. https://doi.org/10.1186/1471-2261-6-43

Lee, C. S., Westland, H., Faulkner, K. M., Iovino, P., Thompson, J. H., Sexton, J., Farry, E., Jaarsma, T., & Riegel, B. (under review). Meta-analysis of randomized controlled trials in self-care of chronic illness.

Lee, S. (2021). *Understanding the heart failure symptom perception process.* [Dissertation]. University of Pennsylvania.

Lemon, N. (2021). Illuminating five possible dimensions of self-care during the COVID-19 pandemic. *International Health Trends and Perspectives, 1*(2), 161–175. https://doi.org/10.32920/ihtp .v1i2.1426

Linton, M., & Koonmen, J. (2020). Self-care as an ethical obligation for nurses. *Nursing Ethics, 27*(8), 1694–1702. https://doi.org/ 10.1177/0969733020940371.

Luciani, M., De Maria, M., Page, S. D., Barbaranelli, C., Ausili, D., & Riegel, B. (2022). Measuring self-care in the general population: Development and psychometric testing of the Self-Care Inventory. *BMC Public Health, 22,* 598. https://doi.org/10.1186/s12289-022-12913-7

Matarese, M., Clari, M., De Marinis, M. G., Barbaranelli, C., Ivziku, D., Piredda, M., & Riegel, B. (2020). The self-care in chronic obstructive pulmonary disease inventory: Development and psychometric evaluation. *Evaluation and the Health Professions, 43*(1), 50–62. https://doi .org/10.1177/0163278719856660

McAlister, F. A., Stewart, S., Ferrua, S., & McMurray, J. J. (2004). Multidisciplinary strategies for the management of heart failure patients at high risk for admission: A systematic review of randomized trials. *Journal of the American College of Cardiology, 44*(4), 810–819. https://doi .org/10.1016/j.jacc.2004.05.055

Mehling, W. E., Acree, M., Stewart, A., Silas, J., & Jones, A. (2018). The multidimensional assessment of interoceptive awareness, version 2 (MAIA-2). *PLoS ONE, 13*(12), e0208034. https:// doi.org/10.1371/journal.pone.0208034

Miller, A. L., Gearhardt, A. N., Fredericks, E. M., Katz, B., Shapiro, L. F., Holden, K., Kaciroti, N., Gonzalez, R., Hunter, C., & Lumeng, J. C. (2018). Targeting self-regulation to promote health behaviors in children. *Behaviour Research and Therapy, 101,* 71–81. https://doi.org/10.1016/j .brat.2017.09.008

National Institute of Nursing Research. (2021). *Self-management: Improving quality of life for individuals with chronic illness.* https://www.ninr.nih.gov/newsandinformation/iq/self-management -workshop

Osokpo, O., & Riegel, B. (2021). Cultural factors influencing self-care by persons with cardiovascular disease: An integrative review. *International Journal of Nursing Studies, 116,* 103383. https://doi.org/10.1016/j.ijnurstu.2019.06.014

Osokpo, O. H., Lewis, L. L., Ikeaba, U., Chittams, J., Barg, F. K., & Riegel, B. (2021). Self-care of African immigrant adults with chronic illness. *Clinical Nursing Research, 31* (1), 413. https:// doi.org/10.1177/10547738211056.168

Pandria, N., Athanasiou, A., Konstantara, L., Karagianni, M., & Bamidis, P. D. (2020). Advances in biofeedback and neurofeedback studies on smoking. *Neuroimage: Clinical, 28,* 102397. https:// doi.org/10.1016/j.nicl.2020.102397

Parke, H. L., Epiphaniou, E., Pearce, G., Taylor, S. J. C., Sheikh, A., Griffiths, C. J., Greenhaigh, T., & Pinnock, H. (2015). Self-management support interventions for stroke survivors: A systematic meta-review. *PLoS ONE, 10*(7), e0131448. https://doi.org/10.1371/journal.pone.0131448

Qin, J., Chen, Y., Guo, S., You, Y., Xu, Y., Wu, J., Liu, Z., Huang, J., Chen, L., & Tao, J. (2020). Effect of tai chi on quality of life, body mass index, and waist-hip ratio in patients with type 2 diabetes mellitus: a systematic review and meta-analysis. *Frontiers of Endocrinology (Lausanne), 11,* 543627. https://doi.org/10.3389/fendo.2020.543627

Riegel, B. (2021). *Self-care vs self-soothing: The hijacking of science by the marketing industry.* http:// www.selfcareresearch.org/2021/01/28/self-care-vs-self-soothing-the-hijacking-of-science -by-the-marketing-industry/

Riegel, B., Barbaranelli, C., Carlson, B., Sethares, K. A., Daus, M., Moser, D. K., Miller, J., Osokpo, O. H., Lee, S., Brown, S., & Vellone, E. (2019a). Psychometric testing of the revised self-care of heart failure index. *Journal of Cardiovascular Nursing, 34*(2), 183–192. https://doi.org/10.1097/ JCN.0000000000000543

Riegel, B., Barbaranelli, C., Sethares, K. A., Daus, M., Moser, D. K., Miller, J. L., Haaedtke, C. A., Feinberg, J. L., Lee, S., Stromberg, A., & Jaarsma, T. (2018). Development and initial testing of the self-care of chronic illness inventory. *Journal of Advanced Nursing, 74*(10), 2465–2476. https://doi.org/10.1111/jan.13775

Riegel, B., & Dickson, V. (2008). A situation-specific theory of heart failure self-care. *Journal of Cardiovascular Nursing, 23*(3), 190–196. https://doi.org/10.1007/978-3-030-63223-6_11

Riegel, B., Dickson, V. V., & Faulkner, K. M. (2016). The situation-specific theory of heart failure self-care: Revised and updated. *Journal of Cardiovascular Nursing, 31*(3), 226–235. https://doi .org/10.1097/JCN.0000000000000244

Riegel, B., Dickson, V. V., & Topaz, M. (2013). Qualitative analysis of naturalistic decision making in adults with chronic heart failure. *Nursing Research, 62*(2), 91–98. https://doi.org/10.1097/ NNR.0b013e318276250c

Riegel, B., Dunbar, S. B., Fitzsimons, D., Freedland, K. E., Lee, C. S., Middleton, S., Stromberg, A., Vellone, E., Webber, D. E., & Jaarsma, T. (2021a). Self-care research: Where are we now? Where are we going? *International Journal of Nursing Studies, 116,* 103402. https://doi.org/10.1016/j .ijnurstu.2019.103402

Riegel, B., Jaarsma, T., Lee, C. S., & Stromberg, A. (2019b). Integrating symptoms into the middle-range theory of self-care of chronic illness. *ANS Advances in Nursing Science, 42*(3), 206–215. https://doi.org/10.1097/ANS.0000000000000237

Riegel, B., Jaarsma, T., & Stromberg, A. (2012). A middle-range theory of self-care of chronic illness. *ANS: Advances in Nursing Science, 35*(3), 194–204. https://doi.org/10.1097/ANS.0b013e318261b1ba

Riegel, B., Moser, D. K., Buck, H. G., Dickson, V. V., Dunbar, S. B., Lee, C. S., Lennie, T. A., Lindenfeld, J., Mitchell, J. E., Treat-Jacobson, D. T., & Webber, D. E. for the American Heart Association Council on Cardiovascular and Stroke Nursing, Council on Peripheral Vascular Disease, and Council on Quality of Care and Outcomes Research. (2017). Self-care for the prevention and management of cardiovascular disease and stroke: A scientific statement for healthcare professionals from the American Heart Association. *Journal of the American Heart Association, 6*(9). https://doi.org/10.1161/JAHA.117.006997

Riegel, B., Westland, H., Iovino, P., Barelds, I., Bruins Slot, J., Stawnychy, M. A., Osokpo, O., Tarbi, E., Trappenburg, J. C. A., Vellone, E., Strömberg, A., & Jaarsma, T. (2021b). Characteristics of self-care interventions for patients with a chronic condition: A scoping review. *International Journal of Nursing Studies, 116*, 103713. https://doi.org/10.1016/j.ijnurstu.2020.103713

Spreckley, M., Seidell, J., & Halberstadt, J. (2021). Perspectives into the experience of successful, substantial long-term weight-loss maintenance: A systematic review. *International Journal of Qualitative Studies of Health and Well-Being, 16*(1), 1862481. https://doi.org/10.1080/17482631.2020.1862481

Tang, H. J., McCurry, S. M., Pike, K. C., Riegel, B., & Vitiello, M. V. (2021). Open-loop Audio-Visual Stimulation for sleep promotion in older adults with comorbid insomnia and osteoarthritis pain: Results of a pilot randomized controlled trial. *Sleep Medicine, 82*, 37–42. https://doi.org/10.1016/j.sleep.2021.03.025

Tang, H. J., McCurry, S. M., Riegel, B., Pike, K. C., & Vitiello, M. V. (2019). Open-loop audiovisual stimulation induces delta EEG activity in older adults with osteoarthritis pain and insomnia. *Biological Research for Nursing, 21*(3), 307–317. https://doi.org/10.1177/1099800419833781

Taylor, C. (2019). *A brief history of self-care, and the OG (original guru), Socrates.* https://mashable.com/article/self-care-history

Tinoco, J. M. V. P., Figueiredo, L. D. S., Flores, P. V. P., Padua, B. L. R., Mesquita, E. T., & Cavalcanti, A. C. D. (2021). Effectiveness of health education in the self-care and adherence of patients with heart failure: A meta-analysis. *Revista Latino Americana Enfermagem, 29*, e3389. https://doi.org/ 10.1590/1518.8345.4281.3389

Vaughan Dickson, V., Lee, C. S., Yehle, K. S., Mola, A., Faulkner, K. M., & Riegel, B. (2017). Psychometric testing of the Self-Care of Coronary Heart Disease Inventory (SC-CHDI). *Research in Nursing & Health, 40*(1), 15–22. https://doi.org/10.1002/nur.21755

Vellone, E., Barbaranelli, C., Pucciarelli, G., Zeffiro, V., Alvaro, R., & Riegel, B. (2020a). Validity and reliability of the caregiver contribution to self-care of heart failure index version 2. *Journal of Cardiovascular Nursing, 35*(3), 280–290. https://doi.org/10.1097/jcn.0000000000000655

Vellone, E., Fida, R., D'Agostino, F., Mottola, A., Juarez-Vela, R., Alvaro, R., & Riegel, B. (2015). Self-care confidence may be the key: A cross-sectional study on the association between cognition and self-care behaviors in adults with heart failure. *International Journal of Nursing Studies, 52*(11), 1705–1713. https://doi.org/10.1016/j.ijnurstu.2015.06.013

Vellone, E., Lorini, S., Ausili, D., Alvaro, R., Di Mauro, S., De Marinis, M. G., Matarese, M., & De Maria, M. (2020b). Psychometric characteristics of the caregiver contribution to self-care of chronic illness inventory. *Journal of Advanced Nursing, 76*(9), 2434–2445. https://doi.org/10.1111/jan.14448

Vellone, E., Pancani, L., Greco, A., Steca, P., & Riegel, B. (2016). Self-care confidence may be more important than cognition to influence self-care behaviors in adults with heart failure: Testing a mediation model. *International Journal of Nursing Studies, 60*, 191–199. https://doi.org/10.1016/j.ijnurstu.2016.04.016

Wood, W., Labrecque, J., Lin, P., & Runger, D. (2014). Habits in dual process models. In J. W. Sherman, B. Gawronski, & Y. Trope (Eds.), *Dual process theories of the social mind* (pp. 371–385). Guilford.

Yu, D. S., De Maria, M., Barbaranelli, C., Vellone, E., Matarese, M., Ausili, D., Rejane, R. E, Osokpo, O. H., & Riegel, B. (2021). Cross-cultural applicability of the self-care self-efficacy scale in a multi-national study. *Journal of Advanced Nursing, 77*(2), 681–692. https://doi.org/10.1111/jan.14617

Zsambok, C. E., & Klein, G. (1997). *Naturalistic decision making.* Lawrence Erlbaum Associates.

Mind–Body–Spirit Therapies

LINDA CHLAN AND MARY FRAN TRACY

The National Center for Complementary and Integrative Health (NCCIH) at the National Institutes of Health (NIH) classifies complementary health approaches by how a specific therapy is delivered or taken (NCCIH, 2021). Among these complementary health approaches is a broad category of Mind and Body Practices. According to the NCCIH, mind and body practices include a large and diverse group of procedures or techniques often administered or taught by a trained practitioner or teacher (NCCIH, 2017). Deep breathing, yoga, and tai chi are among the most popular mind and body practices according to the 2012 National Health Interview Survey (NHIS; Clarke et al., 2015).

NCCIH has designated four broad categories of complementary health approaches including nutritional (dietary supplements, herbs), psychological (meditation, music therapies), physical (acupuncture, massage), as well as combinations that encompass mind and body practices. The editors of this text have elected to use the classification categories of previous editions. Thus, a number of the therapies NCCIH includes in mind and body practices we have placed in the categories of manipulative and body-based therapies.

Not only does the mind affect the body and the body the mind, but the spiritual aspect also has an impact on a person's overall functioning. Nursing has moved away from the Cartesian philosophy in which the body and mind (and spirit) were seen as functioning independently of each other. Cartesian philosophy has for centuries dominated Western medicine. Refuting this dichotomy can be seen in the impact that a severe headache has on one's ability to think, to move, and to pray. The nursing philosophy of holistic care embraces the interconnectedness of mind, body, and spirit.

Imagery is one of these therapies that can bring about change in physical, spiritual, and emotional aspects. Imagery (Chapter 7) can be learned by individuals without the physical presence of a practitioner. Many CDs, DVDs, and smartphone apps for guided imagery exist and allow for learning and guided use at the convenience of the user. Use of music (Chapter 8) is another intervention that has become increasingly accessible for distraction and relaxation during procedures as well as for periods of increased anxiety and stress. Music is available through smartphones, mobile devices, tablets and computers. Research is expanding to determine the benefits of music beyond patients to healthcare workers themselves.

The body of supporting research for therapies in this section is increasing including yoga (Chapter 9), which can benefit anyone with the aim of healing body and mind, and biofeedback (Chapter 10), with its particular use in reduction of anxiety as well as muscle strengthening. Use of and research on meditation (Chapter 11) has substantially increased in the last decade, but especially so during the COVID-19 pandemic. Millions of new users subscribed to meditation apps or participated in live streaming meditation sessions during the pandemic to manage stress and anxiety (Miller, 2021). Much of the research for these three therapies has been done by non-nurse researchers, but the findings provide direction to nurses in selecting and implementing therapies.

Journaling (Chapter 12) and storytelling (Chapter 13) are therapies in which less formal research has been conducted. It is interesting to contrast these two therapies—with journaling being more accepted by people whose culture has a written history, while storytelling has a greater appeal to oral cultures. In addition, research on animal-assisted therapies (Chapter 14) is increasing. Animal-assisted therapy has found a niche in care centers and living facilities for elders, hospitals, and many other settings including on university campuses for students. Although many think of dogs and cats as the animals used in animal-assisted therapy, horses, dolphins, fish, birds, and other creatures are also used. The therapeutic benefits of animals in the United States has never been more evident as during the COVID-19 pandemic when record numbers of dogs and cats were adopted from animal shelters (ASPCA, 2021).

Of particular help in determining the impact of mind–body–spirit therapies on physical, mental, and spiritual well-being has been the development of instruments not only to measure the outcomes of specific therapies, but also to demonstrate the areas of the brain that might be involved. A growing number of researchers are also examining holistic effects of these therapies on outcomes such as resilience, satisfaction with care, and improvement of quality of life. However, as could be said for many complementary therapies, more research needs to be done, especially with populations for whom specific therapies hold promise.

Many of the therapies in this category such as imagery, music, journaling, and meditation have been and continue to be a part of nursing's armamentarium of interventions. The integration of mind–body–spirit is an integral part of healing practices in many non-Western and indigenous healthcare systems. The spirit realm characterizes many healing practices in Native American tribes/nations. Thus, nurses need to be attentive to therapies that are not discussed in this section of the book but are an integral part of the healthcare of people from other cultures who may be receiving care in Western healthcare facilities.

In revising this edition, it became apparent that we need to broaden our perspective beyond patient and client use to promote even more so the use of these therapies for caregivers themselves. Due to the rising incidence of burnout in healthcare workers (National Academies of Sciences, Engineering, and Medicine, 2019), it is becoming more evident that personal use of mind-body-spirit and other therapies can be a means for nurses and nursing students to reduce stress, mitigate burnout, and support resilience.

REFERENCES

ASPCA. (2021). *New ASPCA survey shows overwhelming majority of dogs and cats acquired during the pandemic are still in their homes.* https://www.aspca.org/about-us/press-releases/new-aspca-survey-shows-overwhelming-majority-dogs-and-cats-acquired-during

Clarke, T., Black, L., Stussman, B., Barnes, P., & Nahin, R. (2015, February 10). Trends in the use of complementary health approaches among adults: United States, 2002–2012. *National Health Statistics Reports, 79,* 1–16.

Miller, M. (2021). Is meditation the new therapy? *Verywell Health.* https://www.verywellhealth.com/meditation-pandemic-trend-5201997

National Academies of Sciences, Engineering, and Medicine. (2019). *Taking action against clinician burnout: A systems approach to professional well-being.* The National Academies Press. https://doi.org/10.17226/25521

National Center for Complementary and Integrative Health. (2017). *Mind and body practices.* https://www.nccih.nih.gov/health/mind-and-body-practices

National Center for Complementary and Integrative Health. (2021). *Complementary, alternative, or integrative health: What's in a name?* https://www.nccih.nih.gov/health/complementary-alternative-or-integrative-health-whats-in-a-name

7

Imagery

MAURA FITZGERALD AND MARY LANGEVIN

Imagery is a mind–body intervention that uses the power of the imagination to bring about change in physical, emotional, or spiritual dimensions. Throughout our daily lives, we constantly see images, feel sensations, and register impressions. A picture of lemonade makes our mouths water; a song makes us happy or sad; a smell takes us back to a past moment. Images evoke physical and emotional responses and help us understand the meaning of events.

Imagery is commonly used in healthcare—most often in the form of guided imagery. It can also be useful if used by nurses and nursing students as part of self-care, especially as they face the stressful circumstances surrounding the delivery of care during the COVID-19 pandemic. Nurses and nursing students can implement imagery with adults and children as part of the treatment plan in managing acute and chronic illness for the relief of symptoms, and for enhancement of wellness as part of patient, family, and personal self-care. Imagery is a hallmark of stress-management programs and has become a standard therapy for alleviating anxiety, promoting relaxation, improving coping and functional status. Imagery can also be applied to gain psychological and spiritual insight to enhance holistic wellness.

DEFINITION

Imagery is the formation of a mental representation of an object, place, event, or situation that is perceived through the senses. It is a cognitive behavioral strategy that uses the individual's own imagination and mental processing, practiced as an independent activity or guided by a professional. Imagery uses all the senses—visual, aural, tactile, olfactory, proprioceptive, and kinesthetic. Although imagery is often referred to as *visualization*, it includes imagining through any sense and is not just being able to see something in the mind's eye.

There are different types of guided imagery including pleasant, physiologically focused, mental rehearsal or reframing, and receptive imagery. When inducing imagery, the individual often imagines seeing, hearing, smelling, tasting, and/or touching something in the image. The image used can be active or passive (e.g., playing volleyball vs. lying on the beach). For many participants, physical and mental relaxation tend to facilitate imagery. However, this is not necessary—particularly for children, who often do not need or prefer to be in a relaxed state. Imagery may be receptive or active (Skeens, 2017). In receptive imagery, the individual pays attention to an area of the body or a symptom and mentally explores thoughts or feelings that arise. In active imagery, the individual evokes thoughts or ideas. Active imagery can be outcome- or end-state-oriented, in which the individual envisions a goal, such as being healthy and well; or it can be process-oriented, in which the mechanism of the desired effect is imagined, such as envisioning a strong immune system fighting a viral infection or tumor.

Imagery and clinical hypnosis are closely related. Clinical hypnosis is a strategy where a professional guides the participant into an altered state of deep relaxation, and suggestions for changes in subjective experience and alterations in perception are made. Both hypnosis and guided imagery incorporate the use of relaxation techniques, such as diaphragmatic breathing or progressive muscle relaxation, to help the participant focus the attention. Guided imagery is often used within the context of hypnosis to further deepen the state of relaxation, and in both techniques, suggestions for positive growth, change, or improvement are often made. Because of the close association between these two processes, selected studies on hypnosis are discussed in this chapter.

SCIENTIFIC BASIS

Imagery can be understood as an activity that generates physiologic and somatic responses. It is based on the cognitive process known as *mental imagery*, which is a central element of cognition that operates when mental representations are created in the absence of sensory input. Functional MRI (fMRI) has demonstrated that the mental construction of an image activates the same neural pathways and central nervous system structures that are engaged when an individual is using one or more of the senses (Djordjevic et al., 2005). For example, if an individual is imagining hearing a sound, the brain structures associated with hearing become activated. Mental rehearsal of movements activates motor areas and can be incorporated into stroke rehabilitation and sports-improvement programs (Di Corrado et al., 2020; Schack et al., 2014; Suso-Martí et al., 2020).

Andrasik and Rime (2007) postulated that cognitive tasks, such as mental imagery, can be conceptualized as neuromodulators. *Neuromodulation* is generally defined as the interaction between the nervous system and electrical or pharmacological agents that block or disrupt the perception of pain. By distraction, imagery alters processing in the central, peripheral, and autonomic nervous systems. The perception of a symptom such as pain or nausea is reduced or eliminated.

A key mechanism by which imagery reduces symptoms and may modify disease is thought to be by reducing the stress response, which is triggered when a situation or event (perceived or real) threatens physical or emotional well-being or when the demands of the situation exceed available resources. It activates complex interactions between the neuroendocrine system and the immune system. Emotional responses to situations trigger the limbic system and signal physiologic changes in the peripheral and autonomic nervous systems, resulting in the characteristic fight-or-flight stress response. Over time, chronic stress results in adrenal and immune suppression and may be most harmful to cellular immune function, impairing the ability to ward off viruses and tumor cells.

The complexity of the human responses to stress is best understood through psychoneuroimmunology, an interdisciplinary field of study that explains the mechanisms by which the brain and body communicate through cellular interactions. Early work was based on research by Robert Ader and Nicholas Cohen, which confirmed that the immune system could be conditioned by expectations and beliefs (Ader & Cohen, 1981. Subsequent research focused on the mechanisms of brain and body communication through cellular interactions and identified receptors for neuropeptides, neurohormones, and cytokines that reside on neural and immune cells and induce biochemical changes when activated by neurotransmitters.

A cascade of signaling events in response to perceived or actual stress results in the release of hormones from the hypothalamus, pituitary gland, adrenal medulla, adrenal cortex, and peripheral sympathetic nerve terminals. Psychosocial and physical stressors have the potential to upregulate this hypothalamic–pituitary–adrenal (HPA) axis. Chronic hyperactivation of the HPA axis and sympathetic nervous system with the associated increased levels of cortisol and catecholamines can deregulate immune function, whereas moderate levels of circulating cortisol may enhance immune function (Langley et al., 2006). Cytokines are secreted by cells participating in the immune response and act as messengers between the immune system and the brain (McCance & Huether, 2002). They also function as neurotransmitters, crossing the blood–brain barrier and affecting sensory neurons. Through these channels, cytokines induce symptoms of fever, increased sensitivity to pain, anorexia, and fatigue, which are adaptive responses that may facilitate recovery and healing (Langley et al., 2006). These interactions between the brain and the immune system are bidirectional, and changes in one system influence the others. The stress response can therefore enhance or suppress optimal immunity (Fleshner & Laudenslager, 2004).

Although immune responses to emotional states are extremely complex, acute stress activates cardiac sympathetic activity and increases plasma catecholamines and natural killer (NK) cell activity, whereas chronic stress (inescapable or unpredictable stress) is associated with suppression of NK cells and interleukin-1-beta and other proinflammatory cytokines (Glaser et al., 2001). These effects appear to be mediated by the influence of stress hormones on T-helper components Th1 and Th2 (Segerstrom, 2010). Imagery, by inducing deep relaxation and reprocessing of stressful triggers, interrupts or alters the stress response and supports the immune system. In a review of guided-imagery studies examining immune system function, Trakhtenberg (2009) concluded that there is evidence to support a relationship between the immune system and stress or relaxation.

The degree of response to stress varies according to many factors, including the nature of the stressor, its magnitude and duration, and a person's degree of control over it (Costa-Pinto & Palermo-Neto, 2010). Individuals who have strong physiological responses to everyday stressors have high stress reactivity and are at greater risk for disease susceptibility, even when coping, performance, and perceived stress are comparable. Imagery has been shown to reduce stress reactivity by reframing stressful situations from negative responses of fear and anxiety to positive images of healing and well-being (Menzies & Jallo, 2011). Thoughts produce physiological responses and activate appropriate neurons. Using imagery to increase emotional awareness and restructure the meaning of a remembered situation by changing negative responses to positive images and meaning alters the physiological response and improves outcomes.

INTERVENTION

TECHNIQUES AND GUIDELINES

Imagery has been used extensively in children, adolescents, and adults. Children as young as 4 years old, who have language skills adequate for understanding suggestions, can benefit from imagery (Kohen & Olness, 2011). Young children often are better at imagery because of the natural, active use of their imaginations. Imagery may be practiced independently, with a coach, or with a DVD, CD, or smartphone app. The most effective imagery intervention is one specific to individuals' personalities, their preferences for relaxation and specific settings, their age or developmental stage, and the desired outcomes. The steps of a general guided imagery session are outlined in Exhibit 7.1.

Imagery sessions for adults and adolescents are usually 10 to 30 minutes in length, whereas most children tolerate 5 to 15 minutes. The session typically

---

Exhibit 7.1 *General Guided-Imagery Technique*

1. **Achieving a relaxed state**
   a. Find a comfortable sitting or reclining position.
   b. Uncross any extremities.
   c. Close your eyes or focus on one spot or object in the room.
   d. Focus on breathing with your abdominal muscles—being aware of the breath as it enters through your nose and leaves through your mouth. With your next breath let the exhalation be longer and notice how the inhalation that follows is deeper. And as you notice that, let your body become even more relaxed. Continue to breathe deeply; if it is comfortable, gradually let the exhalation become twice as long as the inhalation.
   e. If your thoughts roam, bring your mind back to thinking about your breathing and your relaxed body.

2. **Specific suggestions for imagery**
   a. Picture a place you enjoy and where you feel good.
   b. Notice what you see, hear, taste, smell, and feel.
   c. Let yourself enjoy being in this place.
   d. Imagine yourself the way you want to be (describe the desired goal specifically).
   e. Imagine what steps you will need to take to be the way you want to be.
   f. Practice these steps now—in this place where you feel good.
   g. What is the first thing you are doing to help you be the way you want to be?
   h. What will you do next?
   i. When you reach your goal of the way you want to be, notice how you feel.

3. **Summarizing process and reinforcing practice**
   a. Remember that you can return to this place, this feeling, and this way of being any time you want.
   b. Allow yourself to feel this way again by focusing on your breathing, relaxing, and imagining yourself in your special place.
   c. Come back to this place and envision yourself the way you want to be every day.

(continued)

Exhibit 7.1 *General Guided-Imagery Technique (continued)*
4. Returning to present a. Be aware again of the favorite place. b. Bring your focus back to your breathing. c. Become aware of the room you are in (drawing attention to the temperature, sounds, or lights). d. Let yourself feel relaxed and refreshed and be ready to resume your activities. e. Open your eyes when you are ready.

begins with a relaxation exercise that enables the participant to focus or "center." A technique that works well both for children and adults is engaging in slow and expansive breathing, which facilitates relaxation as the breath moves lower into the chest, while the diaphragm and abdominal muscles begin to be used more than the upper chest muscles. Other techniques include progressive muscle relaxation or focusing on a word (mantra) or object. Some children may use their bodies to demonstrate or respond to their image. Although most people close their eyes, some, especially young children, will prefer to keep their eyes open.

Once the participant is in a relaxed or "altered" state, the practitioner suggests an image of a relaxing, peaceful, or comforting place or introduces an image suggested by the participant. Scenes commonly used to induce relaxation include watching a sunset or clouds, sitting on a warm beach or by a fire, or floating on water or a cloud. Some individuals, particularly young children, may prefer active images that involve motion, such as flying or playing a sport. The scene used is one that the participant finds relaxing or engaging. It is often introduced as a favorite place. Huth et al. (2006) interviewed children who were participants in a guided-imagery research study, to determine the content of their imagery. The children reported their favorite images as the park, swimming at a beach, amusement parks, and vacationing. They also visualized a variety of familiar places, such as sports events and places that included pets and other animals.

Although mental relaxation is often accompanied by muscle relaxation, this is not always the goal. People of any age, but particularly preschool and school-age children, may imagine in an active state. For example, a group of 9- to 12-year-old boys with sickle cell disease were being taught guided imagery as a pain-control technique. When asked what special place they would like to go to, they requested a trip to a local amusement park and a ride on the roller coaster. During the imagery, many of them were physically and vocally active, swaying from side to side and moving their arms up and down. At the end of the visualization, they all reported feeling like they had been in the park (absorption) and gave examples of things they felt, saw, heard, or smelled.

For directed imagery, the practitioner guides the imagery, using positive suggestions to alleviate specific symptoms or conditions (outcome or end-state imagery) or to rehearse or walk through an event (process imagery). Images do not need to be anatomically correct or vivid. Symbolic images, such as sweeping away cancer cells or using a dial to turn down pain, may be the most powerful healing images because they are drawn from individual beliefs, cultures, and meanings. In a study of adult patients with chronic pain related to fibromyalgia,

Molinari et al. (2018) asked patients to define what a future best possible self would include and then visualize it.

The ability to use guided imagery is related to the individual's hypnotic ability or the ability to enter an altered state of consciousness and to become involved or absorbed in the imagery (Kwekkeboom, Hau, et al., 2008). Studies have demonstrated that responsiveness to hypnosis increases through early childhood, peaking somewhere between ages 7 and 14 and then leveling off into adolescence and adulthood. However, clinicians have argued that in clinical settings, in which techniques are adjusted to the child's development, preschool children and younger can be quite responsive to hypnosis (Kohen & Olness, 2011).

Some individuals have naturally high hypnotic abilities; they recall pictures more accurately, generate more complex images, have higher dream-recall frequency in the waking state, and make fewer eye movements in imagery than poor visualizers. However, most individuals can use imagery if the experience is adjusted to their needs and preferences (Carli et al., 2007; Olness, 2008). Recognizing individual, cultural, and developmental preferences for settings, situations, and preferences for either relaxation or stimulation can improve the effectiveness of the imagery and reduce time and frustration with learning it.

MEASUREMENT OF OUTCOMES

Evaluating and measuring outcomes are important in determining the effectiveness and value of imagery in clinical practice. The clinical outcomes of imagery are related to the context in which it is used and include physical signs of relaxation; lower levels of anxiety and depression; alteration in symptoms; improved functional performance or quality of life; a sense of meaning, purpose, and/or competency; and positive changes in attitude or behavior. Health services benefits may include reduced costs, morbidity, and length of hospital stay.

The outcomes measured should reflect the client's situation and the conceptual framework providing the rationale for the use of imagery. If imagery is used to facilitate rehabilitation or performance, outcomes would include functional measures such as improved gait or ability to perform a specific task. If imagery is used to control symptoms in patients undergoing chemotherapy for cancer, expected outcomes might include reduced nausea, vomiting, and fatigue; enhanced body image; positive mood states; and improved quality of life. When imagery is used to reduce the stress response and promote relaxation, outcomes may include increased oxygen saturation levels, lower blood pressure and heart rate, warmer extremities, reduced muscle tension, greater alpha waves on electroencephalography, and lower anxiety.

Factors that may influence imagery's success include dose (e.g., duration and frequency of sessions), client characteristics, and condition being treated. Great variability exists in how frequently imagery is recommended. In an attempt to quantify this effect, Van Kuiken (2004) conducted a meta-analysis of 16 published studies going back to 1996. Although the final sample of 10 studies was too small for statistical analysis, Van Kuiken concluded that imagery practice for up to 18 weeks increases the effectiveness of the intervention. A minimum dose was not determined, and further study is needed to explore a dose relationship with outcomes. To help with the standardization of imagery interventions and generalizability, documentation should include a detailed description of the specific interventions used, outcomes affected by the imagery, and factors influencing effectiveness.

Individual differences, such as imaging ability, outcome expectancy, preferred coping style, relationship with the imagery practitioner, and disease state, may all affect the outcome of an imagery experience. In a crossover-design pilot study comparing progressive muscle relaxation (PMR) and imagery to a control, the combined intervention groups demonstrated improved pain control (Kwekkeboom, Wanta, et al., 2008). However, the individual responder analysis revealed that subjects did not respond equally to each therapy and that only half of participants had reduced pain after each intervention. Imagery sessions were more likely to have positive results when participants had greater imaging ability, positive outcome expectancy, and fewer symptoms. A study of 323 adult medical patients who received six interactive guided-imagery sessions with a focus on gaining insight and self-awareness demonstrated that participants' ability to engage in the guided-imagery process and the relationship with the practitioner were strong influences on outcomes (Scherwitz et al., 2005).

One of the most difficult determinations to make is whether the outcomes are the result solely of imagery or of a combination of factors. Learning and practicing imagery often change other health-related behaviors, such as getting more sleep, eating a healthier diet, stopping smoking, or exercising regularly. The provider's presence, attention, and compassion also may constitute an intervention independent of the imagery process.

TECHNOLOGY

Technology can allow imagery to be more accessible and available. This can take the form of telemedicine and telephone sessions (Freeman et al., 2015; Winger et al., 2018), mobile health apps (Armin et al., 2017; Gordon et al., 2017), technology tools such as biofeedback to enhance imagery sessions and skill development (Yijing et al., 2015), CDs or videos, and online training for healthcare providers (Kemper & Khirallah, 2015; Rao & Kemper, 2017). The availability of smartphones has provided a range of options, including applications with background sounds to enhance an imagery session (nature sounds or music), audio of various types of guided-imagery and relaxation sessions, reminders to do a relaxation or imagery technique, and links to interventions (Hansen, 2015; Meinlschmidt et al., 2016). Technology can be especially beneficial when delivering guided-imagery interventions to hard-to-reach or very mobile populations. Freeman et al. (2015) demonstrated a successful telemedicine delivery of imagery-based behavioral interventions to community groups of breast cancer survivors, achieving improvement in outcomes. This is promising for rural areas where individuals need to travel long distances for services or for those who have difficulty with transportation. In order to deliver a self-care intervention to traumatized refugees, Zehetmair et al. (2020) developed audio files on mindful breathing, body scan, and Inner Safe Place guided imagery. This was translated into multiple languages and transferred to participants' phones, enabling them to engage in self-care practices whenever possible.

PRECAUTIONS

Imagery is generally a safe intervention, as noted in a systematic review of guided imagery for persons with cancer, in which there were no reports of adverse events or side effects (Roffe et al., 2005). However, occasionally an individual reacts negatively to relaxation or to the imagery. They may experience anxiety, particularly when using imagery to reduce stress, intrusive thoughts, or feelings of losing control (National Center for Complementary and Integrative Health [NCCIH], 2021). Huth et al. (2004) reported that two children became distressed during guided-imagery practice sessions; hence, the authors encourage prescreening. Prescreening could include assessing individuals for a history of mental health illnesses that can make it challenging for the individual to discern their subjective experiences from objective reality, those who have experienced abuse or trauma, or those who may have an intense emotional reaction (Kubes, 2015). The NCCIH (2021) states rare reports of worsening symptoms in people with a history of seizures, abuse, or trauma. Some individuals have anecdotally reported increased discomfort, airway constriction, or difficulty breathing when they focus on diaphragmatic breathing. This is most likely to occur if the participant is experiencing a symptom such as abdominal pain or dyspnea. Using another centering method, such as focusing on an object in the room or repeating a mantra, can reduce this distressing response and still induce relaxation. Some people may report feeling out of control or "spacey" when deeply relaxed. The guide can help individuals become more grounded by focusing on an image such as a tree with strong roots or doing a more alert relaxation such as having the client keep eyes open and focus on an object. Individuals may report dizziness that is often related to mild hyperventilation and can be relieved by encouraging them to breathe slower and less deeply. In addition, when exploring the use of imagery, some people may worry that their illness was caused by their lack of previous use of mind–body exercises or that healing outcomes may be impacted if they choose not to use imagery; they should be reassured that is not the case (Kubes, 2015).

The expertise and training of the nurse should guide judgment in using imagery in clinical practice. Imagery techniques can be easily applied to managing symptoms (e.g., pain, nausea, vomiting) and facilitating relaxation, sleep, or anxiety reduction (see Case Study 7.1). Advanced techniques often associated with hypnosis—such as age regression and management of depression, anxiety, or posttraumatic stress disorder—require further training.

Case Study 7.1 *Use of Guided Imagery in a Pediatric Oncology Clinic*

Nicole Englebert, Oncology Psychologist, United States

Guided imagery was utilized for a young teenage patient who was diagnosed with cancer and a neurologic condition characterized by progressive neurologic impairment, difficulty coordinating muscle movements (ataxia), and involuntary muscle spasms (myoclonus). She had a vivacious personality but was quite limited by the progressive condition and the side effects of chemotherapy treatment. Eventually, she required 24-hour caregiving assistance and support with most daily living activities due to progressive physical immobility. She often did not feel well enough or have the energy to do many activities, and this greatly impacted her mood.

(continued)

Case Study 7.1 *Use of Guided Imagery in a Pediatric Oncology Clinic (continued)*

She was referred to psychology for treatment for concerns related to depressed mood, but she became fatigued while talking for short periods. For this reason, she often declined to talk in therapy because she felt it was too burdensome. Even though she was physically limited, she loved to paint, so the patient and parents determined that painting may be a great activity for therapy. However, when offered to paint, she declined. During a medical appointment, she indicated that she was not feeling well and declined to meet with the psychologist. In that moment, she was quite emotional, tired, and experiencing intense abdominal discomfort, so the psychologist offered guided imagery for pain management and relaxation, and she choose to try it while waiting for medication to relieve her discomfort.

She was provided options about what she could imagine, including imaging being at a beach, watching clouds fly by, or some other activity; she chose to paint an image. Without a script, she was guided through a painting activity, beginning from choosing the canvas and paint colors to signing the painting and choosing where to hang it. While engaged in the imagery, she noticeably became more relaxed, smiling and giggling at specific moments. It became very clear that this was an ideal strategy for her. She not only experienced relief from discomfort, but she could become an artist without the physical limitations of disease, which seemed quite freeing. Since the initial introduction to guided imagery, she continued to utilize guided imagery as a coping mechanism to support comfort and boost her mood, even as neuromuscular functioning continued to decline.

USES

Imagery has been used therapeutically in a variety of conditions and populations (see Exhibit 7.2). Pain, cancer, and obesity are conditions in which imagery has been investigated in adults and in children.

Exhibit 7.2 *Symptoms and Conditions for Which Imagery Has Been Studied*

CLINICAL CONDITION	SELECTED SOURCES
In Children and Adolescents	
Abdominal Pain	Abbott et al. (2017); Cotton et al. (2010; inflammatory bowel disease); Gottsegen (2011; chronic functional abdominal pain); Gulewitsch et al. (2013; functional abdominal pain, irritable bowel syndrome); Yeh et al. (2017; inflammatory bowel disease)
Headache	Sawni and Breuner (2017)

Exhibit 7.2 *Symptoms and Conditions for Which Imagery Has Been Studied (continued)*

CLINICAL CONDITION	SELECTED SOURCES
In Children and Adolescents	
Perioperative Symptoms	Davidson et al. (2016; postoperative pain); Kuttner (2012; anxiety, pain); Vagnoli et al. (2019; anxiety, pain)
Pregnancy and Stress	Flynn et al. (2016)
Procedural Pain	Alexander (2012) (radiology); Forsner et al. (2014; venipuncture); Nilsson et al. (2015; stress, pain in 11-12-year-old girls receiving vaccinations)
Sickle Cell Anemia Pain	Dobson (2015); Dobson and Byrne (2014)
Spinal Fusion Pain	Charette et al. (2015)
Sports Medicine Performance	Di Corrado et al. (2020)
In Adults	
Cancer Treatment—Physical and Emotional Side Effects	Charalambous et al. (2015); Chen et al. (2015); Guerra-Martin et al. (2021)
Cancer	Tsitsi et al. (2017; anxiety, mood in parents of children with cancer)
Critical Illness Symptoms and Biomarkers	Hadjibalassi et al. (2018; anxiety, pain, hemodynamic measurements, neuropeptides, inflammatory markers, sleep, stress); Meghani et al. (2017; anxiety, insomnia, pain); Spiva et al. (2015; sedation levels, sedative and analgesic consumption, vital signs in mechanically ventilated patients)
Fibromyalgia Symptoms	Menzies et al. (2014; fatigue); Onieva-Zafra et al. (2015; depression, pain); Verkaik et al. (2014; functional status, pain, self-efficacy); Zech et al. (2017; acceptability, efficacy, safety)
Health, Well-Being, and Stress Management	Beck et al. (2015; work-related stress); Boehm and Tse (2013; new graduate registered nurses); Cardeña et al. (2013); Greene and Greene (2012); Kraemer et al. (2016; medical students)
General Medical Condition Symptoms	Elkins et al. (2013; hot flashes in menopausal women); Kwekkeboom and Bratzke (2016; dyspnea, fatigue, pain, sleep, in heart failure patients); Peerdeman et al. (2015; fatigue, itch, pain in healthy people)

(continued)

Exhibit 7.2 *Symptoms and Conditions for Which Imagery Has Been Studied (continued)*

CLINICAL CONDITION	SELECTED SOURCES
In Adults	
Orthopedic Surgery Pain	Carpenter et al. (2017); Fan and Chen (2020)
Arthritis and Rheumatic Disease Symptoms	Giacobbi et al. (2015) (anxiety, depression, function, pain, quality of life)
Pain—Abdominal	Boltin et al. (2015; irritable bowel syndrome); Lindfors et al. (2012; irritable bowel syndrome); Mizrahi et al. (2012; inflammatory bowel disease); Palsson and van Tilburg (2015; gastrointestinal disorders)
Pain—Chronic	Posadzki et al. (2012; nonmusculoskeletal)
Pain—Phantom Limb	Beaumont et al. (2011); Brunelli et al. (2015);
Pain—Procedural	Alam et al. (2016; cutaneous surgery); Armstrong et al. (2014; cardiac catheterization); Shenefelt (2013; dermatology procedures)
Perioperative Symptoms	Acar and Aygin (2019; anxiety, postoperative symptoms, anxiety, satisfaction); Álvarez-García and Yaban (2020; anxiety, pain); Billquist et al. (2018; anxiety, preparation for surgery, satisfaction in female pelvic surgery patients); Draucker et al. (2015; acceptability in total knee replacement surgery patients); Felix et al. (2019; pain); Jacobson et al. (2016; function, gait velocity, hair cortisol levels, pain in total knee replacement surgery patients); Nelson et al. (2013); Sears et al. (2013; anxiety, pain)
Pregnancy Symptoms	Chuang et al. (2015; imagery adherence); Jallo et al. (2013; stress); Jallo et al.(2014; anxiety, fatigue, stress, corticotrophin-releasing hormone)
Rehabilitation	Braun et al. (2011); Ji et al. (2021); Kho et al. (2014);
Sleep	Lam et al. (2015); Loft and Cameron (2013; sleep behaviors); Schaffer et al. (2013; maternal sleep quality)
Sports Medicine Performance and Symptoms	Rodriquez et al. (2019; fear of reinjury, pain); Schuster et al. (2011; motor imagery training)
Stress and Trauma	Zehetmair et al. (2020; concentration, empowerment, mood, sleep, tension in traumatized refugees)

PAIN

Pain is a uniquely subjective experience, and proper management depends on individualizing interventions that recognize determinants affecting the pain response. Age, temperament, gender, ethnicity, and stage of development are all considerations when developing a pain management plan. Whether pain is from illness, a side effect of treatment, injury, or physical stress on the body, emotional factors contribute to pain perception, and mind–body interventions such as imagery can help make pain more manageable. Stress, anxiety, and fatigue decrease the threshold for pain, making the perceived pain more intense. Imagery can break this cycle of pain–tension–anxiety–pain. Relaxation with imagery decreases pain directly by reducing muscle tension and related spasms and indirectly by lowering anxiety and improving sleep. Imagery also is a distraction strategy; vivid, detailed images using all senses tend to work well for pain control. In addition, cognitive reappraisal/restructuring used with imagery can increase a sense of control over the ability to reframe the meaning of pain.

There is a considerable body of research examining the efficacy of guided imagery as a therapy to treat pain in adults. Studies have explored the effectiveness of guided imagery in treating cancer pain (De Paolis et al., 2018), orthopedic pain (Carpenter et al., 2017; Charette et al., 2015; Draucker et al., 2015; Jacobson et al., 2016), and fibromyalgia (Zech et al., 2017). Results have been variable but indicate that guided imagery might help relieve some forms of pain, especially when used as an adjunct to standard care measures. Subjects report positive and negative experiences with guided-imagery interventions. Subjects who find guided imagery useful describe it as enjoyable, relaxing, or interesting, whereas subjects who reported negative experiences describe it as unrealistic or annoying (Draucker et al., 2015). Subjects have reported an increased sense of self-efficacy in managing pain, symptoms, and functional status with fibromyalgia (Menzies et al., 2014).

There are many causes of chronic pain, but whatever the underlying etiology, it is generally challenging and costly to treat and has an impact on many aspects of an individual's life. Analgesic therapy often falls short of achieving adequate pain relief, and successful management frequently depends on using cognitive behavioral techniques such as imagery. Two conditions leading to chronic pain in adults are arthritis and fibromyalgia. A systematic review of studies of guided imagery for arthritis found a statistically significant reduction in pain and, in some studies, anxiety (Giacobbi et al., 2015). All studies used audiotapes, but the number of exposures was variable, ranging from 1 to 16. The subjects were predominately women with an average age of 62.

Fibromyalgia is a condition of chronic widespread pain and tenderness accompanied by fatigue, functional disability, disturbed sleep, cognitive impairment, and mood disorders (American College of Rheumatology, 2021; Molinari et al., 2018). Guided imagery and hypnosis have both been studied for pain and symptom management. Menzies and colleagues did a series of investigations on the effect of guided imagery on fibromyalgia symptoms (Menzies et al., 2006, 2014; Menzies & Kim, 2008). In a randomized control trial of 72 female subjects with fibromyalgia, subjects were randomized into usual care or usual care plus guided imagery (Menzies et al., 2014). The intervention group received CDs with a 20-minute guided-imagery audiotaped script and were instructed to use them daily. When compared with the usual-care control group, there was an improvement in self-efficacy for managing other symptoms, perceived stress and levels of fatigue, pain severity, and depression in the intervention group. There was no difference in biomarkers (C-reactive protein, cytokine). Onieva-Zafra et al. (2015) found improvement in pain relief in a guided-imagery group over a control group; however, Verkaik et al. (2014) found no differences in pain, self-efficacy, or functional status between groups. Two systematic reviews endorse the use of guided imagery for fibromyalgia but note that the evidence is not of high quality and that studies use a variety of techniques, treatment types (audiotapes, group sessions), number of sessions, and outcomes measured, making it difficult to compare studies (Meeus et al., 2015; Zech et al., 2017).

Evaluating and treating pain in children offer unique challenges due to age and developmental issues. Multimodal analgesia that includes pharmacology, regional anesthesia, rehabilitation, psychological approaches, spirituality, and integrative modalities are recommended for pain management in children (Friedrichsdorf & Goubert, 2020). Mind–body therapies, including guided imagery, are noted to be safe and effective for children and adolescents (American Academy of Pediatrics Section on Integrative Medicine, 2016). Hypnosis, which includes the use of imagery, can successfully be paired with other integrative strategies such as mindfulness and acupuncture to achieve improved clinical outcomes (Kaiser et al., 2018)

There are adverse short-term and long-term effects of inadequate pain management in children, including hypoxemia, immobility, altered pulmonary function, posttraumatic stress, and adverse psychological and behavioral patterns (Friedrichsdorf & Goubert, 2020). Distraction imagery is particularly helpful in getting a child through a medical procedure with a safe and effective level of sedation/analgesia and as little movement as possible. Suggestions to breathe deeply and to relax or be comfortable are combined with vivid images of a favorite place or pleasant experience that draw the attention away from the pain. It is best to introduce the child to breathing techniques and explore favorite images prior to the procedure. However, in critical or emergency situations, imagery has been successfully used without previous experience. Birnie et al. (2018) updated a previous systemic review of controlled trials of interventions for needle-related procedural pain and distress. In this review, distraction, combined cognitive behavioral interventions, and hypnosis continued to demonstrate efficacy in the management of procedural pain in children. However, two studies using imagery for venipuncture and vaccination in older children (11–12 years old) found no difference between imagery and standard care groups (Forsner et al., 2014; Nilsson et al., 2015). Current guidelines on the management of needle pain (procedures, vaccinations, etc.) in children recommend a bundle of topical anesthesia, sucrose or breastfeeding(for infants 0–12 months), comfort positioning, and age-appropriate distraction, which can include imagery (Friedrichsdorf & Goubert, 2020).

Chronic pain in childhood can be challenging to treat and has a significant impact on the child's quality of life and engagement in school and social activities. Common chronic pain conditions in childhood are musculoskeletal pain, headaches, and abdominal pain. Gulewitsch et al. (2013) assigned children with functional abdominal pain and irritable bowel syndrome (and their parents) to a hypnotherapeutic behavioral treatment or wait-list control. The intervention consisted of group sessions in which the participants learned about stress and were taught hypnotic techniques (relaxation, imagery, and suggestions directed at increasing wellness and managing pain). Children in the treatment group reported a significantly greater reduction in pain scores and pain-related disability.

Parents and children are open to the use of integrative strategies, including imagery, to manage symptoms during hospitalization (Misra et al., 2019). Guided imagery and relaxation as a treatment for preoperative anxiety and postoperative pain were studied in a randomized control trial of 60 children, ages 6 to 12. All participants were undergoing minor surgery under general anesthesia. The experimental group received routine care and a relaxation-guided imagery intervention whereas the control group received routine care alone. In both groups, parents accompanied the child to the operating room and stayed with them during the anesthesia induction process. Children in the experimental group had a significant reduction in preoperative anxiety and postoperative pain (Vagnoli et al., 2019). In a systematic review of psychological interventions for postoperative pain, Davidson et al. (2016) found interventions such as imagery to be at least moderately effective in managing short-term postoperative pain in children.

OBESITY

Obesity in children and young adults has been described as a health emergency due to rising rates and prevalence across the globe. Childhood obesity is a serious problem in the United States, putting children and adolescents at risk for poor health. Obesity prevalence among children and adolescents is high. The Centers for Disease Control and Prevention (CDC, 2021) reports that in 2018, the prevalence rate of obesity, which is defined as body mass index at or above 95% for children aged 2 to 19 years, was 19.3% and affected about 14 million children in the United States. Chronic stress has been linked to obesity in children. A recent study conducted at the University of Athens Medical School in Greece evaluated the effectiveness of a stress management program to address obesity using biomarkers of stress. This intervention study evaluated the effectiveness of a stress management program that included progressive muscle relaxation, breathing, guided imagery, dietary guidance, and physical training. Guided imagery was included in a CD that was given to participants with instructions to use the techniques once a day and record their efforts for 8 weeks. The waist–hip ratio was significantly reduced in the intervention group (Emmanouil et al., 2018). Stress management interventions that include guided imagery for children and adolescents may provide another opportunity for addressing obesity in this population.

CANCER TREATMENT

Imagery interventions in oncology have focused on physiological and psychological responses to cancer treatment. The effectiveness of complementary therapies in cancer patients was reported in a review article by Guerra-Martin et al. (2021). Guided imagery was found to be an effective intervention. As cancer is the second-leading cause of death worldwide, these therapies are increasingly used by patients. Guided imagery research over the past few years has evolved to include more randomized clinical trials and larger sample sizes. Areas that have been investigated are efficacy in managing symptoms (e.g., pain, nausea), influence on surgical outcomes, improvement in quality of life, and changes in immunity (Roffe et al., 2005).

A more recent review by Kapogiannis et al. (2018) investigated the effects of combination therapy utilizing progressive muscle relaxation (PMR) and guided imagery. Eight studies were reviewed. Seven of the eight studies included only breast cancer patients and one study had a sample of breast and prostate patients. Positive results included an improvement in mental state in seven of the eight studies. Three of the eight studies reported significant improvements in nausea and vomiting. The results indicated that a combined intervention with PMR and guided imagery may be a useful addition to supportive care strategies for patients receiving chemotherapy. Earlier studies have also indicated the effectiveness of combining PMR and guided imagery. A study by Charalambous et al. (2016) explored the effectiveness of guided imagery combined with PMR on this cluster of side effects in a randomized control trial. Patients in the intervention group experienced less fatigue, a better quality of life, and less nausea and vomiting. There was also more depression in the control group compared to the intervention group.

Guided imagery is a recognized intervention for women receiving treatment for breast cancer. Serra et al. (2012) studied the effect of a guided-imagery intervention during radiation therapy. A convenience sample of 61 women received a guided-imagery session in the radiation oncology setting immediately before their radiation treatment. Physiological and psychological measurements were evaluated. There was a statistically significant improvement in pulse rate, respiratory rate, and blood pressure between the first and second sessions. There was also a rise in skin temperature, indicating increased peripheral blood flow and decreased sympathetic response. The guided-imagery intervention was determined to be helpful by 86% of the participants.

Another randomized control trial from Italy examined a combination of PMR and guided imagery for pain reduction in hospice patients (De Paolis et al., 2018). It is estimated that one third of cancer patients receiving terminal care suffer from moderate to severe pain. The intervention involved guiding patients to visualize positive and pleasant images encouraging multiple sensory images. Patients were invited to choose their imagery script from several options that included walking on a beach, through fields, into the woods, or on a mountain. The session lasted 20 minutes with a progressive muscle relaxation exercise at the beginning of the session. Pain intensity scores using a numeric scale were obtained at four time points. Pain scores improved in the intervention group. Patients reported improved quality of life and greater control of their pain.

Quality of life for breast cancer survivors is of concern, especially for women with limited access to psychosocial interventions. An earlier study by Freeman et al. (2015), conducted in Alaska, compared in-person group sessions, telemedicine delivery group sessions, and a wait list as a control group. The intervention group sessions included education on mind–body connections, including mental imagery and sensory experiences. Both the in-person group and the telemedicine group experienced significant changes in cognitive function, sleep disturbance, and quality of life. This research invites new methods for delivering guided-imagery interventions for women with breast cancer who have limited abilities to attend in-person sessions.

A randomized controlled trial conducted in Cyprus included subjects with breast cancer and prostate cancer. A total of 236 patients were randomized to receive either a combined guided-imagery and PMR intervention, which included both supervised and unsupervised sessions, or standard care with computer-based education about their specific cancer. Measurement included anxiety and depression scales and saliva biomarkers. Results included significant decreases in anxiety and depression scores in the intervention group (Charalambous et al., 2015).

A breast cancer diagnosis and subsequent treatment can have devastating effects on a woman's body image and quality of life. Cancer therapy can have adverse effects that may include loss of breasts, hair loss, scarring, infertility, early menopause, and sexual function impairments. Researchers from the University of Toronto developed a small-group, 8-week intervention, Restoring Body Image After Cancer (ReBIC). There are two published articles relating to this study. The first article describes the prospective randomized control trial design and reports the results of the trial (Esplen et al., 2018) The second article describes the group therapy intervention with a qualitative focus (Esplen et al., 2020). This intervention utilized acceptance group therapy principles. Outcome measures were body image, sexual dysfunction, and quality of life. The intervention included guided-imagery exercises and education. Guided-imagery sessions in session one provided relaxation and self-nurturing and progressed to future self-images by the eighth session. Results of the trial included significantly less distress about body appearance, decreased body stigma, lower levels of breast cancer-related concerns, and better quality of life. There was no significant group difference in sexual functioning. Several of the participants' vignettes are included as an appendix in the second article and provide insight regarding the success of the intervention. The researchers recommend using this intervention for other cancer diagnoses.

Childhood malignancy has a profound effect on the whole family, including parents. A randomized control trial by Tsitsi et al. (2017) explored guided imagery combined with PMR as an intervention during their child's treatment aimed at reducing parental anxiety and improving mood. Several measurement tools were used. The results supported a statistically significant decrease in tension in the intervention group. Parents in the intervention group also were less sad and had decreased anxiety compared with the control group.

The NCCIH (2021) describes relaxation techniques, including guided imagery, on its website, acknowledging that while more research is needed to fully determine the effectiveness of this therapy, it is generally viewed as safe for healthy people. The improved quality of the studies suggests that there is good evidence for guided imagery as an intervention for cancer patients. The Society for Integrative Oncology published a clinical practice guideline for the use of integrative therapies as supportive care for breast cancer patients and reported that guided imagery can be considered for improving quality of life for breast cancer patients (Greenlee et al., 2014).

CULTURAL APPLICATIONS

Current imagery intervention owes its roots to the use of imagery in many healing systems, including Chinese Medicine and Native American traditions (Krau, 2020). The use of imagery is foundational to shamanic healing, a centuries-old practice in which imagery is used within an ecstatic or altered state to access the patient's subconscious mind and belief system (Reed, 2007). This opens communication among mind, body, and spirit to cure, alleviate suffering, and facilitate spiritual transformation.

The interest in imagery as part of a therapeutic treatment plan is widespread (see Sidebar 7.1). In past decades, studies in imagery were predominately from the United States. However, a review of the recent literature reveals that research on the use and effectiveness of imagery is prevalent globally. Some examples are clinical trials and systematic reviews from Spain (Álvarez-García & Yaban, 2020; Molinari et al., 2018); Brazil (Felix et al., 2019), Italy (Di Corrado et al., 2020; Vagnoli et al., 2019), China (Fan & Chen, 2020), and Greece (Emmanouil et al., 2018).

In the area of oncology, international research on guided imagery is growing. Nurses are at the forefront of this research, seeking new, effective interventions to mitigate the side effects of treatment (see Sidebar 7.2). The global rise in breast cancer incidence has contributed to the search for integrative options, such as guided imagery, to control and manage symptoms. A nursing research study in Taiwan evaluated the effects of cancer treatment on women with breast cancer. The researchers found that guided imagery paired with relaxation had a positive effect on mediating the side effects of anxiety and depression (Chen et al., 2015). In Iran, breast cancer is the most common cancer found in women. A group of nurse researchers studied guided imagery for chemotherapy-induced nausea and vomiting, one of the most distressing side effects of chemotherapy. If not adequately controlled, it can lead to many other serious side effects, such as weight loss, malnutrition, social isolation, depression, insomnia, and dehydration. The intervention was delivered at clinic appointments, and the participants also listened to a guided-imagery CD at home. Guided imagery as an intervention reduced the severity and frequency of chemotherapy-induced nausea and vomiting (Hosseini et al., 2016).

Thyroid cancer incidence is also increasing worldwide. In Korea, thyroid cancer is the most common cancer. A group of nurse researchers observed significant stress in patients who were receiving radioactive iodine treatments post-thyroidectomy. They provided guided imagery CDs to the intervention group and had them view the CD daily for 4 weeks. The control group received standard education about radioactive iodine therapy. There were significant decreases in stress and fatigue in the intervention group (Lee et al., 2013).

Cultures are broadly categorized as tending toward either individualism or collectivism. La Roche et al. (2010) investigated guided imagery scripts to determine their level of idiocentrism versus allocentrism. Idiocentrism is the tendency to define oneself in isolation from others and would be found in individualistic societies; allocentrism is the tendency to define oneself in relation to others and would be seen in cultures valuing collectivism. The authors reviewed 123 guided imagery scripts and found that they tended to be more idiocentric. This indicates that guided imagery scripts may need to be adapted depending on the user's cultural ethnicity.

When directing a guided imagery experience, the practitioner should be aware of individual preferences and use images that are understandable and acceptable to the participant. As a rule, the most powerful and meaningful image is one that the participant creates rather than one that is supplied by the guide. Individuals are more likely to choose images that are congruent with their cultural, spiritual, and personal beliefs. The guide or therapist is there to help them use those images.

Sidebar 7.1 *Using Imagery Online: New Zealand*

Theresa Fleming and Matthew Shepherd

New Zealand or—in the words of the Indigenous Maori people—Aotearoa includes Maori as well as Pacific, Asian, New Zealand European, and other peoples. Our team set out to develop a computerized therapy to help extend the reach of psychological therapies to teenagers with unmet needs, particularly untreated depression and anxiety. We focused on computerized therapies because face-to-face services are limited, sometimes costly, inconvenient, or not preferred by adolescents. Computerized, or online, therapies have been tested and shown to be effective; however, often these have high dropout rates; many are very text-heavy and may not reflect the interests of diverse peoples.

Over several years, we worked with young people, therapists, learning technologists, researchers, and game developers to develop and test a computer program called SPARX (smart, positive, active, realistic, x-factor) thoughts. This was shown to be effective in a large randomized controlled trial and is now freely available in New Zealand, funded through the Ministry of Health (www .fmhs.auckland.ac.nz/assets/fmhs/faculty/ABOUT/newsandevents/docs/SPARX%20 Fact%20sheet.pdf).

SPARX uses cognitive behavioral therapy techniques, storytelling, and metaphor- and play-based learning. These strategies were selected based on evidence and on appeal to Maori and other youth. The program has seven levels or modules that young people can do on their own or with support. SPARX uses both explicit instructional learning and play-based, first-person experiential learning. Each level begins with "the guide," a virtual therapist who welcomes the user, explains what the session is about, and discusses how it relates to real life (instructional learning). The users then go into a game world, where they complete quests and challenges to "right the balance" and reduce negativity in the game world. In general, this is exploratory, play-based learning in the context of a rich visual environment. There is an overarching narrative and metaphors are often used. At the end of each level, users come back to the guide, who invites them to reflect and develop strategies to use skills from the game in real life. For example, in the volcano province, users must negotiate with angry fire spirits and lift blocks from volcanic vents to prevent explosions. When they return to the guide, they consider what causes them to explode with anger and how to deal with these challenges in real life. In another example, users release the "Bird of Hope" from a chest where it has been trapped. From there, the Bird of Hope follows them and helps them throughout the game; again, this is explicitly linked to how one develops and maintains hope in real life.

The imagery in SPARX was created with input from youth, as well as cultural, learning, and computer game experts. The team included Maori and non-Maori health researchers, clinicians, and youth. The computer game company

(continued)

Sidebar 7.1 *Using Imagery Online: New Zealand (continued)*

that developed the software was Maori-led, and cultural experts ensured that the content was appropriate and powerful. Evaluations have shown SPARX to be effective among young people seeking help for depression. There were no differences in its effectiveness between Maori and non-Maori or between males and females. This is exciting because many therapeutic interventions are more appealing to girls and/or majority-culture persons, which may inadvertently increase disparities. Youth feedback has highlighted that the imagery and narrative helped increase the appeal of SPARX and made it easy to understand, remember, and use new skills:

"The Bird of Hope is encouraging, it's like having someone next to you, by your side, it will be in my memory."
"I learnt from the game. It was interesting and fun, you do learn from game stuff."
"It felt personal, you know, like he [the guide] was talking to you, like you got to know him."

FUTURE RESEARCH

The quality of research testing guided imagery in clinical conditions has improved. There are more randomized, controlled trials noted in recent years, however, there remain a number of issues to resolve. Testing the effectiveness of guided imagery and other mind–body interventions remains challenging as it is not possible to blind the participants and many clinical trials have small numbers of participants. While meta-analysis and systematic reviews have been completed, the evidence is often limited by the heterogeneity of the studies regarding the intervention (mixed interventions, single or multiple imagery sessions, methods of delivery) and disparate outcomes measured with different instruments.

Sidebar 7.2 *Comparison of the Use of Guided Imagery Versus Mindful Attention With Children in Thailand With Cancer*

Kesanee Boonyawatanangkool

In Thailand, as elsewhere, children with a life-threatening illness such as cancer experience multiple types of distress. These can range from disease symptoms, procedures, and treatments to the psychological discomfort of living with a potentially terminal illness. Indeed, there are numerous challenges inherent to the provision of holistic nursing care to these children throughout their illness trajectory. Guided imagery is an independent nursing

Sidebar 7.2 *Comparison of the Use of Guided Imagery Versus Mindful Attention With Children in Thailand With Cancer (continued)*

intervention that uses psychoneuroimmunological principles to help manage distress symptoms such as pain, anxiety, and fear by directing attention away from difficult events. Conversely, mindfulness involves devoting attention to one's experience in an accepting and nonjudgmental way; however, the effect of this instruction on distress symptoms—including pain and other outcomes—is unknown.

The objective we addressed in our clinical work was to examine whether mindful attention could help children focus on pain, anxiety, or fear without increasing their distress symptoms or decreasing their symptom tolerance. In this clinical evaluation, we compared the effects of mindful attention to a well-established intervention for reducing difficult symptoms (i.e., guided imagery/self-hypnosis)—an intervention that is designed to take attention away from uncomfortable events.

Anxiety and fear were monitored in children ($N = 58$) 5 to 18 years of age who were hospitalized and receiving chemotherapy. Each child attended and completed a session of guided imagery. Participants then received either mindful-attention or guided-imagery instructions designed to direct attention to focus on or away from their pain, anxiety, and fear, respectively.

Our clinical evaluation revealed that children who received the mindful attention instructions demonstrated more awareness of the physical sensations of pain, anxiety, and fear—including thoughts about those sensations—without decreasing tolerance levels. Some of them said, "I am now feeling better; can you help me do this again please?" (e.g., a 14-year-old boy with palliation of rhabdomyosarcoma pain). There were no interactions observed between baseline characteristics of the children and the specific intervention used to address their symptoms.

Based on our clinical observations, we concluded that mindful (trance) attention—compared with guided imagery—was successful in helping the children focus attention on experiences of pain, anxiety, and fear without increased pain intensity or decreased symptom tolerance.

These conclusions were based solely on the clinical experience in my practice setting in Thailand. Factors that we know to be important to the implementation of either intervention with children include the children's knowledge, their developmental stage, trust and rapport, gender and age, pain and other uncomfortable experiences, coping strategies, disease status, religious and cultural beliefs, and family background. Both interventions appeared to be beneficial in reducing distress in children and included shared strategies such as eye-fixation techniques, deep breaths, and progressive muscle relaxation through guided instruction.

Imagery has been shown to be a key component to stress and symptom management in many situations and conditions; however, key questions remain to be answered regarding specific physiological responses to imagery, the influence of imagery on clinical outcomes and quality of life, and the effect of individual factors. As a low-cost, noninvasive intervention, imagery has the potential to be effective in reducing symptoms and distress across several conditions. Questions to be pursued include the following:

- What is the role of imagery in maintaining health and wellness? Should imagery be a component of preventive medicine? Over time, can imagery reduce stress, improve coping, enhance well-being, create healthier lifestyles, and reduce illness in individuals?
- What is the effect of imagery on clinical outcomes relevant to quality-of-life and health/illness states, and does it have an impact on cost-effectiveness and quality of care?
- What is the relationship between imagery and other relaxation strategies? Are they more effective when paired or should they be used alone?
- Does the type of imagery produce different outcomes? What imagery protocols or processes are most appropriate in specific conditions (use of recording/app or session with a practitioner; duration and number of sessions)?
- Is it possible to predict the usefulness of an imagery intervention in specific individuals? Are there certain characteristics of individuals that determine their ability to respond to imagery and produce desired outcomes? Are there certain individuals or conditions for which imagery should not be recommended?
- What are the long-term effects of imagery?
- What is the role of practitioner characteristics (type of training, practitioner style, number of different practitioners) and their relationship with the imagery recipient in outcomes?

WEBSITES

The following websites contain additional information on guided imagery:

- American Holistic Nurses Association. (2021). (www.ahna.org)
- American Society of Clinical Hypnosis. (2021). Certification, workshops, and resources (www.asch.net)
- Association for Music and Imagery. (2021). Bonny method of guided imagery and music therapy (www.ami-bonnymethod.org)
- Imagery International. (2021). (www.imageryinternational.org)
- National Center for Complementary and Integrative Health Practices. (2021). Relaxation techniques for health (https://nccih.nih.gov/health/relaxation-techniques-for-health.htm)
- National Pediatric Hypnosis Training Institute. (2021). Training in pediatric hypnosis (www.nphti.org)

REFERENCES

Acar, K., & Aygin, D. (2019). Efficacy of guided imagery for postoperative symptoms, sleep quality, anxiety, and satisfaction regarding nursing care: A randomized controlled study. *Journal of PeriAnesthesia Nursing, 34*(6), 1241–1249. https://doi.org/10.1016/j.jopan.2019.05.006

Abbott, R. A., Martin, A. E., Newlove-Delgado, T. V., Bethel, A., Thompson-Coon, J., Whear, R., & Logan, S. (2017). Psychosocial interventions for recurrent abdominal pain in childhood. *Cochrane Database Systematic Review, Jan*(1). https://doi.org/10.1002/14651858CD10971.pub2

Ader, R., & Cohen, N. (1981). Conditioned immunopharmacologic responses. In R. Ader (Ed.), *Psychoneuroimmunology* (pp. 281–319). Academic Press.

Alam, M., Roongpisuthipong, W., Kim, N., Goyal, A., Swary, J. H., Brindise, R. T., Iyenagar, S., Pace, N., West, D. P., Polavarapu, M., & Yoo, S. (2016). Utility of recorded guided imagery and relaxing music in reducing patient pain and anxiety, and surgeon anxiety, during cutaneous surgical procedures: A single-blinded randomized and controlled trial. *Journal of the American Academy Dermatology, 75*, 585–589. https://doi.org/10.1016/j.jaad.2016.02.1143

Alexander, M. (2012). Managing patient stress in pediatric radiology. *Radiologic Technology, 83*(6), 549–560. http://www.radiologictechnology.org/content/83/6/549.short

Álvarez-García, C., & Yaban, Z. S. (2020). The effects of preoperative guided imagery interventions on preoperative anxiety and postoperative pain: A meta-analysis. *Complementary Therapies in Clinical Practice, 38*. https://doi.org/10.1016/j.ctcp.2019.101077

American Academy of Pediatrics Section on Integrative Medicine. (2016). Mind-body therapies in children and youth. *Pediatrics, 138*(3), e20161896. https://doi.org/10.1542/peds.2016-1896

American College of Rheumatology. (2021). *Fibromyalgia.* https://www.rheumatolgy.org/I-Am-A/Patient-Caregiver/disease-condidions/fibromyalgia

Andrasik, F., & Rime, C. (2007). Can behavioural therapy influence neuromodulation? *Neurological Sciences, 28*(Suppl. 2), S124–S129. https://doi.org/10.1007/s10072-007-0764-6

Armin, J., Johnson, T., Hingle, M., Giacobbi, Jr., P., & Gordon, J. S. (2017). Development of a multi-behavioral mHealth app for women smokers. *Journal of Health Communication, 22*(2), 153–162.

Armstrong, K., Dixon, S., May, S., & Patricolo, G. E. (2014). Anxiety reduction in patients undergoing cardiac catheterization following massage and guided imagery. *Complementary Therapies in Clinical Practice, 20*(2014), 334–338. https://doi.org/10.1016/j.ctcp.2014.07.009

Beaumont, G., Mercier, C., Michon P. E., Malouin, F., & Jackson, P. L. (2011). Decreasing phantom limb pain through observation of action and imagery: A case series. *Pain Medicine, 12*, 289–299. https://doi.org/10.1111/j.1526-4637.2010.01048.x

Beck, B. D., Hansen, A. M., & Gold, C. (2015). Coping with work-related stress through guided imagery and music (GIM): Randomized controlled trial. *Journal of Music Therapy, 52*(3), 323–352. https://doi.org/10.1093/jmt/thv011

Billquist, E. J., Michelfelder, A., Brincat, C., Brubaker, L., Fitzgerald, C. M., & Mueller, E. R. (2018) Pre-operative guided imagery in female pelvic medicine and reconstructive surgery: A randomized trial. *International Urogynecology Journal, 29*, 1117–1122. https://doi.org/10.1007/s00192-017-3443-z

Birnie, K. A., Noel, M., Chambers, C. T., Uman, L. S., & Parker, J. A. (2018). Psychological interventions for needle-related procedural pain and distress in children and adolescents. *Cochrane Database Systematic Reviews, Oct*(10). https://doi.org/10.1002/14651858CD005179.pub4

Boehm, L. B., & Tse, A. M. (2013). Application of guided imagery to facilitate the transition of new graduate registered nurses. *Journal of Continuing Education in Nursing, 44*(3), 113–119. https://doi.org/10.3928/00220124-20130115-16

Boltin, D., Sahar, N., Gil, E., Aizic, S., Hod, K., Levi-Drummer, R., Niv, R., & Dickman, R. (2015). Gut-directed guided affective imagery as an adjunct to dietary modification in irritable bowel syndrome. *Journal of Health Psychology, 20*(6), 712–720. https://doi.org/10.1177/1359105315573450

Braun, S. M., Wade, D. T., & Beurskens, A. J. (2011). Use of movement imagery in neurorehabilitation: Researching effects of a complex intervention. *International Journal of Rehabilitation Research, 34*, 203–208. https://doi.org/10.1097/MRR.0b013e328348b184

Brunelli, S., Giovanni, M., Iosa, M., Ciotti, C., De Giorgi, R., Foti, C., & Traballesi, M. (2015). Efficacy of progressive muscle relaxation, mental imagery, and phantom exercise training on phantom limb: A randomized control trial. *Archives of Physical Medicine and Rehabilitation, 96*, 181–187. https://doi.org/10.1016/j.apmr.2014.09.035

Cardeña, E., Svensson, C., & Hejdström, F. (2013). Hypnotic tape intervention ameliorates stress: A randomized control study. *International Journal of Clinical and Experimental Hypnosis, 61*(2), 125–145. https://doi.org/10.1080/00207144.2013.753820

Carli, G., Cavallaro, F. I., & Santarcangelo, E. L. (2007). Hypnotizability and imagery modality preference: Do highs and lows live in the same world? *Contemporary Hypnosis, 24*(2), 64–75. https://doi.org/10.1002/ch.331

Carpenter, J. J., Hines, S. H., & Lan, V. L. (2017). Guided imagery for pain management in postoperative orthopedic patients. *Journal of Holistic Nursing, 35*(4), 342–351. https://doi.org/10.1177/0898010116675462

Centers for Disease Control and Prevention. (2021, April). *Childhood obesity facts, prevalence of childhood obesity in the United States.* https://www.cdc.gov/obesity/data/childhood.html

Charalambous, A., Giannakopoulou, M., Bozas, E., Marcou, T., Kitslos, P., & Paikousis, L. (2016). Guided imagery and progressive muscle relaxation as a cluster of symptoms management intervention in patients receiving chemotherapy: A randomized control trial. *PLOS ONE, 11*(6). https://doi.org/10.1371/journal.pone.0156911

Charalambous, A., Giannakopoulou, M., Bozas, E., & Paikousis, L. (2015). A randomized controlled trial for the effectiveness of progressive muscle relaxation and guided imagery as anxiety reducing interventions in breast and prostate cancer patients undergoing chemotherapy. *Evidenced-Based Complementary and Alternative Medicine, 2015,* 270876. https://doi.org/10.1155/2015/270876

Charette, S., Fiola, J. L., Charest, M. C., Villeneuve, E., Théroux, J., Joncas, J., Parent, S., & Le May, S. (2015). Guided imagery for adolescent post-spinal fusion pain management: A pilot study. *Pain Management Nursing, 16*(3), 211–220. https://doi.org/10.1016/j.pmn.2014.06.004

Chen, S., Wang, H., Yang, H., & Chung, U. (2015). Effect of relaxation and guided imagery on the physical and psychological symptoms of breast cancer patients undergoing chemotherapy. *Iran Red Crescent Medical Journal, 17*(11), 1–8. https://doi.org/10.5812/ircmj.31277

Chuang, L. L., Liu, S. C., Chen, Y. H., & Lin, L. C. (2015). Predictors of adherence to relaxation guided imagery during pregnancy in women with preterm labor. *Journal of Alternative and Complementary Medicine, 21*(9), 563–568. https://doi.org/10.1089/acm.2013.0381

Costa-Pinto, F., & Palermo-Neto, J. (2010). Neuroimmune interactions in stress. *NeuroImmuno-Modulation, 17,* 196–199. https://doi.org/10.1159/000258722

Cotton, S., Roberts, Y. H., Tsevat, J., Britto, M., Succop, P., McGrady, M. E., & Yi, M. S. (2010). Mind-body complementary alternative medicine use and quality of life in adolescents with inflammatory bowel disease. *Inflammatory Bowel Disease, 16*(3), 501–506. https://doi.org/10.1002/ibd.21045

Davidson, F., Snow, S., Hayden, J. A., & Chomey, J. (2016). Psychological interventions in managing postoperative pain in children: A systematic review. *Pain, 157*(9), 1872–1886. https://doi.org/10.1097/j.pain.0000000000000636

De Paolis, G., Naccarato, A., Cibelli, F., D'Alete, A., Mastroianni, C., Surdo, L., Casala, G., & Magnan, C. (2018). The effectiveness of muscle relaxation and interactive guided imagery as a pain-reducing intervention in advanced cancer patients: A multicenter randomized controlled non-pharmacological trial. *Complementary Therapies in Clinical Practice, 34,* 280–287. https://doi.org/10.1016/j.ctcp.2018.12.014

Di Corrado, D., Guarnera, M., Guerrera, C. S., Maldonato N. M., Di Nuovo, S, Castellano, S., & Coco, M. (2020). Mental imagery skills in competitive young athletes and non-athletes. *Frontiers in Psychology, 11*(633), 1–7. https://doi.org/10.3389/fpsyg.2020.00633

Djordjevic, J., Zatorre, R. J., Petrides, M., Boyle, J. A., & Jones-Gotaman, M. (2005). Functional neuroimaging of odor imagery. *Neuroimage, 24*(3), 791–801. https://doi.org/10.1016/j.neuroimage.2004.09.035

Dobson, C. (2015). Outcome results of self-efficacy in children with sickle disease pain who were trained to use guided imagery. *Applied Nursing Research, 28,* 384–390. https://doi.org/10.1097/01.NAJ.0000445680.06812.6a

Dobson, C. E., & Byrne, M. W. (2014). Using guided imagery to manage pain in young children with sickle cell disease. *American Journal of Nursing, 114*(4), 27–36. https://doi.org/10.1097/01.NAJ.0000445680.06812.6a

Draucker, C. B., Jacobson, A. F., Umberger, W. A., Myerscough, R. P., & Sanata, J. D. (2015). Acceptability of a guided imagery intervention for persons undergoing a total knee replacement. *Orthopedic Nursing, 34*(6), 356–364. https://doi.org/10.1097/NOR.0000000000000193

Elkins, G., Johnson, A., Fisher, W., & Sliwinski, J. (2013). A pilot investigation of guided self-hypnosis in the treatment of hot flashes among postmenopausal women. *International Journal of Clinical and Experimental Hypnosis, 61*(3), 342–350. https://doi.org/10.1080/00207144.2013.784112

Emmanouil, C. C., Pervanidou, P., Charmandari, E., Darviri, C., & Chrousos, G. P. (2018). The effectiveness of a health promotion and stress management program in a sample of obese children and adolescents. *Hormones, 17*, 405–413. https://doi.org/10.1007/s42000-018-0052-2

Esplen, M. J., Warner, E., Boquiren, V., & Wong, J. (2020). Restoring body image after cancer (ReBIC): A group therapy intervention. *Psycho-Oncology, 29*, 671–680. https://doi.org:10.1002/pon.5304

Esplen, M. J., Wong, J., Warner, E., & Toner, B. (2018). Restoring body image after cancer (ReBIC): Results of a randomized control trial. *Journal of Clinical Oncology, 36*(8), 749–756. https://doi.org/10.12/FCO.2017.74.8244

Fan, M., & Chen, Z. (2020). A systematic review of non-pharmacological interventions used for pain relief after orthopedic surgical procedures. *Experimental and Therapeutic Medicine, 20*(36). https://doi.org/10.3892/etm.2020.9163

Felix, M. M. dS, Ferreira, M. B. G., Cruz, L. F. dC., & Barbosa, M. H. (2019). Relaxation therapy with guided imagery for postoperative pain management: An integrative review. *Pain Management Nursing, 20*(1), 3–9. https://doi.org/10.1016/j.pmn.2017.10.014

Fleshner, M., & Laudenslager, M. L. (2004). Psychoneuroimmunology: Then and now. *Behavioral and Cognitive Neuroscience Reviews, 3*(2), 114–130. https://doi.org/10.1177/1534582304269027

Flynn, T. A., Jones, B. A., & Ausderau, K. K. (2016). Guided imagery and stress in pregnant adolescents. *American Journal of Occupational Therapy, 70*(5), 700522002 1–7. https://doi.org/10.5014/ajot.2016.019315

Forsner, M., Norström, F., Nordyke, K., Ivarsson, A., & Lindh, V. (2014). Relaxation and guided imagery used with 12-year-olds during venipuncture in a school-based screening study. *Journal of Child Health Care, 18*(3), 241–252. https://doi.org/10.1177/1367493513486963

Freeman, L., White, R., Ratcliff, M., Sutton, S., Stewart, M., Palmer, J., Link, J., &. Cohen, L. (2015). A randomized trial comparing live and telemedicine delivery of an imagery-based behavioral intervention to breast cancer survivors: Reducing symptoms and barriers to care. *Psycho-Oncology, 24*(8), 1–16. https://doi.org/10.1002/pon.3656

Friedrichsdorf, S. J., & Goubert, L. (2020). Pediatric pain treatment and prevention for hospitalized children. *Pain Reports, 5*, e804. https://doi.org/10.1097/PR9.0000000000000804

Giacobbi, P. R., Stabler, M., Stewart, J., Jaeschke, A., Siebert, J. L., & Kelly, G. A. (2015). Guided imagery for arthritis and other rheumatic diseases: A systematic review of randomized controlled trials. *Pain Management Nursing, 16*(5), 792–803. https://doi.org/10.1016/j.pmn.2015.01.003

Glaser, R., MacCallum, R. C., Laskowski, B. F., Malarkey, W. B., Sheridan, J. F., & Kiecolt-Glaser, J. K. (2001). Evidence for a shift in the Th-1 to Th-2 cytokine response associated with chronic stress and aging. *Journal of Gerontology. A: Biological Science and Medical Science, 56*(8), M477–M482. https://doi.org/10.1093/gerona/56.8.M477

Gordon, J. S., Armin, J., Hingle, M. D., Giacobbi, Jr., P., Cunningham, J. K., Johnson, T., Abbate, K., Howe, C. L., & Roe, D. J. (2017). Development and evaluation of the See Me Smoke-Free multi-behavioral mHealth app for women smokers. *Translational Behavioral Medicine, 7*(2), 172–184. https://doi.org/10.1007/s13142-017-0463-7

Gottsegen, D. (2011). Hypnosis for functional abdominal pain. *American Journal of Clinical Hypnosis, 54*, 56–69. https://doi.org/10.1080/00029157.2011.575964

Greene, C., & Greene, B. A. (2012, May–June). Efficacy of guided imagery to reduce stress via the internet: A pilot study. *Holistic Nursing Practice, 26*(3), 150–163. https://doi.org/10.1097/HNP.0b013e31824ef55a

Greenlee, H., Balneaves, L. G., Carlson, L. E., Cohen, M., Deng, G., Hershman, D., Mumber, M., Perlmutter, J., Seely, D., Sen, A., & Zick, S. M. (2014). Clinical practice guidelines on the use of integrative therapies as supportive care in patients treated for breast cancer. *JNCI Monographs, 50*, 346–358. https://doi.org/10.1093/jncimonographs/lgu041

Guerra-Martín, M. D., Tejedor-Bueno, M. S., & Correa-Casado, M. (2021). Effectiveness of complementary therapies in cancer patients: A systematic review. *International Journal of Environmental Research and Public Health, 18*, 1017. https://doi.org/10.3390/ijerph18031017

Gulewitsch, M. D., Müller, J., Hautzinger, M., & Schlarb, A. A. (2013). Brief hypnotherapeutic-behavioral intervention for functional abdominal pain and irritable bowel syndrome in childhood: A randomized controlled trial. *European Journal of Pediatrics, 172*, 1043–1051. https://doi.org/10.1007/s00431-013-1990-y

Hadjibalassi, M., Lambrinou, E., Papastavrou, E., & Papathanassoglou, E. (2018). The effect of guided imagery on physiological and psychological outcomes of adult ICU patients: A systematic literature review and methodological implications. *Australian Critical Care, 31*, 73–86. https://doi.org/10.1016/j.aucc2017.03.001

Hansen, M. M. (2015). A feasibility pilot study on the use of complementary therapies delivered via mobile technologies on Icelandic surgical patients' reports of anxiety, pain, and self-efficacy in healing. *Complementary and Alternative Medicine, 15*, 92–104. https://doi.org/10.1186/s12906-015-0613-8

Hosseini, M., Tirgari, B., Forouzi, M. A., & Janhani, Y. (2016). Guided imagery effects on chemotherapy induced nausea and vomiting in Iranian breast cancer patients. *Complementary Therapies in Clinical Practice, 25*, 8–12. https://doi.org/10.1016/j.ctcp.2016.07.002

Huth, M. M., Broome, M. E., & Good, M. (2004). Imagery reduces children's postoperative pain. *Pain, 110*(1–2), 439–448. https://doi.org/10.1016/j.pain.2004.04.028

Huth, M. M., Van Kuiken, D. M., & Broome, M. E. (2006). Playing in the park: What school-age children tell us about imagery. *Journal of Pediatric Nursing, 21*(2), 115–125. https://doi.org/10.1016/j.pedn.2005.06.010

Jacobson, A. F., Umberger, W. A. Palmieri, P. A., Alexander, T. S., Myerscough, R. P., Draucker, C. B., Steudte-Schmiedgen, S., & Kirschbaum, C. (2016). Guided imagery for total knee replacement: A randomized, placebo-controlled pilot study. *Journal of Alternative and Complementary Medicine, 22*(7), 563–575. https://doi.org/10.1089/acm.2016.0038

Jallo, N., Cozens, R., Smith, M. W., & Simpson, R. I. (2013). Effects of a guided imagery intervention on stress in hospitalized pregnant women: A pilot study. *Holistic Nursing Practice, 27*(3), 129–139. https://doi.org/10.1097/HNP.0b013e31828b6270

Jallo, N., Ruiz, J., Elswick, R. K. Jr., & French, E. (2014). Guided imagery for stress and symptom management in pregnant African American women. *Evidence-Based Complementary and Alternative Medicine, 2014*, 840923. https://doi.org/10.1155/2014/840923

Ji, E. K., Wang, H. H., Jung, S. J., Lee, K. B., Kim, J. S., Jo, L., Hong, B. Y., & Lim, S. H. (2021). Graded motor imagery training as a home exercise program for upper limb motor function in patients with chronic stroke: A randomized controlled trial. *Medicine, 100*(3), e24351. https://doi.org/10.1097/MD.0000000000024351

Kaiser, P., Kohen, D. P., Brown, M., Kajander, R., & Barnes, A. J. (2018). Integrating pediatric hypnosis with complementary modalities: Clinical perspectives on personalized treatment. *Children, 5*, 108. https://doi.org/10.3390/children5080108

Kapogiannis, A., Tsoli, S., & Chrousos, G. (2018). Investigating the effects of the progressive muscle relaxation-guided imagery combination on patients with cancer receiving chemotherapy treatment: A systemic review of randomized controlled trials. *Explore, 14*(2), 137–142. http://doi.org/10.1016/j.explore.2017.10.008

Kemper, K. J., & Khirallah, M. (2015). Acute effects of online mind-body skills training on resilience, mindfulness, and empathy. *Journal of Evidence-Based Complementary and Alternative Medicine, 20*(4), 247–253. https://doi.org/10.1177/2156587215580882

Kho, A. Y., Liu, K. P. Y., & Chung, R. C. K. (2014). Meta-analysis on the effect of mental imagery on motor recovery of the hemiplegic upper extremity function. *Australian Occupational Therapy Journal, 61*, 38–48. https://doi.org/10.1111/1440-1630.12084

Kohen, D., & Olness, K. (2011). *Hypnosis and hypnotherapy with children* (4th ed.). Routledge.

Kraemer, K. M., Luberto, C. M., O'Bryan E. M., Mysinger, E., & Cotton, S. (2016). Mind-body skills training to improve distress in tolerance in medical students: A pilot study. *Teaching and Learning in Medicine, 28*(2), 219–228. https://doi.org/10.1080/10401334.2016.1146605

Krau, S. D. (2020). The multliple uses of guided imagery. *Nursing Clinics of North America, 55,* 467–474. https://doi.org/10.1016/j.cnur.2020.06.013

Kubes, L. F. (2015). Imagery for self-healing and integrative nursing practice. *The American Journal of Nursing, 115*(11), 36–43. https://doi.org/10.1097/01.NAJ.0000473313.17572.60

Kuttner, L. (2012). Pediatric hypnosis: Pre-, peri-, and post-anesthesia. *Pediatric Anesthesia, 22,* 573–577. https://doi.org/10.1111/j.1460-9592.2012.03860.x

Kwekkeboom, K. L., & Bratzke, L. C. (2016). A systematic review of relaxation, meditation, and guided imagery strategies for symptom management in heart failure. *Journal of Cardiovascular Nursing, 31*(5), 457–468. https://doi.org/10.1097/JCN.0000000000000274

Kwekkeboom, K. L., Hau, H., Wanta, B., & Bumpus, M. (2008). Patients' perceptions of the effectiveness of guided imagery and progressive muscle relaxation interventions used for cancer pain. *Complementary Therapies in Clinical Practice, 14,* 185–194. https://doi.org/10.1016/j.ctcp.2008.04.002

Kwekkeboom, K. L., Wanta, B., & Bumpus, M. (2008). Individual difference variables and the effects of progressive muscle relaxation and analgesic imagery interventions on cancer pain. *Journal of Pain and Symptom Management, 36*(6), 604–615. https://doi.org/10.1016/j.jpainsymman.2007.12.011

Lam, T., Chung, K. F., Yeung, W., Yu, B. Y., Yung, K. P., & Ng, T. H. (2015). Hypnotherapy for insomnia: A systematic review and meta-analysis of randomized controlled trials. *Complementary Therapies in Medicine, 23,* 719–732. https://doi.org/10.1016/j.ctim.2015.07.011

Langley, P., Fonseca, J., & Iphofen, R. (2006). Psychoneuroimmunology and health from a nursing perspective. *British Journal of Nursing, 15*(29), 1126–1129. https://doi.org/10.12968/bjon.2006.15.20.22298

La Roche, M. J., Batista, C., & D'Angelo, E. (2010). A content analyses of guided imagery scripts: A strategy for the development of cultural adaptations. *Journal of Clinical Psychology, 67*(1), 45–57. https://doi.org/10.1002/jclp.20742

Lee, M. H., Kim, D., & Yu, H. S. (2013). The effect of guided imagery on stress and fatigue in patients with thyroid cancer undergoing radioactive iodine therapy. *Evidence-Based Complementary and Alternative Medicine, 2013,* 130324. https://doi.org/10.1155/2013/130324

Lindfors, P., Unge, P., Arvidsson, P., Nyhlin, H., Björnsson, E., Abrahamsson, H., & Simrén, M. (2012). Effects of gut-directed hypnotherapy on IBS in different clinical settings: Results from two randomized, controlled trials. *American Journal of Gastroenterology, 107,* 276–285. https://doi.org/10.1038/ajg.2011.340

Loft, M. H., & Cameron, L. D. (2013). Using mental imagery to deliver self-regulation techniques to improve sleep behaviors. *Annals of Behavioral Medicine, 46,* 260–272. https://doi.org/10.1007/s12160-013-9503-9

McCance, K. L., & Huether, S. E. (2002). *Pathophysiology: The biologic basis for disease in adults and children* (4th ed.). Mosby.

Meeus, M., Nijs, J., Vanderheiden, T., Baert, I., Descheemaeker, F., & Struyf, F. (2015). The effect of relaxation therapy on autonomic functioning, in patients with chronic fatigue syndrome or fibromyalgia: A systematic review. *Clinical Rehabilitation, 29*(3), 221–233. https://doi.org/10.1177/0269215514542635

Meghani, N., Tracy, M. F., Hadidi, N. N., & Lindquist, R. (2017). Part II: The effects of aromatherapy and guided imagery for the management of anxiety, pain, and insomnia in critically ill patients. *Dimensions of Critical Care Nursing, 36*(6), 334–348. https://doi.org/10.1097/DCC0000000000000272

Meinlschmidt, G., Lee, J. H., Stalujanis, E., Belardi, A., Oh, M., Jung, E. K., Kim, H., Alfano, J., Yoo, S., & Tegethoff, M. (2016). Smartphone-based psychotherapeutic micro-interventions to improve mood in a real-world setting. *Frontiers in Psychology, 7,* 1112. https://doi.org/10.3389/fpsyg.2016.01112

Menzies, V., & Jallo, N. (2011). Guided imagery as a treatment option for fatigue. *Journal of Holistic Nursing, 29*(4), 279–286. https://doi.org/10.1177/0898010111412187

Menzies, V., & Kim, S. (2008). Relaxation and guided imagery in Hispanic persons diagnosed with fibromyalgia: A pilot study. *Family and Community Health, 31*(3), 204–212. https://doi .org/10.1097/01.FCH.0000324477.48083.08

Menzies, V., Lyon, E. E., Elswick, R. K., McCain, N. L., & Gray, D. P. (2014). Effects of guided imagery on biobehavioral factors in women with fibromyalgia. *Journal of Behavioral Medicine, 37*(1), 70–80. https://doi.org/10.1007/s10865-012-9464-7

Menzies, V., Taylor, A. G., & Bourguignon, C. (2006). Effects of guided imagery on outcomes of pain, functional status, and self-efficacy in persons diagnosed with fibromyalgia. *Journal of Alternative and Complementary Medicine, 12*(1), 12–30. https://doi.org/10.1089/acm.2006.12.23

Misra, S. M., Monico, E., Kao, G., Guffey, D., Kim, E., Khatker, M., Gilbert, C., Biard, M., Marcus, M., Roth, I., & Giardino, A. P. (2019). Addressing pain with inpatient integrative medicine at a large children's hospital. *Clinical Pediatrics (Phila), 58*(7), 738–745. https://doi .org/10.1177/0009922819839232

Mizrahi, M. C., Reicher-Atir, R., Levy, S., Haramati, S., Wengrower, D., Israeli, E., & Goldin, E. (2012). Effects of guided imagery with relaxation training on anxiety and quality of life among patients with inflammatory bowel disease. *Psychology and Health, 27*(12), 1463–1479. https://doi.org/10.1080/08870446.2012.691169

Molinari, G., Garcia-Palacios, A.,Engique, A., Comella, N. F., & Botella, C. (2018). The power of visualization: Back to the future of pain management in fibromyalgia syndrome. *Pain Medicine, 19*, 1451–1468. https://doi.org/10.1093/pm/pnx298

National Center for Complementary and Integrative Health. (2021). *Relaxation techniques: What you need to know.* U.S. Department of Health and Human Services. https://www.nccih.nih .gov/health/relaxation-techniques-what-you-need-to-know

Nelson, E. A., Dowsey, M. M., Knowles S. R., Castle, D. J., Salzberg, M. R., Monshat, K., Dunin, A. J., & Choong, P. F. M. (2013). Systematic review of the efficacy of pre-surgical mind-body based therapies on post-operative outcome measures. *Complementary Therapies in Medicine, 21*, 697–711. https://doi.org/10.1016/j.ctim.2013.08.020

Nilsson, S., Forsner, M., Finnström, B., & Mörelius, E. (2015). Relaxation and guided imagery do not reduce stress, pain, and unpleasantness for 11 to 12 year-old girls during vaccinations. *ACTA Paediatrica, 104*, 724–729. https://doi.org/10.1111/apa.13000

Olness, K. (2008). Helping children and adults with hypnosis and biofeedback. *Cleveland Clinic Journal of Medicine, 75*(Suppl. 2), S39–S43. https://doi.org/10.3949/ccjm.75.Suppl_2.S39

Onieva-Zafra, M. D., Garcia, L. H., & del Valle, M. G. (2015, January–February). Effectiveness of guided imagery relaxation on levels of pain and depression in patients diagnosed with fibromyalgia. *Holistic Nursing Practice, 29*, 13–21. https://doi.org/10.1097/HNP.000000000 0000062

Palsson, O. S., & van Tilburg, M. (2015). Hypnosis and guided imagery treatment for gastrointestinal disorders: Experience with scripted protocols developed at the University of North Carolina. *American Journal of Clinical Hypnosis, 58*(1), 5–21. https://doi.org/10.1080/00029157 .2015.1012705

Peerdeman, K. J., van Laarhoven, A. I. M., Donders, A. R. T., Hopman, M. T. E., Peters, M. L., & Evers, A. W. M. (2015). Inducing expectations for health: Effects of verbal suggestion and imagery on pain, itch, and fatigue as indicators of physical sensitivity. *PLOS ONE, 10*(10), e0139563. https://doi.org/10.1371/journal.pone.0139563

Posadzki, P., Lewandowski, W., Terry, R., Ernst, E., & Stearns, A. (2012). Guided imagery for non-musculoskeletal pain: A systematic review of randomized clinical trials. *Journal of Pain and Symptom Management, 44*(1), 95–104. https://doi.org/10.1016/j.jpainsymman.2011.07.014

Rao, N., & Kemper, K. J. (2017). The feasibility and effectiveness of online guided imagery training for health professionals. *Journal of Evidence-Based Complementary & Alternative Medicine, 22*(1), 54–58. https://doi.org/10.1177/2156587216631903

Reed, T. (2007). Imagery in the clinical setting: A tool for healing. *Nursing Clinics of North America, 42*, 261–277. https://doi.org/10.1016/j.cnur.2007.03.006

Rodriquez, R. M., Marroquin, A., & Cosby, N. (2019). Reducing fear of reinjury and pain perception in athletes with first-time anterior cruciate ligament reconstructions by implementing imagery training. *Journal of Sport Rehabilitation, 28*, 385–389. https://doi.org/10.1123/jsr.2017-0056

Roffe, L., Schmidt, K., & Ernst, E. (2005). A systematic review of guided imagery as an adjuvant cancer therapy. *Psycho-Oncology, 14*, 607–617. https://doi.org/10.1002/pon.889

Sawni, A., & Breuner, C. C. (2017). Clinical hypnosis, an effective mind-body modality for adolescents with behavioral and physical complaints. *Children, 4*(4), 19. https://doi.org/10.3390/children4040019

Schack, T., Essig, K., Frank, C., & Koester, D. (2014). Mental representation and motor imagery training. *Frontiers in Human Neuroscience, 8*(328), 1–10. https://doi.org/10.3389/fnhum.2014.00328

Schaffer, L., Jallo, N., Howland, L., James, K., Glaser, D., & Arnell, K. (2013). Guided imagery: An innovative approach to improving maternal sleep quality. *Journal of Perinatal and Neonatal Nursing, 27*(2), 151–159. https://doi.org/10.1097/JPN.0b013e3182870426

Scherwitz, L. W., McHenry, P., & Herrero, R. (2005). Interactive guided imagery therapy with medical patients: Predictors of health outcomes. *Journal of Alternative and Complementary Medicine, 11*(1), 69–83. https://doi.org/10.1089/acm.2005.11.69

Schuster, C., Hilfiker, R., Amft, O., Scheidhauer, A., Andrews, B., Butler, J., Kischka, U., & Ettlin, T. (2011). Best practice for motor imagery: A systematic literature review on motor imagery training elements in five different disciplines. *BMC Medicine, 9,* 75. http://www.biomedcentral.com/1741-7015/9/75

Sears, S. R., Bolton, S., & Bell, K. (2013). Evaluation of "Steps to Surgical Success" (STEPS): A holistic perioperative medicine program to manage pain and anxiety related to surgery. *Holistic Nursing Practice, 27*(6), 349–357. https://doi.org/10.1097/HNP.0b013e3182a72c5a

Segerstrom, S. (2010). Resources, stress, and immunity: An ecological perspective on human psychoneuroimmunology. *Annals of Behavioral Medicine, 40*, 114–125. https://doi.org/10.1007/s12160-010-9195-3

Serra, D., Parris, C. R., Carper, E., Homel, P., Fleishman, S. B., Harrison, L. B., & Chadha, M. (2012). Outcomes of guided imagery in patients receiving radiation therapy for breast cancer. *Clinical Journal of Oncology Nursing, 16*(6), 617–623. https://doi.org/10.1188/12.CJON.617-623

Shenefelt, P. D. (2013). Anxiety reduction using hypnotic induction and self-guided imagery for relaxation during dermatologic procedures. *International Journal of Clinical and Experimental Hypnosis, 61*(3), 305–318. https://doi.org/10.1080/00207144.2013.784096

Skeens, L. M. (2017). Guided imagery: A technique to benefit youth at risk. *National Youth-At-Risk Journal, 2*(2). https://doi.org/10.20429/nyarj.2017.020207

Spiva, L., Hart, P. L., Gallagher, E., McVay, F., Garcia, M., Malley, K., Kadner, M., Segars, M., Brakovich, B., Horton, S. Y., & Smith, N. (2015). The effects of guided imagery on patients being weaned from mechanical ventilation. *Evidence-Based Complementary and Alternative Medicine, 2015*, 802865. https://doi.org/10.1155/2015/802865

Suso-Martí, L., La Touche, R., Angulo-Diaz-Parreño, S., & Cuenca-Martínez, F. (2020). Effectiveness of motor imagery and action observation training on musculoskeletal pain intensity: A systematic review and meta-analysis. *European Journal of Pain, 24*, 886–901. https://doi.org/10.1002/ejp.1540

Trakhtenberg, E. C. (2009). The effects of guided imagery on the immune system: A critical review. *International Journal of Neuroscience, 118*, 839–855. https://doi.org/10.1080/00207450701792705

Tsitsi, T., Charalambous, A., Papastavrou, E., & Raftopoulos, V. (2017). Effectiveness of a relaxation intervention (progressive muscle relaxation and guided imagery) to reduce anxiety and improve mood of parents of hospitalized children with malignancies: A controlled trial in the Republic of Cyprus and Greece. *European Journal of Oncology Nursing, 26*, 9–18. https://doi.org/10.1016/j.ejon.2016.10.007

Vagnoli, L., Bettini, A., Amore, E., De Masi, S., & Messeri, A. (2019). Relaxation-guided imagery reduces perioperative anxiety and pain in children: A randomized study. *European Journal of Pediatrics, 178*, 913–921. https://doi.org/10.1007/s00431-019-03376-x

Van Kuiken, D. (2004). A meta-analysis of the effect of guided imagery practice on outcomes. *Journal of Holistic Nursing, 22*(2), 164–179. https://doi.org/10.1177/0898010104266066

Verkaik, R., Busch, M., Koeneman, T., Van Den Berg, R., Spreeuwenberg, P., & Francke, A. L. (2014). Guided imagery in people with fibromyalgia: A randomized controlled trial of effects on pain, functional status and self-efficacy. *Journal of Health Psychology, 19*(5), 678–688. https://doi.org/10.1177/1359105313477673

Winger, J. G., Rand, K. L., Hanna, N., Jalal, S. I., Einhorn, L. H., Birdas, T. J., Ceppa, D. P., Kesler, K. A., Champion, V. L., & Mosher, C. E. (2018). Coping skills practice and symptom change: A secondary analyis of a pilot telephone symptom management intervention for lung cancer patients and their family caregivers. *Journal of Pain and Symptom Management, 55*(5), 1341–1349. https://doi.org/10.1016/j.jpainsymman.2018.01.005

Yeh, A. M., Wren, A., & Golianu, B. (2017). Mind-body interventions for pediatric inflammatory bowel disease. *Children, 4,* 22. https://doi.org/10.3390/children4040022

Yijing, Z., Xiaoping, D., Fang, L., Xiaolu, J., & Bin, W. (2015). The effects of guided imagery on heart rate variability in simulated spaceflight emergency tasks performers. *BioMed Research International, 2015,* 687020. https://doi.org/10.1155/2015/687020

Zech, N., Hansen, E., Bernardy, K., & Häuser, W. (2017). Efficacy, acceptability and safety of guided imagery/hypnosis in fibromyalgia—A systematic review and meta-analysis of randomized controlled trials. *European Journal of Pain, 21,* 217–227. https://doi.org/10.1002/ejp.933

Zehetmair, C., Nagy, E., Leetz, C., Cranz, A., Kindermann, D., Reddemann, L., & Nikendei, C. (2020). Self-practice of stabilizing and guided imagery techniques for traumatized refugees via digital audio files: Qualitative study. *Journal of Medical Internet Research, 22*(9), e17906. https://doi.org/10.2196/17906

8

Music Intervention

LINDA L. CHLAN AND ANNIE HEIDERSCHEIT

Music has been used throughout history as a healing and treatment modality by shamans and Indigenous healers. Preliterate and ancient cultures throughout the world, such as Egypt, China, India, and Greece understood the healing nature of music and linked practices of medicine to music (Heiderscheit & Jackson, 2018). Nursing pioneer Florence Nightingale (1860/1969) recognized the healing power of music. Today, nurses can use music in a variety of settings to benefit patients and clients.

DEFINITIONS

Music has been simply described as sound organized with silence, designed for the purpose of human expression. It is the unique combination of different sounds with silence that allows music to express our range of emotions and experiences (Bruscia, 2014; Heiderscheit & Jackson, 2018;).

Several elements serve as the building blocks of music that are combined in an infinite number of ways to compose a song or piece of music. The combination of these elements is what allows a listener to recognize a song or piece of music as a unique entity. Exhibit 8.1 defines the specific elements and the functions of each element.

Exhibit 8.1 *Definitions and Functions of Musical Elements*		
MUSICAL ELEMENT	**DEFINITION**	**FUNCTION OF THE ELEMENT**
Rhythm	The systematic arrangement of patterns in music that allows it to be perceived as occurring in a particular relationship in time.	Provides the movement in the music and reveals the amount of energy expressed. Rhythm influences motor skills and activates muscles. Faster and intense rhythms create a sense of more intense energy; slow(er) rhythms can invoke a feeling of slowing down, peace, or calm.

(continued)

MUSICAL ELEMENT	DEFINITION	FUNCTION OF THE ELEMENT
Melody	The sequence of pitches and tones in time that create a "musical sentence." The frequency of a pitch is produced by the number of vibrations of the musical tone. Higher pitches have more rapid vibrations.	A tonal element used to express specific feelings. It is often the element a listener follows; it can serve to focus and engage the listener, providing distraction.
Harmony	A combination of pitches in relationship to each other and the melody, as the sounds are played or sung simultaneously. Adds richness and support; can be consonant (pleasing sound) or dissonant (sound of tension, conflict, or unpleasant).	A tonal element that communicates the connection or relationship between pitches. Cultural norms determine what a listener deems enjoyable and pleasant. Different tonal systems may sound dissonant in one culture.
Timbre	The characteristic and unique sounds of an instrument or voice. The construction, shape, materials, and technique impact the timbre of an instrument; voice is impacted by the vocalist's technique.	An expressive element that holds psychological significance. A listener often has associations of feelings, memories, and/or events with the sound.
Dynamics	The change(s) in sound intensity and volume in music; a full range of loudness to softness that remains consistent or changes throughout a piece.	Influence a listener's experience with music. Softer/quieter dynamics create a sense of calm, closeness, and intimacy; louder dynamics create feelings of energy and power.
Form	The structure of the musical piece; how music is structurally organized. Symphonies follow a form of four movements, whereas a song will include verses and a chorus.	Provides the listener a sense of comfort and predictability. A listener can become acquainted with the structure of a song or even a genre or style of music. Allows a listener to anticipate, predicate, and know what to expect.

Exhibit 8.1 *Definitions and Functions of Musical Elements (continued)*

Source: Heiderscheit, A., & Jackson, N. (2018). *Introduction to music therapy practice.* Barcelona Publishers; Rutherford-Johnson, T., Kennedy, M., & Kennedy, J. (2013). *The Oxford dictionary of music* (6th ed.). Oxford University Press.

Music therapists understand the functions of musical elements and are well versed in utilizing them to meet specific, individualized patient needs (Heiderscheit & Jackson, 2018). In the United States and around the world, music therapists are employed in a wide variety of healthcare facilities and clinical settings (American Music Therapy Association [AMTA], 2021; World Federation of

Music Therapy, 2014). Although music therapists are specifically trained to use music in various therapeutic ways, there are many situations in which nurses can implement music listening into a patient's plan of care. So as not to confuse the practice of music therapy by a board-certified music therapist (MT-BC), the use of music from a nursing perspective is represented by the term *music intervention* in this chapter.

SCIENTIFIC BASIS

Music is a complex auditory stimulus that affects the physiological, psychological, and spiritual dimensions of human beings (Bruscia, 2014). Individual responses to music can be influenced by personal preferences, experiences, demographic characteristics, the environment, education, and cultural factors (Heiderscheit, 2013). Processing of musical stimuli by the brain's auditory cortex includes musical perception, recognition, and emotion (Okumura et al., 2014). Musical elements such as melody, harmony, and consonance activate the brain bilaterally (Okumura et al., 2014). Listening to music that is perceived to be personally pleasurable can elicit an emotional response associated with dopamine activity in the brain's mesolimbic reward system (Salimpoor et al., 2011).

Entrainment, a physics principle, is a process whereby two objects vibrating at similar frequencies tend to cause mutual sympathetic resonance, resulting in their vibrating at the same frequency (Dissanayake, 2009). Entrainment also refers to the synchronization of body rhythms to an external rhythm (Bruscia, 2014; Hodges & Sebald, 2011). Music and physiological processes (including heartbeat, respiratory rate, blood pressure, brain waves, body temperature, digestion, and adrenal hormones) involve rhythms and vibrations that occur in a regular, periodic manner and consist of oscillations (Crowe, 2004). The rhythm and tempo of music can be used to synchronize or entrain body rhythms (e.g., heart rate and respiratory pattern) with resultant changes in physiological states. Certain properties of music (less than 80 beats per minute with fluid, consistent tempi) can be used to promote relaxation by causing body rhythms to slow down or entrain with the slower beat and regular, repetitive rhythm (Bradt et al., 2010; Davies et al., 2016; Pelletier, 2004).

The tempo of music also influences the parasympathetic and sympathetic nervous systems (Bernardi et al., 2006; Ooishi et al., 2017). Listening to relaxing, slow tempo music can increase salivary oxytocin and high-frequency components of heart rate variability, as well as decrease heart rate and cortisol levels, providing biomarkers of the relaxation response (Ooishi et al., 2017).

Likewise, music can decrease anxiety by occupying attention channels in the brain with meaningful, distractive auditory stimuli (Heiderscheit, 2013). Music intervention provides a patient with a familiar, comforting stimulus that can evoke pleasurable sensations (memories, feelings, experiences, etc.) while focusing the individual's attention on the music (distraction) instead of pain, discomfort, or other environmental stimuli (Heiderscheit, 2013). Music can also provide emotional support and help to combat loneliness when the listener feels a connection to the music or that the music or lyrics resonates with their own experience(s). This can allow music to function as a "social surrogate," helping a patient to feel a "sense of empathic company" (Schäfer et al., 2020, p. 1) impacting mood and fostering a feeling of comfort (Schäfer & Eerola, 2020; Schäfer et al., 2020).

INTERVENTION

Determining a patient's music preferences through assessment is essential; among the tools developed for this purpose is an assessment instrument by Chlan and Heiderscheit (2009) that elicits information on how frequently music is listened to; the type of music selections, artists, groups, and genres preferred; and the individual's reasons for listening to music. A brief music assessment tool is also available (Heiderscheit, 2021). For some people, the purpose of listening to music may be to relax, whereas others may prefer music that distracts, stimulates, and invigorates. After assessment data have been gathered, appropriate techniques with specific music can then be implemented (Heiderscheit et al., 2011, 2014).

MUSIC INTERVENTION

The use of music for intervention can take many forms such as listening, singing or playing, improvising, and composing music. While some of these methods require specialized training and specific equipment to facilitate, music listening is a viable and accessible intervention. There are a number of factors that should be kept in mind when considering the specific method: the type of music and personal preferences, active music-making versus passive listening, length of time involved with the music, and desired outcomes.

MUSIC LISTENING

Providing the means for patients to listen to music is the intervention technique most frequently implemented by nurses. Listening to music is very accessible given the available technologies. Music is available through mobile devices, smartphones, tablets, and computers (Krause et al., 2015). Advancements in digital technologies provide immediate access to a wide array of music (Anderson et al., 2021). Music can be purchased and downloaded from reputable internet sources (www.MyMusicInc.com or iTunes®) or accessed through streaming services (Spotify, Amazon Prime Music, Tidal, Qobuz, etc.). Access to many different platforms makes it easy to provide music intervention for patients in a wide range of healthcare settings. Mobile devices are relatively inexpensive; they are small and can be used in even the most crowded confines, such as critical care units. Digital music files have superior sound clarity and track selection that allows a patient to make an immediate choice of a desired piece of music. Tablets and mobile devices can be used to provide a menu of music choices. Comfortable headphones allow patients private listening that does not disturb others. Equipment selected for music intervention should be easy for patients to use with minimal effort or with assistance. Patients may or may not have familiarity with various technologies, therefore the method of music delivery should be considered. It is important to consider patient dexterity and visual acuity to determine what method of music listening will be most appropriate.

Nurses can encourage patients and their family members to bring their own music from home to use while hospitalized. Patients may already have their own preferred music available on a mobile device or tablet. The Public Radio Music Source (n.d.) offers diverse music for purchase. It is also easy to individualize a digital music library or playlists to accommodate the preferences of each patient. Attention to copyright laws is necessary when downloading music (www .copyright.gov).

Although various musical genres are available on the radio, the internet, or music-streaming services, commercial messages and talking are deterrents to their use for music listening interventions. Likewise, the quality of the radio signal reception or the specific music selections cannot be controlled. Premium options without commercial messages are available for purchase through music streaming services.

MUSIC LISTENING FOR INTERVENTIONS

Careful attention to the selection of the music contributes to its therapeutic effect. For example, music to induce relaxation has a consistent and steady rhythm (less than 80 beats per minute); a melody that is smooth, flowing, and predictable, with a small range of interval dynamics; and a harmonic structure that is consonant and pleasing, with instrumentation that the individual enjoys (Ghetti, 2012; Grocke & Wigram, 2006). It is important to note that past experiences can influence one's response to music and that music can elicit a powerful emotional response or reaction at times. Refer to Exhibit 8.1 for details.

GUIDELINES

Music intervention for relaxation uses music as a pleasant stimulus to block out feelings of anxiety, fear, and attenuate stress (Khan et al., 2018; Yue et al., 2021). Although the definition of relaxing music may vary by individual, factors affecting responses to music include individual musical preferences (Heiderscheit, 2013), a familiarity with selections, and cultural background. Relaxing music should have a tempo at or below a resting heart rate (less than 80 beats per minute), predictable dynamics, fluid melodic movement, pleasing harmonies, regular rhythm without sudden changes, and tonal qualities that include strings, flute, piano, or specially synthesized music (Ghetti, 2012). One of the most widely used classical music selections for relaxation is Pachelbel's Canon in D Major. In the last several years, many music companies have been producing recordings specifically packaged as music for relaxation. There are many recordings available in various genres and styles that can also include various instrumentation and environmental sounds. Exhibit 8.2 outlines the basic steps for implementing music listening intervention for promoting relaxation in patients.

TECHNOLOGY

Advances in digital technology make music accessible and a viable option for patient self-directed listening. Mobile devices and streaming services provide immediate access to music and music libraries (Anderson et al., 2021), changing the way we interact and use music (Fricke et al., 2019; Krause et al., 2015). Newer digital technologies and delivery platforms allow listeners to have individual control over music and allow access to music in various places and spaces (Heiderscheit, 2021; Krause et al., 2105). These include a compact disc player or a digital device such as a tablet or personal mobile smartphone. Music can be accessed through streaming platforms (Spotify™, Apple Music™) or an internal platform (GetWell Network™).

There are a number of factors to consider when selecting a delivery platform for music listening. The method of delivery needs to be accessible to patients, and the operation of the equipment needs to be feasible based on their abilities. The funds

Exhibit 8.2 *Guidelines for Music Intervention for Relaxation*

1. Ascertain that patient has adequate hearing
2. Ascertain the patient's like/dislike for music
3. Assess music preferences and previous experience with music for relaxation
4. Provide a choice of relaxing selections; assist with CD/MP3/tablet selections as needed
5. Determine mutually agreed-upon goals for music intervention with the patient
6. Complete all nursing care prior to intervention; allow for a minimum of 20 minutes of uninterrupted listening time
7. Gather equipment (CD or MP3 player, smartphone, tablet device, CDs, headphones, fresh batteries) and ensure all are in good working order
8. Test volume and comfort of volume level with the patient prior to intervention
9. Assist patient to a comfortable position as needed; ensure call light is within easy reach and assist patient with equipment as needed
10. Enhance environment as needed (e.g., draw blinds, close door, turn off lights)
11. Post a "Do Not Disturb" sign to minimize unnecessary interruptions
12. Encourage and provide the patient with opportunities to practice relaxation with music
13. Document patient responses to music intervention
14. After using music intervention, discuss the patient's experience and any emotions they noticed as they listened. Discuss the usefulness of the intervention with the patient. Identify whether they encountered any challenges or problems with the equipment
15. Revise intervention plan and goal(s) as needed

Note: Initiating music intervention without first assessing a person's likes and dislikes may produce deleterious effects. Because of music's effect on the limbic system, it can bring about intense emotional responses. Using portable players with headphones may be inappropriate or prohibited for patients in psychiatric settings, who may use the equipment cords for self-harm.

available to provide music and purchase equipment need to be considered, as this may impact which method of delivery is feasible; maintaining the listening platform is also important. Institutions need to be aware of copyright laws and restrictions that may apply regarding the use of music (Heiderscheit, 2021). It is also important to consider the use of headphones for music listening. Using headphones can help enhance the listening experience by blocking out extraneous noises and avoid adding additional sound in busy patient care areas. Finally, it can be helpful to consider more than one platform. For example, an institution may provide music for patients using a streaming platform as well as encourage patients to bring their own personal music from a mobile device.

MEASUREMENT OF OUTCOMES

The outcome indices for evaluating the effectiveness of music intervention vary, depending on the purpose for which the music is used. Results may be physiological and/or psychological alterations and include a decrease in anxiety or stress arousal, promotion of relaxation, increase in social interaction, reduction in the need for medications, and increase in overall well-being. The nurse should carefully consider the goals of intervention and select outcome measurements and appropriate instruments accordingly.

PRECAUTIONS

It is imperative that music preferences be assessed prior to initiating a music-listening intervention. Everyone has "musical memories" and listening to a piece of music can bring up a myriad of emotions, even negative emotions that can be detrimental to an individual's well-being and also negatively impact the goals of intervention. Likewise, using music for diversion in patients with tenuous or unstable cardiovascular status should be done with extreme caution. Patients should be closely monitored for any untoward cardiovascular responses.

AGE-RELATED IMPLICATIONS OR ADJUSTMENTS NEEDED FOR OPTIMAL IMPLEMENTATION

Older adults may require additional precautions prior to music listening interventions. Older adults may enjoy patriotic and popular songs from an earlier era or hymns with slower tempos played with familiar instruments. Religious music may be preferred by those unable to attend spiritual services, and for whom faith is important. Volume and bass may need to be adjusted to accommodate and match hearing acuity. Headphones are ideal for masking background noise that can interfere with hearing acuity. Careful selection of equipment for music-listening interventions requires special attention to comfort, dexterity, and/or vision impairments. Diminishing dexterity or vision may impact the frequency or use of individual music listening.

USES

Music has been tested as a therapeutic intervention with many different patient populations; a majority of the nursing literature focuses on individualized music listening. Exhibit 8.3 highlights selected patient populations, clinical settings, and purposes for which music listening has been tested.

Exhibit 8.3 *Uses of Music Intervention*

Decreasing Anxiety: Reducing the physiological and emotional effects of anxiety
Awaiting dental treatment (Thoma et al., 2015)
Surgical patients (Ames et al., 2017; Kuhlmann et al., 2018; Ugras et al., 2018)
Endoscopy procedure (Wang et al., 2014)
Persons with end-stage renal disease on maintenance hemodialysis (Kim et al., 2015)
Ventilator-dependent intensive care unit (ICU) patients (Chlan et al., 2013; Davis & Jones, 2012; Heiderscheit et al., 2011)
Coronary angiogram (Çetinkaya et al., 2018)
Anxiety reduction for nurses (Zamanifar et al., 2020)

Decreasing Pain: Pain Management Adjuvant
Acute pain (Feneberg et al., 2020; Huang et al., 2010; Ko et al., 2019; Koelsch et al., 2011); post-operative pain (Kuhlmann et al., 2018); reducing perioperative medication requirements (Fu et al., 2020)

(continued)

> **Exhibit 8.3** *Uses of Music Intervention (continued)*
>
> Chronic pain management (Garza-Villarreal et al., 2017; Guetin et al., 2012; Hunt et al., 2021)
> Interventional radiological procedures (Kulkarni et al., 2012)
>
> **Stress Reduction and Relaxation**
> Mechanically ventilated ICU patients (Conrad et al., 2007)
> Hospitalized psychiatric patients (Yang et al., 2012)
> Sleep enhancement for medical ICU patients (Su et al., 2013)
>
> **Distraction**
> Bone marrow biopsy and aspiration (Shabanloei et al., 2010)
> Discomfort with noninvasive ventilation (Messika et al., 2019)
> Emergency department brief intervention pain and anxiety (Chai et al., 2020)
> Hemodialysis-associated pain and anxiety (Kim et al., 2015; Lin et al., 2012)
>
> **Mood Management/Quality of Life**
> Cancer radiotherapy treatment–associated symptoms and quality of life (Alcantara-Silva et al., 2018)
> Managing negative or depressive mood states (Heiderscheit & Madson, 2015)
> Reduction of sadness, worry, tiredness, and fear in healthcare workers (Giordano et al., 2020)

DECREASING ANXIETY AND STRESS

One of the strongest effects of music is anxiety reduction (Chlan et al., 2013; Kuhlmann et al., 2018). Music can enhance the immediate environment, provide distraction, and lessen the impact of potentially disturbing sounds (Heiderscheit, 2013) during recovery from surgical procedures (Ebneshahidi & Mohseni, 2008; Ghetti, 2012; Kuhlmann et al., 2018). The effect of music intervention on the stress response has been documented in ventilator-dependent ICU patients (Almerud & Peterson, 2003; Chlan, 1998; Chlan et al., 2013; Conrad et al., 2007; Heiderscheit et al., 2011; Wong et al., 2001). Empowering ICU patients receiving mechanical ventilatory support to self-manage their anxiety levels with preferred relaxing music results in the need for less intense sedative medication regimens (Chlan et al., 2013). Likewise, music intervention during the postoperative recovery period can reduce the need for opioid and sedative medications (Fu et al., 2020). Listening to specially composed slow-tempo piano music has been found to induce relaxation and promote sleep in a small sample of patients in a medical ICU (Su et al., 2013).

DECREASING PAIN

Patients typically experience pain after any given surgical procedure. Music listening is effective in reducing pain both during general anesthesia as well as during postoperative recovery (Kuhlmann et al., 2018). Furthermore, self-selected music can reduce pain associated with chronic conditions (Garza-Villarreal et al., 2017). It is imperative to keep in mind that music intervention should never be used in place of pharmacological therapy for the management of acute or severe pain. Music can, however, serve as an adjunctive intervention for pain management, particularly when individuals are empowered to select their own music (Garza-Villarreal et al., 2017).

DISTRACTION

Music is an effective adjunctive intervention for creating distraction, particularly for procedures that induce untoward symptoms and distress, such as pain and anxiety with hemodialysis (Kim et al., 2015; Lin et al., 2012) and in distracting patients from the discomfort of receiving noninvasive ventilation (Messika et al., 2019). A brief music listening experience can distract patients from the distress of the emergency department setting (Chai et al., 2020).

MUSIC LISTENING FOR NURSES

The COVID-19 pandemic has intensified and highlighted the stress that nurses experience as they address the needs of patients and families. Recent research has indicated healthcare workers are reporting higher levels of stress, anxiety, depression, and post-traumatic stress disorder (PTSD) (Gilleen et al., 2021; Hammond et al., 2021; Jagiasi et al., 2021; Shaukat et al., 2020). The effectiveness of music listening in patient populations has led researchers to utilize this music intervention to help nurses and healthcare workers manage stress and cope during this unprecedented time. Catlin et al. (2019) found that nurses demonstrated statistically significant improvements in centering themselves, calmness, peacefulness, and connecting with patients after listening to a capella music. Zamanifar et al. (2020) found that music listening paired with aromatherapy significantly decreased nurses' levels of anxiety. Giordano et al. (2020) found that as healthcare workers listened to music from research-created playlists over a 4-week period, they reported significantly decreased intensity of perceived sadness, worry, tiredness, and fear.

HOW TO LOCATE A BOARD-CERTIFIED MUSIC THERAPIST FOR CONSULTATION OR COLLABORATION

Given the importance of music preference assessment and knowledge of the physiological and psychological influences of music on a listener, it may be appropriate for a nurse to consult or collaborate with a professional music therapist prior to instituting music-listening interventions. One source to locate a music therapist in the United States is the American Music Therapy Association (www.musictherapy .org). For international needs contact the World Federation of Music Therapy (www.wfmt.info.org).

CULTURAL ASPECTS

Although music may indeed be considered a universal phenomenon, there is no universal language to music. Various cultures structure music differently from what is usual to the average Western listener. For example, music from Eastern cultures contains very different rhythmic, tonal structures and timbre, which can be foreign to the Western listener. Likewise, individuals from a non-Western culture may find the classical music of Mozart or Beethoven foreign-sounding and irritating. These structural differences in what various cultures consider music are crucial to consider when implementing music-listening interventions. These cultural aspects of music highlight the importance of music preference assessment.

There is interest in music for clinical applications around the world. Investigators in their clinical settings are exploring the benefits of music to address patient conditions that they encounter. Sidebar 8.1 provides a theoretical and clinical example of music therapy in India.

Sidebar 8.1 *Music Therapy as a Salutogenic Approach Into Medical Care: Indian Perspectives*

Sumathy Sundar

Setting the Scene

In India, in recent times music therapy has been introduced as an innovative method of patient care service in regular medical care with an interest in shifting from the pathogenic approach of focusing on factors causing the diseases to a salutogenic approach of focusing on factors influencing health (Sundar, 2016). This is supported by a steady surge of empirical evidence in understanding the mechanisms underlying the therapeutic effects of music. On one hand, the scientific aspect of music therapy is understood in a universal music therapy language. On the other hand, the "field of play" (Kenny, 2013) in music therapy is explained and understood in terms of the indigenous cultural practices and healing traditions with the use of the unique microtonal Indian music. Both the strengths and the challenges faced in integrating these two paradoxes of science and traditions in music therapy practice from the Indian context are explained in this sidebar.

Hospital-Based Clinical Practice

The "field of play" for music therapy in India is a beautiful reconciliation of science and tradition.

While the scientific aspects of understanding the benefits of music and understanding the therapeutic processes remain in the global framework, traditional healing practices used in the "field of play" are scientifically validated wherever possible in understanding the benefits of music therapy applications. This is the most challenging part, as traditional healing practices are inherent not so much with words but by the "feeling in one's body, heart and soul," as well as one's belief in these practices. It is important to recognize that these practices require validation. Relevant musicological and spiritual theories are also integrated into practice and research. A few popular healing applications utilized in the Indian music therapy field of play are *Raga Cikitsa*, Ayurveda, and Time Theory of *Ragas*. As there is increasing evidence suggesting the role of emotional factors in diseases, the beneficial effects of different *ragas* (*Raga Cikitsa*) are explained by eliciting positive emotions in the listener. These emotional responses to music

Sidebar 8.1 *Music Therapy as a Salutogenic Approach Into Medical Care: Indian Perspectives (continued)*

can be explained by several mechanisms like (a) brain stem reflexes, (b) rhythmic entrainment, (c) evaluative conditioning, (d) contagion, (e) visual imagery, (f) episodic memory, or (g) musical expectancy (Juslin et al., 2010). Time Theory of *Ragas* is another interesting concept in Indian classical music in that each *raga* is assigned a specific time of the day/night for performing/listening. It is believed that the effects of a *raga* are best produced when it is performed or listened to during the specific time period assigned to it. This perspective can be tested by integrating concepts of the Time Theory of *Ragas* and the chronobiological Ayurvedic concepts of assigning the biological energies of *Vata, Pitha,* and *Kapha* humors, divided into different 24-hour-a-day time zones in accordance with their active and inactive functional states (Sundar et al., 2016).

In India, music therapists work in many hospital clinical departments including pediatrics, nephrology, obstetrics and gynecology, respiratory medicine, cardiology, oncology, dermatology, surgery, and psychiatry. Likewise, music therapists work in the areas of procedural support (both diagnostic and interventional), pain management, neurological rehabilitation, in community settings serving psychiatric and transgender individuals, older adults, and children with special needs in outreach programs. Some common reasons for music therapy referral include pre-procedural anxiety, pain perception, sleep quality, clinical depression, quality of life, emotional regulation, attention, and behavioral and communication issues. Music therapists also work with pregnant women to help them through a healthy pregnancy and deliver a healthy baby through a traditional *Garbh-Sanskar* (learning in the womb) program and to reduce their delivery anxiety.

Conclusion

Music therapy practice in India is strongly influenced by its cultural practices and musical traditions. Efforts are being made by music therapist researchers to explore, evaluate, understand, apply, and integrate concepts of Indian music healing traditions into current music therapy practice.

References

Juslin, P., Liljestrom, S., Vastfjall, D., & Lundqvist, L. (2010). How does music evoke emotions? Exploring underlying mechanisms. In P. Juslin & J. Sloboda (Eds.), *Handbook of music and emotion: Theory research, applications* (pp. 605–642). Oxford University Press.

Kenny, C. (2013). *Music therapy theory: Yearning for beautiful ideas. Voices Resources.* https://voices.no/community/index.html?q=fortnightly-columns%252F2001-music-therapy-theory-yearning-beautiful-ideas

Sundar, S. (2016). Can interdisciplinary collaborative research result in newer understandings towards therapeutic effects of music? *Annals of Sri Balaji Vidyapeeth, 5*(2), 6. https://doi.org/10.5005/jp-journals-10085-5203

Sundar, S., Durai, P., & Parmar, P. (2016). Indian classical music as receptive music therapy improves *tridoshic* balance and major depression in a pregnant woman. *International Journal of Ayurveda and Pharma Research, 4*(9), 8–11. https://ijapr.in/index.php/ijapr/article/view/414

FUTURE RESEARCH

Although the evidence base is increasing, the following are areas in which research is needed to further build the science of music listening intervention:

■ Meta-analyses have been published on the consistent effects of music intervention on preoperative anxiety (Bradt, Dileo, & Shim, 2013), anxiety reduction in critically ill patients receiving mechanical ventilatory support (Bradt & Dileo, 2014; Bradt et al., 2010), coronary heart disease patients (Bradt, Dileo, & Potvin, 2013), oncology patients (Bradt et al., 2016), and managing the interconnected symptoms of anxiety and pain during the postoperative period (Kuhlmann et al., 2018). Whereas music consistently induces favorable outcomes, investigations are needed that build on the findings of these meta-analyses through the consistent use of instruments to measure important clinical outcomes and the conduct of multisite clinical trials. One source for obtaining valid and reliable instruments to measure a variety of health outcomes is from the Patient-Reported Outcomes Measurement Information System (PROMIS®; www .healthmeasures.net/explore-measurement-systems/promis).   Furthermore, identifying a core set of instruments to consistently measure common symptoms would build the scientific basis of music listening interventions.

■ Additional exploration into the management of co-occurring symptoms and symptom clusters would enhance the scientific base of music intervention. For example, persons with cancer typically experience nausea, vomiting, distress, and fatigue with treatments. Can the implementation of carefully selected music and its delivery improve a constellation of symptoms? Can persons experiencing cancer treatment be empowered to engage in symptom self-management through the initiation of preferred music for anxiety reduction?

■ Much of the evidence in the available literature focuses on immediate or short-term effects of music intervention. To advance science, investigators should consider longitudinal research designs to begin to address important questions such as whether music listening interventions improve outcomes and quality of life in individuals with chronic health conditions.

■ There is an urgent need for the utilization of innovative research designs and more rapid integration of music listening into clinical practice. Music listening has been documented to be a safe nonpharmacological intervention that holds great benefit in numerous patient populations. Implementation of music listening interventions into clinical settings is needed to ensure rapid uptake of these research findings into clinical practice in a more expedient manner through the conduct of pragmatic clinical trials. Whether music listening is a cost-effective or cost-neutral intervention and, if cost-effective, which patient care settings or specific symptom(s) could be included in pragmatic trial designs.

Although an intervention study itself is labor-intensive, there is a need for additional investigation on music intervention. The knowledge base about music intervention for promoting patient/client health and well-being can be expanded through high-quality research and by dissemination of those findings in a timely manner. To further build a strong body of knowledge surrounding the implementation and outcomes of music intervention, the authors of this chapter recommend an interdisciplinary approach, including nurses and music therapists conducting collaborative research. From quality evidence, music-intervention implementation guidelines can then be integrated into patient care.

REFERENCES

Alcantara-Silva, T. R., de Freitas-Junior, R., Aires Freitas, N. M., de Paula Junior, W., da Silva, D. J., Pinhero Machado, G. D., Alves Ribeiro, M. K., Paiva Carneiro, J., & Ribeiro Soares, L. (2018). Music therapy reduces radiotherapy-induced fatigue in patients with breast or gynecological cancer: A randomized trial. *Integrative Cancer Therapies, 17*(3), 628–635. https://doi .org/10.1177/1534735418757349

Almerud, S., & Peterson, K. (2003). Music therapy—A complementary treatment for mechanically ventilated intensive care patients. *International Critical Care Nursing, 19*(1), 21–30. https://doi .org/10.1016/s0964-3397(02)00118-0

American Music Therapy Association. (2021). *AMTA member and workforce analysis.*

Ames, N., Shuford, R., Yang, L., Moriyama, B., Frey, M., Wilson, F., Sundaramurthi, T., Gori, D. Mannes, A., Ranucci, A., Koziol, D., & Wallen, Q. (2017). Music listening among postoperative patients in the intensive care unit: A randomized controlled trial with mixed-methods analysis. *Integrative Medicine Insights, 12*, 1–13. https://doi.org/10.1177/1178633717716455.

Anderson, I., Santiago, G., Gibson, C., Wolf, S., Shapiro, W., Semerci, O., & Greenberg, D. (2021). "Just the way you are": Linking music listening to Spotify and personality. *Social Psychology and Personality Science, 12*(4), 561–572. https://doi.org/10.1177/1948550620923228

Bernardi, L., Porta, C., & Sleight, P. (2006). Cardiovascular, cerebrovascular, and respiratory changes induced by different types of music in musicians and non-musicians: The importance of silence. *Heart, 92*, 445–452. https://doi.org/10.1136/hrt.2005.064600

Bradt, J., & Dileo, C. (2014). Music interventions for mechanically ventilated patients. *Cochrane Database of Systematic Reviews, 2014*(12), CD006902. https://doi.org/10.1002/14651858 .CD006902.pub3

Bradt, J., Dileo, C., & Grocke, D. (2010). Music interventions for mechanically ventilated patients. *Cochrane Database of Systematic Reviews,* (12), CD006902. https://doi.org/10.1002/14651858 .CD006902.pub2

Bradt, J., Dileo, C., Magill, L., & Teague, A. (2016). Music interventions for improving psychological and physical outcomes in cancer patients. *Cochrane Database of Systematic Reviews,* (8), CD006911. https://doi.org/10.1002/14651858.CD006911.pub3

Bradt, J., Dileo, C., & Potvin, N. (2013). Music for stress and anxiety reduction in coronary heart disease patients. *Cochrane Database of Systematic Reviews,* (12), CD006577. https://doi .org/10.1002/14651858.CD006577.pub3

Bradt, J., Dileo, C., & Shim, M. (2013). Music interventions for preoperative anxiety. *Cochrane Database of Systematic Reviews,* (6), CD006908. https://doi.org/10.1002/14651858.CD006908 .pub2

Bruscia, K. (2014). *Defining music therapy* (3rd ed.). Barcelona Publishers.

Catlin, A., Cobbina, M., Dougherty, R., & Laws, D. (2019). Music, spirituality, and caring science: The effect of a cappella song on healthcare staff in medical–surgical Units. *International Journal for Human Caring, 23*(3), 234–241. https://doi.org/10.20467/1091-5710.23.3.234

Çetinkaya, F., Asiret, G., Yilmaz, C., & Inci, S. (2018). Effect of listening to music on anxiety and physiological parameters during coronary angiography: A randomized clinical trial. *European Journal of Integrative Medicine, 23*, 37–42. https://doi.org/10.1016/j.eujim.2018 .09.004

Chai, P. R., Schwartz, E., Hasdianda, M. A., Azizoddin, D. R., Kikut, A., Jambaulikar, G. D., Edwards, R., Boyer, E., & Schriber, K. (2020). A brief music app to address pain in the emergency department: Prospective study. *Journal of Medical Internet Research, 22*(5), e18537. https://doi.org/10.2196/18537

Chlan, L. (1998). Effectiveness of a music therapy intervention on relaxation and anxiety for patients receiving ventilatory assistance. *Heart & Lung, 27*(3), 169–176. https://doi.org/10.1016/s0147-9563(98)90004-8

Chlan, L., & Heiderscheit, A. (2009). A tool for music preference assessment in critically ill patients receiving mechanical ventilatory support: An interdisciplinary approach. *Music Therapy Perspectives, 27*(1), 42–47. https://doi.org/10.1093/mtp/27.1.42

Chlan, L., Weinert, C., Heiderscheit, A., Tracy, M. F., Skaar, D., Guttormson, J., & Savik, K. (2013). Effects of patient directed music intervention on anxiety and sedative exposure in critically ill patients receiving mechanical ventilatory support. *JAMA: Journal of the American Medical Association, 309*(22), 2335–2344. https://doi.org/10.1001/jama.2013.5670

Conrad, C., Niess, H., Jauch, K. W., Bruns, C., Hartl, W., & Welker, L. (2007). Overture for growth hormone: Requiem for interleukin-6? *Critical Care Medicine, 35*(12), 2709–2713. https://doi.org/10.1097/01.ccm.0000291648.99043.b9

Crowe, B. (2004). *Music and soul making: Toward a new theory of music therapy.* The Scarecrow Press.

Davies, R., Baker, F., Tamplin, J., Bajo, E., Bolger, K., Sheers, N., & Berlowitz, D. (2016). Music-assisted relaxation during transition to non-invasive ventilation in people with motor neuron disease: A qualitative case series. *British Journal of Music Therapy, 30*(2), 74–82. https://doi.org/10.1177/1359457516669153

Davis, T., & Jones, P. (2012). Music therapy: Decreasing anxiety in the ventilated patient: A review of the literature. *Dimensions of Critical Care Nursing, 31*(3), 159–166. https://doi.org/10.1097/DCC.0b013e31824dffc6

Dissanayake, W. (2009). Bodies swayed to music: The temporal arts as integral to ceremonial ritual. In S. Malcok & C. Trevarthen (Eds.), *Communicative musicality: Exploring the basis of human companionship* (pp. 17–30). Oxford University Press.

Ebneshahidi, A., & Mohseni, M. (2008). The effect of patient-selected music on early postoperative pain, anxiety, and hemodynamic profile in cesarean section surgery. *Journal of Alternative and Complementary Medicine, 14*(7), 827–831. https://doi.org/10.1089/acm.2007.0752

Feneberg, A., Kappert, M., Maldhof, R., Doering, B., Olbrich, D., & Nater, U. (2020). Efficacy, treatment characteristics and biopsychological mechanisms of music-listening interventions in reducing pain (MINTREP): Study protocol of a three-armed pilot randomized controlled trial. *Frontiers in Psychiatry, 11*, 1–18. https://doi.org/10.3389/fpsyt.2020.518316.

Fricke, K., Greenberg, D., Rentfrow, P., & Herzberg, P. (2019). Measuring musical preferences from listening behavior: Data from one million people and 200,000 songs. *Psychology of Music, 49*(3), 371–381. https://doi.org/10.1177/0305735619868280

Fu, V. X., Oomens, P., Klimek, M., Verhofstad, M. H. J., & Jeekel, J. (2020). The effect of perioperative music on medication requirement and hospital length of stay. *Annals of Surgery, 272*(6), 961–972. https://doi.org/10.1097/SLA.0000000000003506

Garza-Villarreal, E. A., Pando, V., Vuust, P., & Parsons, C. (2017). Music-induced analgesia in chronic pain conditions: A systematic review and meta-analysis. *Pain Physician, 20*, 597–610. https://doi.org/10.1101/105148

Ghetti, C. (2012). Music therapy as procedural support for invasive medical procedures: Toward the development of music therapy theory. *Nordic Journal of Music Therapy, 21*(1), 3–35. https://doi.org/10.1080/08098131.2011.571278

Gilleen, J., Santaolalla, A., Valdearenas, L., Salice, C., & Fusté, M. (2021). Impact of the COVID-19 pandemic on the mental health and well-being of UK healthcare workers. *BJPsych Open, 7*(3), e88. https://doi.org/10.1192/bjo.2021.42

Giordano, F., Scarlata, E., Baroni, M., Gentile, E., Puntillo, F., Brienza, N., & Gesualdo, L. (2020). Receptive music therapy to reduce stress and improve wellbeing in Italian clinical staff involved in COVID-19 pandemic: A preliminary study. *The Arts in Psychotherapy, 70*, 101688. https://doi.org/10.1016/j.aip.2020.101688

Grocke, D., & Wigram, T. (2006). *Receptive methods in music therapy: Techniques and clinical applications for music therapy clinicians, educators and students.* Jessica Kingsley Publishers.

Guetin, S., Ginies, P., Siou, D. K., Picot, M. C., Pommie, C., Guldner, E., Ostyn, K., Coudeyre, E., & Touchon, J. (2012). The effects of music intervention in the management of chronic pain: A single-blind, randomized, controlled trial. *Clinical Journal of Pain, 28*(4), 329–337. https://doi .org/10.1097/AJP.0b013e31822be973

Hammond, N. E., Crowe, L., Abbenbroek, B., Elliott, R., Tian, D. H., Donaldson, L. H., Fitzgerald, E., Flower, O., Grattan, S., Harris, R., Sayers, L., & Delaney, A. (2021). Impact of the corona-virus disease 2019 pandemic on critical care healthcare workers' depression, anxiety, and stress levels. *Australian Critical Care, 34*(2), 146–154. https://doi.org/10.1016/j.aucc.2020.12.004

Heiderscheit, A. (2013). Music therapy in surgical and procedural support for adult medical patients. In J. Allen (Ed.), *Guidelines for music therapy with adult medical patients* (pp. 17–34). Barcelona Publishers.

Heiderscheit, A. (2021). Non-pharmacological management of symptoms during mechanical ventilation and chronic obstructive pulmonary disease in critical care: Patient directed music listening. In K. Chung Ong (Ed.), *Chronic obstructive pulmonary disease—A current conspectus*. IntechOpen. https://doi.org/10.5572/intechopen.95889

Heiderscheit, A., Breckenridge, S., Chlan, L., & Savik, K. (2014). Music preferences of mechani-cally ventilated patients participating in a randomized controlled trial. *Music and Medicine, 6*(2), 29–38. https://doi.org/10.47513/mmd.v6i2.177

Heiderscheit, A., Chlan, L., & Donely, K. (2011). Instituting a music listening intervention for critically ill patients receiving mechanical ventilation: Exemplars from two patient cases. *Music and Medicine, 3*(4), 239–245. https://doi.org/10.1177/1943862111410981

Heiderscheit, A., & Jackson, N. (2018). *Introduction to music therapy practice*. Barcelona Publishers.

Heiderscheit, A., & Madson, A. (2015). Use of the iso principle as a central method in mood man-agement: A music psychotherapy clinical case study. *Music Therapy Perspectives, 33*(1), 45–52. https://doi.org/10.1093/mtp/miu042

Hodges, D., & Sebald, D. (2011). *Music in the human experience: An introduction to music psychology.* Routledge.

Huang, S., Good, M., & Zauszniewski, J. (2010). The effectiveness of music in relieving pain in cancer patients: A randomized controlled trial. *International Journal of Nursing Studies, 47*(11), 1354–1362. https://doi.org/10.1016/j.ijnurstu.2010.03.008

Hunt, A. M., Fachner, J., Clark-Vetri, R., Raffa, R. B., Rupnow-Kidd, C., Maidhof, C., & Dileo, C. (2021). Neuronal effects of listening to entrainment music versus preferred music in patients with chronic cancer pain as measured via EEG and LORETA imaging. *Frontiers in Psychology, 12*, 390. https://doi.org/10.3389/fpsyg.2021.588788

Jagiasi, B. G., Chanchalani, G., Nasa, P., & Tekwani, S. (2021). Impact of COVID-19 pandemic on the emotional well-being of healthcare workers: A multinational cross-sectional survey. *Indian Journal of Critical Care Medicine, 25*(5), 499–506. https://doi.org/10.5005/ jp-journals-10071-23806

Khan, S., Kitsis, M., Golovyan, D., Wang, S., Chlan, L., Boustani, M., & Khan, B. (2018). Effects of music intervention on inflammatory markers in critically ill and post-operative patients: A systematic review of the literature. *Heart & Lung, 47*(5), 489–496. https://doi.org/10.1016/j .hrtlng.2018.05.015

Kim, Y., Evangelista, L., & Park, Y. G. (2015). Anxiolytic effects of music interventions in patients receiving incenter hemodialysis: A systematic review and meta-analysis. *Nephrology Nursing Journal, 42*(4), 339–347.

Ko, S., Leung, D., & Wong, E. (2019). Effects of easy listening music intervention on satisfaction, anxiety, and pain in patients undergoing colonoscopy: A pilot randomized controlled trial. *Clinical Interventions in Aging, 14*, 977–986. https://doi.org/10.2147/CIA.S207191

Koelsch, S., Fuermetz, J., Sack, U., Bauer, K., Hohenadel, M., Wiegel, M., & Heinke, W. (2011). Effects of music listening on cortisol levels and propofol consumption during spinal anes-thesia. *Frontiers in Psychology, 2*, 58. https://doi.org/10.3389/fpsyg.2011.00058

Krause, A., North, A., & Hewitt, L. (2015). Music-listening in everyday life: Devices and choice. *Psychology of Music, 43*(2), 155–170. https://doi.org/10.1177/0305735613496860

Kuhlmann, A. Y. R., de Rooij, A., Krouese, L. F., van Dijk, M., Hunink, M. G. M., & Jeekel, J. (2018). Meta-analysis evaluating music interventions for anxiety and pain in surgery. *BJS, 105,* 773–783. https://doi.org/10.1002/bjs.10853

Kulkarni, S., Johnson, P. C., Kettles, S., & Kasthuri, R. S. (2012). Music during interventional radiological procedures, effect on sedation, pain and anxiety: A randomized controlled trial. *British Journal of Radiology, 85*(10), 1059–1063. https://doi.org/10.1259/bjr/71897605

Lin, Y. J., Lu, K. C., Chen, C., & Chang, C. C. (2012). The effects of music as therapy on the overall well-being of elderly patients on maintenance hemodialysis. *Biological Research for Nursing, 14*(3), 277–285. https://doi.org/10.1177/1099800411413259

Messika, J., Martin, Y., Maquigneau, N., Puechberty, C., Henry-Lagarrigue, M., Stoclin, A., Panneckouke, N., Villard, S., Dechanet, A., Lafourcade, A., Dreyfuss, D., Hajage, D., & Ricard, J. D., on behalf of the MUS-IRA team. (2019). A musical intervention for respiratory comfort during non-invasive ventilation in the ICU. *European Respiratory Journal, 53*(1), 1801873. https://doi.org/10.1183/13993003.01873-2018

Nightingale, F. (1969). *Notes on nursing.* Dover. (Original work published 1860)

Ooishi, Y., Mukai, H., Watanabe, K., Kawato, S., & Kashino, M. (2017). Increase in salivary oxytocin and decrease in salivary cortisol after listening to relaxing slow-tempo and exciting fast-tempo music. *PLoS ONE, 12*(12), e0189075. https://doi.org/10.1371/journal.pone.0189075

Okumura, Y., Asano, Y., Takenaka, S., Fukuyama., S., Yonezawa, S., Kasuya, Y., & Shinoda, J. (2014). Brain activation by music in patients in a vegetative or minimally conscious state following diffuse brain injury. *Brain Injury, 28*(7), 944–950. https://doi.org/10.3109/02699052.2014.888477

Pelletier, C. (2004). The effect of music on decreasing arousal due to stress: A meta-analysis. *Journal of Music Therapy, 41,* 192–214. https://doi.org/10.1093/jmt/41.3.192

Public Radio Music Source. (n.d.) *The current.* www.prms.org

Rutherford-Johnson, T., Kennedy, M., & Kennedy, J. (2013). *The Oxford dictionary of music* (6th ed.). Oxford University Press.

Salimpoor, V., Benovoy, M., Larcher, K., Dagher, A., & Zatorre, R. (2011). Anatomically distinct dopamine release during anticipation and experience of peak emotion to music. *Nature Neuroscience, 14*(2), 257–262. https://doi.org/10.1038/nn.2726

Schäfer, K., & Eerola, T. (2020). How listening to music and engagement with other media provide a sense of belonging: An exploratory study of social surrogacy. *Psychology of Music, 48*(2), 232–251. https://doi.org/10.1177/0305735618795036

Schäfer, K., Saarikallio, S., & Eerola, T. (2020). Music may reduce loneliness and act as a social surrogate for a friend: Evidence from an experimental listening study. *Music & Science, 3,* 1–16. https://doi.org/10.1177/2059204320935709

Shabanloei, R., Golchin, M., Esfani, A., Dolatkhah, R., & Rasoulian, M. (2010). Effects of music therapy on pain and anxiety in patients undergoing bone marrow biopsy and aspiration. *AORN Journal, 91*(6), 746–751. https://doi.org/10.1016/j.aorn.2010.04.001

Shaukat, N., Ali, D. M., & Razzak, J. (2020). Physical and mental health impacts of COVID-19 on healthcare workers: A scoping review. *International Journal of Emergency Medicine, 13*(1), 40. https://doi.org/10.1186/s12245-020-00299-5

Su, C. P., Lai, H. L., Chang, E. T., Yiin, L. M., Perng, S. J., & Chen, P. W. (2013). A randomized controlled trial of the effects of listening to non-commercial music on quality of nocturnal sleep and relaxation indices in patients in medical intensive care unit. *Journal of Advanced Nursing, 69*(6), 1377–1389. https://doi.org/10.1111/j.1365-2648.2012.06130.x

Thoma, M., Zemp, M., Kreienbuhl, L., Hofer, D., Schmidlin, P., Attin, T., Ehlert, U., & Nater, U. (2015). Effects of music listening on pre-treatment anxiety and stress levels in a dental hygiene recall population. *International Journal of Behavioral Medicine, 22,* 498–505. https://doi.org/10.1007/s12529-014-9439-x

Ugras, G., Yilddirim, G., Yüksel, S., Özturkcu, Y., Kuzdere, M., & Özteekin, S. (2018). The effect of different types of music on patients' preoperative anxiety: A randomized controlled trial. *Complementary Therapies in Clinical Practice, 31,* 158–163. https://doi.org/10.1016/j.ctcp.2018.02.012

Wang, M., Zhang, L., Zhang Y., Zhang Y., Xu, X., & Zhang, Y. (2014). Effect of music in endoscopy procedures: Systematic review and meta-analysis of randomized controlled trials. *Pain Medicine, 15*(10), 1786–1794. https://doi.org/10.1111/pme.12514

Wong, H., Lopez-Nahas, V., & Molassiotis, A. (2001). Effects of music therapy on anxiety in ventilator-dependent patients. *Heart & Lung, 30*(5), 376–387. https://doi.org/10.1067/mhl.2001.118302

World Federation of Music Therapy. (2014). *WFMT strategic plan.* http://www.wfmt.info/resource-centers/publication-center/wfmt-documents/

Yang, C. Y., Chen, C. H., Chu, H., Chen, W. C., Lee, T. Y., Chen, S. G., & Chou, K. R. (2012). The effect of music therapy on hospitalized psychiatric patients' anxiety, finger temperature, and electroencephalography: A randomized clinical trial. *Biological Research for Nursing, 14*(2), 197–206. https://doi.org/10.1177/1099800411406258

Yue, W., Han, X., Luo, J., Zeng, Z., & Yang, M. (2021). Effect of music therapy on preterm infants in neonatal intensive care unit: Systematic review and meta-analysis of randomized controlled trials. *Journal of Advanced Nursing, 77*(2), 635–652. https://doi.org/10.1111/jan.14630

Zamanifar, S., Bagheri-Saveh, M. I., Nezakati, A., Mohammadi, R., & Seidi, J. (2020). The effect of music therapy and aromatherapy with chamomile-lavender essential oil on the anxiety of clinical nurses: A randomized and double-blind clinical trial. *Journal of Medicine and Life, 13*(1), 7. https://doi.org/10.25122/jml-2019-0105

9

Yoga

MIRIAM E. CAMERON AND CORJENA K. CHEUNG

Yoga is an ancient spiritual, mental, physical discipline based on Indian philosophy. Although classical yoga began as a spiritual practice, millions of people around the world use yoga for physical and mental well-being. Anyone can benefit from yoga, regardless of health, beliefs, age, or culture. The systematic practice of yoga heals the body and mind. Yoga's "do-it-yourself" prescription for stress management and well-being, if done properly, has little or no side effects and does not require expensive training or equipment (National Center for Complementary and Integrative Health [NCCIH], 2021c; Natural Medicines, 2021b).

However, yoga has a deeper dimension. Yoga is an ethical, spiritual way of life to transform consciousness, as yogis for millennia have advocated, and Western researchers are affirming. Yoga teaches that self-centeredness underlies suffering and most disease (or "lack of ease"). Practitioners who let go of ego realize they are linked to every being, the environment, and larger forces in the universe. Grateful for this vast interconnectedness, they reach out to relieve suffering (DiNardo & Pearce-Hayden, 2018).

This chapter explores how nurses—and nursing students—can use yoga for self-care and integrative nursing (Earl E. Bakken Center for Spirituality & Healing, University of Minnesota, 2021a). The systematic practice of yoga will help nurses distinguish between conventional reality and ultimate reality, allowing their true nature to shine through. Their inner wisdom will flow spontaneously through all the cells of the body, promoting optimal health, peace, and joy (DiNardo & Pearce-Hayden, 2018).

DEFINITION

Yoga means "to yoke" or unite mind, body, and universe. According to tradition, two millennia ago Patanjali, a sage in India, systematized yoga into the *Yoga Sutra*. The book consists of 196 precise, concise statements called *sutras*. This unique blend of theoretical knowledge and practical application is the foundational textbook for all schools of yoga. In the *Yoga Sutra*, Patanjali analyzed how we know what we know and why we suffer. He explained that the primary purpose of consciousness is to see things as they *really* are and to make choices that bring about freedom from suffering. Yoga helps us rein in our tendency to seek happiness through external phenomena. By turning inward and developing mindfulness of our true nature, we can come to understand how to cultivate happiness and wisdom. By becoming still inside, we can abide in this deep, absorptive knowing (DiNardo & Pearce-Hayden, 2018).

Patanjali described yoga as eight interconnected limbs, like limbs of a tree. Doing all eight limbs simultaneously leads to higher stages of ethics, spirituality, and healing. The first five limbs still the mind and body to prepare for the last three limbs. Exhibit 9.1 lists the eight limbs, Sanskrit names, and definitions (DiNardo & Pearce-Hayden, 2018). The *Bhagavad Gita* (Prime, 2021), another ancient, sacred text from India, described eight kinds of yoga and their focus, as listed in Exhibit 9.2.

HATHA YOGA AND YOGA THERAPY

Hatha yoga, which is popular around the world, consists primarily of physical poses, breathing techniques, and relaxation (Muktibodhananda, 2016). Although Hatha yoga focuses on the body, classes open the door to the deeper ethical, spiritual dimension of yoga. Hatha styles include Himalayan Tradition, Tibetan Yoga, Iyengar, Ashtanga, Viniyoga, Sivananda, Kripalu, and Kundalini (Natural Medicines, 2021b).

Exhibit 9.1 *The Eight Limbs of Yoga in Patanjali's Yoga Sutra*

1. Ethical behavior (*yama*)—nonharming, truthfulness, nonstealing, responsible sexuality, and nonacquisitiveness
2. Personal behavior (*niyama*)—purity, commitment, contentment, self-study, and surrender to the whole; *niyama* includes *sattvic* (pure) mind, food, beverages, air, and environment
3. Posture (*asana*)—physical poses that stretch, condition, and massage the body
4. Breath expansion (*pranayama*)—refinement of the breath to expand *prana* (life force) and get rid of toxins
5. Sensory inhibition (*pratyahara*)—temporary withdrawal of the senses from the external environment to the inner self (e.g., by closing the eyes and looking inward)
6. Concentration (*dharana*)—locking attention on the breath, mantra, image, or something else
7. Meditation (*dhyana*)—increasingly sustained attention, leading to a profound state of peace and awareness
8. Integration (*samadhi*)—a transcendent state of oneness, wisdom, and ecstasy

---

Exhibit 9.2 *Kinds of Yoga and Their Focus, as Described in the Bhagavad Gita*

- *Kundalini yoga:* energy
- *Jnana yoga:* knowledge
- *Mantra yoga:* recitation of sacred syllables
- *Tantra yoga:* technique
- *Bhakti yoga:* devotion
- *Karma yoga:* action, good deeds
- *Raja yoga:* control of mind and body through the Eight Limbs of Patanjali
- *Hatha yoga:* willpower to do physical exercises and expand the breath

Frequently, yoga is practiced together with Ayurveda, a traditional healing system from India (Natural Medicines, 2021a; NCCIH, 2021a). Furthermore, Tibetan yoga is integral to Tibetan medicine, a traditional healing system from Tibet, which is similar to Ayurveda (Cameron & Namdul, 2020; Earl E. Bakken Center for Spirituality & Healing, University of Minnesota, 2020; 2021b).

The Yoga Alliance (2021) developed standards for Hatha yoga teachers and teacher training (see website link for the organization at the end of this chapter). The Yoga Alliance offers six Registered Yoga Teacher (RYT) credentials, as well as specialty-level RYT credentials in children's yoga and prenatal yoga. Moreover, the Yoga Alliance offers five school-based Registered Yoga School (RYS) credentials for yoga teacher training programs of various lineages, styles, and methodologies.

Yoga therapists practice therapeutic yoga on a professional level. The International Association of Yoga Therapists (IAYT, 2020) defines *yoga therapy* as the professional application of the principles and practices of yoga to promote health and well-being within a safe, therapeutic relationship. IAYT certifies (C-IAYT) members who graduated from an IAYT accredited yoga therapist training program.

Yoga is evolving into a profession based on yoga's time-tested philosophy and scientific evidence. To ensure safe, informed practice, yoga education is moving from community centers to academia with more rigorous standards about ethics, anatomy, physiology, and evidence-based practice. For example, at one university, undergraduate and graduate students can take academic courses to become Hatha yoga teachers (Earl E. Bakken Center for Spirituality & Healing, University of Minnesota, 2021b), and graduate students can earn a master's degree in yoga therapy. These courses and degree are popular among nursing and health science students. Coursework focused on yoga can be taken as a focus or concurrent with courses within a degree program. Furthermore, University of Minnesota faculty and PhD students conduct yoga research. Teaching yoga and conducting yoga research in academia promote standardization, professionalism, and evolution of yoga.

SCIENTIFIC BASIS

Yoga is based on ancient observations, principles, and theories of the mind/body connection. For millennia, yogis have passed down this knowledge from one generation to the next (DiNardo & Pearce-Hayden, 2018). Now researchers are validating many of these health claims. Systematic reviews and meta-analyses report that yoga generally is safe and feasible for healthy adults, children (Anusuya et al., 2021; NCCIH, 2021b), and older adults (Bhattacharyya et al., 2021).

Studies found that yoga treats symptoms and/or prevents their onset and recurrence. Yoga improves wellness by relieving anxiety and depression; improving mental health, sleep, and balance; and supporting good health habits. Individuals practice Yoga to decrease pain in the low back and neck, tension headaches, and knee osteoarthritis. Yoga can help overweight people to lose weight, assist smokers to quit smoking, and relieve menopause symptoms. People with chronic illness can use yoga to manage symptoms and improve quality of life (Jakicic et al., 2021; Natural Medicines, 2021b; NCCIH, 2021b). Laughter yoga reduced stress in first-year nursing students (Ozturk & Tezel, 2021) and healthy adults (Meier et al., 2021).

INTERVENTION

TECHNIQUES

Each of Patanjali's eight limbs is a potential intervention that nurses can implement with children, adults, older adults, pregnant women, people with disabilities and illnesses, and individuals who are dying (DiNardo & Pearce-Hayden, 2018; Natural Medicines, 2021b; NCCIH, 2021c). Nurses can encourage clients to behave with nonviolence and compassion toward themselves, others, and our planet (Limb 1) and to engage in cleanliness, nutritious eating, and self-discipline (Limb 2). Moreover, nurses can suggest yoga postures (Limb 3) and breathing techniques (Limb 4) for relaxation and harmony.

Exhibit 9.3 explains how to do Corpse Pose and relax deeply. Exhibit 9.4 lists steps for doing Alternate Nostril Breathing to harmonize mind and body. Doing Corpse Pose and Alternate Nostril Breathing can reduce stress before and after treatments and surgery.

Exhibit 9.3 *Corpse Pose (Savasana; Yoga Limb 3)*

- Lie on your back with your arms relaxed near your sides, palms up, and head, trunk, and legs straight. If you are uncomfortable, put a pillow or blanket under your head and/or knees.
- Close your eyes, relax, and let your body sink.
- Breathe in a circular manner: slowly, evenly, deeply through your nostrils, from your abdomen, with your in-breath the same length as your out-breath, and no break between.
- When you are ready, open your eyes, bend your knees, turn to your right, and get up.

Corpse Pose promotes deep relaxation and can reduce hypertension, anxiety, insomnia, stress, and fatigue.

Exhibit 9.4 *Alternate Nostril Breathing (Nadi Shodhana; Yoga Limb 4)*

- Sit comfortably with a straight back.
- Breathe in a circular manner: slowly, evenly, deeply through your nostrils, from your abdomen, with the in-breath the same length as the out-breath, and no break between.
- Place your right thumb on your right nostril, ring finger on your left nostril, and inhale through both nostrils.
- Use the thumb to close your right nostril; exhale slowly through your left nostril, and then inhale slowly through your left nostril.
- Use your ring finger to close your left nostril; exhale slowly through your right nostril, and then inhale slowly through your right nostril.
- This sequence constitutes one round; repeat for five more rounds.

Pranayama promotes balance, gives equal time to both sides of the body, and strengthens the breath in the weaker nostril.

Exhibit 9.5 *Withdrawal of Senses, Concentration, Meditation (Limbs 5–8)*

- Lie in Corpse Pose or sit comfortably with a straight back in a chair or on a meditation cushion; close your eyes, relax, and look inward.
- Breathe in a circular manner: slowly, evenly, deeply through your nostrils, from your abdomen, with the in-breath the same length as the out-breath, and no break between.
- Focus on your breath.
- Inhale through your nose. Silently count "one." Exhale. Inhale again and count, "two," and so on.
- When your mind wanders away, bring it back to your breath and start with one again.
- At 10, go back to one again.
- When you are deeply relaxed and focused, open up to your inner experience; simply observe and let go of whatever arises, without attachment, judgment, or direction.

Limbs 6 through 8 promote deep relaxation, healing, balance, replenishment, focus, insight, and joy.

Nurses can encourage clients to let go of external stimuli, relax, and sleep through yoga with selected Pantanjali Limbs 5 through 8 as presented earlier (Limb 5). Learning to concentrate and meditate can create meaning in suffering and motivation to develop optimal health (Limb 6 and Limb 7). Through integration or *samadhi*, individuals can experience oneness and joy, even when seriously ill and dying (Limb 8). Exhibit 9.5 explains a breathing exercise to apply Limbs 5 to 8. Meditating on the breath for even 2 minutes can transform anger and fear into compassion and wisdom.

GUIDELINES

There are a number of resources available to properly learn yoga. Yoga publications, videos, online postings, and modules describe guidelines for beginning through advanced levels. Some individuals use these resources to learn yoga on their own. Other people benefit from yoga classes and individual instruction. Qualified, experienced teachers can assist nurses to do yoga themselves and to use yoga as a nursing intervention.

MEASUREMENT OF OUTCOMES

Nurses can determine the effectiveness of yoga by asking themselves and clients how they feel before and after doing it. Most health problems develop over time, and yoga may not alleviate them immediately. Minor health issues may improve quickly, but chronic conditions may require sustained practice. Yoga advocates gradual change. Optimal benefits occur from systematic practice. Short-term outcomes, however—including a more relaxed attitude, decreased anxiety, optimism, improved balance, better sleep, and increased musculoskeletal flexibility—are notable. Dedicated practice can produce long-term outcomes of better physical, spiritual, and mental health (Natural Medicines, 2021b).

PRECAUTIONS

Generally, yoga is safe for healthy people, when performed properly under the guidance of a qualified teacher. Even so, injuries can occur, although serious injuries are rare. The most common injuries are sprains and strains, particularly of the shoulder, knee, lower leg, and back. Older adults need to be cautious because the rate of yoga-related injuries treated in emergency departments is higher for individuals age 65 and older than for younger people. Hot yoga can lead to dehydration, profuse sweating, dizziness, and headaches. Individuals may need modifications in yoga if they have preexisting health conditions, such as a knee injury, shoulder inflammation, hip replacement, lumbar spine deterioration, severe high blood pressure, balance issues, and glaucoma (NCCIH, 2021b, 2021c).

Precautions are needed to avoid doing yoga in a manner that causes harm. Pregnant women should talk with their healthcare providers and yoga instructors about their individual needs. New practitioners are best off avoiding extreme practices such as hot yoga, headstands, shoulder stands, lotus position, and forceful breathing. Yoga discourages anything unnatural, competitive, and hurtful. To avoid injury, nurses can encourage clients to be mindful of their own inner wisdom and do yoga with gentleness, self-compassion, and moderation. Exhibit 9.6 lists additional guidelines (NCCIH, 2021b).

Before working with Hatha yoga teachers or yoga therapists, nurses are advised to review their education, credentialing, and experience. Ideally, Hatha yoga teachers have RYT credentials (Yoga Alliance, 2021), and yoga therapists are certified by IAYT (2020). Many American states, such as Minnesota, have passed statutes to regulate unlicensed practitioners of complementary and alternative therapies. Chapter 146A of the Minnesota Statutes (2020) states that unlicensed practitioners cannot call themselves a doctor, refer to clients as patients, and

---

Exhibit 9.6 *Precautions Involving Yoga*

- Practice yoga under the guidance of a qualified instructor; doing yoga by self-study without supervision is associated with increased risks.
- Relax and enjoy yoga rather than being tense while doing yoga practices.
- Do not use yoga to replace conventional healthcare or to postpone seeing a health professional.
- If you have a health problem, talk with your trusted health professionals before starting yoga.
- Choose a beneficial style of yoga; for example, hot yoga may not be good for you.
- Select a qualified Hatha yoga teacher or yoga therapist to modify yoga so that you practice safely.
- Give your health professionals a full picture of your health, including your yoga practice.
- Trust your inner wisdom in doing yoga and working with a Hatha yoga teacher and/or yoga therapist.

use treatments covered by other licensing boards. They must give each client a detailed bill of rights about their qualifications and the client's rights and responsibilities. Hatha yoga teachers and yoga therapists must follow these laws. Nurses who integrate yoga into their care are required to adhere to the higher standards of their state boards of nursing.

USES

Yoga and nursing are an excellent fit. Both disciplines treat the whole person. By doing yoga and using yoga as an intervention, nurses promote nonreactivity of the mind and inner calmness that embraces, rather than denies, challenging situations (DiNardo & Pearce-Hayden, 2018). Researchers around the world have published hundreds of studies about the benefits of yoga. Exhibit 9.7 lists a sample of recent studies.

CULTURAL APPLICATIONS

All over the world, individuals adapt yoga to their culture and values. Yoga is integral to many traditional healing systems, such as Ayurveda (Natural Medicines, 2021a; NCCIH, 2021a) and Tibetan medicine (Cameron & Namdul, 2020; Earl E. Bakken Center for Spirituality & Healing, University of Minnesota, 2020, 2021b). These ancient, holistic healing traditions teach the importance of creating a healthy body and mind in order to live a yogic life (DiNardo & Pearce-Hayden, 2018). In Sidebar 9.1, an Australian yoga instructor in Hong Kong describes his experience with yoga.

Exhibit 9.7 *Studies Demonstrating Benefits of Yoga for Persons With Selected Health Issues*

Anxiety: Simon et al. (2021)
Anxiety in children: Shreve et al. (2021)
Cancer: Patel et al. (2021); Song et al. (2021); Sullivan et al. (2021); Yi et al. (2021)
Chronic respiratory disease: Ozer et al. (2021)
Cognitive function in older adults: Bhattacharyya et al. (2021); Hoy et al. (2021)
Depression, anxiety: Clarke et al. (2021); La Rocque et al. (2021); Ravindran et al. (2021)
Hypertension: Dhungana et al. (2021); Makhija et al. (2021)
Intellectual/developmental disabilities: Acabchuk et al. (2021); Allison et al. (2021); Ullas et al. (2021)
Low back pain: Roseen et al. (2021)
Parkinson's disease: Cherup et al. (2021)
Posttraumatic stress: Kysar-Moon et al. (2021)
Psychiatric disorders: Bhargav et al. (2021)
Severe traumatic brain injury: Wen et al. (2021)
Stress: Ciezar-Andersen et al. (2021); Divya et al. (2021); Park et al. (2021)
Stress during the COVID-19 lockdown: Sahni et al. (2021)
Type 2 diabetes: Viswanathan et al. (2021)
Urgency urinary incontinence in women: Tenfelde et al. (2021)

Sidebar 9.1 *Yoga in Australia and Hong Kong*

George Dovas

I went to my first yoga class in Sydney, Australia in 1999. My friend had given me a black-and-white leaflet for an Iyengar Yoga school. Not knowing anything about yoga, I enrolled in a beginner's course. From the first class, I experienced something compelling. I was not being asked to "do" or "copy" the instructor. I was being taught, not told.

In each yoga posture, the teacher asked us to become aware of one body part and then another. As the teacher guided our awareness, I started to notice parts of my body that I previously hadn't seen. I thought, "I have been inhabiting my body for so many years, why didn't I notice these things before?" It was a revelation! Later, the teacher brought our attention to one body part, the knee for instance, and then asked us to compare the front of the knee with the back of the knee. My attention was obligated to see more details about the knee. Furthermore, in the process of comparing, intelligence (discernment) was being employed. Through yoga I learned that my awareness and attention are like a spotlight. I realized that I have control over where I show the spotlight—I have control over my attention. As time passed, my ability to focus improved and I developed a greater sense of responsibility for my life. My impatience diminished. My sense of contentment grew.

In 2001, I moved to Hong Kong to work for a global fitness chain. Here, in Hong Kong, I embarked on a 3-year training program to become a yoga teacher. During my apprenticeship, I learned that yoga postures are tools to study ourselves. We need to become attentive and sensitive to ourselves and our needs. What matters is not "doing the posture" but "what you are doing *in* the posture." In recent years, science increasingly has understood the brain, and particularly its ability to change and adapt as a result of experience (brain plasticity). As I studied yoga more, I became aware that yoga was helping me to rewire my brain. The experiences I was having in my yoga practice were molding me.

In 2010, I became the proprietor of the Iyengar Yoga Centre of Hong Kong. I teach yoga to help people understand themselves. I teach yoga to help people cope with the vicissitudes of the mind by improving their level of attention and awareness. People say that yoga is holistic, but because it has changed the "whole" of my life, I say that yoga is "whole-istic!"

FUTURE RESEARCH

More research is needed to understand yoga and the ways that systematic yoga practice can contribute to integrative nursing. Research studies about yoga generally report positive effects. The results of each study may be influenced by the participants' characteristics (age, gender, health status, diagnosis), study entry criteria, type and duration of the yoga intervention, compliance, attrition, and related factors. Although more systematic reviews and meta-analyses are being published, many yoga studies are pilot studies with small sample sizes, short study periods, methodological flaws, inadequate control groups, and other limitations. Strong evidence of yoga efficacy for people with various health conditions has yet to be established. The lack of standardized practices and the variety of yoga styles further complicate the applicability of the findings (Natural Medicines, 2021b; NCCIH, 2021b, 2021c).

Yoga's holistic approach poses challenges for conducting scientific research. Yoga practices affect body and mind in a manner that may not be reproducible and quantifiable. Teasing out specific aspects of yoga is challenging and may not produce statistically significant results. Even so, the NCCIH (2021c) is funding yoga studies with promising results. Because yoga treats both the body and the mind, research involving biology, physiology, neurology, genetics, psychology, and other disciplines can add to the understanding of yoga. Interdisciplinary science has a vital role to play in yoga nursing research.

Nursing would benefit from well-designed studies that address these and other research questions:

- Which yoga practices are therapeutic for individuals with which health issues?
- What yoga practices are best for managing stress among nurses and nursing students?
- How can nurses, nursing students, and clients be encouraged to use yoga for self-care?
- What are effective strategies for teaching nurses how to use yoga as part of integrative nursing?

In summary, new qualitative methodologies may be needed to study yoga as a holistic healing system. Investigating the deeper dimension of yoga, instead of focusing on poses and breathing, will enrich the findings. Research will encourage nurses—and nursing students—to use yoga for self-care and integrative nursing (Earl E. Bakken Center for Spirituality & Healing, University of Minnesota, 2021b).

WEBSITES

- Example of graduate courses about Yoga and Tibetan Medicine at the University of Minnesota: www.csh.umn.edu/education/focus-areas/yoga -tibetan-medicine
- Example of a State (Minnesota) Statute regulating Hatha Yoga Teachers and Yoga Therapists in the United States: www.revisor.mn.gov/statutes/ cite/146A#stat.146A.001
- International Association of Yoga Therapists: www.iayt.org/
- Yoga Alliance: www.yogaalliance.org/

REFERENCES

Acabchuk, R. L., Brisson, J. M., Park, C. L., Babbott-Bryan, N., Parmelee, O. A., & Johnson, B. T. (2021). Therapeutic effects of meditation, yoga, and mindfulness-based interventions for chronic symptoms of mild traumatic brain injury: A systematic review and meta-analysis. *Applied Psychology Health and Well-Being, 13*, 34–62. https://doi.org/10.4103/ijoy.IJOY_32_18

Allison, C. K., Van Puymbroeck, M., Crowe, B. M., Schmid, A. A., & Townsend, J. A. (2021). The impact of an autonomy-supportive yoga intervention on self-determination in adults with intellectual and developmental disabilities. *Complementary Therapies in Clinical Practice, 43,* 101332. https://doi.org/10.1016/j.ctcp.2021.101332

Anusuya, U. S., Mohanty, S., & Saoji, A. A. (2021). Effect of mind sound resonance technique (MSRT – a yoga-based relaxation technique) on psychological variables and cognition in school children: A randomized controlled trial. *Complementary Therapies in Medicine, 56,* 102606. https://doi.org/10.1016/j.ctim.2020.102606

Bhargav, H., George, S., Varambally, S., & Gangadhar, B. N. (2021). Yoga and psychiatric disorders: A review of biomarker evidence. *International Review of Psychiatry, 33,* 162–169. https://doi.org/10.1080/09540261.2020.1761087

Bhattacharyya, K. K., Andel, R., & Small, B. J. (2021). Effects of yoga-related mind-body therapies on cognitive function in older adults: A systematic review with meta-analysis. *Archives of Gerontology and Geriatrics, 93,* 104319. https://doi.org/10.1016/j.archger.2020.104319

Cameron, M. E., & Namdul, T. (2020). *Tibetan medicine and you: A path to wellbeing, better health, and joy (Blessing by His Holiness the Dalai Lama).* Rowman & Littlefield.

Cherup, N. P., Strand, K. L., Lucchi, L., Wooten, S. V., Luca, C., & Signorile, J. F. (2021). Yoga meditation enhances proprioception and balance in individuals diagnosed with Parkinson's disease. *Perceptual & Motor Skills, 128,* 304–323. https://doi.org/10.1177/0031512520945085

Ciezar-Andersen, S. D., Hayden, K. A., & King-Shier, K. M. (2021). A systematic review of yoga interventions for helping health professionals and students. *Complementary Therapies in Medicine, 58,* 1–8. https://doi.org/10.1016/j.ctim.2021.102704

Clarke, R. D., Morris, S. L., Wagner, E. F., Spadola, C. E., Bursac, Z., Fava, N. M., & Hospital, M. (2021). Feasibility, acceptability, and preliminary impact of mindfulness-based yoga among Hispanic/Latinx adolescents. *Explore, 18*(3), 299–305. https://doi.org/10.1016/j.explore.2021.03.002

Dhungana, R. R., Pedisic, Z., Joshi, S., Khanal, M. K., Kalauni, O. P., Shakya, A., Bhurtel, V., Panthi, S., Ramesh Kumar, K. C., Ghimire, B., Pandey, A. R., Bista, B., Khatiwoda, S. R., McLachlan, C. S., Neupane, D., & de Courten, M. (2021). Effects of a health worker-led 3-month yoga intervention on blood pressure of hypertensive patients: A randomised controlled multicentre trial in the primary care setting. *BMC Public Health, 21,* 550. https://doi.org/10.1186/s12889-021-10528-y

DiNardo, K., & Pearce-Hayden, A. (2018). *Living the Sutras: A guide to yoga wisdom beyond the mat.* Shambhala Publications, Inc.

Divya, K., Bharathi, S., Somya, R., & Darshan, M. H. (2021). Impact of a yogic breathing technique on the well-being of healthcare professionals during the COVID-19 pandemic. *Global Advances in Health & Medicine, 10,* 2164956120982956. https://doi.org/10.1177/2164956120982956

Earl E. Bakken Center for Spirituality & Healing, University of Minnesota. (2020). *Tibetan medicine.* https://www.takingcharge.csh.umn.edu/tibetan-medicine

Earl E. Bakken Center for Spirituality & Healing, University of Minnesota. (2021a). *Integrative nursing.* https://www.csh.umn.edu/education/focus-areas/integrative-nursing

Earl E. Bakken Center for Spirituality & Healing, University of Minnesota. (2021b). *Yoga and Tibetan medicine.* https://www.csh.umn.edu/education/focus-areas/yoga-tibetan-medicine

Hoy, S., Osth, J., Pascoe, M., Kandola, A., & Hallgren, M. (2021). Effects of yoga-based interventions on cognitive function in healthy older adults: A systematic review of randomized controlled trials. *Complementary Therapies in Medicine, 58,* 102690. https://doi.org/10.1016/j.ctim.2021.102690

International Association of Yoga Therapists. (2020). *Eligibility of applying for IAYT certification (C-IAYT).* https://www.iayt.org/page/CertEligibility

Jakicic, J. M., Davis, K. K., Rogers, R. J., Sherman, S. A., Barr, S., Marcin, M. L., Collins, K. A., Collins, A. M., Yuan, N., & Lang, W. (2021). Feasibility of integration of yoga in a behavioral weight-loss intervention: A randomized trial. *Obesity, 29,* 512–520. https://doi.org/10.1002/oby.23089

Kysar-Moon, A., Vasquez, M., & Luppen, T. (2021). Trauma-sensitive yoga interventions and post-traumatic stress and depression outcomes among women: A systematic review and analysis of randomized control trials. *International Journal of Yoga Therapy, 3*(1), Article _23. https://doi.org/10.17761/2021-D-20-00005

La Rocque, C. L., Mazurka, R., Stuckless, T. J. R., Pyke, K., & Harkness, K. L. (2021). Randomized controlled trial of Bikram Yoga and aerobic exercise for depression in women: Efficacy and stress-based mechanisms. *Journal of Affective Disorders, 280,* 457–466. https://doi.org/10.1016/j.jad.2020.10.067

Makhija, A., Khatik, N., & Raghunandan, C. (2021). A randomized control trial to study the effect of integrated yoga on pregnancy outcome in hypertensive disorder of pregnancy. *Complementary Therapies in Clinical Practice, 43,* 101366. https://doi.org/10.1016/j.ctcp.2021.101366

Meier, M., Wirz, L., Dickinson, P., & Pruessner, J. C. (2021). Laughter yoga reduces the cortisol response to acute stress in healthy individuals. *Stress, 24,* 44–52. https://doi.org/10.1080/10253890.2020.1766018

Minnesota Statutes. (2020). *Chapter 146A. Complementary and alternative health care practices.* https://www.revisor.mn.gov/statutes/cite/146A#stat.146A.001

Muktibodhananda, S. (2016). *Hatha Yoga Pradipika.* Yoga Publications Trust.

National Center for Complementary and Integrative Health. (2021a). *Ayurvedic medicine: In depth.* https://www.nccih.nih.gov/health/ayurvedic-medicine-in-depth

National Center for Complementary and Integrative Health. (2021b). *Yoga: What you need to know.* https://www.nccih.nih.gov/health/tips/things-you-should-know-about-yoga?nav=govd

National Center for Complementary and Integrative Health. (2021c). *Yoga.* https://nccih.nih.gov/health/yoga

Natural Medicines. (2021a). *Ayurveda.* https://naturalmedicines-therapeuticresearch-com.ezp3.lib.umn.edu/databases/health-wellness/professional.aspx?productid=1201

Natural Medicines. (2021b). *Yoga.* https://naturalmedicines-therapeuticresearch-com.ezp3.lib.umn.edu/databases/health-wellness/professional.aspx?productid=1241

Ozer, Z., Bahcecioglu Turan, G., & Aksoy, M. (2021). The effects of yoga on dyspnea, sleep and fatigue in chronic respiratory diseases. *Complementary Therapies in Clinical Practice, 43,* 101306. https://doi.org/10.1016/j.ctcp.2021.101306

Ozturk, F. O., & Tezel, A. (2021). Effect of laughter yoga on mental symptoms and salivary cortisol levels in first-year nursing students: A randomized controlled trial. *International Journal of Nursing Practice, 27,* e12924. https://doi.org/10.1111/ijn.12924

Park, C. L., Finkelstein-Fox, L., Sacco, S. J., Braun, T. D., & Lazar, S. (2021). How does yoga reduce stress? A clinical trial testing psychological mechanisms. *Stress & Health, 37,* 116–126. https://doi.org/10.1002/smi.2977

Patel, S. R., Zayas, J., Medina-Inojosa, J. R., Loprinzi, C., Cathcart-Rake, E. J., Bhagra, A., Olson, J. E., Couch, F. J., & Ruddy, K. J. (2021). Real-world experiences with yoga on cancer-related symptoms in women with breast cancer. *Global Advances in Health & Medicine, 10,* 2164956120984140. https://doi.org/10.1177/2164956120984140

Prime, R. (2021). *The Bhagavad Gita: Talks between the soul and God.* Mandala Publishing.

Ravindran, A. V., McKay, M. S., Silva, T. D., Tindall, C., Garfinkel, T., Paric, A., & Ravindran, L. (2021). Breathing-focused yoga as augmentation for unipolar and bipolar depression: A randomized controlled trial. *Canadian Journal of Psychiatry—Revue Canadienne de Psychiatrie, 66,* 159–169. https://doi.org/10.1177/0706743720940535

Roseen, E. J., Gerlovin, H., Felson, D. T., Delitto, A., Sherman, K. J., & Saper, R. B. (2021). Which chronic low back pain patients respond favorably to yoga, physical therapy, and a self-care book? Responder analyses from a randomized controlled trial. *Pain Medicine, 22,* 165–180. https://doi.org/10.1093/pm/pnaa153

Sahni, P. S., Singh, K., Sharma, N., & Garg, R. (2021). Yoga an effective strategy for self-management of stress-related problems and wellbeing during COVID19 lockdown: a cross-sectional study. *PLoS ONE [Electronic Resource], 16,* e0245214. https://doi.org/10.1371/journal.pone.0245214

Shreve, M., Scott, A., McNeill, C., & Washburn, L. (2021). Using yoga to reduce anxiety in children: exploring school-based yoga among rural third- and fourth-grade students. *Journal of Pediatric Health Care, 35,* 42–52. https://doi.org/10.1016/j.pedhc.2020.07.008

Simon, N. M., Hofmann, S. G., Rosenfield, D., Hoeppner, S. S., Hoge, E. A., Bui, E., & Khalsa, S. B. S. (2021). Efficacy of yoga vs cognitive behavioral therapy vs stress education for the treatment of generalized anxiety disorder: A randomized clinical trial. *JAMA Psychiatry, 78,* 13–20. https://doi.org/10.1001/jamapsychiatry.2020.2496

Song, J., Wang, T., Wang, Y., Li, R., Niu, S., Zhuo, L., Guo, Q., & Li, X. (2021). The effectiveness of yoga on cancer-related fatigue: A systematic review and meta-analysis. *Oncology Nursing Forum, 48,* 207–228. https://doi.org/10.1188/21.ONF.207-228

Sullivan, D. R., Medysky, M. E., Tyzik, A. L., Dieckmann, N. F., Denfeld, Q. E., & Winters-Stone, K. (2021). Feasibility and potential benefits of partner-supported yoga on psychosocial and physical function among lung cancer patients. *Psycho-Oncology. 30*(5), 789–793. https://doi.org/10.1002/pon.5628

Tenfelde, S., Tell, D., Garfield, L., Mathews, H., & Janusek, L. (2021). Yoga for women with urgency urinary incontinence: a pilot study. *Female Pelvic Medicine & Reconstructive Surgery, 27,* 57–62. https://doi.org/10.1097/SPV.0000000000000723

Ullas, K., Maharana, S., Metri, K. G., Gupta, A., & Nagendra, H. R. (2021). Impact of yoga on mental health and sleep quality among mothers of children with intellectual disability. *Alternative Therapies in Health & Medicine, 27*(S1), 128–132. http://ovidsp.ovid.com/ovidweb.cgi?T=JS&PAGE=reference&D=medp&NEWS=N&AN=33421039

Viswanathan, V., Sivakumar, S., Sai Prathiba, A., Devarajan, A., George, L., & Kumpatla, S. (2021). Effect of yoga intervention on biochemical, oxidative stress markers, inflammatory markers, and sleep quality among subjects with type 2 diabetes in South India: Results from the Satyam Project. *Diabetes Research & Clinical Practice, 172,* 108644. https://doi.org/10.1016/j.diabres.2020.108644

Wen, P. S., Herrin, I., & Pittman, A. (2021). Feasibility of yoga to improve symptoms in individuals with severe, chronic traumatic brain injury: A mixed-methods case series. *Alternative Therapies in Health & Medicine. 28*(1), 32–37.http://ovidsp.ovid.com/ovidweb.cgi?T=JS&PAGE=reference&D=medp&NEWS=N&AN=33421043

Yi, L. J., Tian, X., Jin, Y. F., Luo, M. J., & Jimenez-Herrera, M. F. (2021). Effects of yoga on health-related quality, physical health, and psychological health in women with breast cancer receiving chemotherapy: A systematic review and meta-analysis. *Annals of Palliative Medicine, 10,* 1961–1975. https://doi.org/10.21037/apm-20-1484

Yoga Alliance. (2021). *Member overview.* https://www.yogaalliance.org/Credentialing

Biofeedback

JACLENE A. ZAUSZNIEWSKI AND ELIZABETH A. WILLIAMS

Biofeedback is a technique that teaches people how to gain more control of involuntary bodily functions. Electronic sensors applied to the body allow a person to become more aware (feedback) of processes in their body (bio). Many different types of healthcare professionals rely on biofeedback to help their patients cope with a variety of conditions such as chronic pain, regain movement in paralyzed muscles, and learn to relax. Patients who suffer from migraine headaches, high blood pressure, and incontinence are just a few examples of those who can benefit from biofeedback therapy. This chapter provides an overview of biofeedback, its scientific basis, health conditions in which it is useful, and a technique that can be used by nurses trained in its practice.

DEFINITION

Biofeedback is based on holistic self-care perspectives in which (a) the mind and body are not separated and (b) people can learn ways to improve their health and performance. Biofeedback therapists use instruments and teach self-regulation strategies to help individuals increase voluntary control over their internal physiological and mental processes. Biofeedback instruments measure physiological activity, such as muscle tension, skin temperature, cardiac activity, and brainwaves, and then provide immediate and real-time feedback to people in the form of visual and/or auditory signals that increase their awareness of internal processes. The biofeedback therapist then teaches individuals to change these signals and to take a more active role in maintaining the health of their minds and bodies. The holistic and self-care philosophies underlying biofeedback and its focus on helping people gain more control over personal functioning make the intervention an appropriate one for nurses to use. Over time, a person can learn to maintain these changes without the continued use of a feedback instrument (Association for Applied Psychophysiology and Biofeedback [AAPB], 2016).

SCIENTIFIC BASIS

Biofeedback has been around for some time. The following data provide the basis for the use of biofeedback:

■ Biofeedback originated from research in the fields of psychophysiology, learning theory, and behavioral theory. It has been used by nurses for decades and is consistent with self-care nursing theories.

■ For centuries, it was believed that responses such as heart rate were beyond the individual's control. In the 1960s, scientists found that the autonomic nervous system (ANS) had an afferent system as well as a motor system that revealed control of ANS functioning was possible with instrumentation and conditioning.

■ For years, many researchers have used electromyography (EMG) feedback of muscle tension to measure states of relaxation, anxiety, and muscular strength.

■ Heart rate variability (HRV) biofeedback was first studied by Soviet scientists in the 1980s. HRV is the amount of fluctuation from the mean heart rate. It represents the interaction between the sympathetic and the parasympathetic systems and specifically targets ANS reactivity. HRV biofeedback is based on the premise that slowed breathing increases HRV amplitude, strengthens baroreflexes, and improves ANS functioning (McKee, 2008). HRV biofeedback is easy to learn and can be used with inexpensive, user-friendly devices, some of which can be used independently in the home.

■ Neurofeedback uses electroencephalogram (EEG) feedback to show people their actual patterns in cortical functioning. It also makes use of the brain's ability to change and can train the brain to function better (Neurodevelopment Center Inc., 2016).

The model for biofeedback is a skills-acquisition model in which individuals explore the relationship between ANS functioning and their voluntary muscle or cognitive/affective activities. They learn skills to control these activities, which are then reinforced by a visual and/or auditory display on the biofeedback instrument. The display informs the person whether control has been achieved, reinforcing learning. The following are conditions in which biofeedback has been used:

■ Behavioral strategies, such as relaxation or muscle strengthening, are often part of biofeedback treatment to modify physiological activity.

■ Biofeedback with relaxation strategies can be used to control autonomic responses that affect brain waves, peripheral vascular activity, heart rate, blood glucose, and skin conductance.

■ Biofeedback combined with exercise can strengthen muscles weakened by conditions such as chronic pulmonary disease, knee surgery, or age.

BIOFEEDBACK RESOURCES

Nurses are the ideal professionals to provide biofeedback because of their knowledge of physiology, psychology, and health and illness states. However, to use biofeedback they need to acquire special information, skills, and equipment. It is recommended that information be gained from classes and workshops available in many locations in the United States, a few other countries, and online. Nurses using biofeedback should become certified by the Biofeedback Certification International Alliance (BCIA, www.bcia.org), which offers certifications in general biofeedback, neurofeedback, HRV biofeedback, and pelvic muscle dysfunction biofeedback. People across the globe have received BCIA certificates, including the countries of Australia, Austria, Brazil, Canada, China, Egypt, El Salvador, Germany, Greece, Ireland, Israel, Jamaica, Japan, Mexico, the Netherlands, Poland, the Republic of Korea, the Republic of Singapore, Slovakia, South Africa, Taiwan, Turkey, the United Kingdom, the United States, and Venezuela. The AAPB (www.aapb.org) is also an excellent resource for information.

For professionals in Europe, North and South America, Asia, and Africa, the Biofeedback Foundation of Europe (BFE) sponsors education, training, and research activities in biofeedback. On its website (www.bfe.org), the BFE lists these opportunities in the form of conferences, workshops, internet courses, courseware, and other materials. Both AAPB and BFE recommend the book *Biofeedback Mastery: An Experiential Teaching and Self-Training Manual*, which can be used for teaching and self-directed learning (Peper et al., 2009).

Another organization, Biofeedback Resources International (BRI; www .biofeedbackinternational.com), offers self-directed online courses that meet the didactic requirements for BCIA certification and offers software, books, and CDs of biofeedback treatment programs for anxiety, addiction, anger, and pain. Face-to-face training programs with hands-on training and mentoring, however, are strongly recommended. Biofeedback equipment for purchase can also be found on the AAPB and the BRI websites.

The International Society for Neurofeedback and Research (ISNR) is a non-profit member organization for health professionals, researchers, educators, and other individuals who are interested in the promotion of self-regulation of brain activity for healthier functioning. The major mission of the society is "to promote excellence in clinical practice, educational applications, and research in applied neuroscience in order to better understand and enhance brain function" (www. isnr.org). Although it is located in McLean, Virginia, Society members gather from around the globe for their annual scientific meetings.

INTERVENTIONS

Although different forms of biofeedback exist, biofeedback interventions commonly involve the use of an electrical sensor that is attached to the body to detect physiological activity. These sensors may measure such physiological parameters as muscle tension, body temperature, heart rate, brain waves, or skin responses. The physiological activity detected by these sensors is transmitted to an electronic auditory or visual display to provide the intervention recipient feedback regarding their physiological activity. On receiving this feedback, intervention recipients can work towards modifying their thoughts, feelings, or behavior, which will, in turn, affect their physiological processes.

Biofeedback provides information about changes in a physiological parameter when specific strategies are used by the intervention recipient. For example, the heart rate can be lowered through breathing exercises, relaxation techniques, and mental activities. Directed relaxation or listening to music can help relax muscles and affect body temperature. As muscles relax, circulation improves, and the fingers and toes become warmer. When exercises are used to strengthen perineal muscles in preventing urinary incontinence in women, success in contracting the correct muscles may be monitored by a pressure sensor inserted into the vagina. In health conditions exacerbated by stress, biofeedback is often combined with stress management counseling.

Although biofeedback is typically used in an office or clinic setting, with the increasing availability of remote physiological measures, biofeedback is also being used in home and community settings. However, regardless of the setting in which the biofeedback intervention occurs, both the behavioral and feedback aspects of the intervention should be explained to the intervention recipients. The length and number of sessions depend on the condition for which the person is being treated. If the intervention recipient is unable to achieve mastery or control of a physiological parameter by the end of an agreed-on number of sessions, the reasons and the need for further sessions should be discussed.

The first session is devoted to assessing the intervention recipient, choosing the appropriate mode of biofeedback, discussing the roles of the nurse and the intervention recipient, and obtaining baseline measurements. Measuring several parameters helps in obtaining valid baseline data. Because success is determined by changes from baseline, it is essential that these are accurate and reflect the true status of the parameter being used. The first session is typically longer than subsequent ones, perhaps lasting 1 to 2 hours. Behavioral exercises, which may involve breathing and relaxation, are provided.

The nurse as the interventionist plays a key role in the success of biofeedback. It is helpful for the nurse to have advanced training in relaxation, guided imagery, breathing exercises, and stress management counseling. Because practicing behavioral techniques is vital, the nurse who succeeds in motivating intervention recipients to practice at home is most likely to see them achieve or exceed their goals.

The final sessions focus on integrating the learning into the person's life. The intervention recipient is connected to the feedback system but does not receive feedback while practicing the technique; the nurse monitors the degree of control achieved. Descriptions of stressful situations are provided, and the person is asked to practice the procedure as if in those situations. Final measurements are taken. Follow-up sessions at 1 month and 6 months are usually recommended.

GUIDELINES FOR BIOFEEDBACK-ASSISTED RELAXATION

A sample protocol for using biofeedback with cognitive behavioral interventions for relaxation and stress management is found in Exhibit 10.1. This technique could be used for hypertension, anxiety, asthma, headache, or pain because muscle relaxation improves these conditions. The protocol should be tailored to the patient, condition, and type of feedback.

Various types of relaxation exercises, such as autogenic phases or systematic relaxation, may be used. To increase patient awareness of the relaxed state versus the state of tension, progressive muscle relaxation with alternate contraction and relaxation may be helpful. Imagery may relax patients by distracting the mind and reducing negative or stressful thoughts. Hypnosis and self-hypnosis also produce an alternative state of mind. Soft music relaxes and distracts and may be used with relaxation or imagery. Slow-paced deep breathing facilitates relaxation, reduces stress, and promotes overall health.

Exhibit 10.1 *Biofeedback Protocol*

1. **Before first session**
   - Determine health problem for which biofeedback treatment is sought.
   - Ask for physician's name so that care can be coordinated. Give information on location, time commitment, and cost.
   - Request a 2-week patient log with medications and the frequency and severity of the health problem (e.g., number, intensity, time of headaches).
   - Answer questions.

2. **First session**
   - Interview patient for a health history; include the specific health condition.
   - Assess abilities for carrying out current medical regimen and behavioral intervention. Assess cultural preferences for behavioral treatments.
   - Discuss rationale for biofeedback, type of feedback, and behavioral intervention.
   - Explain that the role of the nurse is to provide ten 50-minute sessions once a week, using the biofeedback instrument to supply physiological information.
   - Explain that the patient is the major factor in the successful use of biofeedback and that it is important to continue to keep a log of the health problem, including home practice sessions. The patient should consult the physician if other health problems occur.
   - Explain the procedure. If using frontalis muscle tension EMG feedback, apply three sensors to the forehead after cleaning the skin with soap and water and applying gel. Set the biofeedback machine and operate according to instructions.
   - Obtain baseline EMG readings of frontalis muscle tension for 5 minutes while the patient sits quietly with closed eyes.
   - Instruct the patient to practice taped relaxation instructions for 20 minutes while the EMG sensors are on the forehead. Ask the patient to watch the biofeedback display for information on the decreasing level of muscle tension.
   - Review the 2-week record of the health problem and set mutual goals.
   - Provide an electronic sound file with instructions for practicing relaxation at home. Provide a log to record practice and responses. Discuss timing, frequency, length, and setting for practice.
   - Discuss self-care for any possible side effects to the behavioral intervention.

3. **Subsequent sessions**
   - Open the session with a 20-minute review of the health-problem log, stressors, and ways used for coping in the past week; provide counseling for adaptive coping.
   - Apply sensors and earphones and let the patient practice relaxation for 20 minutes while watching the display. Quietly leave the room after the patient masters the technique.
   - Vary relaxation techniques to maintain interest and increase skill.
   - Give instructions for incremental integration of relaxation into daily life. For example, add 30-second mini relaxation exercises for busy times of the day (e.g., touch thumbs to middle fingers, close eyes, and feel relaxation spreading through the body).

(continued)

Exhibit 10.1 *Biofeedback Protocol (continued)*

4. Final session
- Conduct the session as described; obtain final EMG readings.
- Discuss a plan for ongoing practice and stress management after treatment ends.

Exhibit 10.2 *Parameters Used for Feedback to Patients*	
Airway resistance	Gastric pH
Blood pressure	Heart rate
Blood volume	Heart rate variability
Bowel sounds	Peripheral skin temperature
EEG neurofeedback	Pneumography
EMG muscle feedback	Tidal volume
Forced expiratory volume	Tracheal noise
Galvanic skin response	Vagal nerve stimulation

It is important to keep the requirements for home practice simple, interesting, and meaningful. For example, boredom with the same relaxation instructions, failure to find a convenient time to practice, and a lack of noticeable improvements may decrease adherence to home practice. Changing to a new relaxation technique can revive interest. To integrate new skills into daily life, patients can progress from mini-relaxation and using cues (thoughts, positions, activities) to signal relaxation. In women caregivers experiencing stress who received HRV biofeedback training, Zauszniewski and colleagues examined six parameters for evaluating self-management interventions from the women's perspectives. The findings from that study provided evidence that the women caregivers believed the biofeedback intervention was necessary, appropriate, manageable, easy to learn, safe, and beneficial in ameliorating their stress (Zauszniewski et al., 2017).

Although some patients have multiple symptoms that may benefit from treatment, biofeedback training should be focused on one symptom at a time. Other symptoms can be addressed sequentially after mastery of the first biofeedback method is attained. The intervention recipient can decide which symptom will be treated first.

MEASUREMENT OF OUTCOMES

Feedback parameters that reflect mastery of the behavioral intervention are listed in Exhibit 10.2. Frequently used mastery parameters include heart rate, muscle tension, peripheral temperature, blood pressure, HRV, and EEG neurofeedback. For learning purposes, it is important that the nurse interventionist be clear about (a) mastery parameters that consist of ongoing feedback to the intervention recipient and (b) outcome parameters that reflect the desired health improvement.

For example, temperature feedback is used for peripheral vascular problems, but healthcare outcomes may result in fewer episodes of painful vasoconstriction. Both EMG feedback and temperature feedback are learning modalities used in those with diabetes mellitus, tension headache, and chronic pain. Outcomes may include decreased glycosylated hemoglobin, fewer and/or less severe headaches, cessation of urinary incontinence, and relief of pain.

PRECAUTIONS

Biofeedback should be used cautiously, if at all, in persons with depression, psychosis, seizures, and hyperactive conditions. Those with rigid personalities may be unwilling to change their mode of functioning. The nurse interventionist should consider that negative reactions may be related to relaxation rather than to biofeedback. Relaxation-related reactions may be avoided by means of patient education and the type of relaxation used (Schwartz & Andrisik, 2016).

Biofeedback-assisted relaxation is expected to lower blood pressure and heart and respiratory rates. Excessive decreases should be avoided in persons with cardiac conditions, hemodynamic instability, or multiple illnesses. Using relaxation therapies may also reduce the amount of medication needed to control diabetes mellitus, hypertension, and asthma. This should be discussed with potential intervention recipients and their physicians, and responses to therapy should be carefully monitored. For example, in individuals with diabetes, there is the potential for hypoglycemic reactions if appropriate education is not provided or if adjustments in insulin or diet are not made. Persons with diabetes should be taught to manage hypoglycemia and blood glucose. The nurse interventionist should have simple carbohydrates, glucagon, and a blood glucose monitor readily available and have the expertise to administer them. Home practice can be timed to avoid low blood glucose (McGrady & Lakia, 2016).

Nurses should therefore consider the person, the health problem, any known adverse reactions to the behavioral intervention used, and negative reactions to the biofeedback itself. For example, perineal muscle strengthening exercises for stress incontinence carry the risk of urinary leakage during the muscle strengthening process, which can be managed with a pad. Pharyngeal muscle exercises for dysphagia following stroke carry a more serious risk of aspiration as strength is slowly regained. Although there are generally few side effects associated with biofeedback with relaxation or exercises to improve function, ineffectiveness is always possible. Nurses should be cautioned to consider the risks of using a mild intervention with variable effectiveness and assess for age- and culturally related acceptability and effectiveness as the patient tries both biofeedback and the nonpharmacological treatment. On the other hand, both the nurse interventionist and the intervention recipient should consider the benefits of learning to use a nondrug method, such as biofeedback, in relation to the individual's efforts in improving body functioning.

Electric shock is a potential hazard when any electrical equipment is used. Dangerous levels of current flow may arise from equipment malfunction or operator error. Patients who have devices such as pacemakers or implantable cardiac defibrillators should consult with their healthcare provider and the device manuals prior to using biofeedback. Zauszniewski et al. (2017) studied the perceived safety of an HRV biofeedback intervention from the perspective of caregivers who were the biofeedback recipients. In the case of electricity, objective evaluation of safety is highly important. The AAPB publishes a list of companies whose products have met their safety code.

Although biofeedback is noninvasive, cost-effective, and promising in the treatment of many conditions, it is not a miracle intervention. It requires that the nurse interventionist is knowledgeable about the health problem, intervention, and medication effects and has a sincere interest in the intervention recipient's outcome. It requires the intervention recipient to contribute time, attention, and motivation for the success of the biofeedback practice. Ongoing use of the behavioral technique may be needed to control the condition after biofeedback sessions end. This should be made very clear before training is initiated.

USES

Biofeedback has been used in the treatment of a wide range of medical and psychological problems. However, empirical studies have shown varying levels of efficaciousness related to biofeedback modality and the condition that is being treated. Specific criteria for the levels of efficacy of biofeedback, ranging from level 1 (not empirically supported) to level 5 (efficacious and specific), have been defined (see Yucha, 2016). In addition, the AAPB website lists a number of conditions in which biofeedback has been empirically studied with efficacy ratings between 3 (probably efficacious) to 5 (efficacious and specific). Biofeedback has been shown to be efficacious in multiple observational, clinical, and wait-list controlled studies, including replications. A visitor to the AAPB website can click on the health condition of interest and obtain information on the level of evidence, the reason biofeedback would help, and the supporting evidence (www.aapb.org/i4a/pages/index.cfm?pageID=3404)

The most recent edition of *Evidence-Based Practice in Biofeedback and Neurofeedback* (Tan et al., 2016) provides up-to-date information regarding the efficacy of biofeedback or neurofeedback for use in treating forty different conditions. Considering the most recent empirical evidence, the highest efficacy rating (5: efficacious and specific) has been determined for attention-deficit/hyperactivity disorder (ADHD). A Level 4 rating (efficacious) was determined for anxiety, constipation, depression, epilepsy, erectile dysfunction, fecal incontinence, headache, hypertension, irritable bowel syndrome, pre-eclampsia, Raynaud's disease, temporomandibular muscle and joint disorder, some forms of chronic pain, and glycemic control associated with diabetes mellitus. Biofeedback is probably efficacious (Level 3) for treating alcohol and substance abuse disorders, arthritis, asthma autism, facial palsy, fibromyalgia, effects of chemotherapy, insomnia, motion sickness, posttraumatic stress disorder, tinnitus, traumatic brain injury, and urinary incontinence. Biofeedback is possibly efficacious (Level 2) for treating cerebral palsy, chronic obstructive pulmonary disease, coronary heart disease, function recurrent abdominal pain hyperhidrosis, immune functioning, repetitive strain injury, stroke, and vasovagal syndrome (Tan et al., 2016).

SYSTEMATIC REVIEWS AND META-ANALYSES

Over the past decade, nurse authors have published five systematic reviews or meta-analyses of studies of biofeedback within nursing journals that include the *International Journal of Nursing Studies, Pain Management Nursing, and the Journal of Holistic Nursing, and Urologic Nursing.* Three of these reviews involved the use of biofeedback in pelvic floor muscle training for urinary incontinence, two involved men (Hsu et al., 2016; Nahon et al., 2014), and one focused on women (McIntosh et al., 2015). Hsu and colleagues (2016) studied pelvic floor muscle training with and without biofeedback in men with urinary incontinence following prostatectomy and found significant immediate, intermediate, and long-term effects in those who received biofeedback compared with those who did not. However, Nahon and colleagues (2014) reported that adding biofeedback to pelvic muscle floor training in men preoperatively had little effect in improving their continence. In a scoping review of studies of women with stress incontinence, pelvic floor muscle training with biofeedback emerged as one of the most frequently described treatment modalities (McIntosh et al., 2015).

The other two reviews authored by nurses examined biofeedback in persons with fibromyalgia (Reneau, 2020) and in peripartum women experiencing psychological stress (Herbell & Zauszniewski, 2018). Both of these reviews focused on evaluating the effectiveness of HRV biofeedback. While Reneau (2020) reported that HRV biofeedback was effective in reducing chronic pain, Herbell and Zauszniewski (2018) found that peripartum women who completed HRV biofeedback experienced a reduction in psychological stress compared with women who did not receive HRV biofeedback.

TECHNOLOGY

Technological advancements in biofeedback are constant. Wearable biofeedback technology has expanded into clothing garments, watches, and patches. Many devices have not been tested in studies; only 5% have been formally validated (Peake et al., 2018). In addition, smartphone apps for biofeedback are emerging. A game-based smartphone app for HRV biofeedback training has been developed and has shown success in physiological stress recovery in young adults (Hunter et al., 2019). More studies need to be done to validate newer technology for biofeedback.

SPECIAL POPULATIONS

Family Caregivers. Stress accompanies many life experiences. For example, the stress experienced by grandmothers who are raising grandchildren in the absence of the parents has been found to have adverse effects on the grandmother's health. HRV biofeedback has been examined in that population in four small studies in which the grandmothers were taught slow-paced breathing to increase their HRV using a portable biofeedback device in their homes for 4 weeks (Zauszniewski et al., 2013, 2015, 2017; Zauszniewski & Musil, 2014).

Biofeedback focused on HRV has also been used with family caregivers of persons with cancer (Hasuo et al., 2020), In addition, HRV biofeedback is currently being studied as a health self-management intervention in studies of family caregivers of patients with bipolar disorder (Zauszniewski et al., 2016–2021) and family caregivers of persons with dementia (Zauszniewski et al., 2020–2024); both studies were funded by the National Institutes of Health (NIH).

CHILDREN AND ADOLESCENTS

Biofeedback can be used for children and adolescents for treating a variety of conditions, including autism, ADHD, anxiety, depression, headache, and urinary incontinence. However, compared to biofeedback studies in adults, there are fewer studies examining the usefulness and effectiveness of biofeedback in children and adolescents. For children and adolescents, the biofeedback modality and training must be tailored to be age-appropriate and appealing in order to be effective (Olness, 2008). Video game–based biofeedback training has been used successfully to enhance exercise and improve gait training, indicated by EMG patterns changes in children with cerebral palsy (Booth et al., 2019; Flux et al., 2020; MacIntosh et al., 2020). A spirometry game for helping children with cystic fibrosis to achieve airway clearance has been developed (Bingham et al., 2012). In addition, game-based biofeedback has been used to decrease anxiety and depression in children (Knox et al., 2011). The use of virtual reality in feedback is being explored in children with ADHD and with those requiring gait training (Blume et al., 2017; Booth et al., 2019).

A recent systematic review and meta-analysis identified a number of studies conducted in pediatric populations that demonstrated significant effects of biofeedback indicated by changes in symptoms associated with specific conditions or changes in physiological functioning (Darling et al., 2019). However, their findings require caution because the studies reviewed were of low quality (Darling et al., 2019). Continued research and rigorous testing of various biofeedback modalities in children and adolescents experiencing diverse medical and psychological conditions are needed.

GENDER CONSIDERATIONS

Women are more likely to use complementary and alternative therapies to improve health and well-being while men are more likely to use alternative therapies to improve athletic or sports performance (Zhang et al., 2015). The use of HRV biofeedback has shown positive effects on health and athletic performance in men and women (Lehrer et al., 2020). Further research is needed to explore outcomes by gender.

RACIAL AND ETHNIC CONSIDERATIONS

African Americans and Hispanic and Latino Americans, the largest racial minority groups in the United States, are the least likely to use complementary and alternative therapies, including biofeedback (Rhee et al., 2017; Su & Li, 2011). Furthermore, racial/ethnic minorities often experience a great amount of psychological stress, have less access to health services, and experience poor health outcomes.

Few studies have been conducted to establish the feasibility and effectiveness of biofeedback in these racial groups. Biofeedback has been examined as a home-based, 8-week complementary therapy to reduce blood pressure in a small sample of hypertensive African Americans (Frankfurt, 2016). HRV biofeedback has been examined as a complementary therapy for depression in Latinos (Thode, 2020). In addition, HRV biofeedback has been implemented as a complementary therapy in a culturally adapted intervention for comorbid asthma and panic disorder in Latino adults (Feldman et al., 2016). Feldman and colleagues (2016) reported a 40% attrition rate. More research on biofeedback in racial/ethnic minority groups is warranted.

Biofeedback practitioners must understand cultural barriers and ensure vulnerable populations have adequate information before performing biofeedback.

Multicultural and diversity training considerations for professionals who teach biofeedback have been published (Harvey et al., 2015).

NURSES AND HEALTHCARE PROVIDERS

There are few studies in which the use of biofeedback has been studied in nurses; however, initial results have been promising in terms of reducing stress, anxiety, and depression symptoms and improving resilience (Cutshall et al., 2011; Hsieh et al., 2020). In light of the pandemic and the stress within and external to healthcare settings, biofeedback could be an area of fruitful exploration to improve the well-being of healthcare providers.

CULTURAL APPLICATIONS

Biofeedback therapy has been used and studied around the world. In Thailand, for example, it has been used for a variety of conditions, as shown in Sidebar 10.1

Sidebar 10.1 *Use of Biofeedback in Thailand*

Nutchanart Bunthumporn

Many kinds of biofeedback—including galvanic skin response, electromyography, electroencephalography, and heart rate variability—are used in Thailand. However, electromyography feedback is used most widely. Biofeedback is most often used with relaxation techniques to decrease stress and anxiety in students, staff nurses, and patients with chronic diseases. Along with autogenic training, it has also helped decrease aggressive behaviors in drug abusers and improve behaviors in children with attention-deficit/hyperactivity disorder. In a randomized study, an HRV biofeedback training program with support for paced breathing decreased older patients' depressive symptoms, negative affect, and depressive cognitions and enhanced their resourceful behaviors ($N = 100$; Bunthumporn, 2012). The first of three biofeedback studies by nurse researchers in Thailand reported that progressive relaxation and group supportive psychotherapy reduced depressive symptoms and muscle tension in older adults with chronic illness (Muijeen et al., 2012). The second found that meditation training with biofeedback training reduced stress in patients with chronic disease (Thongkhum et al., 2015). The third study showed that heart rate variability biofeedback significantly decreased depressive symptom scores in adults with depressive disorders (Ngamlers et al., 2018).

The benefits of biofeedback are limited by practitioner issues such as complexity of use, availability of training, and overall cost of some devices. To improve training issues, biofeedback concepts have been integrated into courses for nursing and psychology graduate students. Interestingly, the challenges of biofeedback technology did not deter Thai older adults, as there was no attrition during the Bunthumporn study (2012).

Sidebar 10.1 *Use of Biofeedback in Thailand (continued)*

There are national biofeedback associations in 15 countries in North and South America, Europe, Asia, the Middle East, and Russia (Biofeedback Certification International Alliance, https://www.bcia.org/international-bf-nf-associations). Although the number of articles published outside the United States cannot be easily estimated, the PubMed database identifies scientific articles about biofeedback that have been written in Japanese, German, Dutch, French, Spanish, Chinese, Norwegian, Finnish, Czech, Hebrew, Korean, Russian, and other languages. In the Russian and Japanese languages, for example, there are studies using biofeedback for many different health problems, including epilepsy, asthma, itch, sleep, and mandibular dysfunction. Many of these studies are written in English.

Using their native languages, nurses have authored or coauthored research reports on biofeedback for a variety of health problems of interest to nurses. Nurses in England reviewed how biofeedback is used to treat bowel dysfunction in adults with constipation (Burch & Collins, 2010). In the Chinese language, nurses reported that biofeedback training in adults with functional constipation improved bowel symptoms, quality of life, and psychological status (Zhu et al., 2011). Nurse researchers in Taiwan used a quasi-experimental design and demonstrated that biofeedback relaxation reduced the pain associated with continuous passive motion after total knee arthroplasty (Wang et al., 2015).

References

Bingham, P. M., Lahiri, T., & Ashikaga, T. (2012). Pilot trial of spirometer games for airway clearance practice in cystic fibrosis. *Respiratory Care, 57*(8), 1278–1284. https://doi.org/10.4187/respcare.01263

Bunthumporn, N. (2012). *Effects of biofeedback training on negative affect, depressive cognitions, resourceful behaviors, and depressive symptoms in Thai elders.* OhioLINK ETD Center. https://etd .ohiolink.edu/!etd.send_file?accession=case1333479530&disposition=inline

Burch, J., & Collins, B. (2010). Using biofeedback to treat constipation, Faecal incontinence, and other bowel disorders. *Nursing Times, 106*(37), 20–21. https://www.nursingtimes.net/clinical-archive/ continence/using-biofeedback-to-treat-constipation-faecal-incontinence-and-other-bowel -disorders-19-09-2010/#:~:text=Biofeedback%20therapy%20is%20used%20in,bowel%20 disorders%2C%20such%20faecal%20incontinence.

Muijeen, K., Ruchiwit, M., & Somprasert, C. H. (2012). The effect of progressive muscular relaxation program and group supportive psychotherapy on the depression level of the elderly with chronic illness. *The Journal of Psychiatric Nursing and Mental Health, 26*(1), 19–34. https://he02.tci-thaijo .org/index.php/JPNMH/article/view/17995/15908

Ngamlers, D., Bunthumporn, N., & Somprasert, C. (2018, September–December). The effects of a heart rate variability biofeedback training program on depression symptoms of adults with depression disorder. *Journal of Psychiatric Nursing and Mental Health, 32*(3), 61–74. https://he02.tci-thaijo .org/index.php/JPNMH/article/view/163105/117849

Thongkhum, K., Ruchiwity, M., & Somprasert, C. (2015). The effect of meditation training together with a biofeedback training program on the stress levels of chronic disease setting. *Nursing Journal, 42*(1): 24-37.

Wang, T-J., Chang, C-F., Lou, M-F., Ao, M-K., Liu, C-C, Liang, S-Y., Wu, S-F. V., & Tung, H-H. (2015). Biofeedback relaxation for pain associated with continuous passive motion in Taiwanese patients after total knee arthroplasty. *Research in Nursing & Health, 38*(1), 39–50. https://doi.org/10.1002/nur.21633

Zhu, F., Lin, Z., & Wang, M. (2011). Changes in quality of life during biofeedback for people with puborectalis dyssynergia: Generic and disease-specific measures. *Journal of Advanced Nursing, 67*(6), 1285–1293. https://doi.org/10.1111/j.1365-2648.2010.05593.x

FUTURE RESEARCH

There continues to be a great need for randomized controlled clinical trials to determine the effectiveness, acceptability, and sustainability of biofeedback in treating physiological and psychological conditions in adults, children, and minorities worldwide. Biofeedback studies of prevalent local health problems are needed in developing countries. However, large multicenter studies with similar inclusion criteria, biofeedback protocol, and research methods are needed to show overall efficacy (Yucha, 2002). In addition, the perspective of biofeedback recipients regarding factors that are needed for ongoing self-care practice needs further study. Nurses can address the following questions:

- What is the availability of biofeedback training in various countries?
- What culturally acceptable behavioral treatments can be provided with biofeedback?
- What are the predictors of improvement in using biofeedback for managing health?
- Do potential biofeedback recipients believe that biofeedback is necessary, acceptable, feasible, effective, and safe and that it can be performed by following a specified protocol (i.e., fidelity)?

REFERENCES

Association for Applied Psychophysiology and Biofeedback. (2016). *2018 AAPB 49th Annual Scientific Meeting.* http://www.aapb.org

Bingham, P. M., Lahiri, T., & Ashikaga, T. (2012). Pilot trial of spirometer games for airway clearance practice in cystic fibrosis. *Respiratory Care, 57*(8), 1278–1284. https://doi.org/10.4187/respcare.01263

Blume, F., Hudak, J., Dresler, T., Ehlis, A., Kühnhausen, J., Renner, T. J., & Gawrilow, C. (2017). NIRS-based neurofeedback training in a virtual reality classroom for children with attention-deficit/hyperactivity disorder: Study protocol for a randomized controlled trial. *Trials, 18*, 41. https://doi.org/10.1186/s13063-016-1769-3

Booth, A. T. C., van der Krogt, M. M., Buizer, A. I., Steenbrink, F., & Harlaar, J. (2019). The validity and usability of an eight marker model for avatar-based biofeedback gait training. *Clinical Biomechanics, 70*, 146–152. https://doi.org/10.1016/j.clinbiomech.2019.08.013

Bunthumporn, N. (2012). *Effects of biofeedback training on negative affect, depressive cognitions, resourceful behaviors, and depressive symptoms in Thai elders.* OhioLINK ETD Center. http://rave.ohiolink.edu/etdc/view?acc_num=case1333479530

Cutshall, S. M., Wentworht, L. J., Wahner-Roedler, D. L., Vincent, A., Schmidt, J. E., Loehrer, L. L., Cha, S. S., & Bauer, B. A. (2011). Evaluation of a biofeedback-assisted meditation program as a stress management tool for hospital nurses: A pilot study. *Explore: The Journal of Science & Healing, 7*(2), 110–112. https://doi.org/10.1016/j.explore.2010.12.004

Darling, K. E., Benore, E. R., & Webster, E. E. (2019). Biofeedback in pediatric populations: A systematic review and meta-analysis of treatment outcomes. *Translational Behavioral Medicine, 10*(6), 1436–1449. https://doi.org/10.1093/tbm/ibz124

Feldman, J. M., Matte, L., Interian, A., Lehrer, P. M., Lu, S.-E., Scheckner, B., Steinberg, D. M., Oken, T., Kotay, A., Sinha, S., & Shim, C. (2016). Psychological treatment of comorbid asthma and panic disorder in Latino adults: Results from a randomized controlled trial. *Behaviour Research and Therapy, 87*, 142–154. https://doi.org/10.1016/j.brat.2016.09.007

Flux, E., Atteveld, O. A., Bar-On, L., Buizer, A. I., Harlaar, J., & van der Krogt, M. M. (2020). Biofeedback-driven gaming to improve EMG patterns during gait in children with cerebral palsy. *Gait & Posture, 81*, 97–98. https://doi.org/10.1016/j.gaitpost.2020.07.082

Frankfurt, P. A. (2016). *A home-based biofeedback intervention in a hypertensive African American sample: A pilot study.* ProQuest Dissertations & Theses Global (1884347034).

Harvey, R., Lin, I.-M., & Booiman, A. (2015). Multicultural and diversity training considerations for biofeedback practitioners. *Biofeedback, 43*(4), 163–167. https://doi.org/10.5298/1081-5937-43.4.05

Hasuo, H., Kanbara, K., & Fukunaga, M. (2020). Effect of heart rate variability biofeedback sessions with resonant frequency breathing on sleep: A pilot study among family caregivers of patients with cancer. *Frontiers in Medicine, 7,* 61–69. https://doi.org/10.3389/fmed.2020.00061w

Herbell, K., & Zauszniewski, J. A. (2018). Reducing psychological stress in peripartum Women with heart rate variability biofeedback: A systematic review. *Journal of Holistic Nursing, 37*(3), 273–285. https://doi.org/10.1177/0898010118783030

Hsieh, H. F., Huang, I. C., Liu, Y., Chen, W. L., Lee, Y. W., & Hsu, H. T. (2020). The effects of biofeedback training and smartphone-delivered biofeedback training on resilience, occupational stress, and depressive symptoms among abused psychiatric nurses. *International Journal of Environmental Research & Public Health [Electronic Resource], 17*(8), 4. https://doi.org/10.3390/ijerph17082905

Hsu, L.-F., Liao, Y.-M., Lai, F.-C., & Tsai, P.-S. (2016). Beneficial effects of biofeedback-assisted pelvic floor muscle training in patients with urinary incontinence after radical prostatectomy: A systematic review and metaanalysis. *International Journal of Nursing Studies, 60,* 99–111. https://doi.org/10.1016/j.ijnurstu.2016.03.013

Hunter, J. F., Olah, M.S., Williams, A. L., Parks, A. C., & Pressman, S. D (2019). Effect of brief biofeedback via a smartphone app on stress recovery: Randomized experimental study. *JMIR Serious Games, 7*(4), e15974. https://doi.org/10.2196/15974

Knox, M., Lentini, J., Cummings, T. S., McGrady, A., Whearty, K., & Sacrant, L. (2011). Game-based biofeedback for pediatric anxiety and depression. *Mental Health in Family Medicine, 8*(3), 195–203.

Lehrer, P., Kaur, K., Sharma, A., Shah, K., Huseby, R., Bhavsar, J., & Zhang, Y. (2020). Heart rate variability biofeedback improves emotional and physical health and performance: A systematic review and meta-analysis. *Applied Psychophysiology and Biofeedback, 45*(3), 109–129. https://doi.org/10.1007/s10484-020-09466-z

MacIntosh, A., Desailly, E., Vignais, N., Vigneron, V., & Biddiss, E. (2020). A biofeedback-enhanced therapeutic exercise video game intervention for young people with cerebral palsy: A randomized single-case experimental design feasibility study. *PLOS ONE, 15*(6), 1–22. https://doi.org/10.1371/journal.pone.0234767

McGrady, A., & Lakia, D. M. (2016). Diabetes mellitus. In M. S. Schwartz & F. Andrisik (Eds.), *Biofeedback: A practitioner's guide* (4th ed., pp. 400–422). Guilford Press.

McIntosh, L., Andersen, E., & Reekie, M. (2015). Conservative treatment of stress urinary incontinence in women: A 10-year (2004–2013) scoping review of the literature. *Urologic Nursing, 35*(4), 179–186. https://doi.org/10.7257/1053-816x.2015.35.4.179

McKee, M. G. (2008). Biofeedback: An overview in the context of heart-brain medicine. *Cleveland Clinic Journal of Medicine, 75*(Suppl. 2), S31–S34. https://doi.org/10.3949/ccjm.75.Suppl_2.S31

Nahon, I., Martin, M., & Adams, R. (2014). Pre-operative pelvic floor muscle training – A review. *Urologic Nursing, 34*(5), 230–237. https://doi.org/10.7257/1053-816x.2014.34.5.230

Neurodevelopment Center Inc. (2016, December 14). *What is neurofeedback?* https://neurodevelopmentcenter.com/neurofeedback-2

Ngamlers, D., Bunthumporn, N., & Somprasert, C. (2018, September–December). The effects of a heart rate variability biofeedback training program on depression symptoms of adults with depression disorder. *Journal of Psychiatric Nursing and Mental Health, 32*(3), 61–74. https://he02.tci-thaijo.org/index.php/JPNMH/article/view/163105/117849

Olness, K. (2008, March). Helping children and adults with hypnosis and biofeedback. *Cleveland Clinic Journal of Medicine, 75*(Suppl. 2), S39–S43. https://doi.org/10.3949/ccjm.75.Suppl_2.S39

Peake, J. M., Kerr, G., & Sullivan, J. P. (2018). A critical review of consumer wearables, mobile applications, and equipment for providing biofeedback, monitoring stress, and sleep in physically active populations. *Frontiers in Physiology, 9,* 743. https://doi.org/10.3389/fphys.2018.00743

Peper, E., Tylova, H., Gibney, K. H., Harvey, R., & Combatalade, D. (2009). *Biofeedback mastery—An experiential teaching and self-training manual.* Association for Applied Psychophysiology and Biofeedback.

Reneau, M. (2020). Heart rate variability biofeedback to treat fibromyalgia: An integrative literature review. *Pain Management Nursing, 21*(3), 225–232. https://doi.org/10.1016/j.pmn.2019.08.001

Rhee, T. G., Evans, R. L., McAlpine, D. D., & Johnon, P. J. (2017). Racial/ethnic differences in the use of complementary and alternative medicine in US adults with moderate mental distress. *Journal of Primary Care & Community Health, 8*(2), 43–54. https://doi.org/10.1177/2150131916671229

Schwartz, M. S., & Andrisik, F. (Eds.). (2016). *Biofeedback: A practitioner's guide* (4th ed.). Guilford Press.

Su, D., & Li, L. (2011). Trends in the use of complementary and alternative medicine in the United States: 2002–2007. *Journal of Health Care for the Poor and Underserved, 22*(1), 296–310. https://doi.org/10.1353/hpu.2011.0002

Tan, G., Shaffer, F., Lyle, R., & Teo, I. (2016). *Evidence-based practice in biofeedback and neurofeedback* (3rd ed.). Association for Applied Psychophysiology and Biofeedback.

Thode, L. C. (2020). Heart rate variability biofeedback as a complementary treatment for depression in Latinos. *Dissertation Abstracts International Section A: Humanities and Social Sciences, 81*(7–A).

Yucha, C. (2016). Clinical efficacy of biofeedback therapy: Explanation of efficacy levels. In G. Tan, I. Teo, R. Lyle, & F. Schaffer (Eds.), *Evidence-based practice in biofeedback and neurofeedback* (pp. 5–6). Association for Applied Psychophysiology and Biofeedback.

Yucha, C. B. (2002). Problems inherent in assessing biofeedback efficacy studies. *Applied Psychophysiology and Biofeedback, 27*(1), 99–106. https://doi.org/10.1023/a:1014528622061

Zauszniewski, J. A., Au, T.Y., & Musil, C. M. (2013). Heart rate variability biofeedback in grandmothers raising grandchildren: Effects on stress, emotions, and cognitions. *Biofeedback, 41*(2), 144–149. https://doi.org/10.5298/1081-5937-41.3.06

Zauszniewski, J. A., Kahana, E., & Burant, C. J. (2020–2024). *Self-management interventions: Considering needs and preferences of dementia caregivers* (RO1-NR018476). National Institute of Nursing Research.

Zauszniewski, J. A., & Musil, C. M. (2014). Interventions for grandmothers: Comparative effectiveness of resourcefulness training, HRV biofeedback, and journaling. *Biofeedback, 42*(3), 131–129. https://doi.org/10.5298/1081-5937-42.3.03

Zauszniewski, J. A., Musil, C. M., Herbell, K., & Givens, S. (2017). Heart rate variability in grandmothers: Evaluation of intervention parameters. *Issues in Mental Health Nursing, 38*(6), 493–499.

Zauszniewski, J. A., Musil C. M., & Variath, M. (2015). Biofeedback in grandmothers raising grandchildren: Correlations between subjective and objective measures. *Biofeedback, 44*(4), 193–199. https://doi.org/10.5298/1081-5937-43.4.01

Zauszniewski, J. A., Sajatovic, M., & Burant, C. J. (2016–2021). *Tailored health self-management interventions for highly distressed family caregivers* (,RO1-NR16817). National Institute of Nursing Research.

Zhang, Y., Leach, M. J., Hall, H., Sundberg, T., Ward, L., Sibbritt, D., & Adams, J. (2015). Differences between male and female consumers of complementary and alternative medicine in a national US population: A secondary analysis of 2012 NIHS Data. *Evidence-based Complementary and Alternative Medicine:eCAM, 2015,* 413173. https://doi.org/10.1155/2015/413173

11

Meditation

MICHAEL CHRISTOPHER, DANA DHARMAKAYA COLGAN,
AND AKEESHA SIMMONS

Meditation is the quintessential mind–body practice and the foundation for a number of widely used training programs, each with a rapidly growing evidence base to support health benefits (Rose et al., 2020). Between 2012 and 2017, the number of U.S. adults turning to meditation for health reasons significantly increased, and in 2017, an estimated 14% of U.S. adults practiced meditation—over 29 million people (National Center for Complementary and Integrative Health [NCCIH], 2022). The primary reasons for meditating among a large nationally representative sample were to reduce stress, enhance well-being, mitigate symptoms such as anxiety or pain, and self-manage chronic conditions (Upchurch & Johnson, 2019). Among the most widely used and well-researched meditation programs are mindfulness-based stress reduction (MBSR; Kabat-Zinn, 1990) and its various derivatives (e.g., mindfulness-based cognitive therapy [MBCT] Segal et al., 2002). This chapter focuses on these and closely related programs and includes experimental findings on the structural, physiological, cognitive, and emotional effects of meditation training. Although some definitions of *mindfulness meditation* consider practices such as yoga, tai chi, qi gong, and meditation within the context of religious observance and prayer, some of these practices are covered elsewhere in this book and are therefore not included in this chapter.

Over the past decade, there has been a substantial increase in research on meditation. Whereas in 2007 a major evidence report concluded that no firm conclusions could be drawn regarding the therapeutic impacts of any meditative practice or program based on the available evidence (Ospina et al., 2007), recent meta-analyses have confirmed benefits for a wide variety of health outcomes (Goldberg et al., 2021; Krittanawong et al., 2020; Schutte et al., 2020). There are many indications that this field is rapidly maturing. These include the development of academic journals devoted to meditation research (e.g., *Mindfulness*), increased National Institutes of Health funding for meditation research, and publication of recent guidelines regarding training and certification of meditation teachers to ensure rigor and quality in clinical and research endeavors (e.g., Crane et al., 2017). Currently, funded clinical trial research grants have heeded calls for rigorously designed and adequately powered clinical trials, in-depth and replicable investigations of mechanisms of change, and tailored interventions.

DEFINITION

For thousands of years, and in many civilizations, meditation practices have played an important role in religious observances and as a means of cultivating well-being. *Meditation* can be defined as a family of self-regulation practices that focus on training attention and awareness to bring mental processes under greater voluntary control, thereby, self-regulating the body, mind, and emotions and fostering general mental and physical well-being (Walsh & Shapiro, 2006). Meditation characteristically contains three essential processes: awareness of the present moment, attentional allocation, and the cultivation of specific qualities pertaining to attention and awareness.

The first and foremost process of meditation is a deliberate, present moment awareness of one's internal or "personal" experiences, including thoughts, emotions, sensations, and behaviors, as well as awareness of sensory perceptions (e.g., sights, sounds, smells). This can be contrasted with "automatic" cognitive and behavioral reactions that occur without conscious awareness.

A second inherent process of meditation is attentional allocation that involves sustained attention, the monitoring of attention, and attentional shifting (Lutz et al., 2008). As an individual attempts to deliberately attend to the present moment (sustained attention), one also acknowledges discursive thoughts and emotions that may arise (monitoring of attention). The ability to notice when one is getting "caught up" in thoughts or emotions, and the subsequent returning of attention to the present moment, requires disengaging from distractions, negative emotions, rumination, or worry via a purposeful and fluid shifting of attention (attentional shifting).

A third, and perhaps most important, process of meditation is the cultivation of particular qualities of awareness. Attitudes that exemplify this quality include kindness, curiosity, acceptance, nonreactivity, and equanimity. A kind, curious, and nonreactive awareness is developed so that one simply notices the object, or series of emerging objects, and the secondary evaluations and appraisals that occur (Bishop et al., 2004). With continued practice, this nonreactive awareness eventually allows for the de-automatization of habitual reactions to the present moment and the associated secondary appraisals, predictions, analyses, critics, or judgments about what has or is taking place (Keng et al., 2011; Olendzki, 2011). Together, these three processes are thought to lead to the development of mindfulness, defined as the "awareness that emerges by way of paying attention on purpose, in the present moment, and nonjudgmentally to the unfolding of experience, moment by moment" (Kabat-Zinn, 2003, p. 145). Mindfulness can be understood as a stable trait or a more temporary state and is characterized by an expanded awareness, a greater presence, and a more integrated sense of self (Davis et al., 2009).

Although historically intimately interwoven, the scientific community has categorized meditation practices into three groups based on neuroscientific conceptions and orientation of attention allocation: focused attention (FA), open monitoring (OM), and contemplative meditation (CM; Lutz et al., 2008; Vago & Silbersweig, 2012). FA is considered a "concentrative practice," which requires restricting and sustaining one's attention to a single object, such as the breath, a subvocal repeated sound or word (mantra), or an imagined mental image. When the mind wanders during FA practice, attention is brought back to the object of attention with little or no investigation of the distraction. A concentration practice is thought to calm and stabilize the wandering and distracted mind and has historically been considered a prerequisite for more advanced OM practice. Neural correlates of FA meditation include activation of brain regions associated with selective attention (e.g., ventrolateral prefrontal cortex), sustained attention (e.g., thalamus, right frontal lobes), conflict monitoring (e.g., dorsolateral prefrontal cortex and the anterior cingulate cortex; Manna et al., 2010), and deactivation and functional connectivity in regions associated with the default mode, a network associated with mind-wandering (Mason et al., 2007).

In contrast, OM meditation, frequently described as *mindfulness meditation*, does not involve any specific object of focus. OM meditations expand awareness to monitor all content of present moment experience (i.e., thoughts, emotions, sensations, sights, sounds) while cultivating a curious, accepting, and nonreactive stance. Every arising sensation, thought, or feeling is attended to in an equal manner; therefore, mind wandering is simply another event to witness (Olendzki, 2011). OM meditations are thought to foster a greater detachment from autobiographical memories, counteract the tendency toward experiential avoidance, and alter the relationship and interaction with one's internal content to create a sense of spaciousness around whatever is being experienced or observed (Fujino et al., 2018). An individual becomes familiar with, and perhaps even friendly toward, the habits of the mind, affording a broader and more skillful behavioral repertoire in response to the present moment (Alex Brake et al., 2016; Uusberg et al., 2016). Neural correlates of OM meditation include activation of brain regions associated with conscious awareness of thoughts and emotions (e.g., left frontoparietal and insular regions), decreased connectivity among regions associated with attention regulation and autobiographical memories, and deactivation of regions associated with the default mode network.

In comparing these two types of meditation, Germer et al. (2013) noted that FA meditation practice is like a laser light beam that highlights whatever object on which it is directed, whereas OM is akin to a searchlight that illuminates a wider range of objects as they arise in awareness, one at a time. FA practice develops the capacity to cultivate attentional allocation in a more direct and deliberate manner and can be likened to the sharpening of the blade of a knife. The subsequent practice of OM meditation, then, uses the sharpened knife to understand the nature and habits of the mind, increasing one's ability to skillfully respond to the present moment. It has been hypothesized that meditators pass through stages, from effortful to effortless maintenance of a meditative state (Tang & Posner, 2013). Consistent with this conceptualization, the concentrative and guided-meditation techniques taught to novices have been termed "scaffolding" by Kabat-Zinn (2003).

Finally, Vago and Silbersweig (2012) suggested a third group of practices that are largely based on the Buddhist principle, the Four Immeasurables: loving-kindness, compassion, empathic joy, and equanimity. *Loving-kindness* is defined as the wish for all sentient beings to have happiness and its causes (Salzberg, 2011). *Compassion* is defined as the wish for all sentient beings to be free from suffering and its causes. *Empathic joy* is the celebrating and finding joy in the happiness and success of others. *Equanimity* has been defined as an even-minded mental state that cannot be swayed by biases or preferences (Bodhi, 2011). These four interrelated attitudes are generated and then directed toward self and eventually all other sentient beings. Two examples of a CM are loving-kindness and compassion. Loving-kindness meditation (LKM) aims to develop an affective state of unconditional kindness to self and all people, while compassion meditation involves techniques to cultivate a deep and genuine compassion for self and others. CM practices entail elements of both FA and OM styles of practice. Neural correlates of CM practices may include brain regions associated with emotional processing, empathy, and theory of mind (e.g., amygdala, right temporo-parietal junction, anterior cingulate cortex, and lateral prefrontal cortex; Lee et al., 2012).

SCIENTIFIC BASIS

Understanding how meditation works is the basis for groundbreaking research by leading scientists. The scientific literature on meditation has virtually exploded in recent years. A search of PubMed.gov from January 2016 to July 2021 found 439 systematic reviews or meta-analyses addressing the impact of meditation on health (e.g., pain, heart disease, anxiety, depression, diabetes, multiple sclerosis), harmful health behaviors (e.g., binge eating, smoking, substance abuse), across populations (e.g., cancer survivors, healthcare workers, older adults), and settings (e.g., schools, prisons, workplaces).

A common denominator of many mindfulness-based interventions (MBIs), including MBSR, is the goal of mitigating the deleterious impact of stress on health, and chronic stress in particular. Chronic stress is often defined as the response to emotional pressure suffered for a prolonged period of time in which individuals perceive that they have no control (American Psychological Association [APA], 2020). It derives from persistent feelings of despair and hopelessness and can be related to a number of factors, such as poverty, family dysfunction, racial discrimination, and traumatic early-childhood experiences (APA, 2020). Stress influences the pathogenesis of physical disease by causing negative affective states (e.g., feelings of anxiety and depression), which, in turn, exert direct effects on biological processes or behavioral patterns that influence disease risk (Cohen et al., 2019). Chronic stress influences changes in the brain structurally and chemically. Furthermore, chronic early-life stressful events have the potential to inflict permanent changes in physiology that adversely impact development and can lead to stress-related diseases and unhealthy lifestyles (McEwen, 2017). Chronic stress is also associated with an increased risk of developing psychological illness and poorer immune functioning (Cohen et al., 2012). In turn, these changes in biological processes and the immune system can impact cognitive functioning and mood, which may increase maladaptive behaviors (Morgado & Cerqueira, 2018). The economic cost of chronic disease is staggering. It is estimated that chronic disease and mental health conditions account for more than 90% of the $3.8 trillion healthcare costs in the United States annually (Martin et al., 2021).

Creswell and Lindsay (2014) developed the mindfulness stress-buffering hypothesis to explain how mindfulness can improve stress perceptions and mitigate its impact on health. The mindfulness stress-buffering hypothesis posits that mindfulness mitigates stress appraisals and reduces stress reactivity responses and that these stress reduction effects partly or completely explain how mindfulness affects mental and physical health outcomes. In support of this model, a recent systematic review (Morton et al., 2020) examined existing studies that used an empirically validated laboratory protocol, the Trier Social Stress Test (Kirschbaum et al., 1993), to elicit stress reactivity to examine the buffering capacity of mindfulness. A majority of studies included in the review demonstrated the stress-buffering effects of mindfulness training on stress induction. In the following, we review a number of recent meta-analyses that provide further support for mindfulness and related meditations in improving stress reactivity, health outcomes, and harmful health behaviors across a variety of populations.

Similar to the Morton et al. (2020) review, Pascoe et al. (2017) conducted a systematic review and meta-analysis to examine the impact of mindfulness on physiological markers of stress. Forty-five randomized controlled trials (RCTs) that used an active control condition and meditation condition were included in the meta-analysis. Meditation interventions were classified into one of three different conditions: OM (including Integrative Body-Mind Training, qi gong, and MBIs), FA (including Kirtan Kriya, walking meditation, Omkar mantra meditation, integrated amrita meditation, mindfulness-based social-emotional learning program, and one novel intervention), or automatic self-transcending (AST; including transcendental meditation and primordial sound meditation). The meta-analysis included 10 primary outcomes across the various studies: blood cortisol, immune outcomes, norepinephrine, interleukin-6, tumor necrosis factor–alpha, blood pressure, heart rate, heart rate variability, lipids, and fasting blood glucose. Pascoe et al. found the AST interventions reduced systolic blood pressure, FA interventions reduced blood cortisol and resting systolic blood pressure, and OM interventions reduced ambulatory systolic blood pressure, systolic blood pressure after a stress-induction task, and resting heart rate. The level of evidence for these reductions was low to moderate, likely impacted by methodological limitations among the individual studies (i.e., small sample sizes and publication bias). When all three meditation subtypes were grouped together, reductions were found in blood cortisol, c-reactive protein, resting blood pressure and heart rate, ambulatory blood pressure, systolic blood pressure, triglycerides, and tumor necrosis factor-alpha. This meta-analysis of RCTs supported the general hypothesis that physiological measures of stress are an important potential mechanism in MBIs.

There is a dearth of evidence regarding the effects of MBIs on people of color (POC; people who identify as being a member of an ethno-racial minority group), as the majority of extant research has utilized primarily non-Hispanic White samples. There has been a slow, but steady, increase in the number of studies that recruit samples with a wider array of ethno-racial diversity. In a meta-analysis of 24 studies composed predominantly of POC, the first of its kind, Sun et al. (2021) found modest support for MBIs. They utilized data from 22 RCTs, accounting for a sample size of 2,156 participants. More than 94% identified as POC (63.6% Black), 50.8% as male, 63.6% low income, and the average participant age was 23.2 years old. The majority of the MBIs were either MBCT or MBSR. All studies utilized a random design and either active or inactive control group. Outcomes included psychological, mindfulness, biomarkers, coping, behavioral and well-being variables. There were no demographic moderators of treatment effects among studies that used an active control group, but in those that used an inactive group, clinical populations and non-POC had smaller effects for MBIs than the general population and POC. MBIs largely produced superior results compared to both active control conditions ($k = 16$, $g = 0.11$, 95% confidence interval [CI; 0.04, 0.18], $p = .002$) and inactive control conditions ($k = 8$, $g = 0.26$, 95% CI [0.07, 0.45], $p = .007$). In studies that used an active control condition, MBIs were found to provide the most benefit in improving psychosomatic health ($g = 0.26$, 95% CI [0.06, 0.46]) and reducing psychological symptoms ($g = 0.13$, 95% CI [0.02, 0.24]). However, the groups did not differ regarding biomarker shifts, cognitive outcomes, mindfulness, coping skills, well-being, or behavioral outcomes. In studies that used an inactive control group, MBIs had a larger impact on cognitive outcomes (g = 0.25, 95% CI [0.02, 0.48]), coping (g = 0.52, 95% CI [0.10, 0.93]), and mindfulness (g = 0.63, 95% CI [0.04, 1.21]), but not psychological outcomes, biomarkers, or behavioral outcomes. The effect sizes found across all studies were smaller in magnitude (g = 0.11 in active control comparisons and g = 0.26 inactive control comparisons) than those found in other populations but were promising. The authors concluded that sociocultural structural challenges may play a role in MBI efficacy and improvements can be made to existing MBIs to make them efficacious for POC (e.g., cultural adaption, use of homogeneous groups, multilevel intervention, trauma-sensitive practices).

High-quality research has also been conducted to compare the impact of MBIs specifically on clinical populations. Goldberg et al. (2018) conducted a comprehensive systematic review and meta-analysis of 171 RCTs across 12,005 participants that were published between 2000 and 2016. The sample was 64.4% female, with an average age of 43.6, and 61.37% completed some postsecondary education. Over half of the studies used no treatment comparison group and 30.4% studied depression. Assessments were made postintervention and at follow-up. They included all interventions that had a mindfulness component and home-meditation practice but excluded mindfulness-informed interventions, such as acceptance and commitment therapy and dialectical behavior therapy (a type of cognitive behavior therapy that develops several skills, including mindfulness) and practices such as mantra and other forms of meditation. MBIs were found to be superior to other treatment conditions: no treatment (k = 89, d = 0.55, 95% CI [0.47, 0.63]), minimal treatment (e.g., very brief or minimal intensity interventions; k = 4, d = 0.37, 95% CI [0.03, 0.71]), nonspecific treatment (e.g., conversational discussions; k = 9, d = 0.35, 95% CI [0.09, 0.62]), and specific treatment (e.g., treatments with rationale; k = 42, d = 0.23, 95% CI [0.12, 0.34]) at postintervention, except for evidence-based treatments (EBTs; e.g., cognitive behavioral therapy), in which they did not differ (k = 28, d = −0.004, 95% CI [−0.15, 0.14]). MBIs evidenced superior (medium to large) effects for anxiety, depression, pain, schizophrenia, and weight/eating-related disorders (ds = 0.45–0.89) when compared to no treatment groups. Likewise, MBIs exert small to medium effects on depression and addictions when compared to active control groups (ds = 0.27–0.38). MBIs were also superior to EBTs for smoking (d = 0.42). At follow-up, MBIs performed better than no treatment conditions (k = 37, d = 0.50, 95% CI [0.36,0.65]), nonspecific treatment conditions (k = 4, d = 0.52, 95% CI [0.05, 0.99]), and specific active controls (k = 29, d = 0.29, 95% CI [0.13, 0.45]). On average, MBIs led to a moderate drop in psychiatric symptoms. The authors concluded that MBIs performed similar to standard evidence-based psychological interventions and better than active control comparison conditions for various clinical populations, gathering the most support for reducing symptoms of depression, pain, smoking, and addictions.

Scott-Sheldon et al. (2020) conducted a recent systematic review and meta-analysis to assess the impact of MBIs on psychological (anxiety, depression, distress, and perceived stress) and physiological (systolic and diastolic blood pressure) outcomes among individuals with cardiovascular disease (CVD). Data from 16 RCTs and 14 supplemental manuscripts spanning 1,476 participants (40% women, 76% White, and 71% married) were included. The MBIs included in this review and meta-analysis were specifically adapted for adults with CVD. MBIs outperformed control groups in reducing psychological outcomes (ds = 0.49–0.64) and systolic blood pressure (d = 0.89, 95% CI[0.26, 1.51]; k = 7) at postintervention, but no differences were found at follow-up. No differences in diastolic blood pressure were found between groups at either time point. These results lend evidence (*Class IIB*) for the beneficial effects of MBIs for adults with CVD in the short term.

There is very promising evidence that mindfulness meditation can benefit people with chronic pain. Hilton et al. (2017) conducted a systematic review and meta-analysis to investigate the efficacy and safety of mindfulness meditation for patients with chronic pain due to headache, migraine, back pain, arthritis, irritable bowel syndrome, cancer, or neuralgias. They examined evidence from 38 RCTs representing 3,536 randomized participants who had pain for at least 3 months. Interventions were MBSR (21 trials), MBCT (six trials), or other programs that included some formal mindfulness meditation practices. Mindfulness interventions were used as an adjunct therapy (18 trials), used as monotherapy (13 trials), or did not specify other pain therapies. Outcomes included pain (primary outcome), depression, the use of analgesics, and overall quality of life. Comparison groups included treatment as usual, education, support groups, or waiting lists. A statistically significant, small effect on pain was found for meditation compared with all controls (standardized mean difference = 0.32, 95% CI [0.09, 0.54]). Although substantial heterogeneity of effects was found across trials, there was no evidence of publication bias. Hilton et al. concluded that the quality of the evidence for pain reduction is low for both short- (less than 12 weeks) and longer term outcomes. Additional analyses confirmed impacts on secondary outcomes of depression (a small impact with a high level of evidence) and quality of life (small impact with moderate evidence for mental health–related quality of life, low evidence for physical health–related quality of life). No impact of meditation on the use of analgesics was found. Based on these findings, one can be cautiously optimistic about the value of mindfulness training for chronic pain, associated symptoms of depression, and quality of life.

Morone et al. (2016) conducted one of the largest and most recent RCTs of MBSR for low back pain included in the Hilton et al. (2017) review. This trial provides a useful exemplar of meditation for pain research, as the meta-analysts rated this trial as good quality with low risk of bias. The purpose of this RCT was to determine the effectiveness of MBSR on improving functioning and reducing pain among older adults with chronic low back pain. Participants were 282 adults aged 65 or older experiencing daily chronic pain and related functional limitations for at least the past 3 months. Over 66% of participants were women, 28% were Black, and the average age was 75. The intervention was an 8-week MBSR program followed by 6 monthly booster sessions, and the control was a health education program delivered in a similar format to MBSR. The primary outcome was the Roland–Morris Disability Questionnaire score for functional limitations caused by lower back pain. Secondary outcomes included pain (present, average, most severe assessed by a numeric rating scale), quality of life, and pain self-efficacy. At the end of the 8-week program, the MBSR group had significantly improved function (fewer pain limitations) compared with controls (effect size −0.23, p = .01), and more clinically meaningful reductions in limitations, defined as greater than 2.5 points on the Roland–Morris Disability Questionnaire (57% vs.

45%, $p = .051$). Ratings of current and most severe pain in the past week at 6-month follow-up were also better in the MBSR group than in the control group. No serious adverse events related to the interventions were reported. Morone et al. (2016) concluded that mindfulness training resulted in short-term improvements in physical functioning and encouraged more work to improve the durability of meditation's benefit to functioning.

Cillessen et al. (2019) recently completed a comprehensive systematic review and meta-analysis of the effects of MBIs on psychological distress and health outcomes in cancer patients and survivors. Participants ($N = 3,274$) across 29 RCTs were included in the analyses. They used only interventions in which mindfulness meditation was the primary component; nearly half of the studies used MBSR. All of them included a non-MBI control condition. The majority of the sample were women (86%) and 70% had breast cancer. The overall quality of evidence was moderate. Significant pooled effects of MBIs on psychological distress were found at postintervention (Hedges's $g = 0.32$, 95% CI: [0.22, 0.41], $p <. 001$), including self-reported symptoms of anxiety, depression, fear of cancer recurrence, and fatigue (gs = 0.29–0.51). Significant effects of MBIs were found for overall psychological distress at follow-up ($g = 0.19$, 95% CI [0.07, 0.30], $p < .002$) and for depression, sleep disturbance, pain, and anxiety symptoms (gs = 0.20–0.36). The effects were primarily small, but robust, and reductions in psychological distress were related to increases in mindfulness over time. No effects were found on measures of posttraumatic stress symptoms or cancer-related quality of life. The authors noted that adhering to original MBI manuals, utilizing passive control conditions, and shorter follow-up periods evidenced the largest effect sizes.

Burnout among healthcare professionals is commonplace and can lead to emotional exhaustion and reduced quality of patient care. Suleiman-Martos et al. (2020) conducted a systematic review and meta-analysis to determine whether mindfulness training was effective in reducing burnout in frontline nursing staff. All 17 studies included data among a nursing sample, were either an RCT or a quasi-experimental study, and used burnout as the primary outcome of interest. To determine which dimensions of burnout were impacted, they analyzed emotional exhaustion (EE), depersonalization (D), and personal accomplishment (PA) separately. The participant sample ($N = 632$) was composed of primarily women (87% or greater) who worked in hospitals, in medical or surgical areas, or performed supervisory functions. The programs assessed were either MBSR or mindfulness-based self-care and resilience (MBSCR). Their meta-analytic results aligned with prior research on MBIs for healthcare personnel: MBIs led to reductions in EE and D and an increase in PA. The mean difference between the intervention and control groups was 1.32 (95% CI [−9.41, 6.78]) for EE, 1.91 (95% CI [−4.50, 0.68]) for D, and 2.12 (95% CI [−9.91, 14.14]) for PA. However, Sulimen-Martos et al. indicated that although EE was substantially reduced across all studies from pre- to postintervention, there was considerable variation among studies in the results for D and PA. While this study provided a preliminary analysis of MBIs to reduce burnout in nurses, the results should be interpreted with caution. The meta-analysis included only two RCTs, thereby reducing its quality. A body of rigorous RCTs with consistent measures of salient, core outcomes using the same instruments will need to be conducted in order to produce higher quality meta-analytic evidence for the reduction of burnout in frontline nursing staff via mindfulness training.

In summary, there is solid evidence from rigorous RCTs of the benefits of meditation, particularly regarding psychological functioning and well-being across diverse groups, including clinical and healthy populations. There is rapidly mounting evidence of specific benefits to a wide array of outcomes, including pain, addictive disorders, cancer-related outcomes, and cardiovascular risk factors. However, without exception, authors of meta-analyses have called for improved designs, larger samples, longer follow-up, and more rigorous methods to strengthen the evidence base (e.g., Goldberg et al., 2018; Hilton et al., 2017; Pascoe et al., 2017; Sun et al., 2021). These authors also cite issues such as waitlist control groups, no measurement of meditation adherence, no blinding or no blinded assessment of outcomes, and limited follow-up to assess the durability of benefit. Finally, they also call for greater attention to optimizing intervention impacts in terms of type and duration of meditation training. We outline these issues and suggestions for improving the rigor of meditation studies in the Future Research section later.

INTERVENTION

There are many forms of meditation practice, including formal and informal practice. Formal meditations are considered "formal" because they are typically practiced by setting aside and dedicating a period of time in one's day to engage in the practice. Breath awareness, mantra meditation, and body scan are three examples of formal focused attention (FA) meditations. During a breath awareness meditation, the chosen target of attention is sensations that arise in the body as breathing occurs. The intention differs from "breathing exercises" or deep breathing in that participants are instructed not to attempt to change or control breathing but to allow the body to breathe naturally and to bring a curious and kind attention to the associated sensations. Practitioners may direct attention to the rhythm, depth, and speed of the breath. A practitioner may take a narrower focus and attend to particular sensations of breath such as those experienced at the tip of the nose or those associated with the rise and fall of the belly. Aligned with the Zen Buddhist tradition, the practitioner may simply count the breaths (e.g., one, two, three) up to 10 and restart again at one. The practitioner chooses one object, or anchor, of attention and maintains attention to this one object throughout the duration of the practice. Mantra meditation involves continually repeating a chosen word, phrase, or set of syllables (silently or aloud) while disregarding any internal or external distractions. The repeated sound or subvocalized word is proposed to act as an effective vehicle for overriding mental speech, considered a predominant form of conscious thinking for many people, and thereby, may stabilize the distracted mind. In these practices, when the mind wanders, attention is brought back to the object of attention with little or no investigation of the distraction.

The body scan is a somatically oriented FA practice. The body scan practice has been described as an "affectionate, openhearted [and] interested" attention to the body (Dreeben et al., 2013; Kabat-Zinn, 2018). Practitioners are instructed to notice bodily sensations that are present in a particular region with an attitude of curiosity and acceptance. When the mind wanders, practitioners kindly return attention back to the sensations present in the particular body region. Walking and movement meditations are two other somatically oriented FA practices. During walking meditation, the eye gaze is generally soft and straight ahead. Attention is directed to sensations of movements, shifts of weight and balance, and sensations in the feet and legs associated with walking. As in other meditation exercises, participants are encouraged to notice when their minds wander off and gently bring their attention back to the physical sensations of walking. Walking meditation often is practiced slowly. To emphasize the absence of a destination, participants typically walk back and forth across a room; however, a mindful walking practice can also occur outdoors. Similarly, movement meditation cultivates an individual's awareness of bodily sensations while slowly and gently moving, stretching, or holding a position. When one notices that the mind has drifted away from the sensations of the body, the practitioner draws attention back to the sensations arising in the body.

A common OM practice is sitting meditation, often described as *mindfulness meditation*. During a sitting meditation practice, the practitioner maintains a comfortable seated position and cultivates soft awareness of present-moment sensations in the body. The practitioners then expand awareness to monitor all content of present moment experience (i.e., thoughts, emotions, sensations, sights, sounds) while cultivating a curious, accepting, and nonreactive stance. Every arising sensation, thought, or feeling is attended to in an equal manner. When the mind wanders to concerns about the future, ruminations about events that occurred in the past, or evaluative secondary appraisals of the present moment, the meditation practitioner simply notices these processes with a curious, nonreactive, and nonjudgmental stance. A sitting meditation cultivates an ability to "take a step back" and observe the contents of their mind and associated bodily sensations. When the practitioner recognizes that they are no longer observing the internal experience but rather interacting with the thoughts or has "gotten carried away" with a story line, the practitioner may identify the experience (e.g., planning, remembering, evaluating, itching) and draw the attention back again to simply observe (Britton et al., 2018).

LKM and *compassion meditation* are CM terms that are often used interchangeably and sometimes incorporate similar methodology; however, at the heart of each is the cultivation of separate constructs, or qualities. LKM is practiced to develop kindness and warmth, whereas compassion meditation is used to develop sensitivity to suffering and a commitment to its alleviation in self and others (Graser & Stangier, 2018). Both are used to cultivate an affective state of increased feelings of warmth and caring for the self and others (Salzberg, 2002). Like other meditation practices, LKM involves quiet contemplation in a seated posture, often with eyes closed and an initial focus on the breath. It can also be practiced while slowly walking with the eyes open. Whereas mindfulness and similar types of meditation encourage nonjudgmental awareness of experiences in the present moment by focusing on bodily or other sensorial experiences, affective states, thoughts, or images, LKM focuses on loving and kind concern for well-being. During LKM, the meditator typically repeats four phrases as they proceed through a number of stages that differ in focus and generally become more challenging. The phrases commonly used (with subtle variations included in parentheses) are (a) May I be free from danger (may I be safe), (b) May I have mental happiness (may I be happy), (c) May I have physical happiness (may I be healthy/healed), and (d) May I have ease of well-being (may I live with ease). These phrases are sometimes differentiated from those used in compassion meditation, which often directly refer to the alleviation of suffering and its causes (Sirotina & Shchebetenko, 2020). As LKM practice advances, the focus of the phrase changes, such that the meditator moves through a series of stages. These include (a) focus on self, (b) focus on a good friend (i.e., a person who is still alive and who does not invoke sexual desires), (c) focus on a neutral person (i.e., a person who typically does not elicit either particularly positive or negative feelings but who is commonly encountered during a normal day), (d) focus on a difficult person (i.e., a person who is typically associated with negative feelings), and, eventually, (e) focus on the entire universe (Salzberg, 2002). As can be seen from this sequence, typically warm feelings are initially directed toward oneself and then extended to an ever-widening circle of others, ultimately radiating them in all directions (e.g., north, south, east, west), although the order can be changed to accommodate individual preferences. In LKM, people cultivate the intention to experience positive emotions during the meditation itself, as well as in their life more generally. Within traditional Buddhist practice, LKM is considered particularly helpful for people who have a strong tendency toward hostility or anger (Anālayo, 2003). Although there are no training requirements or guidelines for LKM, a number of Buddhist and secular resources are available to help develop practice.

The cultivation of empathic joy and equanimity are two contemplative attitudes that are developed under the umbrella of contemplative practice. Empathic joy refers to the cultivation of joy and pleasure through witnessing the prosperity, good fortune, and genuine happiness of others. Empathic joy meditations may utilize visualizations and the repetition of one or more phrases related to the joy of others. Similar to LKM, the focus (i.e., self, friend, neutral person, difficult person, universe) of this meditation changes throughout its course (Salzberg, 2002). Equanimity, the fourth component of the interconnected Four Immeasurables, refers to an even-minded mental state or dispositional trait characterized by the development of an impartial attitude, emotional detachment and balance, and acceptance of experience, regardless of the affective valence of the source or situation. Importantly, the cultivation of equanimity does not incorporate indifference or emotional suppression and is a skill that is developed through intentional practice (Desbordes et al., 2014). Equanimity can be developed during FA or OM practices by maintaining a sense of nonjudgmental awareness of one's experience. It can also be developed through reflecting on a series of contemplations about one's automatic thoughts, assumptions, schemas, and habituated responses to difficult situations.

Informal practice involves applying OM styles, or mindfulness meditation practice, to daily activities or situations, such as eating, cleaning, walking, or interpersonal interactions (Kabat-Zinn, 1990). Increased awareness of daily experiences is believed to lead to increased self-awareness and enhanced ability to make real-time, adaptive decisions during difficult and problematic situations as they arise. Furthermore, applying mindfulness to daily living can increase the frequency and enjoyment of pleasant moments. Mindful awareness of breathing in daily life also is encouraged and promotes the generalization of self-awareness of the constantly fluctuating internal states experienced in ordinary activities. Turning one's attention to one's breathing at any moment of the day is intended to increase self-awareness, develop insight and familiarity with the nature of the mind, and is thought to reduce habitual, automatic, and maladaptive behaviors.

TECHNIQUES AND GUIDELINES

Although there are numerous meditation programs, the most widely used and well-researched meditation programs in Western healthcare are MBSR and its related programs. These programs incorporate different combinations of formal FA, OM, and CM practices, as well as informal practice.

MBSR and Related Programs

MBSR was developed by Jon Kabat-Zinn at the Stress Reduction Clinic at the University of Massachusetts Medical Center (www.umassmed.edu/cfm) more than 30 years ago. It is a particular way of learning mindfulness meditation that emerged in a hospital system and was fashioned as a complement to traditional medical care for patients with chronic pain conditions (Kabat-Zinn, 1990). The program is theoretically grounded in secularized Buddhist meditation practices, mind–body medicine, and the transactional model of stress that suggests people can be taught to manage their stress by adjusting their cognitive perspective and increasing their coping skills to build self-confidence in handling external, stressful situations. MBSR is an 8-week, generic skills–based program led by an instructor in a classroom format. The course comprises eight weekly 2.5-hour classes, one 7.5-hour meditation retreat, and 30 to 45 minutes of daily homework practicing the techniques learned in the course. Sessions include information about stress, cognition, and health but primarily concentrate on learning to focus attention through a variety of meditative techniques, such as focusing on the breath, body scan, sitting and walking meditations, and gentle yoga. Participants are trained to perceive their immediate emotional and physical state, including pain or discomfort, and to let thoughts come and go into awareness with no attempt to change, suppress, or ruminate on them.

Through mindfulness training, participants come to view their thoughts as temporary mental events. In this way, they become exposed to the positive and negative content of their thoughts but do not get absorbed in thought—caught up in planning for the future or worrying about the past. By incorporating mindfulness techniques into their daily lives, practitioners learn to find breathing space to respond skillfully to stressors with appropriate action, as opposed to reacting on automatic pilot with conditioned responses that can be emotionally arousing or unhelpful. The goal of MBSR is lifelong self-management. Although MBSR was originally developed for people with chronic pain, it was later applied to patients with a variety of conditions, such as cancer (Hoffman et al., 2012), diabetes (Hartmann et al., 2012), fibromyalgia (Schmidt et al., 2011), and irritable bowel syndrome (Schmidt et al., 2011). Moreover, MBSR has expanded beyond medical settings, and courses are now widely available in community settings, at universities, and in the workplace. Referral by a health provider and medical oversight are not required. Becoming a certified MBSR instructor (for details, see www.ummhealth.org/center-mindfulness) requires intensive experiential and didactic training, including a practicum and supervised work.

Over the past two decades, a number of similar programs have been developed that integrate core elements of mindfulness practices with existing evidence-based therapies. Unlike MBSR, which is a generic stress-reduction program, most of these programs target a specific physical or mental illness. One of the first of these to emerge was MBCT (Segal et al., 2002). MBCT is an 8-week group intervention that integrates elements of cognitive therapy (CT) with the MBSR program to prevent depressive relapse in patients with a history of major depressive disorder. Unlike CT, there is no attempt to challenge or change the content of thoughts; rather, the emphasis is on changing the awareness of and relationship to thoughts, feelings, and bodily sensations. Aspects of CT included in MBCT are primarily those designed to facilitate a detached or decentered view, such as "thoughts are not facts" and "I am not my thoughts." Increased mindfulness allows early detection of relapse-related patterns of negative thinking, feelings, and bodily sensations, allowing them to be stopped at a stage when this may be much easier than if such warning signs were noticed later or ignored (Segal et al., 2002). The MBCT program has added several techniques to MBSR that have been widely disseminated, including the 3-minute breathing space (see Exhibit 11.1). In addition, the MBCT protocol is clear and concise and includes all necessary materials to begin an MBCT group.

Exhibit 11.1 *MBSR and MBCT Sample Intervention Techniques*

Breath Awareness
Breath awareness is a practice in which passive breathing is carefully observed. Breath awareness may be used as needed or can be practiced as a technique to promote awareness and health. Continued practice of breath awareness is an anchor for mindfulness, which helps the practitioner to remain in the moment, bringing calm and creativity to situations requiring perspective (Kabat-Zinn, 1990). The practice of breath awareness requires a beginner's mind being open to observation without attempts to change the breath. Kabat-Zinn (1990) describes a simple process that can be used to teach breath awareness to patients:

1. Sit or lie in a comfortable position. If sitting, keep a straight spine and let the shoulders drop.
2. Close your eyes if that is comfortable, or gaze ahead without focusing.
3. Bring attention to your full in-breath and out-breath. Notice the sensation of the breath, especially in the rising and falling abdomen.
4. Don't try to change the breath, just notice the waves of your own breathing.
5. When your mind wanders away from the breath (e.g., you notice that you are thinking of something else) just return your focus to the breath.

Body Scan
Body scan is a technique that promotes the mind's ability to focus and adapt and is a powerful tool for reconnecting with the body. This practice involves lying down or sitting comfortably in a chair and focusing attention through the parts of the body, noticing the sensations, both pleasant and unpleasant, with an attitude of curiosity and acceptance. The typical sequence for the scan follows: toes of left foot, left foot, left ankle, leg, pelvis, then toes of the right foot progressing up to the right hip, pelvis, low back and belly, high back and chest, fingers of both hands (simultaneously), and then both arms, shoulders, neck, face, back of the head, and top of the head (Kabat-Zinn, 1990). At the end of the body scan, one visualizes that the breath goes through

---

(continued)

Exhibit 11.1 *MBSR and MBCT Sample Intervention Techniques (continued)*

the whole body, through the toes, and in and out of an imaginary blowhole at the top of the head. As in other mindfulness practices, unrelated thoughts or interruptions are noted and let go, and the practitioner brings attention back to the scan. The body scan may be deeply relaxing for some, and so taking some time to move slowly afterward is helpful. Meditation novices may find that they fall asleep while practicing body scan or have concerns they are not doing it right. These are normal responses, and practitioners may be encouraged to continue practicing and to bring themselves back to the scan with awareness and acceptance when they notice that their minds have wandered.

Breathing Space
Breathing space can be used routinely to cultivate awareness and self-compassion, or it can be used as needed when experiencing unwanted thoughts or feelings. A three-step, 3-minute Breathing Space practice designed by Segal and colleagues (2002) is part of MBCT.

1. Awareness: Bring awareness to the breath and thoughts, feelings, and sensations of this moment, observing carefully and describing the experience silently, in words (e.g., "Noticing tension in the body and feeling anxious").
2. Redirecting attention: Bring your attention to the breath and experience it fully.
3. Expanding attention: Let awareness grow to include the whole body, breathing into areas of discomfort (thoughts, feelings, sensations), breathing out discomfort, and making accepting statements (e.g., "Whatever it is, it's okay").

MBCT, mindfulness-based cognitive therapy; MBSR, mindfulness-based stress reduction.

Similar to MBCT, mindfulness-based relapse prevention (MBRP; Witkiewitz et al., 2005) was developed to integrate mindfulness into cognitive behavioral treatment (CBT) of substance use and the prevention of relapse. In MBRP, mindfulness practices provide a unique opportunity to decrease habitual responding and avoidance by cultivating an attitude of curiosity and attention to ongoing cognitive, affective, and physical stimuli (Bowen et al., 2011). The goal of MBRP is to develop an awareness of thoughts, feelings, and sensations (including urges or cravings) by developing mindfulness skills that can be applied in high-risk situations for relapse.

Mindfulness-based eating awareness training (MB-EAT; Kristeller & Hallett, 1999) was developed by integrating elements from MBSR and CBT with guided-eating meditations. The program draws on traditional mindfulness meditation techniques, as well as guided meditation, to address specific issues pertaining to shape, weight, and eating-related self-regulatory processes, such as appetite as well as both gastric and taste-specific satiety (Kristeller & Hallett, 1999). The meditative process is integrated into daily activity related to food craving and eating. Similar to MBCT and MBRP, mindfulness meditation is conceptualized as a way of training attention to help individuals first to increase awareness of automatic patterns and then to disengage from undesirable reactivity.

Adaptations of MBSR or MBCT have also been developed or are in the developmental process for specific populations, such as adolescents, pregnant women, and couples, and for health conditions, such as cancer, diabetes, insomnia, and posttraumatic stress disorder. It is now possible to find MBI materials and homework assignments designed specifically for children or teenagers, as well as curricula for delivery of MBSR in schools, prisons, rehabilitation centers, and other settings.

Mindfulness-Based Resilience Training

MBRT (Christopher et al., 2016, 2018) is designed to enhance resilience and reduce aggression and use of force errors among law enforcement and other first responders. Based on an MBRP framework, it is an 8-week course with experiential and didactic exercises, including body scan, sitting and walking meditations, mindful movement, and other MBRP practices (Bowen et al., 2011). Weekly classes last 2 hours, and the seventh week is an extended 6-hour class.

Each class contains experiential and didactic exercises, as well as discussion and homework. The content and language of experiential exercises were altered to be more relevant to first responders, and much of the curriculum is focused on learning strategies to manage stressors inherent to this type of work. These include critical incidents, chronic stress, and public scrutiny, as well as interpersonal, affective, and behavioral challenges in first responders' personal lives. Didactic learning is much more prominent than in most other MBIs. This was found to be very helpful for first responders as they sought to enhance their intention to endure the challenges of the training. An additional adaptation, in the tradition of typical first responder meetings, is the inclusion of a debriefing at the conclusion of each class, in which participants ask questions and give frank feedback about the class. The mindful encounters exercise is a derivation of the martial arts exercises (e.g., conversational jujitsu) used in the MBSR curriculum to practice mindful interpersonal conflict. The exercise is framed as an important skill to be used when interacting with others. In another exercise, reactivity awareness, participants settle into a sustained, reclined breath-awareness practice, and then with verbal instruction to sustain awareness, a 911 call center recording with an emergency audio tone is played for 60 seconds and then turned off. Participants are cued to continue sustained attention to body sensation and breath for a few more minutes, helping them gain an experiential sense of stress physiology. In addition, participants are invited to include a component of mindfulness during their regular exercise regimen, such as running, swimming, or biking, as part of their mindful movement homework.

While exposure to trauma and stressors is an inherent part of a police officer's job, programs that teach them to relate to these experiences more skillfully may help reduce the harmful effects of stress on their behaviors with the diverse citizens they serve. An important training practice is LKM, through which officers develop kindness and warmth for themselves and members of the communities they serve. In a recent study, we administered a computerized measure assessing weapon identification, an aspect of force response decision-making, and implicit racial bias (specifically, implicit stereotype reliance) to police officers before and after mindfulness training. Although there was no change in the role of implicit race bias in force response decision-making after the intervention, we are hopeful that increased sensitivity of measurement will allow us to better identify these potential subtle changes in future research (Hunsinger et al., 2019). Given the injustices communities of color are suffering, it is important for police officers to develop connections and an understanding of the humanness of people in these communities.

Mindfulness-Based Wellness and Resilience Training

Mindfulness-Based Wellness and Resilience (MBWR; Colgan et al., 2019) was designed to increase resilience and team cohesion and reduce burnout among multidisciplinary medical providers. MBWR is grounded in the evidence-based practices of MBSR (Kabat-Zinn et al., 1985) and the Mindful Practice (Epstein et al., 2007) curriculum. MBWR was initially delivered on-site in eight, 60-minute weekly sessions to multidisciplinary primary care teams, typically consisting of one to three physicians, physician assistants, nurses and nurse practitioners, medical assistants, social workers, pharmacists, and community coordinators. Weekly MBWR sessions include "formal" mindfulness practices, such as body scan, mindful breathing, sitting meditation, and LKM. Brief didactics on mindfulness, resilience, self-compassion, and relevant scientific research are presented weekly. Class discussions explore how to integrate informal practices into the workday and create the structure and consistency needed to develop and maintain new skillful responses to stress and adversity in the workplace. Informal practices are used prior to entering an examination room, during patient–provider communication, professional consultation or team meetings, or at the beginning or end of the workday. For example, a provider may incorporate pausing before entering an examination room to intentionally scan the body, breath, and mind state before walking into a room. Adaptations of MBWR have been developed for diverse healthcare providers in various medical clinics and settings. Alternative dosing effects are currently being investigated.

MEASUREMENT OF OUTCOMES

Meditation training with programs such as MBSR or LKM is a low-risk activity that supports well-being and complements regular medical treatments, diet, exercise, and other lifestyle changes prescribed for known health conditions. Because these meditation practices have no known serious adverse effects, recommendations for monitoring patients who engage in meditation are consistent with general practice guidelines. Regular assessments to screen for depression, pain, and changes in disease-specific symptoms are warranted. In research studies, meditation has been found to have impacts on mood, perceived stress, physiological markers of stress, and global indicators of health-related quality of life. Due to meditation's physiological effects, meditators with hypertension should be regularly monitored for possible dose adjustments. Also, nurses should be alert to changes in other conditions because preliminary evidence suggests that meditation practice enhances medication adherence (Çetin & Aylaz, 2018) and enables practitioners to better tolerate intrusive treatments such as continuous positive airway pressure for obstructive sleep apnea (Li et al., 2020). One would speculate that present-moment attention and awareness lead to better symptom awareness, attention to cues to treating symptoms that wax and wane, and recognizing health changes in conditions such as asthma and diabetes. Brief, valid, and reliable self-report instruments appropriate for measuring patient outcomes in clinical practice or research are available at no cost through the Patient-Reported Outcomes Measurement Information System (PROMIS) project of the National Institutes of Health (www.healthmeasures.net/explore-measurement-systems/promis). Additionally, a current study is underway to develop a self-report mindfulness measure using the PROMIS methodology (https://clinicaltrials.gov/ct2/show/NCT03510117).

PRECAUTIONS

Meditation practices are considered generally safe as a complementary therapy. They are appealing in medical settings because they are inherently portable, do not require a prescription, and can be personalized to meet the needs of the individual. However, meditation-related side effects and adverse events can occur across different domains (e.g., cognitive, perceptual, affective somatic, conative, sense of self, social; Lindahl et al., 2017). Transient unpleasant sensations are commonly experienced during and shortly after meditation, including in focused attention and open monitoring practices. These may include physical discomfort, heightened awareness of unpleasant emotions, sleepiness, dizziness, hyperarousal, and emotional blunting. Some meditators may experience one or more of these sensations for a longer duration, which can impact well-being. Long-term iatrogenic effects are rare but can occur (Baer et al., 2021; Britton et al., 2021; Goldberg et al., in press). Importantly, the interpretation of meditation-related side effects varies by context. Some traditions perceive unpleasant experiences and adverse events as a natural component of the developmental process among meditators (Compson, 2018). It is important for meditation students to have access to a knowledgeable practitioner who can help them skillfully respond to and navigate these experiences. There are a few conditions for which we do not recommend meditation at the bedside, including delirium, psychosis, drug or alcohol intoxication, and mania. Additionally, people experiencing symptoms of posttraumatic stress or grief may find it difficult to practice awareness exercises because meditation might intensify their negative experiences. Research in this area is ongoing, so consultation with a mental health provider is encouraged. People who practice meditation may experience decreased blood pressure and need for insulin or cardiovascular medications. Patients with low blood pressure or who are dizzy or light-headed should not meditate, and medication dose and levels should be considered if their effects could be potentiated by the relaxation response. In studies of organ transplant recipients, kidney transplant candidates, and people with chronic insomnia, no adverse events related to meditation were encountered (Gross et al., 2011, 2017). Additional resources can be found at Cheetah House, a nonprofit organization that provides resources about meditation-related difficulties (www.cheetahhouse.org/)

USES

DOSAGE

Regular home meditation practice is considered a core element of most meditation interventions. Frequency and consistency of home practice have been positively related to levels of mindfulness (Carmody & Baer, 2008), resilience (Jha et al., 2017), and well-being (Parsons et al., 2017) and negatively related to levels of anxiety, stress, and poor mental health outcomes (Hoge et al., 2017); however, other studies, including systematic reviews, have not found a statistically significant relationship between frequency, duration, or type of home practice and clinical outcomes (Lloyd et al., 2018; Quach et al., 2017; Ribeiro et al., 2018). These mixed results highlight the need for further investigation into the dose effects needed to achieve and maintain clinical benefits. Dosing effects are likely to vary based on personal characteristics such as age, gender, personality traits, and genetics, as well as social and cultural differences.

MECHANISMS

Mounting evidence suggests that meditation may improve a range of stress-related and disease-specific outcomes. Research now aims to understand the underlying causes, or mechanisms, that explain *how* meditation fosters wellbeing. The development of more efficacious, better targeted treatments requires a greater understanding of the mechanisms that mitigate the harmful effects of stress. While this research is still in its relative infancy, there are promising psychological, cognitive, neurological, and behavioral mechanisms that link mindfulness interventions with physical health.

Meditation training appears to modify two psychological mechanisms that contribute to an individual's susceptibility to stress-related illness: perceived stress and negative affect (Colgan et al., 2019; Creswell et al., 2019). Negative affect refers to undifferentiated, subjective distress and subsumes a broad range of aversive mood states, such as worry, anxiety, anger, self-criticism, and life dissatisfaction (Van Diest et al., 2005). Negative affect is associated with more health complaints, lower levels of health perception (Barlow et al., 2014), and greater levels of perceived stress. More specifically, when individuals appraise that a situational demand is stressful or threatens to overwhelm their ability to successfully cope, (i.e., perceived stress), they may be more likely to meet this demand with negative affect (Lazarus, 2006). These affective responses may be the most proximal determinants for engaging in healthy or unhealthy behaviors to seek relief from stress (Epel et al., 2018).

Stein and Witkiewitz (2020) conducted a systematic review of mechanistic studies of mindfulness-based programs for adults with psychological conditions. These studies dismantled MBSR, MBCT, unified mindfulness, and core mindfulness processes. Across eight studies, a total of 758 participants were enrolled. Largely congruent with the mindfulness stress buffering hypotheses (Creswell & Lindsay, 2014), two proposed mechanisms were revealed to be promising active ingredients of these meditation interventions: awareness of the present moment (i.e., the capacity to observe and experience internal reactions to a stressor as they arise) and acceptance and/or nonreactivity to the internal landscape of the present moment. Awareness paired with nonreactivity may buffer initial threat appraisals and, subsequently, reduce negative affect or emotional reactivity, leading to greater health (Colgan et al., 2019; Creswell & Lindsay, 2014). Meditation training may enhance awareness of the habitual and potentially historically influenced evaluations and appraisals that occur in reaction to a stressor. With continued practice, the cultivated nonreactive awareness may eventually allow for the de-automatization of maladaptive appraisal and affective reactivity patterns, promoting more adaptive responses to stress and buffering the individual from stress-related illness, and preventing the harmful cycle of stress reactivity.

Stress-related health behaviors are also considered potential mechanisms of meditation. Stress is associated with negative health behaviors such as greater tobacco use (Kassel et al., 2003), poor diet and unhealthy eating behaviors (Hill et al., 2021), and impaired sleep quality (Åkerstedt, 2006). Meditation training may reduce stress-related physical symptoms and sleep disturbances through improvements in perseverative cognition and emotion regulation processes. Nonreactivity, or acceptance of the present moment, acts as a protective factor. Increases in awareness may contribute to heightened psychological distress and stress and reduced sleep quality, but the ability to remain nonreactive reduces the intensity of this relationship (Greeson et al., 2018). Indeed, the acceptance of emotions is likely a key mechanism, explaining how meditation contributes to enhanced mental health (Burzler et al., 2019).

Enhancements in attention processing may also explain the cognitive benefits of meditation, particularly in OM and FA practices. When practiced separately and combined, both OM and FA meditations lead to improvements in generalized attention, its alerting and executive control networks, and both the inhibition and updating components of executive functioning (Sumantry & Stewart, 2021). The alerting network allows for the initial capture of attention and is characterized by a state of readiness to respond to novel stimuli whereas the executive control network is implicated in attentional shifting between competing stimuli. Both attentional components are needed in OM and FA practices, in which attention is maintained on a stimulus of choice or continually shifts while filtering out unneeded, external information. These modest increments in attention processing may further impact a wide array of mental health and psychological outcomes, but more research is needed to determine the potential mechanistic role of attentional network enhancements from meditation on outcomes of interest.

Contemplative practices that specifically target empathy, compassion, and prosocial behavior contain their own set of mechanisms, but also overlap with mindfulness mechanisms. Luberto et al. (2018) conducted a systematic review and meta-analysis assessing the effects of primarily LKM and compassion meditation on these constructs and behavior. They included 26 RCTs across 1,714 participants. A subset of these trials conducted mediation analyses in which increased social and emotional connectedness explained the effects of compassion meditation on prosocial behaviors. Stress and affect also played an important role. Increased positive affect and decreased stress mediated the impact of LKM on interpersonal bias and greater home practice and decreased stress explained the impact of meditation on compassion levels. It has been suggested that these meditative practices strengthen one's socio-emotional well-being, which drives the enhancement of prosocial outcomes.

Finally, two neurological mechanisms that may explain the effects of meditation on mitigating the harmful effects of stress include increasing activity and functional connectivity in regions of the prefrontal cortex and decreasing activity and functional connectivity in regions of the limbic system. That is, meditation may increase the connectivity of prefrontal regulatory regions (e.g., ventral and dorsal regions of the lateral prefrontal cortex) to inhibit activity in stress processing regions (Modinos et al., 2010; Taren et al., 2017), thereby turning down the activity and functional connectivity of regions associated with the brain's fight-or-flight response under stress, including the central nucleus of the amygdala (Hölzel et al., 2011).

All these mechanisms have been proposed to account for the impact of meditation on health outcomes (Gu et al., 2015; Tang et al., 2015). Varying levels of evidence support each of these mechanisms, derived mostly from longitudinal intervention trials using self-report scales to measure mechanisms. Causal modeling of self-report data using structural equation models is another source of support for some of these mechanisms. Finally, a growing number of qualitative studies contribute to our understanding of the effects of meditation as perceived by patients and offer insights into how patients used meditative practices to benefit their health (Colgan et al., 2017; Hubbling et al., 2014)

PORTABLE RESOURCES—IS THERE AN APP FOR THAT?

A majority (97%) of U.S. citizens report owning a cellphone, and 85% of these are smartphones (Pew Research Center, 2021). As smartphone ownership has increased over the years, so has the interest in digital mental health among the public. Tools for meditation instruction and practice are widely available as portable applications. These electronic resources enhance accessibility and can be useful for introducing patients to the principles of various meditation practices. Mani et al. (2015) conducted a systematic review of 700 mindfulness meditation apps for smartphones and tablets. Narrowing to those in the English language, relevance, mindfulness training, and education (not merely a timer, relaxation, music, or guided imagery) resulted in only 23 unique apps in English with mindfulness training that were accessible and inexpensive. The systematic review identified only one mindfulness meditation app, Headspace, that is high in quality and has efficacy data; it is included in Exhibit 11.2 with selected resources. The mindfulness meditation app Calm is also highly rated and widely available. Of note, the scientific evidence on the effectiveness of mobile meditation apps is

Exhibit 11.2 *Portable Resources for Meditation*

RESOURCE	TOOL, TECHNOLOGY, SOURCE	DESCRIPTION
Mindfulness meditation and contemplative practice tracks	MARC Mindfulness Meditation (podcasts and iTunes downloads); UCLA Mindful Awareness Center (marc.ucla.edu); UCSD Center for Mindfulness (guided audio and live practice sessions) (https://cih.ucsd.edu/mindfulness)	Instructions, 5-minute breathing meditation, LKM, body scan, mindful movement. Free.
MBSR information, training, and classes	CFM at the University of Massachusetts Medical School (www.umassmed.edu/cfm)	Search engine identifies MBSR programs worldwide, by state, or country. CFM offers MBSR teacher training, annual scientific conferences, and MBSR courses.

Exhibit 11.2 *Portable Resources for Meditation (continued)*		
RESOURCE	**TOOL, TECHNOLOGY, SOURCE**	**DESCRIPTION**
Mindfulness meditation	Headspace (portable app); Andy Puddicombe (www.headspace. com; available in Apple App Store, GooglePlay, and Amazon)	Instruction and guidance through mindfulness meditation practices. Ten 10-minute practices are free.
Mindfulness meditation	Calm (portable app) (https:// www.calm.com/; available in Apple App Store and GooglePlay)	Instruction and guidance through mindfulness meditation practices.
Mindfulness meditation, contemplative practice recordings	Insight Timer (portable app) (https://insighttimer.com/; available in Apple App Store and Google Play)	Instruction and guidance through various meditation practices.

CFM, Center for Mindfulness; LKM, loving-kindness meditation; MARC, Mindfulness Awareness Research Center; MBSR, mindfulness-based stress reduction; UCLA, University of California, Los Angeles; UCSD, University of California, San Diego

lacking. Effect sizes range from small to medium on a range of health outcomes (e.g., stress, depression, life satisfaction, affect; Gál et al., 2021). There is some concern regarding the high number of low-quality apps that may provide users with misinformation (see Schultchen et al., 2020, for a review). Portable app developers may not be experts in the content, apps are frequently mislabeled, and user reviews do not provide enough information to gauge their content or quality. Thus, it is recommended that meditation apps be vetted by knowledgeable practitioners prior to patient utilization.

CULTURAL APPLICATIONS

The practice of meditation, and mindfulness, in particular, has its roots in Eastern contemplative traditions and constitutes a core element of Buddhism (Hanh, 1998). In the Buddhist context, mindfulness (Pāli: *sati*) has often been defined as remembering and the quality of bearing in mind or bringing to mind; the state of recollecting, remembering, nonfading, and nonforgetting (Payutto, 1995). Buddhadāsa (1988) notes that "to practice mindfulness is thus a matter not so much of doing but of undoing: not thinking, not judging, not associating, not planning, not imagining, not wishing" (p. 72).

Nearly 20 years ago, Kabat-Zinn (2003) noted that mindfulness has been adapted to ensure a fit with Western ideals and to enhance its palatability to Westerners, and further suggested that if the prevailing kinds of mindfulness research and theorizing are continued exclusively, they may prove limiting, distorting, and ethnocentric. Although a number of MBI programs exist, few have been designed for or adapted to account for the specific stressors faced by cultural minorities and international communities. Most MBIs are developed by, with, and for White Americans, and the bulk of the extant MBI literature has been based on a fit with the larger White community. Two recent systematic reviews, Waldron et al. (2018) and DeLuca et al. (2018), highlight the dearth of diverse and international samples in MBI research (particularly RCTs). This underrepresentation reduces the cultural validity of clinical trial outcomes, which are critical for the development, evaluation, and customization of MBIs, and underscores the need for more diverse participants. Failure to include POC and international communities in clinical MBI trial research will ultimately mean even greater economic and social burdens for marginalized populations.

In response, a number of researchers and clinicians have recently offered suggestions to answer the call to diversify and adapt MBIs for different cultural contexts e.g., (Biggers et al., 2020; Burnett-Zeigler et al., 2019; Proulx et al., 2018; Spears, 2019; Woods-Giscombe et al., 2019). These have included delivering programs in the preferred language of participants and patients, with solid preliminary evidence to support Spanish-language adaptations in Latinx communities (Castellanos et al., 2020; Lopez-Maya et al., 2019) Similarly, Proulx et al. (2018) found that for many Native Americans, incorporating traditional approaches to healing (e.g., medicine wheel, talking circles, healers) that align with Native culture increased their initial engagement and also fostered longer term engagement. Traditional elements should constitute the core values of MBI practices, and facilitators should consider where such practices overlap or conflict with indigenous traditions through a culture-focused approach. For example, Proulx et al. (2018) noted that many African Americans are reluctant to discuss the terms of mindfulness and meditation because they are associated with Buddhism and Whites in power. Instead, Proulx et al. (2018) found it more helpful to utilize specific terms like "paying attention" or "staying focused," which may increase acceptance in African American communities.

Western MBIs are rooted in East Asian philosophies, and there are many cultural elements that can be integrated to increase the appropriateness and effectiveness for Asian American communities. These elements include enhanced integration of interdependent and allocentric principles, including conceptions of self, interdependent transcendent selves, and values (Hall et al., 2011). This can include the incorporation of compassion meditations that align oneself toward others and facilitate healing from racial discrimination-related stress (Hwang & Chan, 2019). Many diverse groups benefit from integrating religious or spiritual practices into MBIs (Biggers et al., 2020; Olano et al., 2015). This can be achieved by citing religious hymns, ideas, and writings that encourage the basic premises of being mindful (Woods-Giscombe et al., 2019).

Research suggests that POC are hesitant to access mental health services and face a number of contextual barriers, including a lack of insurance coverage, transportation problems, cultural barriers, mistrust of psychological services, and lower accessibility to mental health facilities in the community (Maura & Weisman de Mamani, 2017). Framing MBIs as stress-related coping skills has been associated with increased acceptability in various cultural groups (Fung et al., 2019; Guo et al., 2017). Abbreviated curricula are also beneficial for fitting into the numerous pressures (e.g., long commutes on public transportation, a lack of employment flexibility) that many POC face. Expectations surrounding daily home practice are often unrealistic among lower socioeconomic status groups. For many, such skepticism does not represent "resistance" but reflects the harsh demands of life in marginalized communities. Consequently, it can be helpful to provide childcare to parents enrolled in MBIs and facilitate transportation, make reminder phone calls, and provide snacks/meals during groups (Biggers et al., 2020; Watson-Singleton et al., 2019). Designing specific culturally competent mindfulness strategies (e.g., mindful assertiveness skills) that are responsive to the specific needs of POC is necessary. For example, it may be useful to include mindfulness strategies that can be geared toward addressing unjust sociocultural contexts (e.g., mindfully standing up to discrimination) that are empowering and promote personal agency (Bhambhani & Gallo, 2021; Watson-Singleton et al., 2019). Gleaning information from community-based participatory efforts utilizing direct experiences from POC presents a unique opportunity to learn new strategies to overcome barriers by developing additional culturally competent mindfulness strategies. Relatedly, including more POC MBI instructors has shown to enhance acceptability among diverse groups (Burnett-Zeigler et al., 2019).

At the root of these recommendations lies the need to understand the cultural context in which diverse communities live (Magee, 2019). It is essential to understand the socioeconomic conditions, history, and needs of each community before any intervention is developed or adapted (Proulx et al., 2018). Increasing cultural and international sensitivity into Westernized MBIs requires a bottom-up approach, in which clients and practitioners begin by generating culture-specific solutions to psychological problems evident with different POC and international groups and subsequently incorporate them into Western mindfulness-based approaches (Woods-Giscombe et al., 2019).

An example of a culturally derived nursing meditation intervention in Thailand, a culture in which 94% of people are Buddhists (Klechaya & Glasson, 2017), is described in Sidebar 11.1.

Sidebar 11.1 *Meditation as a Nursing Intervention In Thailand*

Sukjai Charoensuk

Meditation has long been considered to be a religious practice in Thailand. The application of meditation as a nursing intervention was first documented in 1992, when, for her master's thesis, Pattaya Jitsuwan (1992), examined the effects of anapanasati (mindfulness of breathing) training on anxiety and depression in 35 chronic renal failure patients. The effect of anapanasati was found to decrease anxiety and depression, as well as to improve mental health. Since then, there has been a strong trajectory of studies by faculty and students at a number of Thai universities that have added to the evidence base for the use of meditation for a variety of conditions among a variety of populations. These universities include Ramkhamheng University, Mahidol University, Mahasarakham University, Khon Kaen University, Ratchabhut Nakhon Ratchasima University, Phuket Rajabhat University, and Chiangmai University.

Anapanasati has been used to improve the mental state of students, and meditation combined with cognitive behavioral therapy has been used

(continued)

Sidebar 11.1 *Meditation as a Nursing Intervention In Thailand (continued)*

for depressive disorders. Meditation has been studied with Thai youth and adolescents to enhance happiness, improve emotional well-being, and promote self-esteem and self-control. Studies have also used meditative practices to target indicators of poor health, including hypertension, elevated HbA1c, hypercholesterolemia, tachycardia, anxiety, and pain. Meditation has also been used for specific patient groups with conditions such as diabetes, rheumatoid arthritis, end-stage cancer, and depression.

Types of Practice in Thailand

The most common type of meditation examined in Thai research has been anapanasati. In the studies described earlier, meditation practice times ranged from 30 to 90 minutes daily. In Thailand, meditation includes sitting practices, such as anapanasati, and movement meditation, such as qi gong. Recently, meditation interventions have been incorporated into palliative care as a spiritual dimension; meditation has been applied with other medical treatments and complementary therapies in the care of patients with end-stage cancer to improve clinical status and quality of life.

Case Study: Arokaya Sala

Arokaya Sala is a natural recovery center located at Kam Pramong temple in Sakol Nakorn Province, Thailand. It was established to provide help and integrated treatments for cancer patients—including those who are in the final stages of illness—to aid in relief from stress and pain, and to improve patients' quality of life. Religious ceremonies, including chanting, sitting meditation, and walking meditation, are organized to cultivate faith and encourage patients to treat the illness. Arokaya Sala has served more than 3,300 cancer patients from across Thailand and from other countries since it was established.

Reference

Jitsuwan, P. (1992). *Effect of anapanasati practice on anxiety and depression of chronic renal failure patients with dialysis* (Unpublished master's thesis). Mahidol University.

FUTURE RESEARCH

To survey the lines of research being actively pursued, we searched the database of U.S. federally funded grants (https://reporter.nih.gov), using keywords of meditation or mindfulness, and identified 133 and 334, respectively, active grants, a remarkable 78% increase over the number yielded by the same search just 4 years earlier (searched July 2021). Particularly noteworthy was the substantial number of large, multiyear research grants with annual funding over $500,000. Grants included clinical trials of MBSR, MBCT, and other meditation programs in diverse populations (including POC, children, older adults, veterans, persons with disabilities) and for numerous conditions. These grants had the hallmarks of methodological rigor: randomization, adequate statistical power, active comparison groups, an array of self-reported and physiological outcomes, and longer follow-up to establish the durability of impact. There were also experiments and imaging studies to elucidate mechanisms and examine dose effectiveness, intervention-development studies to create or adapt meditation programs to particular populations, and the use of qualitative or mixed-methods approaches to improve understanding of the patient experience.

To maximize the potential for meditation to improve health, more research is needed about *how* it works and to identify *who* it is most likely to benefit. Meditation is unlikely to be "one size fits all." It is not known whether the quality of the meditation state achieved differs by technique (concentration, mindfulness, or other) and to what extent all meditation approaches engage common pathways versus distinct cognitive and physiological systems. This information could form the foundation for matching specific meditative techniques to particular health problems. Specific personality or genetic factors may predict the ability to learn and use each type of meditation. The roles of personal characteristics such as age, gender, personality traits, and other moderators should be evaluated to determine the best meditation training fit or to tailor programs. With this information, it may be possible to match people to the type of meditation training most likely to work best for them.

Given the high prevalence of trauma- and stressor-related exposure and symptomatology in adults, it is also advantageous to determine how these factors impact one's meditation experience. Assessing trauma history, acute trauma-related symptoms, and chronic trauma-related symptoms may provide insightful information regarding for whom meditation-related adverse side effects might occur. Modifications in the approach to meditation, the type of practice, and the dosage could reduce the likelihood of adverse events while promoting its salutary effects in these populations. Trauma-informed meditation interventions (e.g., MBIs and OM, FA, CM practices) may include, but are not limited to, the utilization of trauma-sensitive facilitators, the use of invitational language, maintaining ample physical boundaries and vigilance of posttraumatic stress responses among participants, and providing adequate lighting, options for practice (e.g., focused attention anchors, eye placement, postural modifications) and permission to exit the space at any point. Most importantly, researchers should be equipped with adequate education about trauma and the traumatic stress response, how and when symptoms may arise through the process of meditation, and the ability to skillfully navigate these potentially challenging experiences. As noted earlier, they should also have an understanding of the sociocultural and historical factors that contribute to practice and research barriers. Incorporating these components may enhance the efficacy and effectiveness of meditation interventions by promoting resiliency and posttraumatic growth.

Although research over the last two decades has demonstrated that meditation practices are effective at improving symptoms in conditions such as pain and anxiety, the efficacy of any single-modality treatment is typically modest. Increasing clinical efficacy of meditation interventions is a critically important goal and a core element of the National Center for Complementary and Integrative Health's Strategic Plan for 2021–2025 (www.nccih.nih.gov/about/

nccih-strategic-plan-2021-2025). Multicomponent interventions that combine con-ventional *and* complementary approaches may prove fruitful to increase treatment effects on hard-to-treat clinical outcomes. For example, it may be more effective to combine a mindfulness-meditation intervention with pain neuroscience education for chronic pain populations than either of these two stand-alone interventions.

It is important to recognize that health is on a continuum. To date, research on meditation interventions has largely focused on mitigating disease states (e.g., reducing anxiety, lowering depression, diminishing cardiovascular risk factors); less research, however, has focused on how to quantify, measure, and increase health, health restoration, and resilience. Research is needed to identify the gaps in knowledge regarding if and how meditation interventions play a role in the prevention of disease and the progression from disease to health restoration. This would entail appropriate longitudinal designs with careful thought to retaining participation and strategies to minimize attrition.

REFERENCES

Âkerstedt, T. (2006). Psychosocial stress and impaired sleep. *Scandinavian Journal of Work, Environment & Health, 32*(6), 493–501. http://www.jstor.org/stable/40967601

Alex Brake, C., Sauer-Zavala, S., Boswell, J. F., Gallagher, M. W., Farchione, T. J., & Barlow, D. H. (2016). Mindfulness-based exposure strategies as a transdiagnostic mechanism of change: An exploratory alternating treatment design. *Behavior Therapy, 47*(2), 225–238. https://doi .org/10.1016/j.beth.2015.10.008

American Psychological Association. (2020). *Stress in America™ 2020: A national mental health crisis.*

Anālayo. (2003). *Satipaṭṭhāna: The direct path to realization.* Windhorse.

Baer, R., Crane, C., Montero-Marin, J., Phillips, A., Taylor, L., Tickell, A., Kuyken, W., & The MYRIAD Team. (2021). Frequency of self-reported unpleasant events and harm in a mindful-ness-based program in two general population samples. *Mindfulness, 12*(3), 763–774. https:// doi.org/10.1007/s12671-020-01547-8

Barlow, D. H., Sauer-Zavala, S., Carl, J. R., Bullis, J. R., & Ellard, K. K. (2014). The nature, diagnosis, and treatment of neuroticism: Back to the future. *Clinical Psychological Science, 2*(3), 344–365. https://doi.org/10.1177/2167702613505532

Bhambhani, Y., & Gallo, L. (2021). Developing and adapting a mindfulness-based group inter-vention for racially and economically marginalized patients in the Bronx. *Cognitive and Behavioral Practice.* https://doi.org/10.1016/j.cbpra.2021.04.010

Biggers, A., Spears, C. A., Sanders, K., Ong, J., Sharp, L. K., & Gerber, B. S. (2020). Promoting mindfulness in African American communities. *Mindfulness, 11*(10), 2274–2282. https://doi .org/10.1007/s12671-020-01480-w

Bishop, S. R., Lau, M., Shapiro, S., Carlson, L., Anderson, N. D., Carmody, J., Segal, Z. V., Abbey, S., Speca, M., Velting, D., & Devins, G. (2004). Mindfulness: A proposed operational defi-nition. *Clinical Psychology: Science and Practice, 11*(3), 230–241. https://doi.org/https://doi .org/10.1093/clipsy.bph077

Bodhi, B. (2011). What does mindfulness really mean? A canonical perspective. *Contemporary Buddhism, 12*(1), 19–39. https://doi.org/10.1080/14639947.2011.564813

Bowen, S., Witkiewitz, K., Chawla, N., & Grow, J. (2011). Integrating mindfulness meditation and cognitive behavioral traditions for the long-term treatment of addictive behaviors. *JCOM, 18*(10), 473–479.

Britton, W. B., Davis, J. H., Loucks, E. B., Peterson, B., Cullen, B. H., Reuter, L., Rando, A., Rahrig, H., Lipsky, J., & Lindahl, J. R. (2018). Dismantling mindfulness-based cognitive therapy: Creation and validation of 8-week focused attention and open monitoring interventions within a 3-armed randomized controlled trial. *Behaviour Research and Therapy, 101*, 92–107. https://doi.org/10.1016/j.brat.2017.09.010

Britton, W. B., Lindahl, J. R., Cooper, D. J., Canby, N. K., & Palitsky, R. (2021). Defining and measuring meditation-related adverse effects in mindfulness-based programs. *Clinical Psychological Science*. Advanced online publication. https://doi.org/10.1177/2167702621996340

Buddhadāsa, B. (1988). *Ānāpānasati: Mindfulness with Breathing; Unveiling the Secrets of Life; a Manual for Serious Beginners*. Dhamma Study-Practice Group.

Burnett-Zeigler, I., Satyshur, M. D., Hong, S., Wisner, K. L., & Moskowitz, J. (2019). Acceptability of a mindfulness intervention for depressive symptoms among African-American women in a community health center: A qualitative study. *Complementary Therapies in Medicine, 45*, 19–24. https://doi.org/10.1016/j.ctim.2019.05.012

Burzler, M. A., Voracek, M., Hos, M., & Tran, U. S. (2019). Mechanisms of mindfulness in the general population. *Mindfulness, 10*(3), 469–480. https://doi.org/10.1007/s12671-018-0988-y

Carmody, J., & Baer, R. A. (2008). Relationships between mindfulness practice and levels of mindfulness, medical and psychological symptoms and well-being in a mindfulness-based stress reduction program. *Journal of Behavioral Medicine, 31*(1), 23–33. https://doi.org/10.1007/s10865-007-9130-7

Castellanos, R., Yildiz Spinel, M., Phan, V., Orengo-Aguayo, R., Humphreys, K. L., & Flory, K. (2020). A systematic review and meta-analysis of cultural adaptations of mindfulness-based interventions for Hispanic populations. *Mindfulness, 11*(2), 317–332. https://doi.org/10.1007/s12671-019-01210-x

Çetin, N., & Aylaz, R. (2018). The effect of mindfulness-based psychoeducation on insight and medication adherence of schizophrenia patients. *Archives of Psychiatric Nursing, 32*(5), 737–744. https://doi.org/10.1016/j.apnu.2018.04.011

Christopher, M. S., Goerling, R. J., Rogers, B. S., Hunsinger, M., Baron, G., Bergman, A. L., & Zava, D. T. (2016). A pilot study evaluating the effectiveness of a mindfulness-based intervention on cortisol awakening response and health outcomes among law enforcement officers. *Journal of Police and Criminal Psychology, 31*(1), 15–28. https://doi.org/10.1007/s11896-015-9161-x

Christopher, M. S., Hunsinger, M., Goerling, L. Richard J., Bowen, S., Rogers, Brant S., Gross, C. R., Dapolonia, E., & Pruessner, J. C. (2018). Mindfulness-based resilience training to reduce health risk, stress reactivity, and aggression among law enforcement officers: A feasibility and preliminary efficacy trial. *Psychiatry Research, 264*, 104–115. https://doi.org/https://doi.org/10.1016/j.psychres.2018.03.059

Cillessen, L., Johannsen, M., Speckens, A. E. M., & Zachariae, R. (2019). Mindfulness-based interventions for psychological and physical health outcomes in cancer patients and survivors: A systematic review and meta-analysis of randomized controlled trials. *Psycho-Oncology, 28*(12), 2257–2269. https://doi.org/10.1002/pon.5214

Cohen, S., Janicki-Deverts, D., Doyle, W. J., Miller, G. E., Frank, E., Rabin, B. S., & Turner, R. B. (2012). Chronic stress, glucocorticoid receptor resistance, inflammation, and disease risk. *Proceedings of the National Academy of Sciences, 109*(16), 5995–5999. https://doi.org/10.1073/pnas.1118355109

Cohen, S., Murphy, M. L. M., & Prather, A. A. (2019). Ten surprising facts about stressful life events and disease risk. *Annual Review of Psychology, 70*(1), 577–597. https://doi.org/10.1146/annurev-psych-010418-102857

Colgan, D. D., Christopher, M., Bowen, S., Brems, C., Hunsinger, M., Tucker, B., & Dapolonia, E. (2019). Mindfulness-based wellness and resilience intervention among interdisciplinary primary care teams: A mixed-methods feasibility and acceptability trial. *Primary Health Care Research & Development, 20*, e91. https://doi.org/10.1017/S1463423619000173

Colgan, D. D., Wahbeh, H., Pleet, M., Besler, K., & Christopher, M. (2017). A qualitative study of mindfulness among veterans with posttraumatic stress disorder: Practices differentially affect symptoms, aspects of well-being, and potential mechanisms of action. *Journal of Evidence-Based Complementary & Alternative Medicine, 22*(3), 482–493.

Compson, J. (2018). Adverse meditation experiences: Navigating Buddhist and secular frameworks for addressing them. *Mindfulness, 9*(5), 1358–1369. https://doi.org/10.1007/s12671-017-0878-8

Crane, R. S., Brewer, J., Feldman, C., Kabat-Zinn, J., Santorelli, S., Williams, J. M. G., & Kuyken, W. (2017). What defines mindfulness-based programs? The warp and the weft. *Psychological Medicine*, 47(6), 990–999. https://doi.org/10.1017/s0033291716003317

Creswell, J. D., & Lindsay, E. K. (2014). How does mindfulness training affect health? A mindfulness stress buffering account. *Current Directions in Psychological Science*, 23(6), 401–407. https://doi.org/10.1177/0963721414547415

Creswell, J. D., Lindsay, E. K., Villalba, D. K., & Chin, B. (2019). Mindfulness training and physical health: mechanisms and outcomes. *Psychosomatic Medicine*, 81(3), 224. https://doi.org/10.1097/PSY.0000000000000675

Davis, K. M., Lau, M. A., & Cairns, D. R. (2009). Development and preliminary validation of a trait version of the Toronto Mindfulness Scale. *Journal of Cognitive Psychotherapy*, 3, 185–197. https://doi.org/10.1891/0889-8391.23.3.185

DeLuca, S. M., Kelman, A. R., & Waelde, L. C. (2018). A systematic review of ethnoracial representation and cultural adaptation of mindfulness-and meditation-based interventions. *Psychological Studies*, 63(2), 117–129. https://doi.org/10.1007/s12646-018-0452-z

Desbordes, G., Gard, T., Hoge, E. A., Hölzel, B. K., Kerr, C., Lazar, S. W., Olendzki, A., & Vago, D. R. (2014). Moving beyond mindfulness: Defining equanimity as an outcome measure in meditation and contemplative research. *Mindfulness*, 2014(January), 356–372. https://doi.org/10.1007/s12671-013-0269-8

Dreeben, S. J., Mamberg, M. H., & Salmon, P. (2013). The MBSR body scan in clinical practice. *Mindfulness*, 4(4), 394–401. https://doi.org/10.1007/s12671-013-0212-z

Epel, E. S., Crosswell, A. D., Mayer, S. E., Prather, A. A., Slavich, G. M., Puterman, E., & Mendes, W. B. (2018). More than a feeling: A unified view of stress measurement for population science. *Frontiers in Neuroendocrinology*, 49, 146–169. https://doi.org/10.1016/j.yfrne.2018.03.001

Epstein, R., Quill, T., Krasner, M., & McDonald, S. (2007). *A curriculum in mindful practice for students and residents faculty manual*. University of Rochester, School of Medicine and Dentistry.

Fujino, M., Ueda, Y., Mizuhara, H., Saiki, J., & Nomura, M. (2018). Open monitoring meditation reduces the involvement of brain regions related to memory function. *Scientific Reports*, 8(1). https://doi.org/10.1038/s41598-018-28274-4

Fung, J., Kim, J. J., Jin, J., Chen, G., Bear, L., & Lau, A. S. (2019). A randomized trial evaluating school-based mindfulness intervention for ethnic minority youth: Exploring mediators and moderators of intervention effects. *Journal of Abnormal Child Psychology*, 47(1), 1–19. https://doi.org/10.1007/s10802-018-0425-7

Gál, É., Ştefan, S., & Cristea, I. A. (2021). The efficacy of mindfulness meditation apps in enhancing users' well-being and mental health related outcomes: A meta-analysis of randomized controlled trials. *Journal of Affective Disorders*, 279, 131–142. https://doi.org/https://doi.org/10.1016/j.jad.2020.09.134

Germer, C. K., Siegel, R. D., & Fulton, P. R. (2013). *Mindfulness and psychotherapy*. Guilford Press.

Goldberg, S. B., Lam, S. U., Britton, W. B., & Davidson, R. J. (2022). Prevalence of meditation-related adverse effects in a population-based sample in the United States. *Psychotherapy Research*, 32(3), 291–305. https://doi.org/10.1080/10503307.2021.1933646

Goldberg, S. B., Riordan, K. M., Sun, S., & Davidson, R. J. (2021). The empirical status of mindfulness-based interventions: A systematic review of 44 meta-analyses of randomized controlled trials. *Perspectives on Psychological Science*, 0(0), 1745691620968771. https://doi.org/10.1177/1745691620968771

Goldberg, S. B., Tucker, R. P., Greene, P. A., Davidson, R. J., Wampold, B. E., Kearney, D. J., & Simpson, T. L. (2018). Mindfulness-based interventions for psychiatric disorders: A systematic review and meta-analysis. *Clinical Psychology Review*, 59, 52–60. https://doi.org/https://doi.org/10.1016/j.cpr.2017.10.011

Graser, J., & Stangier, U. (2018). Compassion and loving-kindness meditation: An overview and prospects for the application in clinical samples. *Harvard Review of Psychiatry*, 26(4), 201–215. https://doi.org/10.1097/hrp.0000000000000192

Greeson, J. M., Zarrin, H., Smoski, M. J., Brantley, J. G., Lynch, T. R., Webber, D. M., Hall, M. H., Suarez, E. C., & Wolever, R. Q. (2018). Mindfulness meditation targets transdiagnostic symptoms implicated in stress-related disorders: Understanding relationships between changes in mindfulness, sleep quality, and physical symptoms. *Evidence-Based Complementary and Alternative Medicine, 2018*. https://doi.org/10.1155/2018/4505191

Gross, C. R., Kreitzer, M. J., Reilly-Spong, M., Wall, M., Winbush, N. Y., Patterson, R., Mahowald, M., & Cramer-Bornemann, M. (2011). Mindfulness-based stress reduction versus pharmacotherapy for chronic primary insomnia: a randomized controlled clinical trial. *Explore, 7*(2), 76–87.

Gross, C. R., Reilly-Spong, M., Park, T., Zhao, R., Gurvich, O. V., & Ibrahim, H. N. (2017). Telephone-adapted Mindfulness-based Stress Reduction (tMBSR) for patients awaiting kidney transplantation. *Contemporary Clinical Trials, 57*, 37–43. https://doi.org/10.1016/j.cct.2017.03.014

Gu, J., Strauss, C., Bond, R., & Cavanagh, K. (2015). How do mindfulness-based cognitive therapy and mindfulness-based stress reduction improve mental health and wellbeing? A systematic review and meta-analysis of mediation studies. *Clinical Psychology Review, 37*, 1–12. https://doi.org/10.1016/j.cpr.2015.01.006

Guo, S., Kim, J. J., Bear, L., & Lau, A. S. (2017). Does depression screening in schools reduce adolescent racial/ethnic disparities in accessing treatment? *Journal of Clinical Child & Adolescent Psychology, 46*(4), 523–536. https://doi.org/10.1080/15374416.2016.1270826

Hall, G. C., Hong, J. J., Zane, N. W., & Meyer, O. L. (2011). Culturally competent treatments for Asian Americans: The relevance of mindfulness and acceptance-based psychotherapies. *Clinical Psychology: Science and Practice, 18*(3), 215. https://doi.org/10.1111/j.1468-2850.2011.01253.x

Hanh, T. N. (1998). *The heart of the Buddha's teaching: Transforming suffering into peace, joy, & liberation: The four truths, the noble eightfold path, and other basic Buddhist teachings*. Harmony.

Hartmann, M., Kopf, S., Kircher, C., Faude-Lang, V., Djuric, Z., Augstein, F., Friederich, H.-C., Kieser, M., Bierhaus, A., & Humpert, P. M. (2012). Sustained effects of a mindfulness-based stress-reduction intervention in type 2 diabetic patients: design and first results of a randomized controlled trial (the Heidelberger Diabetes and Stress-study). *Diabetes Care, 35*(5), 945–947. https://doi.org/10.2337/dc11-1343

Hill, D., Conner, M., Clancy, F., Moss, R., Wilding, S., Bristow, M., & O'Connor, D. B. (2021). Stress and eating behaviours in healthy adults: A systematic review and meta-analysis. *Health Psychology Review*, 1–25. https://doi.org/10.1080/17437199.2021.1923406

Hilton, L., Hempel, S., Ewing, B. A., Apaydin, E., Xenakis, L., Newberry, S., Colaiaco, B., Maher, A. R., Shanman, R. M., Sorbero, M. E., & Maglione, M. A. (2017). Mindfulness meditation for chronic pain: Systematic review and meta-analysis. *Annals of Behavioral Medicine, 51*(2), 199–213. https://doi.org/10.1007/s12160-016-9844-2

Hoffman, C. J., Ersser, S. J., Hopkinson, J. B., Nicholls, P. G., Harrington, J. E., & Thomas, P. W. (2012). Effectiveness of mindfulness-based stress reduction in mood, breast-and endocrine-related quality of life, and well-being in stage 0 to III breast cancer: A randomized, controlled trial. *Journal of Clinical Oncology, 30*(12), 1335–1342. https://doi.org/10.1200/JCO.2010.34.0331

Hoge, E. A., Guidos, B. M., Mete, M., Bui, E., Pollack, M. H., Simon, N. M., & Dutton, M. A. (2017). Effects of mindfulness meditation on occupational functioning and health care utilization in individuals with anxiety. *Journal of Psychosomatic Research, 95*, 7–11. https://doi.org/10.1016/j.jpsychores.2017.01.011

Hölzel, B. K., Lazar, S. W., Gard, T., Schuman-Olivier, Z., Vago, D. R., & Ott, U. (2011). How does mindfulness meditation work? Proposing mechanisms of action from a conceptual and neural perspective. *Perspectives on Psychological Science, 6*(6), 537–559. https://doi.org/10.1177/1745691611419671

Hubbling, A., Reilly-Spong, M., Kreitzer, M. J., & Gross, C. R. (2014). How mindfulness changed my sleep: Focus groups with chronic insomnia patients. *BMC Complementary and Alternative Medicine, 14*(1), 1–11. https://doi.org/10.1186/1472-6882-14-50

Hunsinger, M., Christopher, M., & Schmidt, A. M. (2019). Mindfulness training, implicit bias, and force response decision-making. *Mindfulness, 10*(12), 2555–2566. https://doi.org/10.1007/s12671-019-01213-8

Hwang, W.-C., & Chan, C. P. (2019). Compassionate meditation to heal from race-related stress: A pilot study with Asian Americans. *American Journal of Orthopsychiatry, 89*(4), 482. https://doi.org/10.1037/ort0000372

Jha, A. P., Morrison, A. B., Parker, S. C., & Stanley, E. A. (2017). Practice is protective: mindfulness training promotes cognitive resilience in high-stress cohorts. *Mindfulness, 8*(1), 46–58.

Kabat-Zinn, J. (1990). *Full catastrophe living: Using the wisdom of your body and mind to face stress, pain, and illness*. Delta.

Kabat-Zinn, J. (2003). Mindfulness-based interventions in context: Past, present, and future. *Clinical Psychology: Science and Practice, 10*(2), 144–156. https://doi.org/10.1093/clipsy.bpg016

Kabat-Zinn, J. (2018). Proprioception—the felt sense of the body. *Mindfulness, 9*(6), 1979–1980. https://doi.org/10.1007/s12671-018-1028-7

Kabat-Zinn, J., Lipworth, L., & Burney, R. (1985). The clinical use of mindfulness meditation for the self-regulation of chronic pain. *Journal of Behavioral Medicine, 8*(2), 163–190. https://doi .org/10.1007/BF00845519

Kassel, J. D., Stroud, L. R., & Paronis, C. A. (2003). Smoking, stress, and negative affect: correlation, causation, and context across stages of smoking. *Psychological Bulletin, 129*(2), 270. https://doi.org/10.1037/0033-2909.129.2.270

Keng, S.-L., Smoski, M. J., & Robins, C. J. (2011). Effects of mindfulness on psychological health: A review of empirical studies. *Clinical Psychology Review, 31*(6), 1041–1056. https://doi .org/10.1016/j.cpr.2011.04.006

Kirschbaum, C., Pirke, K.-M., & Hellhammer, D. H. (1993). The 'Trier Social Stress Test'–a tool for investigating psychobiological stress responses in a laboratory setting. *Neuropsychobiology, 28*(1–2), 76–81. https://doi.org/10.1159/000119004

Klechaya, R., & Glasson, G. (2017). Mindfulness and place-based education in Buddhist-oriented schools in Thailand. In *Weaving complementary knowledge systems and mindfulness to educate a literate citizenry for sustainable and healthy lives* (pp. 159–170). Brill Sense.

Kristeller, J. L., & Hallett, C. B. (1999). An exploratory study of a meditation-based intervention for binge eating disorder. *Journal of Health Psychology, 4*(3), 357–363. https://doi.org/ 10.1177/135910539900400305

Krittanawong, C., Kumar, A., Wang, Z., Narasimhan, B., Jneid, H., Virani, S. S., & Levine, G. N. (2020). Meditation and cardiovascular health in the US. *The American Journal of Cardiology, 131*, 23–26. https://doi.org/10.1016/j.amjcard.2020.06.043

Lazarus, R. S. (2006). *Stress and emotion: A new synthesis*. Springer Publishing Company.

Lee, T. M. C., Leung, M.-K., Hou, W.-K., Tang, J. C. Y., Yin, J., So, K.-F., Lee, C.-F., & Chan, C. C. H. (2012). Distinct neural activity associated with focused-attention meditation and loving-kindness meditation. *PLOS One, 7*(8), e40054. https://doi.org/10.1371/journal.pone .0040054

Li, Y., Huang, X., Su, J., & Wang, Y. (2020). Mindfulness may be a novel factor associated with CPAP adherence in OSAHS patients. *Sleep and Breathing, 24*(1), 183–190. https://doi .org/10.1007/s11325-019-01858-8

Lindahl, J. R., Fisher, N. E., Cooper, D. J., Rosen, R. K., & Britton, W. B. (2017). The varieties of contemplative experience: A mixed-methods study of meditation-related challenges in Western Buddhists. *PLOS ONE, 12*(5), e0176239. https://doi.org/10.1371/journal.pone.0176239

Lloyd, A., White, R., Eames, C., & Crane, R. (2018). The utility of home-practice in mindfulness-based group interventions: a systematic review. *Mindfulness, 9*(3), 673–692. https://doi.org/ 10.1007/s12671-017-0813-z

Lopez-Maya, E., Olmstead, R., & Irwin, M. R. (2019). Mindfulness meditation and improvement in depressive symptoms among Spanish- and English speaking adults: A randomized, controlled, comparative efficacy trial. *PLOS ONE, 14*(7), e0219425. https://doi.org/10.1371/journal .pone.0219425

Luberto, C. M., Shinday, N., Song, R., Philpotts, L. L., Park, E. R., Fricchione, G. L., & Yeh, G. Y. (2018). A systematic review and meta-analysis of the effects of meditation on empathy, compassion, and prosocial behaviors. *Mindfulness, 9*(3), 708–724. https://doi.org/10.1007/ s12671-017-0841-8

Lutz, A., Slagter, H. A., Dunne, J. D., & Davidson, R. J. (2008). Attention regulation and monitoring in meditation. *Trends in Cognitive Sciences, 12*(4), 163–169. https://doi.org/10.1016/j. tics.2008.01.005

Magee, R. V. (2019). *The inner work of racial justice: Healing ourselves and transforming our communities through mindfulness.* TarcherPerigee.

Mani, M., Kavanagh, D. J., Hides, L., & Stoyanov, S. R. (2015). Review and evaluation of mindfulness-based iPhone apps. *JMIR mHealth and uHealth, 3*(3), e4328. https://doi.org/10.2196/mhealth.4328

Manna, A., Raffone, A., Perrucci, M. G., Nardo, D., Ferretti, A., Tartaro, A., Londei, A., Del Gratta, C., Belardinelli, M. O., & Romani, G. L. (2010). Neural correlates of focused attention and cognitive monitoring in meditation. *Brain Research Bulletin, 82*(1), 46–56. https://doi.org/https://doi.org/10.1016/j.brainresbull.2010.03.001

Martin, A. B., Hartman, M., Lassman, D., Catlin, A., & Team, N. H. E. A. (2021). National health care spending in 2019: Steady growth for the fourth consecutive year: Study examines national health care spending for 2019. *Health Affairs, 40*(1), 14–24. https://doi.org/10.1377/hlthaff.2020.02022

Mason, M. F., Norton, M. I., Van Horn, J. D., Wegner, D. M., Grafton, S. T., & Macrae, C. N. (2007). Wandering minds: The default network and stimulus-independent thought. *Science (New York, NY), 315*(5810), 393–395. https://doi.org/10.1126/science.1131295

Maura, J., & Weisman de Mamani, A. (2017). Mental health disparities, treatment engagement, and attrition among racial/ethnic minorities with severe mental illness: A review. *Journal of Clinical Psychology in Medical Settings, 24*(3), 187–210. https://doi.org/10.1007/s10880-017-9510-2

McEwen, B. S. (2017). Neurobiological and systemic effects of chronic stress. *Chronic Stress, 1,* 247054701769232. https://doi.org/10.1177/2470547017692328

Modinos, G., Ormel, J., & Aleman, A. (2010). Individual differences in dispositional mindfulness and brain activity involved in reappraisal of emotion. *Social Cognitive and Affective Neuroscience, 5*(4), 369–377. https://doi.org/10.1093/scan/nsq006

Morgado, P., & Cerqueira, J. J. (2018). Editorial: The impact of stress on cognition and motivation [Editorial]. *Frontiers in Behavioral Neuroscience, 12*(326). https://doi.org/10.3389/fnbeh.2018.00326

Morone, N. E., Greco, C. M., Moore, C. G., Rollman, B. L., Lane, B., Morrow, L. A., Glynn, N. W., & Weiner, D. K. (2016). A mind-body program for older adults with chronic low back pain. *JAMA Internal Medicine, 176*(3), 329. https://doi.org/10.1001/jamainternmed.2015.8033

Morton, M. L., Helminen, E. C., & Felver, J. C. (2020). A systematic review of mindfulness interventions on psychophysiological responses to acute stress. *Mindfulness, 11*(9), 2039–2054. https://doi.org/10.1007/s12671-020-01386-7

National Center for Complementary and Integrative Health. (2022). *Meditation in depth.* https://www.nccih.nih.gov/health/meditation-in-depth

Olano, H. A., Kachan, D., Tannenbaum, S. L., Mehta, A., Annane, D., & Lee, D. J. (2015). Engagement in mindfulness practices by US adults: Sociodemographic barriers. *The Journal of Alternative and Complementary Medicine, 21*(2), 100–102. https://doi.org/10.1089/acm.2014.0269

Olendzki, A. (2011). The construction of mindfulness. *Contemporary Buddhism, 12*(1), 55–70. https://doi.org/10.1080/14639947.2011.564817

Ospina, M. B., Bond, K., Karkhaneh, M., Tjosvold, L., Vandermeer, B., Liang, Y., Bialy, L., Hooton, N., Buscemi, N., Dryden, D. M., & Klassen, T. P. (2007). Meditation practices for health: State of the research. *Evidence/Report Technology Assessment (Full Rep), 155,* 1–263.

Parsons, C. E., Crane, C., Parsons, L. J., Fjorback, L. O., & Kuyken, W. (2017). Home practice in mindfulness-based cognitive therapy and mindfulness-based stress reduction: A systematic review and meta-analysis of participants' mindfulness practice and its association with outcomes. *Behaviour Research and Therapy, 95,* 29–41. https://doi.org/10.1016/j.brat.2017.05.004

Pascoe, M. C., Thompson, D. R., Jenkins, Z. M., & Ski, C. F. (2017). Mindfulness mediates the physiological markers of stress: Systematic review and meta-analysis. *Journal of Psychiatric Research, 95,* 156–178. https://doi.org/https://doi.org/10.1016/j.jpsychires.2017.08.004

Payutto, P. (1995). *Buddhadhamma: Natural laws and values for life* (G. A. Olson, Trans.). State University of New York Press (Original work published 1971).

Pew Research Center. (2021). *Mobile fact sheet.* https://www.pewresearch.org/internet/fact-sheet/mobile/

Proulx, J., Croff, R., Oken, B., Aldwin, C. M., Fleming, C., Bergen-Cico, D., Le, T., & Noorani, M. (2018). Considerations for research and development of culturally relevant mindfulness interventions in American minority communities. *Mindfulness, 9*(2), 361–370. https://doi .org/10.1007/s12671-017-0785-z

Quach, D., Gibler, R. C., & Mano, K. E. J. (2017). Does home practice compliance make a difference in the effectiveness of mindfulness interventions for adolescents? *Mindfulness, 8*(2), 495–504. https://doi.org/10.1007/s12671-016-0624-7

Ribeiro, L., Atchley, R. M., & Oken, B. S. (2018). Adherence to practice of mindfulness in novice meditators: practices chosen, amount of time practiced, and long-term effects following a mindfulness-based intervention. *Mindfulness, 9*(2), 401–411. https://doi.org/10.1007/s12671 -017-0781-3

Rose, S., Zell, E., & Strickhouser, J. E. (2020). The effect of meditation on health: A metasynthesis of randomized controlled trials. *Mindfulness, 11*(2), 507–516. https://doi.org/10.1007/ s12671-019-01277-6

Salzberg, S. (2002). *Lovingkindness: The revolutionary art of happiness.* Shambhala Publications.

Salzberg, S. (2011). Mindfulness and loving-kindness. *Contemporary Buddhism, 12*(1), 177–182. https://doi.org/10.1080/14639947.2011.564837

Schmidt, S., Grossman, P., Schwarzer, B., Jena, S., Naumann, J., & Walach, H. (2011). Treating fibromyalgia with mindfulness-based stress reduction: results from a 3-armed randomized controlled trial. *PAIN®, 152*(2), 361–369. https://doi.org/10.1016/j.pain.2010.10.043

Schultchen, D., Terhorst, Y., Holderied, T., Stach, M., Messner, E.-M., Baumeister, H., & Sander, L. B. (2020). Stay present with your phone: A systematic review and standardized rating of mindfulness apps in European app stores. *International Journal of Behavioral Medicine.* Advanced online publication. https://doi.org/10.1007/s12529-020-09944-y

Schutte, N. S., Malouff, J. M., & Keng, S.-L. (2020). Meditation and telomere length: a metaanalysis. *Psychology & Health, 35*(8), 901–915. https://doi.org/10.1080/08870446.2019.1707827

Scott-Sheldon, L. A. J., Gathright, E. C., Donahue, M. L., Balletto, B., Feulner, M. M., Decosta, J., Cruess, D. G., Wing, R. R., Carey, M. P., & Salmoirago-Blotcher, E. (2020). Mindfulnessbased interventions for adults with cardiovascular disease: A systematic review and metaanalysis. *Annals of Behavioral Medicine, 54*(1), 67–73. https://doi.org/10.1093/abm/kaz020

Segal, Z. V., Williams, J. M. G., & Teasdale, J. D. (2002). *Mindfulness-based cognitive therapy for depression: A new approach to preventing relapse.* Guilford Press.

Sirotina, U., & Shchebetenko, S. (2020). Loving-kindness meditation and compassion meditation: Do they affect emotions in a different way? *Mindfulness, 11*(11), 2519–2530. https://doi .org/10.1007/s12671-020-01465-9

Spears, C. A. (2019). Mindfulness-based interventions for addictions among diverse and underserved populations. *Current Opinion in Psychology, 30,* 11–16. https://doi.org/10.1016/j .copsyc.2018.12.012

Stein, E., & Witkiewitz, K. (2020). Dismantling mindfulness-based programs: A systematic review to identify active components of treatment. *Mindfulness, 11*(11), 2470–2485. https:// doi.org/10.1007/s12671-020-01444-0

Suleiman-Martos, N., Gomez-Urquiza, J. L., Aguayo-Estremera, R., Cañadas-De La Fuente, G. A., De La Fuente-Solana, E. I., & Albendín-García, L. (2020). The effect of mindfulness training on burnout syndrome in nursing: A systematic review and meta-analysis. *Journal of Advanced Nursing, 76*(5), 1124–1140. https://doi.org/10.1111/jan.14318

Sumantry, D., & Stewart, K. E. (2021). Meditation, mindfulness, and attention: A meta-analysis. *Mindfulness, 12*(6), 1332–1349. https://doi.org/10.1007/s12671-021-01593-w

Sun, S., Goldberg, S. B., Loucks, E. B., & Brewer, J. A. (2021). Mindfulness-based interventions among people of color: A systematic review and meta-analysis. *Psychotherapy Research,* 1–14. https://doi.org/10.1080/10503307.2021.1937369

Tang, Y.-Y., Hölzel, B. K., & Posner, M. I. (2015). The neuroscience of mindfulness meditation. *Nature Reviews Neuroscience, 16*(4), 213–225. https://doi.org/10.1038/nrn3916

Tang, Y.-Y., & Posner, M. I. (2013). Tools of the trade: theory and method in mindfulness neuro-science. *Social Cognitive and Affective Neuroscience, 8*(1), 118–120. https://doi.org/10.1093/scan/nss112

Taren, A. A., Gianaros, P. J., Greco, C. M., Lindsay, E. K., Fairgrieve, A., Brown, K. W., Rosen, R. K., Ferris, J. L., Julson, E., & Marsland, A. L. (2017). Mindfulness meditation training and execu-tive control network resting state functional connectivity: a randomized controlled trial. *Psychosomatic Medicine, 79*(6), 674. https://doi.org/10.1097/PSY.0000000000000466

Upchurch, D. M., & Johnson, P. J. (2019). Gender differences in prevalence, patterns, purposes, and perceived benefits of meditation practices in the United States. *Journal of Women's Health, 28*(2), 135–142. https://doi.org/10.1089/jwh.2018.7178

Uusberg, H., Uusberg, A., Talpsep, T., & Paaver, M. (2016). Mechanisms of mindfulness: The dynamics of affective adaptation during open monitoring. *Biological Psychology, 118*, 94–106. https://doi.org/10.1016/j.biopsycho.2016.05.004

Vago, D. R., & Silbersweig, D. A. (2012). Self-awareness, self-regulation, and self-transcendence (S-ART): A framework for understanding the neurobiological mechanisms of mindfulness. *Frontiers in Human Neuroscience, 6*, 296. https://doi.org/10.3389/fnhum.2012.00296

Van Diest, I., De Peuter, S., Eertmans, A., Bogaerts, K., Victoir, A., & Van den Bergh, O. (2005). Negative affectivity and enhanced symptom reports: Differentiating between symptoms in men and women. *Social Science & Medicine, 61*(8), 1835–1845. https://doi.org/10.1016/j.socscimed.2005.03.031

Waldron, E. M., Hong, S., Moskowitz, J. T., & Burnett-Zeigler, I. (2018). A systematic review of the demographic characteristics of participants in US-based randomized controlled trials of mindfulness-based interventions. *Mindfulness, 9*(6), 1671–1692. https://doi.org/10.1007/s12671-018-0920-5

Walsh, R., & Shapiro, S. L. (2006). The meeting of meditative disciplines and Western psy-chology: A mutually enriching dialogue. *American Psychologist, 61*(3), 227–239. https://doi.org/10.1037/0003-066x.61.3.227

Watson-Singleton, N. N., Black, A. R., & Spivey, B. N. (2019). Recommendations for a culturally-responsive mindfulness-based intervention for African Americans. *Complementary Therapies in Clinical Practice, 34*, 132–138. https://doi.org/10.1016/j.ctcp.2018.11.013

Witkiewitz, K., Marlatt, G. A., & Walker, D. (2005). Mindfulness-based relapse prevention for alcohol and substance use disorders. *Journal of Cognitive Psychotherapy, 19*(3), 211–228. https://doi.org/10.1891/jcop.2005.19.3.211

Woods-Giscombe, C. L., Gaylord, S. A., Li, Y., Brintz, C. E., Bangdiwala, S. I., Buse, J. B., Mann, J. D., Lynch, C., Phillips, P., Smith, S., Leniek, K., Young, L., Al-Barwani, S., Yoo, J., & Faurot, K. (2019). A mixed-methods, randomized clinical trial to examine feasibility of a mindfulness-based stress management and diabetes risk reduction intervention for African Americans with prediabetes. *Evidence-Based Complementary and Alternative Medicine, 2019*, 3962623. https://doi.org/10.1155/2019/3962623

Journaling

KASEY R. BOEHMER

Journal writing is one of a group of therapies that provides an opportunity for individuals to reflect on and analyze their lives, the events and people surrounding them, and to get in touch with their feelings. It is a therapy that requires individuals to be engaged in reflecting on and gaining insights into their lives and experiences. While people have recorded the events of their lives from the beginning of history, first in pictures and then in words, journaling is perhaps best known contemporarily from Anne Frank's journal that detailed her life in hiding during World War II. Frank stated (1947/1994):

> *I want to go on living even after my death! And therefore I am grateful to God for this gift, this possibility of developing myself and of writing, of expressing all that is in me. I can shake off everything if I write; my sorrows disappear; my courage is reborn. (p. 177)*

More recently, scores of people have been using journaling to record memories of and cope with the COVID-19 pandemic (Phadke, 2020; Scimecca, 2021). Less commonly known, however, is that journaling has an evidence base and is utilized as a healthcare intervention across many conditions and contexts.

DEFINITION

The terms *journaling, diary, reflective writing, expressive writing,* and *therapeutic writing* are often used in the literature interchangeably; minor differences exist. Diaries more commonly focus on recording details of an event or tracking symptoms. The other terms instead typically refer to a tool for reflection. For the purposes of this chapter, we focus on these written reflective practices, which are referred to collectively as "journaling."

SCIENTIFIC BASIS

Journaling is a holistic therapy because it involves all aspects of a person–physical (muscular movements), mental (thought processes), emotional (getting in touch with or expressing feelings), and spiritual (finding meaning). Scholars have put forth multiple theoretical mechanisms by which journaling may produce beneficial outcomes. These include self-regulation theory, which purports that patients regulate their emotional and functional responses to stressful healthcare events (Johnson, 1999; Jones et al., 2016; Kim-Godwin et al., 2020); cognitive process theory, which focuses on constructing a written narrative to make sense of and share experiences (Flower & Hayes, 1981; Jones et al., 2016; Williams, 1984); and the cognitive theory of stress and coping, which explains the modes of problem-focused, emotion-focused, meaning-focused coping (Folkman, 1997; Kim-Godwin et al., 2020; Lazarus & Folkman, 1984; Whitney & Smith, 2015).

Two scientific premises advancing journaling as a healthcare intervention exist in the literature today: one grounded in traditional psychology that aims to prompt persons to reflect deeply on past upsetting experiences, traumas, and behaviors. These interventions are grounded in the seminal work of Pennebaker in the 1980s and 1990s (Pennebaker, 1993). More recently, a contemporary view of journaling interventions has emerged grounded in positive psychology (termed "positive journaling" in this chapter), where interventions are intentional activities aimed at improving perceived well-being through the cultivation of positive emotions (Sin & Lyubomirsky, 2009). These interventions focus on writing gratitude, positive thoughts, or turning negative experiences into positive situations through writing (Emmons & McCullough, 2003; Suhr et al., 2017). In both instances, the writing may be facilitated by a trained facilitator present during the writing process or conducted independently in privacy with verbal or written instructions provided prior to the writing process.

The traditional journaling paradigm is built on the idea that inhibiting emotional expression may result in increased stress that can be harmful to the body and disclosure of emotions can instead release tension to improve mental and physical health (Ullrich & Lutgendorf, 2002). In a review of three studies that had explored the efficacy of diary use by families of intensive care unit patients, Ullman et al. (2015) found that the experimental group using diaries had reduced posttraumatic stress symptomatology when compared with the control group, who did not use diaries, although the differences between the groups were small. Likewise, Sayer et al. (2015) reported beneficial effects of journaling on distress in a veterans' group. Emotional disclosure in an online journaling study found that mothers of children with autism manifesting behavior problems had reduced stress compared with the control group (Whitney & Smith, 2015). More recently, Nyssen et al. (2016) conducted a large systematic review of journaling in the context of chronic health conditions. Overall, the meta-analyses found little evidence of benefit in nonfacilitated journaling interventions across several long-term conditions, including HIV, breast cancer, and asthma, noting the only exception in inflammatory arthropathy (Nyssen et al., 2016). However, the authors commented that the majority of the interventions described in the reviewed literature did not reflect the way in which journaling was typically used clinically in the United Kingdom and that their findings were in contrast to benefits typically noted in the general population (Nyssen et al., 2016).

INTERVENTION

As illustrated in the scientific literature, there are a variety of ends to which journaling can be a useful means. To begin journaling, it is useful to first clarify an individual's purpose for journaling. Sometimes, people initially write during a stressful situation or transition in their lives but become comfortable journaling and continue writing after the initial event has ended. Questions to help clarify the best journaling strategy for individuals are shown in Exhibit 12.1. The optimal strategy may change over time through experimentation.

The length of time that journaling is carried out (weeks, months, years) depends on the specific purpose of the journaling. The time spent on daily journaling can vary, with some recommending sessions lasting at least 20 minutes (Pennebaker & Evans, 2014). However, journaling during short spurts of time such as during coffee breaks may be a feasible option.

After determining purpose, one must consider where to write journal entries. Entries can be made in a special notebook. However, some people who write about distressing topics may find this uncomfortable. For example, they may feel a requirement to preserve the writing if is written in a special notebook, even if they do not want to keep the writing. Therefore, in some cases, loose paper that can easily be destroyed or discarded is useful. Exploring what feels most comfortable for the individual is an important step to ensure journaling is not discontinued before an honest start. Should a person want to review their journal entries for self-reflection or legacy writing, a pen should be used. If a person is looking for a disposable option, pencils may be used.

Developments in technology have created many new avenues for journal writing. Some individuals may prefer using a computer to make entries. Using passwords helps ensure privacy. With the advent of tablets and smartphones, it is easy to make entries during short breaks. Some may wish to use blogs to share their reflections with others.

The physical location of the writing can be another important consideration. One should consider where they are most comfortable writing, and if there are any specific locations that trigger discomfort or writer's block. The optimal time for writing will vary between individuals and may also vary within the individual given varying seasons of life. For example, the retiree may find it suiting to start their early morning with journaling, whereas a sleep-deprived new parent may find squeezing in journaling at various downtimes throughout the week more appropriate. Early morning may be a good time to write when information in the unconscious seems closest to the surface, whereas journaling in the evening can resolve pent-up stress or troublesome events of the day.

TECHNIQUES

There are several different types of journaling, and each lends itself to specific goals. Over the course of treatment, individuals may use more than one type to accomplish what they need. Free-flow journaling, topical journaling, and creative writing are effective journaling techniques, and each has a different focus.

Exhibit 12.1 *Questions to Clarify Journaling Methods*

- What purpose is one hoping to fulfill through writing?
  - ○ Catharsis, emotional exploration, improved outlook, etc.
- What method is most appropriate for fulfilling this purpose?
  - ○ Special notebook, scrap paper, computer/tablet
- Where should the writing occur?
- When is the best time to write and for how long?
- Who can the writing be shared with if anyone?

Free-Flow Journaling

Free-flow journaling is the most common type of journaling. The main goal is to put thoughts and feelings on paper. Journaling provides a vehicle for uncovering the wisdom already possessed and the feelings that have been dormant. Sometimes a person writes multiple pages on one topic or event. At other times, the mind flits from topic to topic. The latter may happen when one is distressed and concentrating on one topic is difficult. There is no right or wrong way to journal. The main goal is to put words into written form and then reflect on them.

Topical Journaling

Topical journaling focuses on a specific event or situation. It is often used in groups in which a specific topic is given to the participants. For example, individuals may be asked to write about when they were confronted with a challenge and how they reacted. Patients or family members may be asked to write about the way that a new diagnosis is affecting them, concerns they may have, and their fears and feelings. Instructions may include specific questions to which the person is to respond. For example, in using journaling with people working on stress management, the following are a sampling of questions that could be posed:

- What situations do you notice trigger greater levels of stress?
- How do you know when you're in a high-stress state?
- Where do you hold stress in your physical body?
- What actions do you take when you are stressed?
- How do you currently handle stress?
- How would you like to handle stress in your future?

Creative Writing

Some people may be more comfortable writing in story or poetic form rather than focusing on specific events or emotions in their lives. This type of writing can assist individuals in uncovering deeper thoughts or emotions in a safe manner because a story may have characters saying things that individuals would feel uncomfortable attributing to themselves. Stories allow for feelings to be seen initially in the people in the story and then as they relate to oneself. Pictures may be used as an initiator of a story.

Poetic journaling is another form of creative writing that allows the writer to explore their feelings. Using short lines and spreading the content over a page make it easier to examine thoughts and emotions. Combining journaling and art is another form of creative writing. Several authors have described using scrapbooking and journaling for therapeutic purposes (Davidson & Robison, 2008; Subhani & Kanwal, 2012). Pictures or items used in creating the scrapbook served as the trigger for the journaling for the participants. Digital online pictures could be used for the journaling stimulus. Infinite possibilities exist and can be adapted to the preferences of the patient.

There are websites, apps, and paper-based journaling resources that can help novices begin journaling. Some of these are noted in Exhibit 12.2.

Exhibit 12.2 *Resources for Journaling*

Online/App-Based:
- Penzu (https://penzu.com)
- Reflectly (https://reflectly.app)
- Diaro (https://diaroapp.com)
- Day One (https://dayoneapp.com)
- Conversations Within: Journal Writing & Inner Dialog (www.journal-writing.com)

Paper-based:
- Expressive Writing: Words That Heal by James W. Pennebaker, PhD, and John F. Evans, EdD
- The High Performance Journal by Brendon Burchard, available on amazon.com
- Erin Condren Guided Journals, available at erincondren.com
- Be Unapologetically Who You Are Journal by Jessica Butts, available on amazon.com

---

MEASUREMENT OF OUTCOMES

Many outcomes from journal writing may not be immediately discernible. Possible patient-reported outcome measures include quality of life, illness intrusiveness, anxiety, depression, resilience, pain, and fatigue. Physiological measures such as the immune system, weight loss, and blood pressure have also been used to determine the efficacy of journaling. Unless patients share, nurses are not aware of the content or focus of the journaling. However, in the context of research, qualitative analyses can facilitate the in-depth review of journals kept by participants.

PRECAUTIONS

Fear that others will find and read journal entries is a common concern and may deter people from being open in expressing themselves in a journal. In these situations, as mentioned earlier, scrap paper may be a useful tool. Additional care should be taken for vulnerable populations, for whom a journal's confiscation could have further implications. These situations include, but are not limited to, journaling by incarcerated persons, children under state care, and adults living in elder care facilities. Furthermore, care needs to be taken if individuals appear to be extremely introspective or scrupulous because journaling may deepen this inward focus. In such cases, journaling under the supervision of a therapist as an adjunct to therapy may be more appropriate than unsupervised writing. When technology is used for journaling, passwords are recommended to protect privacy.

USES

Recent research has focused on for whom traditional journaling about traumatic experiences is most beneficial and whether positive journaling interventions are more beneficial than the traditional paradigm clinically. When exploring differences, Mordechay et al. (2019) found that participants with more symptoms of mental health problems experienced greater benefit from expressive writing. They also found that participants with high levels of experiential avoidance were more likely to benefit from expressive writing (Mordechay et al., 2019). It is possible that journaling served as a safe space or a prompted reason to confront normally suppressed emotions. Similar results were reported in another study where individuals with high levels of social inhibition experienced greater benefit from a positive journaling intervention, compared to those with low social inhibition (Allen et al., 2020). Finally, veterans with less complex psychosocial issues were the most likely to benefit from a stand-alone journaling intervention (Frankfurt et al., 2019).

Regarding positive journaling, numerous benefits have been reported, including improved gratitude scores and reduced inflammatory biomarkers in patients with asymptomatic heart failure (Redwine et al., 2016), improved gratitude and optimism amongst mothers of children with troubled lives (Kim-Godwin et al., 2020), and reduced anxiety among individuals with distressed personality type (Smith et al., 2018). Suhr et al. (2017) found positive journaling decreased depression scores and increased the use of reappraisal for emotional regulation in patients who had recently been discharged from psychiatric inpatient treatment. In the inpatient setting, Ducasse (2019) found that positive journaling in the hospital after a suicide attempt reduced patients' depression and anxiety and increased their optimism. As an adjunct to psychotherapy, positive journaling improved self-reported mental health compared to participants receiving psychotherapy alone or psychotherapy plus traditional journaling (Wong, 2018). Benefits of positive journaling appear to extend to healthcare workers as well. A onetime gratitude writing intervention decreased emotional exhaustion and improved perceived happiness and work–life balance among healthcare workers shortly after writing (Adair et al., 2020). This may be particularly useful in light of increasing evidence of burnout in healthcare workers (National Academies of Science, Engineering, and Medicine, 2019), as well as the distress caused by the COVID-19 pandemic.

Overall, these journaling interventions primarily examine short-term outcomes, leaving questions regarding any sustained benefit. It is unclear how long effects persist and what additional impact is incurred with long-term use. Exhibit 12.3 lists some of the situations in which journaling has been used.

Exhibit 12.3 *Uses of Journaling*

- Cope with cancer (Baggs et al., 2013; Chu et al., 2020; Milbury et al., 2014; Wu et al., 2021)
- Cope with posttraumatic stress (Blasio et al., 2015; Glass et al., 2019; Meshberg-Cohen et al., 2014; Sayer et al., 2015)
- Improve health-related quality of life with seizures (Rawlings et al., 2018)
- Decrease jail recidivism (Proctor et al., 2012)
- Cope with intensive care unit (Carley, 2012; Ullman et al., 2015)
- Manage caregiving stress (Butcher et al., 2016; Jones et al., 2016; Kim-Godwin et al., 2020; Toly et al., 2016; Whitney & Smith, 2015)
- Manage pain (Furnes & Dysvik, 2012; Pepe et al., 2014)
- Cope with palliative care (Penz & Duggleby, 2012)
- Manage substance abuse (Proctor et al., 2012; Young et al., 2013)
- Reduce inflammation and increase positive emotions in heart failure (Redwine et al., 2016)
- Improve mental health (Ducasse et al., 2019; Haertl & Ero-Phillips, 2019; Smith et al., 2018; Suhr et al., 2017; Wong et al., 2018)
- Decrease emotional exhaustion in healthcare workers (Adair et al., 2020)
- Cope with grief (Ennis & Cartagena, 2020)
- Cope with assisted reproductive treatment (Renzi et al., 2020)

CULTURAL APPLICATIONS

Although journaling is a therapy that many find helpful, others—particularly those from oral-based cultures—may find it daunting to reflect on their thoughts and experiences in writing. Painting and other forms of art may be alternative mechanisms that can be used to express feelings. The Hmong culture, an Asian ethnic group, has been an oral culture. The embroidered pieces of art created by Hmong women depict the history of the Hmong. This representational embroidery, or "story cloths," is used by members, especially women, to convey their experiences and history to future generations (Arkenberg, 2007). Journaling is commonly used in many cultures and nations. Sidebar 12.1 describes the consideration of the use of journaling in the Philippines.

Sidebar 12.1 *Reflective Journaling Writing in the Philippines*

Marlene Dohm and Leticia S. Lantican

Journal writing in the Philippines takes many forms as used in day-to-day living, educational settings, and therapeutic environments. In any situation, journaling becomes a way used to express thoughts, feelings, and insights. It gives a person a chance to reflect on life events and experiences and give meaning to them.

Before presenting the use of free-flowing journaling by a Filipino man who was diagnosed with cancer, the following statements describe several values, beliefs, and traditions that I believe, as a Filipino myself, are common among Filipinos; these may impact the use of journaling by Filipinos:

- Most Filipinos are modest and nonverbal when it comes to personal matters. Putting things in writing, as in journaling, works best for those who can express their sentiments in writing better than verbalizing them. Many prefer silence, which should be respected in relating with them.
- Many Filipinos are raised as Roman Catholics and have a strong faith in God. They feel strongly supported by the spirituality of their family, friends, church, and the community.
- Acceptance of a diagnosis and prognosis again is centered on a person's strength derived from faith and support from the family, which includes not only the nuclear family but also the extended family, consisting of brothers, sisters, aunts, uncles, and grandparents.

The following details the use of journaling by Mark (not actual name to protect privacy), a man and animation artist who was born and raised in the Philippines. Mark was diagnosed at age 45 with an autoimmune disease that was in an advanced stage. He underwent almost a year of treatment consisting of intensive chemotherapy and bone marrow transplant. During the many times he waited at his clinic visits and during infusion times when he was having chemotherapy treatments that sometimes lasted 8 hours, Mark found time to do free-flow journaling using his tablet. He wrote on a variety of topics such as

Sidebar 12.1 *Reflective Journaling Writing in the Philippines (continued)*

his experiences with treatment and perspectives on life, often punctuated with spiritual and religious themes. He provided periodic/monthly updates throughout his entire treatment duration to his family and close relatives through email. Most emails provided written expressions of his emotions, attitudes, and ways of coping with his treatment and its side effects. Often, these expressive writings reflected his strong faith in God and gratitude for family support and prayers. Even when he seemed to be in remission, Mark continued to engage in reflective writing while riding on a train. An example of his free-flowing journaling follows:

> One thing about being confined in a cancer treatment center (with other patients) is that your range of emotions can run the entire spectrum. Seeing so many people fight the same battle made me feel I am not alone. However, more often than not, I was constantly reminded of one's mortality. I remember weeks prior to my transplant, I was told, due to the high dose chemo, there's a chance I might not make it. I have to admit, that information shook me a bit. It was circling around my head for days. I was restless to say the least.
>
> After a while, I was able to psyche myself up, that ultimately, I am going in that direction anyway. After all, my life is simply borrowed and not mine to keep. And then that started a slew of other questions. Knowing that my life is simply a borrowed one, why would I want an extension? Do I want to earn more money? Do I still want to see the rest of the world?
>
> Do I hunger for more achievements?
>
> As I thought about the answers to these questions, I realized, I've been so blessed to have the career that I have, the same career that allowed me to see the world, a career that allowed me to live comfortably. But most importantly, it's this same career that led me to meeting that very significant person in my life—my dear wife. I had a good run. I couldn't ask for anything more. I have more blessing than I could possibly count.

Mark found journaling to be helpful not only for himself personally but also for his family members.

FUTURE RESEARCH

While the efficacy of journaling in the general population has a considerable evidence base, its use in healthcare settings has historically been limited. However, research on the topic has increased in the past decade. Some of the areas in which research is still needed include the following:

- *Technology-facilitated journaling:* Technology offers numerous possibilities for new avenues for journaling. Few studies have explored the use of technology as a means for journaling. Investigations in this arena are particularly needed with younger populations.

■ *Journaling strategies for vulnerable populations:* Ethical and legal implications for journaling require study and need to be resolved, especially for vulnerable populations. Fears about their journals being "used against them" may inhibit people from being honest. Alternative formats may need to be explored to benefit these populations.

■ *Populations for which journaling is most useful and why:* Research that examines for whom journaling is most beneficial is underway and should continue. Most of this research is being conducted using quantitative analyses alone. However, there are opportunities for mixed methods research on this topic that would add much-needed nuance to this literature.

■ *Positive journaling versus traditional journaling:* The regular use of journaling as a positive psychology intervention in research is relatively new. This promising area of scientific work requires attention to understand which intervention is most efficacious across a variety of conditions and healthcare settings.

■ *Longer term interventions and outcome measurement:* Few studies examined long-term outcomes for short journaling interventions used clinically, nor examined the use of journaling interventions for more than 6 weeks. Both longer term interventions and outcomes should be explored, and fidelity monitoring of the intervention should be a core component of the research plan.

REFERENCES

Adair, K. C., Rodriguez-Homs, L. G., Masoud, S., Mosca, P. J., & Sexton, J. B. (2020). Gratitude at work: Prospective cohort study of a web-based, single-exposure well-being intervention for health care workers. *Journal of Medical Internet Research, 22*(5), e15562. https://doi.org/10.2196/15562

Allen, S. F., Wetherell, M. A., & Smith, M. A. (2020). Online writing about positive life experiences reduces depression and perceived stress reactivity in socially inhibited individuals. *Psychiatry Research, 284,* 112697. https://doi.org/10.1016/j.psychres.2019.112697

Arkenberg, R. (2007). Hmong story cloths. *SchoolArts: The Art Education Magazine for Teachers, 107*(2), 32–33. https://eric.ed.gov/?id=EJ776244

Baggs, C., McKhann, L., Gessert, C. E., & Johnson, B. P. (2013). Healing through reflective writing: Breast cancer survivors' experience. *Minnesota Medicine, 96*(7), 45–47. https://www.ncbi.nlm.nih.gov/pubmed/24133890

Blasio, P. D., Camisasca, E., Caravita, S. C., Ionio, C., Milani, L., & Valtolina, G. G. (2015). The effects of expressive writing on postpartum depression and posttraumatic stress symptoms. *Psychological Reports, 117*(3), 856–882. https://doi.org/10.2466/02.13.PR0.117c29z3

Butcher, H. K., Gordon, J. K., Ko, J. W., Perkhounkova, Y., Cho, J. Y., Rinner, A., & Lutgendorf, S. (2016). Finding meaning in written emotional expression by family caregivers of persons with dementia. *American Journal of Alzheimer's Disorders and Other Dementias, 31*(8), 631–642. https://doi.org/10.1177/1533317516660611

Carley, A. (2012). Can journaling provide support for NICU families? *Journal for Specialists in Pediatric Nursing, 17*(3), 254–257. https://doi.org/10.1111/j.1744-6155.2012.00336.x

Chu, Q., Wu, I. H. C., & Lu, Q. (2020). Expressive writing intervention for posttraumatic stress disorder among Chinese American breast cancer survivors: The moderating role of social constraints. *Quality of Life Research, 29*(4), 891–899. https://doi.org/10.1007/s11136-019-02385-5

Davidson, J. U., & Robison, B. (2008). Scrapbooking and journaling interventions for chronic illness: A triangulated investigation of approaches in the treatment of PTSD. *Kansas Nurse, 83*(3), 6–11. https://www.ncbi.nlm.nih.gov/pubmed/18524339

Ducasse, D., Dassa, D., Courtet, P., Brand-Arpon, V., Walter, A., Guillaume, S., Jaussent, I., & Olié, E. (2019). Gratitude diary for the management of suicidal inpatients: A randomized controlled trial. *Depression and Anxiety, 36*(5), 400–411. https://doi.org/10.1002/da.22877

Emmons, R. A., & McCullough, M. E. (2003). Counting blessings versus burdens: An experimental investigation of gratitude and subjective well-being in daily life. *Journal of Personality and Social Psychology, 84*(2), 377–389. https://doi.org/10.1037//0022-3514.84.2.377

Ennis, N., & Cartagena, G. (2020). Therapeutic writing as a tool to facilitate therapeutic process in the context of living with HIV: A case study examining partner loss. *Psychotherapy (Chic), 57*(1), 68–74. https://doi.org/10.1037/pst0000259

Flower, L., & Hayes, J. R. (1981). A cognitive process theory of writing. *College Composition and Communication, 32*(4), 365–387. https://doi.org/10.1002/da.22877

Folkman, S. (1997). Positive psychological states and coping with severe stress. *Social Science & Medicine, 45*(8), 1207–1221. https://doi.org/10.1016/S0277-9536(97)00040-3

Frank, A. (1947/1994). *Diary of a young girl.* Random House.

Frankfurt, S., Frazier, P., Litz, B. T., Schnurr, P. P., Orazem, R. J., Gravely, A., & Sayer, N. (2019). Online expressive writing intervention for reintegration difficulties among veterans: Who is most likely to benefit? *Psychological Trauma, 11*(8), 861–868. https://doi.org/10.1037/tra0000462

Furnes, B., & Dysvik, E. (2012). Therapeutic writing and chronic pain: Experiences of therapeutic writing in a cognitive behavioural programme for people with chronic pain. *Journal of Clinical Nursing, 21*(23–24), 3372–3381. https://doi.org/10.1111/j.1365-2702.2012.04268.x

Glass, O., Dreusicke, M., Evans, J., Bechard, E., & Wolever, R. Q. (2019). Expressive writing to improve resilience to trauma: A clinical feasibility trial. *Complementary Therapies in Clinical Practice, 34*, 240–246. https://doi.org/10.1016/j.ctcp.2018.12.005

Haertl, K. L., & Ero-Phillips, A. M. (2019). The healing properties of writing for persons with mental health conditions. *Arts & Health, 11*(1), 15–25. https://doi.org/10.1080/17533015.2017.1413400

Johnson, J. E. (1999). Self-regulation theory and coping with physical illness. *Research in Nursing & Health, 22*(6), 435–448. https://doi.org/10.1002/(SICI)1098-240X(199912)22:63.0.CO;2-Q

Jones, C. J., Hayward, M., Brown, A., Clark, E., Bird, D., Harwood, G., Scott, C., Hillemann, A., & Smith, H. E. (2016). Feasibility and participant experiences of a written emotional disclosure intervention for parental caregivers of people with psychosis. *Stress and Health, 32*(5), 485–493. https://doi.org/10.1002/smi.2644

Kim-Godwin, Y. S., Kim, S. S., & Gil, M. (2020). Journaling for self-care and coping in mothers of troubled children in the community. *Archives of Psychiatric Nursing, 34*(2), 50–57. https://doi.org/10.1016/j.apnu.2020.02.005

Lazarus, R. S., & Folkman, S. (1984). *Stress, appraisal, and coping.* Springer Publishing Company.

Meshberg-Cohen, S., Svikis, D., & McMahon, T. J. (2014). Expressive writing as a therapeutic process for drug-dependent women. *Substance Abuse, 35*(1), 80–88. https://doi.org/10.1080/08897077.2013.805181

Milbury, K., Spelman, A., Wood, C., Matin, S. F., Tannir, N., Jonasch, E., Pisters, L., Wei, Q., & Cohen, L. (2014). Randomized controlled trial of expressive writing for patients with renal cell carcinoma. *Journal of Clinical Oncology, 32*(7), 663–670. https://doi.org/10.1200/JCO.2013.50.3532

Mordechay, D. S., Nir, B., & Eviatar, Z. (2019). Expressive writing-Who is it good for? Individual differences in the improvement of mental health resulting from expressive writing. *Complementary Therapies in Clinical Practice, 37*, 115–121. https://doi.org/10.1016/j.ctcp.2019.101064

National Academies of Sciences, Engineering, and Medicine. (2019). *Taking action against clinician burnout: A system approach to professional well-being.* Naitonal Academies Press.

Nyssen, O. P., Taylor, S. J., Wong, G., Steed, E., Bourke, L., Lord, J., Ross, C. A., Hayman, S., Field, V., Higgins, A., Greenhalgh, T., & Meads, C. (2016). Does therapeutic writing help people with long-term conditions? Systematic review, realist synthesis and economic considerations. *Health Technology Assessment, 20*(27), vii–xxxvii, 1–367. https://doi.org/10.3310/hta20270

Pennebaker, J. W. (1993). Putting stress into words: Health, linguistic, and therapeutic implications. *Behaviour Research and Therapy, 31*(6), 539–548. https://doi.org/10.1016/0005-7967(93)90105-4

Pennebaker, J. W., & Evans, J. F. (2014). *Expressive writing: Words that heal: Using expressive writing to overcome traumas and emotional upheavals, resolve issues, improve health, and build resilience.* Idyll Arbor, Incorporated.

Penz, K., & Duggleby, W. (2012). "It's different in the home . . ." The contextual challenges and rewards of providing palliative nursing care in community settings. *Journal of Hospice & Palliative Nursing, 14*(5), 365–373. https://doi.org/10.1097/NJH.0b013e3182553acb

Pepe, L., Milani, R., Di Trani, M., Di Folco, G., Lanna, V., & Solano, L. (2014). A more global approach to musculoskeletal pain: Expressive writing as an effective adjunct to physiotherapy. *Psychology, Health & Medicine, 19*(6), 687–697. https://doi.org/10.1080/13548506.2013.859712

Phadke, M. (2020). *When nothing makes sense, I journal. I'm not the only one.* Vox. https://www.vox .com/the-goods/21542132/journaling-bullet-journal-coronavirus-pandemic

Proctor, S. L., Hoffmann, N. G., & Allison, S. (2012). The effectiveness of interactive journaling in reducing recidivism among substance-dependent jail inmates. *International Journal of Offender Therapy and Comparative Criminology, 56*(2), 317–332. https://doi.org/10.1177/0306624X11399274

Rawlings, G. H., Brown, I., Stone, B., & Reuber, M. (2018). A pilot randomised controlled trial of a home-based writing intervention for individuals with seizures. *Psychology & Health, 33*(9), 1151–1171. https://doi.org/10.1080/08870446.2018.1478974

Redwine, L. S., Henry, B. L., Pung, M. A., Wilson, K., Chinh, K., Knight, B., Jain, S., Rutledge, T., Greenberg, B., Maisel, A., & Mills, P. J. (2016). Pilot randomized study of a gratitude journaling intervention on heart rate variability and inflammatory biomarkers in patients with stage B heart failure. *Psychosomatic Medicine, 78*(6), 667–676. https://doi.org/10.1097/PSY.0000000000000316

Renzi, A., Solano, L., Di Trani, M., Ginobbi, F., Minutolo, E., & Tambelli, R. (2020). The effects of an expressive writing intervention on pregnancy rates, alexithymia and psychophysical health during an assisted reproductive treatment. *Psychology & Health, 35*(6), 718–733. https://doi .org/10.1080/08870446.2019.1667500

Sayer, N. A., Noorbaloochi, S., Frazier, P. A., Pennebaker, J. W., Orazem, R. J., Schnurr, P. P., Murdoch, M., Carlson, K. F., Gravely, A., & Litz, B. T. (2015). Randomized controlled trial of online expressive writing to address readjustment difficulties among U.S. Afghanistan and Iraq war veterans. *Journal of Traumatic Stress, 28*(5), 381–390. https://doi.org/10.1002/jts.22047

Scimecca, A. (2021). How journaling together helped this photo duo make sense of the COVID-19 pandemic. *Fortune.* https://fortune.com/2021/03/09/covid-photos-photographers-shaughn -and-john-coronavirus-pictures-photography-stay-home-the-covid-journal/

Sin, N. L., & Lyubomirsky, S. (2009). Enhancing well-being and alleviating depressive symptoms with positive psychology interventions: A practice-friendly meta-analysis. *Journal of Clinical Psychology, 65*(5), 467–487. https://doi.org/10.1002/jclp.20593

Smith, M. A., Thompson, A., Hall, L. J., Allen, S. F., & Wetherell, M. A. (2018). The physical and psychological health benefits of positive emotional writing: Investigating the moderating role of Type D (distressed) personality. *British Journal of Health Psychology, 23*(4), 857–871. https://doi.org/10.1111/bjhp.12320

Subhani, M. T., & Kanwal, I. (2012). Digital scrapbooking as a standard of care in neonatal intensive care units: Initial experience. *Neonatal Network, 31*(3), 162–168. https://doi .org/10.1891/0730-0832.31.3.162

Suhr, M., Risch, A. K., & Wilz, G. (2017). Maintaining mental health through positive writing: Effects of a resource diary on depression and emotion regulation. *Journal of Clinical Psychology, 73*(12), 1586–1598. https://doi.org/10.1002/jclp.22463

Toly, V. B., Blanchette, J. E., Musil, C. M., & Zauszniewski, J. A. (2016). Journaling as reinforcement for the resourcefulness training intervention in mothers of technology-dependent children. *Applied Nursing Research, 32*, 269–274. https://doi.org/10.1016/j.apnr.2016.08.005

Ullman, A. J., Aitken, L. M., Rattray, J., Kenardy, J., Le Brocque, R., MacGillivray, S., & Hull, A. M. (2015). Intensive care diaries to promote recovery for patients and families after critical illness: A Cochrane Systematic Review. *International Journal of Nursing Studies, 52*(7), 1243–1253. https://doi.org/10.1016/j.ijnurstu.2015.03.020

Ullrich, P. M., & Lutgendorf, S. K. (2002). Journaling about stressful events: Effects of cognitive processing and emotional expression. *Annals of Behavioral Medicine, 24*(3), 244–250. https://doi.org/10.1207/S15324796ABM2403_10

Whitney, R. V., & Smith, G. (2015). Emotional disclosure through journal writing: Telehealth intervention for maternal stress and mother-child relationships. *Journal of Autism and Developmental Disorders, 45*(11), 3735–3745. https://doi.org/10.1007/s10803-014-2332-2

Williams, G. (1984). The genesis of chronic illness: Narrative re-construction. *Sociology of Health & Illness, 6*(2), 175–200. https://doi.org/10.1111/1467-9566.ep10778250

Wong, Y. J., Owen, J., Gabana, N. T., Brown, J. W., McInnis, S., Toth, P., & Gilman, L. (2018). Does gratitude writing improve the mental health of psychotherapy clients? Evidence from a randomized controlled trial. *Psychotherapy Research, 28*(2), 192–202. https://doi.org/10.1080/10503307.2016.1169332

Wu, Y., Liu, L., Zheng, W., Zheng, C., Xu, M., Chen, X., Li, W., Xie, L., Zhang, P., Zhu, X., Zhan, C., & Zhou, C. (2021). Effect of prolonged expressive writing on health outcomes in breast cancer patients receiving chemotherapy: A multicenter randomized controlled trial. *Supportive Care in Cancer, 29*(2), 1091–1101. https://doi.org/10.1007/s00520-020-05590-y

Young, C. M., Rodriguez, L. M., & Neighbors, C. (2013). Expressive writing as a brief intervention for reducing drinking intentions. *Addictive Behaviors, 38*(12), 2913–2917. https://doi.org/10.1016/j.addbeh.2013.08.025

13

Storytelling

MARGARET P. MOSS

The art and science of storytelling are presented in this chapter as a mechanism that can be used in alternative or complementary therapy. Its historical roots in orality (also known as oralism) are defined and explicated through examples from primary oral cultures. These are cultures that do not have a written language system (Sampson, 1980). In direct contrast, taking the art form into the future, digital storytelling is explored. However, in another unexpected twist, orality, oral instruction, and knowledge keepers as the trusted messengers proved not only of interest but also a necessity during a global pandemic in the 21st century for Indigenous health. In this case, innovation is actually stepping back to in-person delivery from orator to receiver for necessary information. Additionally, in this chapter, storytelling is connected to its use as an alternative method in which to affect the path of one's health in terms of education, prevention, and intervention. Finally, recommendations for future research are offered.

DEFINITIONS

ORALITY

"The narratives we live and share everyday are our identity as a storied people and make visible what matters most in our lives" (Heliker, 2007, p. 21). Although there are approximately 3,000 languages in existence today, only 106 have ever been written and less than one half of those are said to have literature (Edmondson, 1971). *Orality* is defined as a mostly verbal communication system employed by whole cultures and devoid of the conventions or use of the written word (Olson & Torrance, 1991). The connection of orality or oralism to storytelling is intuitive. Storytelling is as universal in human communication as "the basic orality of language is permanent" (Ong, 2002, p. 7).

Literate societies evolved from oral societies. Each literate individual evolved from an oral beginning (Olson & Torrance, 1991). That is not to say that the formal and informal rules of orality are not as intricate as those in written communication. However, the vast majority of languages have never been translated into a written language (Edmondson, 1971).

The speaker, the process, and the aesthetics of orality are keys to imparting information (Lord, 1960). The rules concerning who speaks and when are defined by the culture. For instance, in some American Indian tribes, certain stories can only be told in the winter, others in the summer. Some words are not to be spoken at certain times of the day or to certain listeners. The process may be as in a prayer, a dance, or a story and can be in front of a large audience or one on one. Aesthetics may involve the use of masks, rattles, costumes, or specific surroundings. Finally, orality uses postural and gestural tools, as well as silence, as paralinguistic features in the transmission of communication (Tedlock, 1983). "Formulaicness is valued when wisdom is seen as knowledge passed down through generations. Novelty is valued when wisdom is viewed as new information" (Tannen, 1982, p. 6). Therefore, anyone wishing to impart information through purposive oral means, such as through storytelling, needs to understand the key components, rules, and assigned power of oralism.

STORYTELLING

Storytelling is defined as the art or act of telling stories (Dictionary.com, 2021b). A story is "a narrative, either true or fictitious, in prose or verse, designed to interest, amuse, or instruct the hearer or reader; [a] tale." (Dictionary.com, 2021a). Sociolinguist William Labov (as cited in Sandelowski, 1994) states that a complete story typically is composed of the following:

- **abstract:** what the story is about
- **orientation:** the "who, when, where, and what" of the story
- **complicating action:** the "then-what-happened" part of the story
- **evaluation:** the "so-what" of the story
- **resolution:** the "what-finally-happened" portion of the story
- **coda:** the signal a story is over
- return to the present (Sandelowski, 1994, p. 25)

It is the instructive nature of storytelling that is of interest for healthcare as an alternative means to an outcome: improved health. But it must also be understood that lives, including our health, are "shaped by the stories we live" (Heliker, 2007, p. 21). Stories have shaped patients' current selves, and it is through stories that nurses can "interest, amuse, or instruct" them as listeners. Storytelling has paralleled human endeavors and will continue to evolve through future mechanisms.

DIGITAL STORYTELLING

Digital storytelling is "the modern expression of the ancient art of storytelling. Digital stories derive their power by weaving images, music, narrative, and voice together, thereby giving deep dimension and vivid color to characters, situations, experiences, and insights" (Rule, 2011).

Although technology in digital storytelling provides the processes and aesthetics, it can also present some difficulties. For those cultures with restrictions on word use, the 24-hour, 365-day availability of words via computer technology brings uncertainty. Matching the listener and the teller and their implicit contract are of utmost importance when choosing the type of conveyance.

Storytelling, whether traditional or digital, whether oral or written, serves multiple purposes across the life span and can be used by nurses. Nurses listen to stories whenever patients tell them what is going on in their lives, and they tell and retell stories every time they pass on information about patients (Fairbairn & Carson, 2002). Whether it is the person being cared for or the nurse, each individual telling the story "is" the story being told (Sandelowski, 1994). It is in the unfolding, intertwining, and connecting that a story becomes my story, your story, or our story. Stories are woven into the threads of life's fabric in our daily lives (Barton, 2004). We are all connected on a deeper or—if you prefer—higher level and storytelling can take us to these levels.

SCIENTIFIC BASIS

Storytelling "is one of the world's most powerful tools for achieving astonishing results" in almost any industry (Guber, 2007, p. 55). Through an implicit contract between the storyteller and the listener (Guber, 2007), time is always a necessary ingredient. The storyteller must take the time to fully tell a story through all of its parts, using the necessary gestures, processes, and aesthetics. A story, as a sequence of events with discernible relations between those events and culminating in some conclusion, is a cognitive package (Bergner, 2007) that can be given to the listener. The listener must make time available to be present within the story to *hear* the message and absorb it. A successful transmission will allow the listener to repeat the story to others in some form. Repetition, of course, leads to stronger transmission on both sides.

Effective storytellers understand their listener(s) and what they already know, what they care about, and what they want to hear (Guber, 2007). The great storyteller will guide the story through essential elements based on the listener's understanding that the story is larger than the teller (Guber, 2007).

LANGUAGE AND HEALING BEYOND HEALTH LITERACY

"One of the few universals is that humans in all known cultures use language and tell stories" (Ramirez-Esparza & Pennebaker, 2006, p. 216). Storytelling without language is not possible. "Language embodies cultural reality" (Kramsch, 1998, p. 3). Language *itself* and healing may have a connection not yet fully explored or understood, beyond health literacy bounds. Most of the literature involving language and health surround the idea of health literacy, which has been defined as "the degree to which individuals have the capacity to obtain, process, and understand basic health information and services needed to make appropriate health decisions" (Nielsen-Bohlman et al., 2004, p. 4). Although evidence points to greater understanding of health services and all that entails when spoken in the receiver's primary language (Koh et al., 2012), language as a healing tool and force are offered for consideration in this section.

In many Indigenous cultures, for example, medicine and religion lines blur (Moss, 2000). Healing prayers are taken as a means toward optimum health whether in the physical, mental, spiritual, or emotional domain (Moss, 2000). These prayers are likely conducted in the traditional language. A study from South Africa offers that "language creates an image of the unknown to which people attach meaning" (Lourens, 2013, abstract). There is comfort in hearing one's own language. It takes away a struggle and the required energy needed to accept either information or prayer, presumably then allowing more energy to be used for healing.

Whereas Indigenous examples of language use in prayer and healing may be specifically seen as other examples, the dominant cultures also use language in healing and prayer beyond their use as delivery of information only. We see this in the change in tone, speed, earnestness, and length of delivery that exceeds any aesthetic needed to merely deliver information. This can be from a mother to a sick child, a prayer group to a member, or other cultural convention or relationship.

AMERICAN INDIAN EXEMPLAR

The Zuni Indians of New Mexico use storytelling through all parts of their lives. It is used casually and formally. It is used in secular and sacred telling. The teller can be a priest, a *kiva* group, a grandmother, or another person. A *kiva* is a "medicine (i.e., priestly) society" to which men are initiated as youths and remain to carry out the work of the *kiva* (Moss, 2000). The purpose of the dances they perform can be solely to heal listeners from sickness. Through word of mouth, the news may spread that a Rain Dance is called. Unlike what Hollywood portrays, this dance calls listeners to one of the small plazas (flat dirt squares) in the village where they can receive needed healing prayers.

Time is part of the contract. The listener arrives at a loosely determined time and waits. The dancers and the lead teller arrive some time later. The teller knows why the listeners are there: The contract is intact. There is respectful listening and targeted telling. The telling is in the form of prayer, song, and dance. The team is in full regalia, with masks and dress from centuries of performances. A formula is employed in the telling. It can take hours. The teller or tellers, the process, and the aesthetics all come together in dance, silence, and singing to heal the listener.

LANGUAGE REVITALIZATION

So far, this chapter has explored present-day oral languages, written languages, and the use of digital "telling." Each of these modalities will have pros and cons to their uses in storytelling. Oral languages represent millennia of information passed down faithfully from one generation to another. Some members' main roles in society are to "remember" and "store" this information. However, there may be discrepancies over the years in which key pieces of important stories may be lost, much like happens in the "telephone game." The addition of processes and aestheics seeks to temper those losses.

Equally important are the issues with written languages (whether scribed or digital). In this mode, there is a reliance on a place (book, computer drive) rather than a person or persons storing and transmitting language/stories. Although, likely as correct as the author would like at the time it is stored, if the place is destroyed, with no person/organic backup, huge amounts of information will be forever lost.

The digital age is largely described as proliferating anywhere from the 1970s or 1980s and continuing through to the present. Written language is acknowledged from about 3500 to 3000 BC, originating in southern Mesopotamia (Mark, 2011). A best guess on the origin of oralism, that is, language use as a modality of information transmission, is around 100,000 years ago (Bolhuis et al., 2014).

What hasn't been discussed is the loss of language and the need for revitalization of same, especially those languages that were forced out of existence rather than fading naturally. Examples of this can be seen especially throughout the *settler states* of the United States, Canada, Australia, and New Zealand. Similar histories "hurried" Indigenous languages to extinction or near extinction and, with it, the loss of stories so vital to the societies, including their health.

In the United States, the passage of the Native American Languages Act of 1990 was an effort to begin attempts to retain and revitalize language among Indigenous communities (Whalen et al., 2016). Little progress has been made, and these languages are still rapidly losing speakers and the knowledge residing in their languages (Whalen et al., 2016). Some of this knowledge contains healing aspects, whether the words themselves, medicines, or therapies specific to the language and its use.

INTERVENTION

Bergner (2007) writes about the "staying power of stories," which has obvious benefits when delivering therapeutic messages. He tells of stories that patients have recounted as far back as 8 years earlier.

TECHNIQUE

Stories in therapy draw from the general culture of the patient, integrate common knowledge sequences, and therefore do not require the acquisition of new knowledge to participate (Bergner, 2007). Code words can then be used to recall the entire story for the patient at later dates. Stories can be targeted to specific diagnoses in increasing meaning for the patient. This allows taking away aspects that do not apply and bringing in aspects that may be unique to the patient.

GUIDELINES

The following guideline sequence has been presented in the literature for storytelling in therapy: Present the story, elaborate as needed to increase understanding, and then discuss application to this particular patient situation (Bergner, 2007). In some cultures, there are situations in which reality can be "spoken into being." Again, often these are strongest in oral cultures. However, even in the dominant culture in the United States, people will shush a person if they speak about death, cancer, or some bad thing happening.

In primarily oral cultures, such as traditional Indigenous societies, it would be difficult to explain advance directives or informed consent in the manner in which they are presented in Western medical facilities. This applies whether when caring for a patient or when conducting research. As an example, it might be the task of a healthcare provider to tell a traditional American Indian older adult from the Southwest that this individual could die, lose a leg, or get an infection if the suggested traditional treatments were completed. The patient would perceive harm in even hearing this message. The patient certainly would not want to review or sign a consent form that contained these facts. In this case, one would be wise to use a hypothetical story instead. The harm would be taken away from the patient, and instead, the teller would describe to the listener facts about "another" person in a similar situation, drawing from cultural norms and common knowledge and asking the listener whether the hypothetical person would be willing to go through the procedure.

Using the preceding guidelines, there would be elaboration as needed in a context familiar to the patient. For instance, one might describe the following:

> Mr. Vigil was an older Pueblo man who had diabetes. He had it for 20 years and lived fairly comfortably with his family on the pueblo and saw his doctor regularly. There came a time when Mr. Vigil's leg began to bother him more and more. He tried several things with his doctor to increase blood flow and promote nerve health. Even though he did what he could for his health, it became apparent that he might have to lose the leg to continue living and being with his family. The doctor told him that he would still be able to participate in ceremonies and get around after the surgery with the use of a prosthetic leg and physical therapy. Mr. Vigil was worried. What do you think he was worried about? What do you think he might have decided? What questions would you ask if you were Mr. Vigil?

The use of vignettes such as the preceding one has been introduced in research as well as in practice.

When using stories as an intervention, one should use the ideas of orality, where repetition, setting, aesthetics, and process are important in the transmission of information. Implementing these will assist the listener in retaining the information.

SUGGESTIONS FOR IMPLEMENTING STORYTELLING

Suggestions for healthcare practitioners, educators, or researchers contemplating using storytelling include the following:

- Learn the difference between orality and literacy:
  - It is much more than one group reads and the other writes.
  - A whole system of rules for use of each exists.
  - Each uses differing paths to arrive at the desired outcomes.
  - Orality and literacy may be used separately or together.
  - Understand the parts and mechanisms for telling the story
  - The right person tells the right patient the right set of facts at the right time, in the right way, and in the right place.

- Understand differences in response to storytelling by age and culture:
  - Younger *and* older patients may be more attuned to traditional, oral, face-to-face storytelling.
  - The teenage through middle adult patient may be more open and attuned to digital storytelling techniques.
  - Using vignettes and anecdotes in the third person takes the pressure off the listener.

- Use technology as appropriate:
  - Certain cultures may not access the computer for fear of encountering a word deemed inappropriate at certain times or to certain people.
  - Interactive media can be used with almost all persons *if geared specifically to their age, culture, and level of technological proficiency.*

MEASUREMENT OF OUTCOMES

A variety of tools can be used to measure the outcomes of storytelling. Depending on the purpose for which storytelling is being used, instruments that measure anxiety, depression, social isolation, spirituality, caring, and sense of well-being may be appropriate. Qualitative research methods may also be used to measure the effectiveness or changes brought about through storytelling, including an increased understanding of the information.

PRECAUTIONS

Those using storytelling need to be prepared to deal with the strong emotions stories may evoke. Health professionals should be ready to assist and support the participants, as diverse reactions can occur. A list of available resources for making referrals for follow-up will be helpful. Only persons trained in psychotherapy should use storytelling with people who have psychological problems. The health sciences represent disciplines that attempt to understand humans from their various perspectives and philosophies, but these disciplines have grown so specialized in their jargon that the message to the patient may easily be lost (Evans, 2007). The use of storytelling in common vernacular can be an antidote to this loss of message.

USES

The use of storytelling in healthcare settings, healthcare research, and teaching is unlimited. This section will share some examples of the use of orality in general and storytelling specifically. Nurses can use storytelling in multiple situations across the life span for a variety of purposes. Stories can be used in family therapy and can assist members in tapping into the flow of meaning of the past, present, and future, and help patients open up possibilities for "making meaning" and healing (Roberts, 1994).

Another aspect of using storytelling is when the *teller* of the story is the one to benefit from it. In Ramirez-Esparza and Pennebaker's (2006) article "Do Good Stories Produce Good Health?" evidence for a link between expressive writing (storytelling) and markers for both mental and physical health are described. The stories do not even have to be coherent but just the ability of the person to express his or her story is beneficial (Ramirez-Esparza & Pennebaker, 2006). Analysis of the story down to which type of pronoun is used (i.e., first person or not) can point to health indicators around depression, for example (Ramirez-Esparza & Pennebaker, 2006).

This use and resulting phenomena have been seen in digital storytelling as well. The *teller* of the story receives a feeling of greater well-being or other health-related benefits. Sharing experiences, lightening a burden, and helping others allowed participants to report feeling better (www.patientvoices.org.uk; Haigh & Hardy, 2011).

ORALITY IN A GLOBAL PANDEMIC

In March 2020, much of the world came to a halt surrounded by a health emergency and utter uncertainty. COVID-19 had descended globally eventually touching all corners of the world, all populations in the United States, rural, urban, and reservation alike. Black and Brown populations were deemed most at risk for infection and for having bad outcomes with an increased risk of death (IDSA, 2020). At additional risk were those of advanced age, or with underlying conditions such as diabetes, chronic obstructive pulmonary disease, or asthma and those who were immunocompromised. Therefore, for many Black Americans, Latinx, and American Indians, they could be in double and triple jeopardy when facing this disease. Many were older and had compromised health in addition to not enjoying the same privileges and equities of many in the dominant culture. Causal issues included

- higher rates of pre-existing, underlying health conditions,
- lack of environmental and public health infrastructure,
- disproportionate impact of structural racism and socioeconomic factors, and
- limited and poor accessibility to healthcare. (IDSA, 2020, para. 6)

Although these are shared factors across minority populations, one group was hit particularly hard—America's Indigenous population.

Point 1: The Problem

American Indians and Alaska Natives (AIAN) make up less than 3% of the U.S. population (Jones et al., 2021). But it is not small population presence alone that allows others to be ignorant of the inequities put upon them. It has been by design over hundreds of years with the reservation, assimilation, termination, and other federal Indian policies either pushing them out of the way or forcing assimilation. Therefore, non-Indigenous people, including healthcare professionals and acade-micians, largely are not aware of AIAN as people, as patients, or as recipients of years of trauma. Therefore, they do not Indigenize their practices or education. To *Indigenize* is to include and indeed naturalize Indigenous knowledge systems and make them evident in order to truly transform practice, education, government, and other systems (Antoine et al., n.d.). It should be viewed as a deliberate com-ing together of two ways of knowing and not displacing Western knowledge but working in concert with it (Antoine et al., n.d.).

The multiple and ongoing federal policy periods and their continuing effects make AIAN reticent to jump on any federal or health system programs, for example, COVID-19 vaccines, which is not unexpected considering that previous federal programs were specifically aimed at "getting rid of the Indian problem." Assuredly, there was/is a continuum of how AIAN felt/feel about trusting the vaccines as they rolled out. In one scenario, in order to continue working and to protect Elders, many AIAN did get the vaccine. For others, there was great hesitancy.

Point 2: Mitigation—"Trusted Messengers"

This persistent, intergenerational, traumatic targeting of Indigenous people in the United States over hundreds of years is not easily or instantly mitigated. Trust and relationship building is key. But this trust building should have been initiated and nurtured over decades not expected on a dime in a pandemic.

Trusted messenger is a term used by the government, U.S. Surgeon General, and others to get the urgent message of the vaccine out. This is in all vaccine-hesitant populations. These messengers in other populations are seen as "local nurses and doctors, with teachers, with faith leaders and others in local communities . . . that's actually who people want to hear from — their own healthcare provider, their family and their friends" (King, 2021, para. 8). For AIAN populations, it is the Elders, knowledge keepers, and Indigenous-language speakers who will have to continue to be the *trusted messengers*, yet they are often the most affected by the virus.

We lost many Elders, speakers, and knowledge keepers during this pandemic. As it is, AIAN have the smallest number and rate of those older than 65 than other populations, almost half of White populations. Their presence and messaging now are more important than ever. They Indigenize healthcare by their very presence. Higher infection rates and death rates, as well as practical issues, such as no running water, inadequate electricity, and heating available in remote areas, long distances for access, poverty, and trust issues, persist. COVID-19 has hit Indian Country with great force. One young person stated to this author that when he hears it in the language, from an Elder, that's when he will get the vaccine.

OLDER PERSONS: PRACTICE

To increase the reciprocity of care between nursing home staff and residents, *story sharing* has been used as an intervention strategy. To lessen the almost totally task-oriented nature of caring, using story sharing has been shown to increase the quality of life of residents in six different nursing homes (Heliker, 2007). Through story sharing, the staff was encouraged to come to know the patients, their backgrounds, their interests, and their likes. Active listening and expressions of concern are key elements. This is a mutual process in which each learns about the other and trust and shared experiences become evident. The intervention suggested by Heliker used three 1-hour sessions between six nurse aides and a facilitator. In Session 1, staff learn about confidentiality, respectful and attentive listening, and role-playing. In Session 2, staff bring an object that holds personal meaning for themselves, to better understand the residents and what few possessions residents may have with them, and the monumental meaning of these possessions. In Session 3, staff learn about "sharing informs care" practices. Both residents and aides reported being in a better relationship with each other, which can be seen as a "best practice" in the care of older, frail adults (Heliker, 2007).

OLDER PERSONS: EDUCATION

"Many older adults were raised in an era when learning occurred primarily through reading, discussion, and retelling stories" (Cangelosi & Sorrell, 2008, p. 19). Often it is through storytelling, whether formal or informal, that otherwise missed information will be shared. Many older patients detail numerous topics and events until they hit on pertinent information in describing their current problem. Unless this wandering is not only allowed but also encouraged, especially with older subjects, crucial data needed for their care will be missed. When questions requiring only *yes* and *no* answers are asked and are hurried in encounters with older clients, they will not be able to share information with the healthcare professional that is vital to their health story. Probing questions require time, patience, and empathy. In addition, older persons will need time to *hear* and process what the healthcare provider is telling them. One strategy is to share health information in a group setting allowing for support from others in the group (Cangelosi & Sorrell, 2008). But by using storytelling as an intervention for teaching older individuals, unique learning needs will be met (Cangelosi & Sorrell, 2008).

DIGITAL STORYTELLING

Digital storytelling may be an effective way to educate younger people, whether in the classroom or in patient education, in this world of ever-changing technology. Visual and audio media may stimulate deeper learning in this population, which is largely familiar and comfortable with the use of technology (Sandars et al., 2008). Sandars and colleagues (2008) have used digital storytelling with medical students. As a guideline, they suggest the following 12-step sequence of events for digital storytelling:

1. Decide on the topic of the story.
2. Write the story.
3. Collect a variety of multimedia to create a story.
4. Select which to use to create the story.
5. Create the story.
6. Present the digital story.
7. Encourage reflection at each stage of the project.
8. Avoid being too ambitious.
9. Provide adequate technical support.
10. Develop a relevant assessment framework.
11. Embed it within existing teaching and learning approaches.
12. Persuade others of its value.

Building the story encourages active learning and constant reflection for the teller. This process could be used with other populations, such as patient groups. Although the storyteller is in many ways the learner in this situation, the same orality notions are in play. The storyteller, the process, and the aesthetics are of great import. Here, rather than regalia, video and audio supply the aesthetics.

When looking ahead to digital delivery and/or storytelling in the future, it is probable that "growth in technology is actually likely to increase health disparities for those with limited health, computer, and reading literacy, unless effort is devoted to the development of IT [information technology] specifically designed for these disadvantaged groups, and issues of technology access are addressed" (Bickmore & Paasche-Orlow, 2012, p. 23).

CULTURAL APPLICATIONS

In many Indigenous societies, especially when they are described as primarily oral cultures, Western health practices will be seen as the alternative and complementary modalities (Moss, 2000). This is important because the practitioner—or, here, the storyteller—must understand that to patients coming from a basically oral culture, storytelling is already seen as primary to their well-being. There have been a number of health-related studies that use storytelling in various cultures (Crawford O'Brien, 2008; Finucane & McMullen, 2008; Inglebret et al., 2008; Larkey & Gonzalez, 2007; Leeman et al., 2008).

In a narrative analysis of 115 stories of women of African descent, Banks-Wallace (2002) found storytelling useful for learning more about the historical and contextual factors affecting the well-being of these women. The major functions storytelling served were: contextual grounding, bonding with others, validating and affirming experiences, venting and catharsis, resisting oppression, and educating others. See Sidebar 13.1 for a vivid personal account of the use of storytelling in Kenya illustrating these major functions.

Rogers (2004) found storytelling at the heart of 11 Pacific Northwest African American widows, 55 years of age and older, who described their experiences of bereavement after their husbands' deaths. During the interviews, the widows took on various mannerisms and speech patterns of people who were part of the story. These included changed tones, mimicking the voices of those involved, and use of hands, body language, and facial expressions. Nurses should be aware of storytelling as a means to gain in-depth understanding and cultural insight into African American experience.

Sidebar 13.1 *Healing Through the Oral Tradition in Kenya and Beyond*

Eunice M. Areba, Kenya

Presenting health messages in a manner that patients can easily understand and incorporate into their lives is usually challenging. Communicating effectively means *transforming* health messages into pieces of information that are not only easily understood but can also be put into *action* by the recipient to attain mutually agreed-upon health outcomes (Silver, 2001). A cornerstone of effective communication is using mechanisms already familiar to the members of the target community, which also ensures the sustainability of the message. A notable example is the use of oral narratives (folklore) or simply storytelling: an art that has been used for eons in communities across the world. Nurses and other healthcare providers in Kenya and beyond have been great proponents and facilitators of storytelling, especially in chronic disease management. These stories are usually real-life accounts of the patients.

I grew up surrounded by stories depicting characters that I could easily relate to and children were encouraged to participate in the storytelling process through song, dance, and rehearsed phrases such as these roughly translated ones:

Paukwa? Pakawa! (Who wants to be served? Me!)
Sahani? Ya mchele! (A plate? Of rice!)

Needless to say, I vividly remember not just the stories but also the lessons that were imparted. The storyteller is most often an elder who aims to instill a virtue, rectify a vice, and educate the young on the history or origin of a community. Some examples in the Kisii, Luhya, and coastal tribes in Kenya, respectively, include *the prophetess Moraa and Otenyo* (a historical event), *Simbi and Nashikufu* (beauty and humility), and *Abunuwasi* (social justice). Over time, oral narratives—especially from tribes whose mother tongue might soon become extinct—are being recorded both on paper and digital platforms. Storytelling in any form is

Sidebar 13.1 *Healing Through the Oral Tradition in Kenya and Beyond (continued)*

a powerful and versatile health-teaching tool that can easily be implemented by healthcare providers across many settings, as illustrated in these examples.

HIV is not killing anybody unless you close your mouth (Leon, 2012, p. 28). HIV-positive women are healing with the help of their peers whose stories have helped them conquer social stigma, fear, and denial. Participants in the programs organized by the nongovernmental organization (NGO) Women Fighting Aids in Kenya and its affiliates draw strength from one another's stories and, in so doing, develop a shared identity that comforts and assures them that they are not alone (Leon, 2012). Storytelling in this setting takes on a communal nature and encourages them to adhere to treatment programs. Healthcare providers also organize storytelling workshops targeting high-risk groups such as transport workers in specific geographical locations.

Peace building and mental health. No matter where or how it happens, those exposed to violence experience traumatic events that can significantly hamper their psychosocial, emotional, and physical well-being. In war, social institutions are destroyed and the tapestry of shared values in the community is torn. Stories utilized by both perpetrators and victims have been used to try to achieve peace by rebuilding relationships and reestablishing trust. Storytelling occurs in the form of people giving their accounts of atrocities committed in a communal setting (e.g., in Rwanda's gacaca courts post the 1994 genocide). Storytelling is seen as *familiar ground,* a tradition that many are exposed to during their upbringing, and is, in turn, perceived as *safe ground.* Some participants in these traditional setups have expressed feelings of relief, empowerment, and personal and communal healing. In cases of community reintegration, storytelling has been critical in accepting people back into the community. Conversely, there is the danger of retraumatization, and therefore, adequate provisions for mental healthcare have to be instituted.

Creating a space for storytelling empowers patients, creates rapport, is easy to replicate, and places decisions in the hands of the patients—thus building the capacity for a community to identify, acknowledge, and come up with solutions for the problems they face.

References

Leon, K. (2012). *Storytelling and healing: The influence of narrative on identity construction among HIV positive individuals in Kisumu, Kenya* (Unpublished manuscript). http://digitalcollections.sit.edu/isp_collection/1385

Silver, D. (2001). Songs and storytelling: Bringing health messages to life in Uganda. *Education for Health, 14,* 51–60. https://doi.org/10.1080/13576280010015362.

Culturally appropriate communication methods, such as storytelling, have been found to be effective in health-promotion activities. The *talking circle* is one format in which the art of storytelling occurs. Indigenous Ojibwa and Cree women healers use talking circles as instruments of healing and storytelling in their everyday traditional practice (Struthers, 1999). Storytelling was preferred as a natural pattern of communication for Yakima Indians to learn about health promotion related to cervical cancer prevention (Strickland et al., 1999).

FUTURE RESEARCH

Technology will certainly play a larger role in storytelling in the future. However, the orality of storytelling with which we are familiar will always be retained. Therefore, integrating future trends will keep the modality in line with evolving human endeavors. Wyatt and Hauenstein (2008) explore "how technology and storytelling can be joined to promote positive health outcomes" (p. 142). They recognize that although storytelling is widely used to teach children in the classroom, it has been minimally used in the health arena as a teaching–learning tool. With advances in technology—and its ubiquitous presence—interactive, digital storytelling may provide one mechanism to help enhance health promotion.

Explorations are needed to determine the efficacy of vignettes in both research and practice, particularly with individuals from other cultures and older adults. The triangulation of qualitative and quantitative measures will provide a more complete examination of a patient's reflection, understanding, and outcomes. Specific questions that require investigation include the following:

■ What are strategies to use to help nurses become more comfortable using storytelling as an intervention?
■ What are some ways in which vignettes can be used with people from diverse cultures and age groups?

REFERENCES

Antoine, A., Mason, R., Mason, R., Palahicky, S. & Rodriguez de France, C. (n.d.). *Indigenization, decolonization, and reconciliation.* Retrieved February 21, 2022, from https://opentextbc.ca/indigenizationcurriculumdevelopers/chapter/indigenization-decolonization-and-reconciliation/

Banks-Wallace, J. (2002). Talk that talk: Storytelling and analysis rooted in African American oral tradition. *Qualitative Health Research, 12*(3), 410–426. https://doi.org/10.1177/104973202129119892

Barton, S. S. (2004). Narrative inquiry: Locating aboriginal epistemology in a relational methodology. *Journal of Advanced Nursing, 45*(5), 519–526. https://doi.org/10.1046/j.1365-2648.2003.02935.x

Bergner, R. M. (2007). Therapeutic storytelling revisited. *American Journal of Psychotherapy, 61*(2), 149–162. https://doi.org/10.1176/appi.psychotherapy.2007.61.2.149

Bickmore, T. W., & Paasche-Orlow, M. K. (2012). The role of information technology in health literacy research. *Journal of Health Communication: International Perspectives, 17*(Suppl. 3), S23–S29. https://doi.org/10.1080/10810730.2012.712626

Bolhuis, J. J., Tattersall, I., Chomsky, N., & Berwick, R. C. (2014). How could language have evolved? *PLoS Biology, 12*(8), e1001934. https://doi.org/10.1371/journal.pbio.1001934

Cangelosi, P. R., & Sorrell, J. M. (2008). Storytelling as an educational strategy for older adults with chronic illness. *Journal of Psychosocial Nursing and Mental Health Services, 46*(7), 19–22. https://doi.org/10.3928/02793695-20080701-07

Crawford O'Brien, S. (Ed.). (2008). *Religion and healing in Native America: Pathways for renewal.* Praeger.

Dictionary.com. (2021a). *Story.* https://www.dictionary.com/browse/story

Dictionary.com. (2021b). *Storytelling.* https://www.dictionary.com/browse/storytelling

Edmondson, M. E. (1971). *Lore: An introduction to the science of folklore and literature.* Holt, Rinehart, & Winston.

Evans, J. (2007). The science of storytelling. *Astrobiology, 7*(4), 710–711. https://doi.org/10.1089/ast.2007.0145

Fairbairn, G. J., & Carson, A. M. (2002). Writing about nursing research: A storytelling approach. *Nurse Researcher, 10*(1), 7–14. https://doi.org/10.7748/nr2002.10.10.1.7.c5875

Finucane, M. L., & McMullen, C. K. (2008). Making diabetes self-management education culturally relevant for Filipino Americans in Hawaii. *Diabetes Educator, 34*(5), 841–853. https://doi.org/10.1177/0145721708323098

Guber, P. (2007). The four truths of the storyteller. *Harvard Business Review, 85*(12), 52–59, 142. https://hbr.org/2007/12/the-four-truths-of-the-storyteller

Haigh, C., & Hardy, P. (2011). Tell me a story—A conceptual exploration of storytelling in healthcare education. *Nurse Education Today, 31*(4), 408–411. https://doi.org/10.1016/j.nedt.2010.08.001

Heliker, D. (2007). Story sharing: Restoring the reciprocity of caring in long-term care. *Journal of Psychosocial Nursing and Mental Health Services, 45*(7), 20–23. https://doi.org/10.3928/02793695-20070701-07

Inglebret, E., Jones, C., & Pavel, D. M. (2008). Integrating American Indian/Alaska Native culture into shared storybook intervention. *Language, Speech, and Hearing Services in Schools, 39*(4), 521–527. https://doi.org/10.1044/0161-1461(2008/07-0051)

ISDA. (2020). *COVID-19 policy brief: Disparities among Native American communities in the United States version: July 7, 2020.* https://www.idsociety.org/globalassets/idsa/public-health/covid-19/covid19-health-disparaties-in-native-american-communities-final.pdf

Jones, N., Marks, R., Ramirez, R., & Ríos-Vargas, M. (2021). *2020 census illuminates racial and ethnic composition of the country American Indian and Alaska Native population.* https://www.census.gov/library/stories/2021/08/improved-race-ethnicity-measures-reveal-united-states-population-much-more-multiracial.html

King, N. (2021). *Local 'trusted messengers' key to boosting COVID vaccinations, Surgeon General says.* https://www.npr.org/sections/coronavirus-live-updates/2021/05/05/993754369/administration-plan-will-make-it-easier-to-get-access-to-vaccines

Koh, H. K., Berwick, D. M., Clancy, C. M., Baur, C., Brach, C., Harris, L. M., & Zerhusen, E. G. (2012). New federal policy initiatives to boost health literacy can help the nation move beyond the cycle of costly 'crisis care'. *Health Affairs, 31*(2), 434–443. https://doi.org/10.1377/hlthaff.2011.1169

Kramsch, C. (1998). *Language and culture.* Oxford University Press.

Larkey, L. K., & Gonzalez, J. (2007). Storytelling for promoting colorectal cancer prevention and early detection among Latinos. *Patient Education and Counseling, 67*(3), 272–278. https://doi.org/10.1016/j.pec.2007.04.003

Leeman, J., Skelly, A. H., Burns, D., Carlson, J., & Soward, A. (2008). Tailoring a diabetes self-care intervention for use with older, rural African American women. *Diabetes Educator, 34*(2), 310–317. https://doi.org/10.1177/0145721708316623

Lord, A. (1960). *The singer of tales* (2nd ed.). Harvard University Press.

Lourens, M. M. (2013). An exploration of Xhosa-speaking patients' understanding of cancer treatment and its influence on their treatment experience. *Journal of Psychosocial Oncology, 31*, 103–121. https://doi.org/10.1080/07347332.2012.741091

Mark, J. (2011). Writing. *Ancient History Encyclopedia.* http://www.ancient.eu/writing/

Moss, M. P. (2000). *Zuni elders: Ethnography of American Indian aging* [Unpublished doctoral dissertation]. University of Texas Health Science Center at Houston. http://digitalcommons.library.tmc.edu/dissertations/AAI9974591

Nielsen-Bohlman, L., Panzer, A., & Kindig, D. (Eds.). (2004). *Health literacy: A prescription to end confusion* (National Research Council). National Academies Press.

Olson, D. R., & Torrance, N. (Eds.). (1991). *Literacy and orality.* Cambridge University Press.

Ong, W. J. (2002). *Orality and literacy.* Routledge.

Ramirez-Esparza, N., & Pennebaker, J. W. (2006). Do good stories produce good health?: Exploring words, language, and culture. *Narrative Inquiry, 16*(1), 211–219. https://doi.org/10.1075/ni.16.1.26ram

Roberts, J. (1994). *Tales and transformations: Stories in families and family therapy.* Norton.

Rogers, L. S. (2004). Meaning of bereavement among older African American widows. *Geriatric Nursing, 25*(1), 10–16. https://doi.org/10.1016/j.gerinurse.2003.11.012

Rule, L. (2011). *Digital storytelling.* http://electronic portfolios.com/digistory

Sampson, G. (1980). *Schools of linguistics.* Stanford University Press.

Sandars, J., Murray, C., & Pellow, A. (2008). Twelve tips for using digital storytelling to promote reflective learning by medical students. *Medical Teacher, 30*(8), 774–777. https://doi.org/10.1080/01421590801987370

Sandelowski, M. (1994). We are the stories we tell: Narrative knowing in nursing practice. *Journal of Holistic Nursing, 12*(1), 23–33. https://doi.org/10.1177/089801019401200105

Strickland, C. J., Squeoch, M. D., & Chrisman, N. J. (1999). Health promotion in cervical cancer prevention among the Yakima Indian women of the Wa'Shat Long-house. *Journal of Transcultural Nursing, 10*(3), 190–196. https://doi.org/10.1177/104365969901000309

Struthers, R. (1999). *The lived experience of Ojibwa and Cree women healers* [Unpublished doctoral dissertation]. University of Minnesota, Minneapolis.

Tannen, D. (Ed.). (1982). *Spoken and written language: Exploring orality and literacy*. Ablex.

Tedlock, D. (1983). *The spoken word and the work of interpretation*. University of Pennsylvania Press.

Whalen, D. H., Moss, M., & Baldwin, D. (2016). Healing through language: Positive physical health effects of Indigenous language use [version 1; referees: 2 approved with reservations]. *F1000Research, 5*, 852. https://doi.org/10.12688/f1000research.8656.1

Wyatt, T. H., & Hauenstein, E. (2008). Enhancing children's health through digital story. *Computers, Informatics, Nursing: CIN, 26*(3), 142–148; quiz, 149–150. https://doi.org/10.1097/01.NCN.0000304779.49941.44

14

Animal-Assisted Therapy

SUSAN O'CONNER-VON

> One of the most fundamental advantages of animal assisted therapy over other therapeutic modalities is that it provides the patient a much needed opportunity to give affection as well as receive it. It is this reciprocity, rare among medical therapies, that makes animal assisted therapy a unique and valuable route to healing. (Weil, 2021, para. 16).

The domestication of animals began more than 15,000 years ago and continues today because animals play a significant role in human life (Ahmad et al., 2020). Much of what was known about the animal–human bond was anecdotal in nature until recently. Research examining the use of animals as a complementary or alternative therapy is based on studies about pet ownership. It is evident—with approximately 77 million pet dogs and 58 million pet cats in the United States—that pets play an important role in people's lives (American Veterinary Medical Association, 2018). Of note, pet ownership differs among ethnic and racial groups with the highest rates among White households (64.7%), Latino/Hispanic (61.4%) households next and the lowest rates (36.9%) among African American households (American Veterinary Medical Association, 2018). Pets can provide companionship, promote dialogue and social interaction, facilitate exercise, increase feelings of security, mitigate the effects of stress, be a source of consistency, and be a comfort to touch (Arkow, 2015). The healing power of pets is "their capacity to make the atmosphere safe for emotions, the spiritual side of healing; whatever you are feeling, you can express it around your pet and not be judged" (Becker, 2002, p. 80).

In a classic comparative study examining the impact of pet ownership in childhood on young adults' social characteristics and professional choices, those who owned a pet in childhood retrospectively rated their pet higher than television, relatives, and neighbors in terms of social support received during childhood (Vizek et al., 2001). The sample included 356 college students at a mean age of 21 years (68% women, 32% men). A total of 74% of the sample had pets (mostly dogs) during childhood and were found to be more empathetic and expressed more altruistic attitudes than those students who did not own a pet in childhood. Moreover, students who had a pet in childhood were more likely to choose a career in the helping professions.

The role that animals play in healing environments was first documented in records from 9th-century Belgium, where animals were used with individuals with physical disabilities, followed by 18th-century England, where animals were used by people with mental illness (Serpell, 2019). Florence Nightingale wrote of the connection between animals and health in 1860 by suggesting that pets were perfect companions for the sick, especially individuals with chronic health conditions (Nightingale, 1860).

The 1970s launched the beginning of widespread interest in the interaction between animals and humans in the healthcare setting. In 1976, Elaine Smith, an American registered nurse, observed the benefits of pets in the healthcare setting while working in England. She noticed how patients reacted positively to the visits of a chaplain and his golden retriever. On returning to the United States, Smith introduced the concept of pet therapy into healthcare settings and founded Therapy Dogs International (TDI, 2021). The goal of creating TDI was to formally test dogs so that they could be certified, insured, and registered as volunteer therapy dogs. In 1977, the Delta Foundation (now Pet Partners) was established to study the human–animal bond and the potential use of animal-assisted therapy (AAT). Scientific research in this area began in the 1980s when the National Institutes of Health convened a conference in 1987 on the health benefits of pets (Fine & Beck, 2019). During the 1990s, the focus was the establishment of professional standards and guidelines with the development of the *Standards of Practice for Animal-Assisted Activities and Animal-Assisted Therapy* (Delta Society, 1996). In 2008, the National Institute of Child and Human Development convened a conference to discuss the need for clarity and well-designed research examining the animal–human bond (Fine & Beck, 2019). Carefully designed studies continue to provide the evidence needed to increase acceptance of AAT as noted by the recent trend of more substantial randomized controlled trials (Fine & Beck, 2019).

DEFINITION

The International Association of Human-Animal Interaction Organizations (IAHAIO, 2018) is the leading global association of 90 multidisciplinary organizations that engage in practice, research, and/or education in AAT, animal-assisted activity (AAA), and service animal training. In an effort to provide consistency of terminology and guidelines for research and practice, a white paper was developed and approved in 2014 and then reapproved in 2018, with the following definitions.

ANIMAL-ASSISTED INTERVENTION

"An animal-assisted intervention is a goal-oriented and structured intervention that intentionally includes animals in health, education, and human service for the purpose of therapeutic gains in humans" (IAHAIO, 2018, p. 5). AAT, education, and activities are examples of types of animal-assisted interventions (IAHAIO, 2018).

ANIMAL-ASSISTED THERAPY

"Animal-assisted therapy is a goal-oriented, planned and structured therapeutic intervention directed and/or delivered by health, education and human service professionals" (IAHAIO, 2018, p. 5). Some key features of AAT are (a) specific goals and objectives are set for each patient, (b) progress is measured, and

(c) interactions are documented. The goals are designed by a nurse, occupational therapist, physical therapist, counselor, physician, or other healthcare professional who uses AAT in the treatment process (American Veterinary Medical Association, 2021a). A physical goal would include, for example, improved mobility by walking with a dog. Examples of cognitive goals include improved verbal expression (via normal interaction with the animal) and improved short- and long-term memory (via recalling the animal's name and activity at last visit). Social goals could include improved social skills and building rapport with others through the animal. Animals may also help increase socialization by facilitating discussion of pets one may have had in the past. An illustration of an emotional goal would be improved motivation shown by getting dressed or walking to see the animal. Although a variety of animal species and breeds, such as cats, birds, rabbits, horses, and dolphins, are involved in AAT, dogs account for the highest percentage of animals (Grandin et al., 2019).

ANIMAL-ASSISTED ACTIVITY

"Animal-assisted activity (AAA) is a planned and goal-oriented informal interaction and visitation conducted by the human–animal team for motivational, educational, and recreational purposes" (IAHAIO, 2018, p. 5). Some key features of AAA are (a) specific goals and objectives are not planned for each patient, (b) visit activities are spontaneous and last as long as needed, and (c) interactions are not necessarily documented. AAAs are less structured and provide human and animal contact for recreation, education, or pleasure. Examples include an informal visit by a friendly pet to a residential care center, hospice, hospital, school, or prison with the intent to bring joy, comfort, and companionship to the residents (Rivera, 2010).

SERVICE ANIMALS

A service animal was originally defined in the Americans with Disabilities Act of 1990 as any animal trained to do work for the benefit of an individual with a disability, including physical, psychiatric, sensory, intellectual, or mental conditions (American Disabilities Act National Network, 2017). As of March 15, 2011, only dogs are recognized as service animals under Title II (state and local government services) or Title III (public accommodations and commercial facilities) of the Americans with Disabilities Act. Service dogs or guide dogs are trained specifically for the service they are providing: sight, sound, movement, or support. Once service animals are certified, they have federally approved access to accompany their owners anywhere. Service dogs are considered working animals, not pets. Although there is increased awareness and acceptance of therapy dogs in healthcare and public settings, such dogs do not receive federal protection or the same rights as service dogs who assist people with physical or emotional disabilities (American Disabilities Act National Network, 2017).

SCIENTIFIC BASIS

Many studies indicate that there are physical and/or psychological benefits derived from human–animal bonds. Most of the research that has examined the physical benefits of AAT has focused on an animal's ability to attenuate a person's response to stress. When an individual becomes stressed, the sympathetic nervous system releases a cascade of hormones such as cortisol, aldosterone, and adrenaline. Stress-reduction strategies, such as petting an animal, can assist in reducing the build-up of these stress hormones. To illustrate, a meta-analysis was conducted by Ein et al. (2018) examining the effect of pet therapy on a human's physiological and subjective stress response. The sample consisted of 28 studies and 34 individual samples ($N = 1,310$), with the results revealing a significant difference in heart rate, self-reported anxiety, and self-reported stress after pet therapy compared with before pet therapy. These results suggest AAT as an effective modality in helping to reduce stress reactivity. Likewise, the hormone oxytocin can lower blood pressure, lower cortisol levels, increase the pain threshold, and have an antianxiety effect. One of the best ways to increase oxytocin levels is through positive physical touch, such as petting an animal (Chandler, 2017). In turn, research has revealed a similar increased level of oxytocin in dogs after interaction with humans (Odendaal & Meintjes, 2003). Research that has examined the psychological benefits of AAT has explored the stress-reducing outcomes and improved quality of life that the animal provides through social support (Arkow, 2015; Yamamoto & Hart, 2019).

INTERVENTION

AAT has been shown to be a successful intervention for patients of all ages with a variety of physical and psychological conditions. This intervention can be provided in many settings, including private homes, acute care and rehabilitation facilities, long-term and group care homes, schools, and correctional facilities.

GUIDELINES

Selecting an animal for AAT requires careful screening and extensive training (American Veterinary Medical Association, 2021b; IAHAIO, 2018). Although some animals are considered good pets, not all animals are appropriate candidates for AAT. There is no ideal animal for AAT, but the animal must be calm, tolerant, and reliable (Arkow, 2015). Furthermore, all animals must complete yearly veterinary screening to ensure that they are healthy, current on vaccinations, and parasite-free (IAHAIO, 2018). AAT requires that the animal and handler work together as a team. To provide safe and effective AAT, the AAT team should abide by established standards of practice for AAT and the requirements of the healthcare facility (Barker et al., 2019). Examples from the Standards of Practice in Animal–Assisted Interventions (Pet Partners, 2018) for the handler include (a) demonstrating appropriate treatment of people and animals, (b) using appropriate social skills, (c) acting as the animal's advocate, (d) having the ability to read the animal's cues, and (e) maintaining confidentiality.

ANIMAL-ASSISTED TRAINING

Most national therapy dog organizations require the Canine Good Citizen test (American Kennel Club [AKC], 2021) as a basic skill requirement for acceptance into a therapy dog training program. This test, developed by the AKC in 1989, is a certification program that tests dogs in everyday situations and requires a dog to have mastered a basic set of skills. Dogs are tested in 10 areas that include response to a friendly stranger and another dog, ability to walk with a loose leash, and reaction to distraction and separation. For the complete list, see www.akc .org/products-services/training-programs/canine-good-citizen/take-the-test/

Additional requirements may include didactic content for the human partner to understand the theory and research supporting AAT, standards of practice, and ethical considerations. The animal partner receives training in simulated healthcare settings that include activities such as (a) learning how to leave alone an object such as food or medication; (b) being bumped while walking in a crowded space; (c) being comfortable around hospital equipment such as wheelchairs, walkers, or crutches; (d) receiving petting from several people at once; and (e) sitting quietly as paws, ears, and tail are examined.

MEASUREMENT OF OUTCOMES

The effects of AAT have been measured through qualitative and quantitative means. A variety of outcomes, such as cardiovascular benefits, decreased pain, lowered blood pressure, increased socialization and exercise, improved coordination and balance, and decreased stress, have been examined. Positive patient outcomes depend on the qualifications and experience of the AAT team. Specifically, the therapy team should complete adequate training, obtain national registration, and undergo yearly evaluation by a veterinarian and a professional therapy animal organization. The effectiveness of outcomes can be further complicated by the multidisciplinary nature of this intervention, along with the lack of standardized protocols and methods of evaluation. Therefore, frequent communication and collaboration are essential between the AAT team and the healthcare professionals or therapists involved in the patient's treatment plan (American Veterinary Medical Association, 2021b).

PRECAUTIONS

Although research supports the positive benefits and the safety of AAT for patients with various health conditions, the potential risks, such as disease transmission, allergies, and bites must be carefully taken into consideration (Dalton et al., 2020). As noted in the white paper titled *Animals in Healthcare Facilities: Recommendations to Minimize Potential Risks* (Murthy et al., 2015), a major concern for healthcare facilities is the transmission of infectious diseases. These potential risks can be decreased by using trained and registered AAT teams, along with enforcing standard hand hygiene before and after every visit for the handler and anyone who pets the animal (Murthy et al., 2015). Additional guidelines from the Centers for Disease Control and Prevention (2015) require that animals used for AAT be clean, groomed, healthy, fully vaccinated, older than 1 year, free of parasites, and the human handler must be in good health.

To prevent possible risks, a mechanism must be in place for regularly scheduled examinations and preventive care by a veterinarian to assess the physical and behavioral health and well-being of the animal. Results of these examinations must be shared with the appropriate animal regulatory agency and AAT organizations on an annual basis (American Veterinary Medical Association, 2021b; IAHAIO, 2018).

A comprehensive review specifically examining the potential health risks of animals in the healthcare setting found that the potential benefits far outweighed the insignificant risks, and few data confirmed pathogen transmission between therapy animals and humans (Dalton et al., 2020). As research findings continue to be reported in this area, it is important to be aware of potential concerns related to disease transmission if they arise.

USES

PHYSICAL CONDITIONS

The research investigating the impact of AAT on physical conditions has concentrated on cardiovascular disease, seizure disorders, dementia, and pain management.

Cardiovascular Disease

The study of the relationship between pets and their positive health effects on a human's cardiovascular system dates back to 1929 (Wolff & Frishman, 2005). Several studies have demonstrated the effect of pet ownership on survival after myocardial infarction. Friedmann et al. (1980) conducted the seminal longitudinal research examining the effect of pet ownership on survival for 92 adult patients after myocardial infarction. Only 5% of the subjects who owned pets died within 1 year after hospitalization, whereas 28% of those who were not pet owners died during the same interval.

Another study by Friedmann and Thomas (1995), examining pet ownership and 1-year survival after myocardial infarction, included the severity of cardiac disease. For the 368 patients in this investigation, disease severity and pet ownership were found to positively affect survival, whereas marital status and living situations did not.

More recent research (Krause-Parello & Kolassa, 2016) examined cardiovascular wellness in a community setting of 28 subjects including male ($n = 12$) and female ($n = 16$) participants with an age range of 60 to 102 years ($M = 82.9$ years). A crossover design was used to investigate changes in blood pressure and heart rate before and after a pet therapy session with a registered therapy dog team versus a session with a volunteer and no canine. The study's goal was to examine the relationships among pet attitude, stress, social support, and health status using reliable and valid study instruments. Results revealed a significant relationship between systolic blood pressure, health rating (participant's rating of their health at present from (1 = *excellent* to 5 = *poor*), gender, stress, and coping that implied a greater decrease in systolic blood pressure when visited by a therapy dog. There was also a significant relationship between heart rate and health rating that predicted a larger decrease in heart rate with pet therapy. These investigators suggest that the therapy dog visitation provided an opportunity to enhance cardiovascular wellness along with enhancing social support.

Seizure Disorders

Approximately 65 million people around the world have epilepsy, with 3.4 million living in the United States (Epilepsy Foundation, 2019). The use of animals as an important component of the treatment plan for individuals with epilepsy was first documented in 1867 in Germany (Fontaine, 2015). Over the past several decades, a number of investigators have examined the value of dogs in caring for patients with seizure disorders. As dogs have been trained to detect cancer and diabetes, researchers have found promising results with canines detecting a seizure odor. Catala et al. (2019) tested the ability of trained dogs to discriminate an epileptic seizure odor from different body odors of the same person in other contexts. Five dogs from the Medical Mutts program (Indianapolis, IN) were individually tested on a seven-choice task. With each trial, seven scent samples from one patient were presented: one from a seizure, two from a sports session, and four from different days during a calm activity. For each dog, the trials were repeated five times for the odors from the same patient. Results revealed that three of the dogs performed at 100% accuracy and the other two dogs displayed 67% to 95% accuracy in detecting the seizure odor (Catala et al., 2019). More research is needed in this area, plus funding to provide trained seizure-response dogs that can activate an alarm or alert a caregiver and then stay with the person to provide support during and after the seizure (Yamamoto & Hart, 2019).

Dementia

Dementia is a chronic, progressive condition with Alzheimer's disease being the most prevalent type, accounting for 60% to 70% of the cases (Kim et al., 2021). According to the World Health Organization (2020), there are approximately 50 million people worldwide living with dementia. For patients with dementia, interacting with an animal seems to have a positive influence on aggressiveness and anxiety and can improve quality of life (Kim et al., 2021). Moreover, the presence of a therapy dog can improve physical activity and increased episodes of smiling (Wood et al., 2017). The benefits associated with mental and physical health were associated specifically with dogs, as physical activity was encouraged by walking longer distances than if they went on a walk by themselves (Boldig & Butala, 2021).

In a randomized multicenter trial with follow-up at 3 months, Olsen et al. (2016) examined the impact of AAT on quality of life and depression. The sample consisted of a group of 58 individuals (65 years and older) with cognitive impairment. A sample of 28 individuals received AAT twice a week for 12 weeks, each session lasting 30 minutes. The experimental group was compared to a passive control group (n = 30). The results revealed a significant effect on depression and quality of life, especially for those with severe dementia.

Although a variety of studies show promising results for patients with dementia, a recent Cochrane review of 9 randomized controlled trials of AAT for dementia (Lai et al., 2019) revealed only a modest reduction in depressive symptoms, with no clear evidence that AAT affects other outcomes such as quality of life. The implications of these findings call for future research to be adequately powered by enrolling a sufficient number of participants and using validated tools to measure outcomes (Lai et al., 2019).

Pain Management

Nurses are aware of the importance of including complementary therapies in providing pain management for patients. The variety of settings in which AAT can be used is limitless in terms of being a diversion from pain and aiding in relaxation (Erich et al., 2021). Researchers have studied the effects of the use of animals on pain management for both adults and children.

Adult Pain Management

Most studies examining AAT for pain management have been conducted in inpatient care settings. Clark et al. (2020) however conducted a randomized controlled trial in an outpatient fibromyalgia treatment program to examine the physiological and emotional effects of AAA. The sample consisted of 221 participants with fibromyalgia who were randomly assigned to the treatment group (n = 111) or the control group (n = 110). Participants were between the ages of 18 and 76 years. Participants in the treatment group received a 20-minute session with a certified therapy dog and handler; those in the control group had a 20-minute session with a handler only. To better understand the physiological and emotional effects of AAA, noninvasive physiologic-emotional biomarkers, including salivary cortisol and oxytocin concentrations, tympanic temperatures, and cardiac parameters were obtained. Results revealed a decrease in heart rate, increase in heart rate variability, an increase in salivary oxytocin, and an increase in well-being survey scores for those in the treatment group, suggesting a visit with a therapy dog can significantly impact the physical and emotional health of patients with fibromyalgia (Clark et al., 2020).

Rodrigo-Claverol et al. (2019) conducted a randomized controlled study at a primary care clinic with geriatric patients who had chronic joint pain. The aim of the study was to evaluate the effectiveness of a group intervention using AAIs with elderly patients with chronic joint pain and polypharmacy (more than five medications of which two or more were prescribed for pain). The sample consisted of 52 patients with a mean age of 77.5 years. The experimental group had a sample size of 30, and the control group had a sample size of 22. The patients participated in 12 weekly sessions of kinesitherapy, with the experimental group receiving the additional assistance of a therapy dog. Results revealed a decrease in pain scores in both groups based on the Western Ontario and McMaster Universities Osteoarthritis Index, with a significantly higher effect of the AAI on participants with more painful symptoms. The investigators noted that the AAI led to a reduction in pain perception and pain-induced insomnia in individuals with higher baseline severity of pain and increased adhesion to the intervention (Rodrigo-Claverol et al., 2019).

Pediatric Pain Management

Sobo et al. (2006) conducted one of the first studies to examine the effectiveness of canine visitation therapy (CVT) on children's postoperative pain in a pediatric hospital. The convenience sample consisted of 25 English-speaking children, aged 5 to 18 years. Each patient received a onetime visit after surgery by a West Highland terrier named Lizzy and could choose the level of interaction with the dog. At high-interaction levels, the child actively played and walked with the dog; at low-interaction levels, the dog would do an occasional trick for the child; and at passive-interaction levels, the dog would sit quietly with the child. Despite the small sample size, there was a significant decrease in pain perception after the dog visitation. Moreover, post-CVT interviews with each child revealed eight themes: The dog (a) brought pleasure or happiness, (b) provided a distraction from the pain, (c) was fun, (d) provided company, (e) was calming, (f) reminded them of home, (g) was nice to cuddle with, and (h) eased the pain.

More recently, a systematic review and meta-analysis were conducted to examine the impact of AAT on hospitalized children and teenagers (Feng et al., 2021). The review consisted of eight studies, four randomized controlled trials and four quasi-experimental studies for a total of 348 participants, ranging in age from 3 to 18 years. Results indicated a statistically significant reduction in pain and systolic blood pressure, an increase in diastolic blood pressure, and no significant changes in anxiety, depression, stress, or heart rate in hospitalized children and teenagers after receiving AAT. Although a primary goal of AAT is to promote happiness and provide a distraction, the reduction of pain contributes to the child's sense of well-being (Feng et al., 2021).

PSYCHOLOGICAL CONDITIONS

Using animals to treat people with mental conditions dates back to 1792 at the York Retreat in England. It was observed that the farm animals helped enhance the humanity of those with emotional disorders (Altschiller, 2011). The goal was to lessen the use of medications and physical restraints by helping residents learn self-control through the care of animals (Fontaine, 2015). More recently, in 1964, American child psychotherapist Boris Levinson (who is considered to be the father of AAT) coined the term *pet therapy*. Levinson first described the therapeutic effects of companionship with his dog, Jingles, for withdrawn children living in a residential mental health program. The dog served as an icebreaker and opened communication to establish a positive relationship for effective therapy (Altschiller, 2011). Since the 1960s, a number of studies have been conducted to examine the effects of AAT on patients hospitalized in psychiatric units. It has been found that AAT can promote feelings of safety and comfort, along with a nonevaluative external focus for patients who are not fearful of animals or do not have a negative attitude toward them (Odendaal, 2000). Research also suggests having a companion dog can reduce loneliness and improve the mental well-being of those living in the community (Powell et al., 2019).

Military Personnel

Veterans can experience negative physical, emotional, and psychological effects from their experiences in war. As early as the 1940s, the beneficial effect of working with animals was evident in returning World War II veterans who recovered at the Army Air Corps Convalescent Hospital in New York (Fontaine, 2015). Today, there are several million veterans in our country, many of whom suffer from posttraumatic stress disorder (PTSD; U. S. Department of Veterans Affairs, 2021). Over the past decade, AAT has become more commonplace in veterans' hospitals, with the Department of Defense allocating funding to examine the effectiveness of its use. In addition, in March 2011, the Americans with Disabilities Act approved PTSD as a qualification of need for a service dog (Arkow, 2015). Veterans suffering with PTSD can apply for a service dog through organizations such as Veterans Moving Forward (2020). Although research to support the use of a service or therapy dog for individuals with PTSD is at an early stage, veterans report that these dogs help manage their PTSD symptoms such as anxiety, panic attacks, and fear (Arkow, 2015). Moreover, promising research exists regarding the use of equine-assisted activities for veterans with PTSD. Small, nonrandomized studies reveal decreased PTSD symptoms, decreased incidence of depressive symptoms (Arnon et al., 2020), and decreased incidence of guilt (Wharton et al., 2019).

ADDITIONAL USES

In addition to the types of interventions already mentioned, the variety of ways and settings in which AAT can be used are virtually limitless. One only has to be creative in the design of the intervention. The following is a partial list of ways that AAT can be used and the populations in which AAT has been studied (see Exhibit 14.1). See also Exhibits 14.2 and 14.3 for quotes from students and AAT providers who participate in a university-based AAT program.

Exhibit 14.1 *Populations in Which Animals and AAT Have Been Used*

- Adults after joint replacement surgery (Havey et al., 2014)
- Adult female abuse survivors (Porter-Wenzlaff, 2007)
- Adults in a hospital emergency department (Reddekopp et al., 2020)
- Adults in a residential substance-abuse therapy program (Wesley et al., 2009)
- Adults in the community to promote adherence to walking (Johnson & Meadows, 2010)
- Adults undergoing electroconvulsive therapy (Barker et al., 2003)
- Adults with fibromyalgia (Clark et al., 2020)
- Adults with heart failure (Cole et al., 2007)
- Adults in a burn center (Pruskowski et al., 2020)
- Children with pain (Barker et al., 2015; Braun et al., 2009)
- Children with attention-deficit/hyperactivity disorder (Perez-Gomez et al., 2020)
- Children with autism (O'Haire, 2017)
- Children with cancer (Chubak et al., 2017)
- Children with cerebral palsy (de Assis et al., 2021)
- Children with pervasive developmental disorders (Martin & Farnum, 2002)
- Children with special healthcare needs (Gasalberti, 2006)
- College student stress before final exams (Barker et al., 2016)
- Nursing students with test anxiety (Anderson & Brown, 2021)
- Older adults in a rehabilitation facility using psychoactive medications (Lust et al., 2007)
- Older adults in long-term care facilities (Banks & Banks, 2002)
- Older adults with dementia (Yakimicki et al., 2018)
- Older adults with mental illness (Moretti et al., 2011)
- Older men with aphasia (Macauley, 2006)
- U.S. Army soldiers dealing with the stressors of living in a deployed environment (Fike et al., 2012)
- U.S. veterans in an occupational therapy life skills program (Beck et al., 2012)

AAT, animal-assisted therapy.

Exhibit 14.2 *Quotes From University Students Experiencing AAT*

I think the connections made at PAWS (Pet Away Worry and Stress) are the most important thing to me—not only with the animals but also with the handlers and other people who attended. I think the short interaction with something so pure as an animal helps me forget about my problems for a little bit.

Animals genuinely bring so much joy, and from the minute I walked into PAWS, I felt so gleeful, excited, and happy to meet all the animals and pet them. I miss my own pet a lot (it lives with my parents out of state), and I always feel hesitant to pet other people's animals if I see an animal out walking with its owner. I really miss the feeling of hanging out with my own pet, so I was so happy I had a safe place to do this and where it is encouraged.

I enjoyed learning about the goals of the program for the students. And I realized the many different resources for handling stress in healthy ways. I recognized that actually using these resources and attending PAWS were very helpful and that it would be beneficial for me to continue! It was my push toward the right direction.

The simplicity of the animals' behaviors helps to take my mind off of stressors and put things in perspective. It helps me remember the importance of compassionate touch and mindfulness.

When I come to PAWS, no matter how my day has gone, I cannot help but smile and laugh. The animals bring out the best of me no matter what else is going on. They are always the same—loving and lovable, goofy, silly, giving, and dependable.

PAWS is my happy place away from home. It's a place where I can interact with my favorite animals, meet people with the same love for dogs as me, destress, and feel comfortable. It's honestly the best part about this university, and it's one of things that kept me here when I was having doubts about staying at this school due to homesickness.

-- University of Minnesota students

Exhibit 14.3 *Quotes From Providers of AAT*

My interest in the relationship between humans and animals started before I can really remember as animals of all kinds and their environmental surroundings have been integral figures of influence. When I began my professional career as a social worker in children's mental health, partnering with animals to support human well-being—also known as animal-assisted interactions (AAI) or animal-assisted therapy (AAT)—was a very recent modality of practice. Intuitively, my personal connection with nature and animals throughout my life helped me have a way of knowing that animals could be very healing, especially regarding trauma, depression, and isolation. I am now grounded in over 30 years of experience as a social worker who has also included and partnered with animals over my entire career. One significant endeavor I am most proud of is a weekly campus-based AAI program for college student mental health that I developed and direct at a large, Midwestern university. Each day, I witness countless students demonstrate many positive emotional states

(continued)

Exhibit 14.3 *Quotes from Providers of AAT (continued)*

when they interact with the AAI teams (handlers and their animal partner), and many of them have also shared verbal and written feedback as to the important—and sometimes lifesaving—impact this program has had in their lives. This campus-based AAI program fills a critical need so many college students have regarding finding connections with others and a sense of belonging, especially in such a large and overwhelming environment that is typical of many college campuses. These students know that this AAI program is available to them on a consistent basis, that it is a safe place, and that they will find animals that are warm, engaging, and accepting of them no matter the circumstances.

Tanya Bailey PhD, LICSW
Animal-assisted Interactions Coordinator, PAWS Program
University of Minnesota

I believe in the magic that is animal-assisted therapy: I witness the relaxation my therapy dog brings to a person living with Parkinson's, the happy distraction my therapy dog creates for a person living with an eating disorder, the gentle laughter and wonder my therapy dog elicits from a person living with persistent mental illness. Dogs bring out the best in us and create a safe space for all of us—handlers included!—to feel welcome and included. It is an honor and a privilege to share the magic of my therapy dog with others.

Sarah Palm
Animal Assisted Interventions Specialist
Nature-Based Therapeutic Services
Minnesota Landscape Arboretum

The calming effect a therapy dog can have on a patient is unmatched. The dog provides an opportunity for diversion from pain, opportunities for emotional expression, and comfortable silence. People often want to fill empty space with words but a therapy dog visit offers moments of quiet relief. As a practitioner, it's important to remain silent and let the visit develop organically.

Molly Johnson, BS, KPA CTP, CHES
Owner, Consultant, & Trainer
Canine Comfort, LLC

CULTURAL APPLICATIONS

There is great diversity in culturally held attitudes about animals, especially pets, both among cultures and within them (Chandler, 2017). To understand the various attitudes about animals, it is important to consider the evolution of the domestication of animals and their role in society. Historically, only royalty and the wealthy were able to keep companion animals. Also significant is the influence of religious beliefs; for example, in some religions, cows are considered to be sacred and dogs are considered to be unclean.

Before implementing AAT, it is vital to be aware of and consider the influence of cultural and personal attitudes about animals. Although one cannot stereotype people's views of animals based on their ethnic or cultural backgrounds, it is important to be aware of the possibility of cultural differences. For example,

Koreans in their native country rarely have cats or dogs as pets because they have been viewed for a long time as a source of food (Chandler, 2017). In contrast, European Americans have integrated cats and dogs into their family system as pets for hundreds of years. Native Americans, on the other hand, may allow their cats and dogs to roam freely, and members of their community share in caring for the animals. Moreover, these animals may never be spayed or neutered, out of respect for the animals' purpose and spirit (Chandler, 2017).

The interest in AAT has grown around the world, following the United States. The Animals Asia Foundation introduced the Dr. Dog program in Hong Kong, China, the Philippines, Japan, India, and Taiwan, with more than 300 dogs visiting hospitals and schools. In Japan, the Companion Animal Partnership Program was developed by the Japan Animal Hospital Association in 1986. It is the most well-known and largest AAT program in Japan with AAT teams visiting schools, nursing homes, and hospitals. In fact, multiple studies examining the impact of AAT and AAA on older patients have been conducted in Japan (Kanamori et al., 2001; Kawamura et al., 2009; Mano et al., 2003).

In India, Saraswathi Kendra—in collaboration with the Blue Cross of India— pioneered the use of AAT for children with autism beginning in 1996; in 2001, Dr. Dog AAT programs were introduced in schools and nursing homes (Krishna, 2009). Also in India, Minal Kavishwar and therapy dog Kutty were the first registered therapy dog team. Kavishwar founded the Animal Angels Foundation of India, the first in the country to consist of mental health professionals who provide AAT for special-needs children in schools, hospitals, and psychiatric settings. This organization is also active in disaster response (Chandler, 2017). Perspectives on the use of AAT in Taiwan are included in Sidebar 14.1 and its use in Brazil is included in Sidebar 14.2.

Sidebar 14.1 *Animal-Assisted Care in Long-Term Care Facilities in Taiwan*

Jing-Jy Sellin Wang and Miaofen Yen

Within the Oriental culture, especially from the older generation's point of view, there are some taboos about the interaction between humans and animals; thus, compared to the West, using animals in the treatment of human health can be restricted. For example, although relationships with cats can be very intimate in the West, many Taiwanese believe that cats have nine lives with negative meanings. Some superstitions say that cats can reduce a person's *yang spirit*. After one's death, the corpse would have a negative resonance with the cat. Moreover, there are legends, such as if a black cat jumps over a dead body, within 7 days, the body will be resurrected. Sometimes these legends make workers or older patients in long-term care facilities fearful. In addition, although a dog is very loyal, Taiwan is an island country, which may cause public environmental health problems due to the humidity, such as when an animal touches human skin. Having dogs is only suitable for the home. As a result, the most widely accepted animals in long-term care facilities are fish and birds. System planning and targeted use of animal

(continued)

Sidebar 14.1 *Animal-Assisted Care in Long-Term Care Facilities in Taiwan (continued)*

intervention can help the older subject, and professionals assist residents in long-term care facilities through breeding fish and birds. This can modestly enhance residents' physiological, psychological, and spiritual well-being.

During her graduate studies, Jing-Yi Lee completed a thesis focused on the use of fish-assisted care in long-term care facilities. In her study, 60 people with normal cognitive function were included. Older residents were selected from the same facility and randomly assigned to an experimental group and a control group of 30 individuals each.

Those in the experimental group were each given a small plastic fish tank containing water, plants, 12 guppies, and a fish feedbox to keep in their rooms. Institutional caregivers assisted residents with changing the water weekly, and residents had to feed the fish, observe them, and record their observations daily. Residents also participated in a weekly half-hour group-sharing session. If caregivers found dead fish, they secretly replaced them with new fish when the resident was not in the room. However, if residents found dead fish by themselves, caregivers helped them replace these with new fish immediately and record the incident. Those in the control group were each given a small plastic fish tank with water and plants to keep in their rooms. They were required to take care of and observe the plants and to record and share their observations. The residents of both groups lived on the same floor but in different rooms. After 3 months of intervention, the measures of quality of life, self-esteem, vitality, and sense of self-control within the experimental group were better than in the control group. In addition, the level of depression was significantly lower in the experimental group than in the control group. Clearly, the experimental group had a meaningful experience of life and expectations in the weekly sharing. According to residents, "Now breeding [these] fish is like raising children, so you have to take care [of] them very carefully, and sometime[s] you will worry that they eat not enough or the water is too dirty . . ."; "Breeding a fish as treating a woman, need attentive care . . ."; "I become very busy since I have [been] breeding fish daily . . ."; "Every day I look at my fish and worry about whether there is a dead fish or not, because it will infect [the] to other fish. Also, I compare with other people to see if I keep them well . . ."; "I am very happy when the fish give birth." A resident of the control group said, "I also want to have fish, because friends who breed fish become more active."

Another example is of an 80-year-old man with dementia who was agitated and aggressive. The resident and caregivers received health services in the Dementia Care Clinic at the university hospital, and the caregiver indicated that the subject had serious problem behaviors. Due to severe delusion, the resident did not sleep at night. After an interview, it was discovered that the resident had loved birds in the past. Therefore, the suggestion was given to the caregiver to purchase a birdcage and help the resident breed a parrot. Because this resident was in a middle stage of dementia, his caregiver had to help with feeding the bird, changing the water, and cleaning up. The birdcage was hung at the resident's eye level, and he was encouraged to speak to the bird and to teach the bird to say "hello" and "thank you." Daily, after breakfast, the music of bird voices was

Sidebar 14.1 *Animal-Assisted Care in Long-Term Care Facilities in Taiwan (continued)*

played so that the subject could listen to this music with the bird. Caregivers were encouraged to write down their observations of interactions between the resident and bird and to note any changes in problem behaviors. After 3 months of the bird-assisted care intervention, it was reported that the subject's problem behaviors had improved, and he had become less irritable. Due to the focus on the interactions with the bird during the day, the resident could fall asleep at night. Clearly, the resident's quality of life was enhanced when he developed a close link with the bird. Thus, it was demonstrated that animal-assisted measures could be useful for older people or those with dementia and problem behaviors.

Sidebar 14.2 *A Pet Therapy Project in a Brazilian Hospital*

Pediatric Oncology Unit

Isabel Rossato[a], Paula Eustáquio[a], Amália de Fátima Lucena[b], Lisiane Pruinelli[b]

In Brazil, as well as in other places in the world, pet therapy has been increasingly used as a way to provide patients with pleasure and happiness and thus enable better conditions for the improvement and recovery of their health challenges. The presence of animals surrounded by adequate health and hygiene care is permitted in several hospitals, such as the Hospital de Clínicas de Porto Alegre, located in southern Brazil. In this hospital, one of several playful therapeutic projects is the Pet Project, which was recently implemented and is offered to pediatric oncology patients. The activities are provided in a therapeutic recreation room for patients and family members once a month. For the Pet Project, a dog that is accompanied by a trainer and up to date with immunizations and a recent bath is transported in a suitable box to the therapeutic recreation room. During the dog visit day, the medical and nursing teams are advised of the visit, and children who have conditions that can receive the dog visit are allowed to interact with the dog.

Once in the therapeutic recreation room, the trainer removes the dog from the box so that children can cuddle and watch and participate in games played by the dog and its trainer. Children are instructed to sanitize their hands with alcohol gel every time they have contact with the dog. Preliminary results of this interaction among the dog, trainer, and patient demonstrate that the hospital environment becomes lighter, happier, and relaxed, reducing solitude and inhibition of patients, with improvement in their interpersonal relationships and social behavior. These benefits also extend to caregivers/family members and health professionals involved in the treatment of these children, who are subjected to suffering caused by witnessing childhood illness.

[a]Pet Therapy Project Developers
[b]Sidebar Writing Collaborators.

Future Considerations: Animal-Assisted Training With Animal Robots

A new frontier in animal robotics opens a vast array of opportunities to implement AAT in diverse populations. Robotic animals may be just as clinically effective as real animals, repeatedly washed with hospital-grade cleaners, and especially useful in limited-resource settings. Recent studies have evaluated the use of animal robots in dementia and long-term care environments. Results indicate that AAT with robots can improve reality orientation, attention span, and communication; eliminate the sense of isolation; reduce stress and anxiety; promote positive social interactions; and enhance the overall quality of life (Hung et al., 2019; Park et al, 2020). Despite early promise, the study of AAT with robots in clinical settings is still in its infancy.

The ICU is one understudied clinical area in which animal robots may be particularly beneficial. Due to the severity of illness associated with critical care, the use of highly technological equipment, and heightened concern for infection control and patient safety, AAT with live animals has not been widely adopted in the ICU (Hetland et al., 2017).

Investigators at the University of Nebraska Medical Center are currently conducting a quasi-experimental, pretest–posttest pilot study to evaluate the feasibility, acceptability, safety, and preliminary therapeutic treatment effects of PARO™, a baby harp seal, during ICU rehabilitation sessions. PARO™ (which means personal robot in the Japanese language) is an advanced interactive medical robot that has five kinds of sensors (tactile, light, audition, temperature, posture) and the ability to perceive people and its environment (Peluso et al., 2018). Preliminary results indicate that PARO™ is feasible and acceptable to use in the ICU, and AAT using robot animals will elicit similar positive effects as AAT with live animals in this population (Wawers et al., 2021). Of note, prior to conducting the study, investigators performed a laboratory bioburden challenge to ensure the robot could be cleaned to appropriate inpatient infection control standards. Results of the challenge showed that the cleaning protocols remarkably decreased the infection risk associated with the clinical use of an animal robot, and therefore, when cleaned correctly, PARO™ is considered safe to use with patients in the ICU (Hetland et al., 2019).

FUTURE RESEARCH

Although there has been great enthusiasm for AAT and a proliferation of therapy teams worldwide, these interventions often lack evidence to support their efficacy (Arkow, 2015). Most research to date supports AAT as making a significant contribution to the quality of life for patients of all ages and a variety of physical and psychological health conditions; however, most studies tend to have small sample sizes and lack adequate control groups (Fine, 2019). Investigations are needed that use random assignment to an AAT intervention group and a standard care group to determine which intervention led to the better outcome. Explorations are also needed to examine the physiological mechanisms contributing to the positive effects of AAT on specific conditions, as well as the duration and frequency of AAT needed to provide maximum improvements. For example, because cardiovascular disease is the leading cause of death in the United States, the role of AAT within cardiovascular disease–prevention programs needs to be examined. Additional research is needed to help identify which patients would most benefit from AAT. Furthermore, it is important that all research results are reported, even nonsignificant findings, as it is critical to know which conditions and contexts do not benefit participants through the use of AAT (Rodriguez et al., 2021).

Studies are needed to examine the relationships among the AAT team, patients, and staff in creating healing environments. Further research is needed in settings such as schools, homeless shelters, outpatient clinics, and community health agencies. Additional work is necessary to examine the ethical use, potential fatigue, and healthcare needs of animals used for AAT. Given that animals have no voice in this intervention, it is imperative that their human companions ensure their physical and emotional well-being (Ng et al., 2019). Nurses can take the lead in advocating for the appropriate use of AAT in their healthcare and school settings.

WEBSITES

ALLIANCE OF THERAPY DOGS

www.therapydogs.com/alliance-therapy-dogs

The Alliance of Therapy Dogs (ATD) is a volunteer organization of dedicated therapy dog handlers and their dogs on a mission of sharing smiles and joy. ATD's goal is to provide registration, support, and insurance for members who are involved in volunteer AAAs. These activities include visits to hospitals, special needs centers, schools, nursing homes, and airports. ATD teams may choose to be members of local therapy dog groups. They may also participate in nationwide therapy dog initiatives with organizations such as the Red Cross and Reading Education Assistance Dogs (R.E.A.D.).

AMERICAN HIPPOTHERAPY ASSOCIATION

www.americanhippotherapyassociation.org

The mission of the American Hippotherapy Association is to educate and promote excellence in the field of equine-assisted therapy. This organization promotes the use of the movement of a horse as a treatment strategy in physical, occupational, and speech therapy sessions for individuals living with disabilities.

AMERICAN VETERINARY MEDICAL ASSOCIATION

www.avma.org/KB/Policies/Pages/default.aspx

Established in 1863, the American Veterinary Medical Association recognizes and promotes the importance of the human–animal bond through clinical practice, service, and research. The policy section of this website includes guidelines for AAA, AAT, and resident animal programs, including key definitions, guiding principles, preventive medical and behavioral strategies, and wellness guidelines.

ANIMAL BEHAVIOR INSTITUTE

www.animaledu.com

The Animal Behavior Institute (ABI) was founded in 2004 by Dr. Gary Fortier and Dr. Janis Hammer to prepare adult students for careers in animal behavior. The ABI provides AAT certificate programs that require the completion of

15 academic credits (online) and 40 hours of hands-on field experience. On graduation, students may use the designation of certified animal-assisted therapy professional (CAATP). The ABI is accredited by the International Association for
Continuing Education and Training.

CENSHARE: CENTER TO STUDY HUMAN–ANIMAL RELATIONSHIPS AND ENVIRONMENTS

www.censhare.umn.edu

Established in 1981, CENSHARE has become a national leader in promoting
health and quality of life for individuals and animals through behavior research,
educational opportunities, and a forum for public policymaking. CENSHARE is a
multidisciplinary group of individuals from the University of Minnesota and the
surrounding community dedicated to studying and improving human–animal
relationships and environments.

EQUINE-ASSISTED GROWTH AND LEARNING ASSOCIATION

www.eagala.org

Equine-Assisted Growth and Learning Association (EAGALA) is dedicated
to improving the mental health of individuals, families, and groups around the
world by setting the standard of excellence in equine-assisted psychotherapy and
equine-assisted learning, also known as *horse therapy* or *equine therapy*. EAGALA
is the largest professional association for equine therapy and has a comprehensive
training and certification program to learn the EAGALA model of equine-assisted
psychotherapy. EAGALA also provides a specialized program for service members, veterans, and their families who are dealing with life challenges, including
the treatment of PTSD, traumatic brain injury, depression, and anxiety.

HUMAN–ANIMAL BOND RESEARCH INSTITUTE

www.habri.org

The Human–Animal Bond Research Institute (HABRI) is a national research
and education nonprofit foundation dedicated to promoting the positive role animals play in the health and well-being of people, families, and communities. This
institute works to educate, inform, advocate, and support research and funding
for human–animal-related initiatives. HABRI is an online hub that archives evidence on the benefits of the human–animal bond and is maintained by Purdue
University under the direction of Dr. Alan Beck. The information focuses on
human and animal health, AAT, and public policy.

PET PARTNERS (FORMERLY DELTA SOCIETY)

www.petpartners.org

In 1977, the Delta Foundation was created in Portland, Oregon, under the
direction of Michael McCulloch, MD. In 1981, the name was changed to Delta
Society, and in 2012 the name Delta Society was changed to Pet Partners to clearly
reflect its mission, which is to improve human health through positive interactions with therapy, service, and companion animals. Pet Partners volunteers visit
hospitals, hospices, schools, and veterans' centers with their animals to provide

comfort to people in need. The Pet Partners Program provides comprehensive standardized training in animal-assisted activities and therapy for volunteers and healthcare professionals. With more than 10,000 registered teams, it is the largest nonprofit organization that registers handlers of multiple species as volunteer teams to provide AAT. Dogs, cats, rabbits, horses, birds, and llamas are eligible for evaluation through Pet Partners.

READING EDUCATION ASSISTANCE DOGS

https://therapyanimals.org/read/

The mission of the R.E.A.D. program is to improve the literacy skills of children through the assistance of a registered therapy team as literacy mentors. The R.E.A.D. program improves a child's reading and communication skills by employing a powerful method—reading to an animal. This program was begun by Intermountain Therapy Animals in 1999 in Salt Lake City, Utah. Today, more than 3,500 therapy teams have been trained and registered with the R.E.A.D. program and work throughout the United States, Canada, Italy, Finland, France, Norway, Slovenia, South Africa, Spain, and Sweden.

THERAPET: ANIMAL-ASSISTED THERAPY

www.therapet.org

Therapet was founded in 1998 by an occupational therapist in Texas to provide AAT in a rehabilitation center. Therapet is a nonprofit foundation whose mission is to use specially trained and certified animals to promote health, hope, and healing. Therapet assists with the establishment of AAT programs throughout the United States and provides education for healthcare professionals, along with AAT training and evaluation of animal and human volunteers.

THERAPY DOGS INTERNATIONAL

www.tdi-dog.org

TDI is the oldest registry for therapy dogs in the United States. In 2012, there were 24,750 dog/handler teams registered with TDI. Founded in 1976 by Elaine Smith—an American RN who observed the benefits of pets in the healthcare setting during a visit to England—TDI is dedicated to the regulation, testing, selection, and registration of qualified dogs and handlers for the purpose of visitations to hospitals, nursing homes, facilities, or any place where therapy dogs are needed. Since the 1995 bombing of the Murrah Federal Building in Oklahoma City, Oklahoma, TDI has provided disaster stress relief dog teams in such places as New York City during the September 11, 2001, attack on the World Trade Center and New Orleans, Louisiana, during Hurricane Katrina in 2005.

WE CAN RIDE

https://www.wecanride.org/

Established in 1982, We Can Ride is the oldest and largest therapeutic riding program in Minnesota. Its mission is to connect humans and horses to transform the lives of individuals with disabilities and to meet the needs of the community.

We Can Ride provides equine-assisted activities such as therapeutic riding, hippotherapy, and equine-assisted therapy for individuals with disabilities or special needs.

ACKNOWLEDGMENT

The author sincerely thanks Breanna Hetland PhD, RN, CCRN-K for her contributions in this chapter addressing the innovative use of animal robots. The author also gratefully thanks her therapy dog, Libby, for showing her the true value of AAT.

REFERENCES

Ahmad, H., Ahmad, M., Jabbir, F., Ahmar, S., Ahmad, N., Elokil, A., & Chen, J. (2020). The domestication makeup: Evolution, survival and challenges. *Frontiers in Ecology and Evolution, 8*(103). https://www.frontiersin.org/articles/10.3389/fevo.2020.00103/full

Altschiller, D. (2011). *Animal-assisted therapy.* Greenwood.

American Disabilities Act National Network. (2017). Service animals. https://adata.org/factsheet/service-animals

American Kennel Club. (2021). *Canine good citizen: The official AKC guide.* Fox Chapel Publishing.

American Veterinary Medical Association. (2018). *U.S. pet ownership & demographics sourcebook.* https://www.avma.org/

American Veterinary Medical Association. (2021a). *Animal-assisted interventions: Definitions.* https://www.avma.org/KB/Policies/Pages/Animal-Assisted-Interventions-Definitions.aspx

American Veterinary Medical Association. (2021b). *Animal-assisted interventions: Guidelines.* https://www.avma.org

Anderson, D., & Brown, S. (2021). The effect of animal-assisted therapy on nursing student anxiety: A randomized control study. *Nursing Education in Practice, 52,* 103042. https://doi.org/10.1016/j.nepr.2021.103042

Arkow, P. (2015). *Animal-assisted therapy and activities: A study and research resource guide for the use of companion animals in animal-assisted interventions* (11th ed.). Animal Therapy.net.

Arnon, S., Fisher, P., Pickover, A., Lowell, A., Turner, J., Hilburn, A., Jacob-McVey, J., Malajian, B., Farber, D., Hamilton, J., Hamilton, A., Markowitz, J., & Neria, Y. (2020). Equine-assisted therapy for veterans with PTSD: Manual development and preliminary findings. *Military Medicine, 185*(5–6), e557–e564. https://doi.org/10.1093/milmed/usz444

Banks, M., & Banks, W. (2002). The effects of animal-assisted therapy on loneliness in an elderly population in long-term care facilities. *Journal of Gerontology, 57*(7), 428–432. https://doi.org/10.1093/gerona/57.7.M428

Barker, S., Barker, R., McCain, N., & Schubert C. (2016). A randomized cross-over exploratory study of the effect of visiting therapy dogs on college student stress before final exams. *Anthrozoos, 29*(1), 35–46. https://doi.org/10.1080/08927936.2015.1069988

Barker, S., Knisely, J., Schubert, C., Green, J., & Ameringer, S. (2015). The effect of an animal-assisted intervention on anxiety and pain in hospitalized children. *Anthrozoos, 28*(1), 101–112. https://doi.org/10.2752/089279315X14129350722091

Barker, S., Pandurangi, A., & Best, A. (2003). Effects of animal-assisted therapy on patients' anxiety, fear, and depression before ECT. *Journal of Electroconvulsive Therapy, 19*(1), 38–44. https://doi.org/10.1097/00124509-200303000-00008

Barker, S., Vokes, R., & Barker, R. (2019). *Animal-assisted interventions in health care settings: A best practices manual for establishing new programs.* Purdue University Press.

Beck, C., Gonzales, F., Sells, C., Jones, C., Reer, T., Wasilewski, S., & Zhu, Y. (2012, April–June). The effects of animal-assisted therapy on wounded warriors in an occupational therapy life skills program. *Army Medical Department Journal, 2012,* 38–45. http://www.cs.amedd.army.mil/amedd_journal.aspx

Becker, M. (2002). *The healing power of pets: Harnessing the amazing ability of pets to make and keep people happy and healthy*. Hyperion.

Boldig, C., & Butala, N. (2021). Pet therapy as a nonpharmacological treatment option for neurological disorders: A review of the literature. *Cureus, 13*(7), e16167. https://doi.org/10.7759/cureus.16167

Braun, C., Stangler, T., Narveson, J., & Pettingell, S. (2009). Animal-assisted therapy as a pain relief intervention for children. *Complementary Therapies in Clinical Practice, 15*, 105–109. https://doi.org/10.1016/j.ctcp.2009.02.008

Catala, A., Grandgeorge, M., Schaff, J., Cousillas, H., Hausberger, M., & Cattet, J. (2019). Dogs demonstrate the existence of an epileptic seizure odour in humans. *Scientific Reports, 9*, 4103. https://doi.org/10.1038/s41598-019-40721-4

Centers for Disease Control and Prevention. (2015). *Guidelines for environmental infection control in healthcare facilities*. https://www.cdc.gov/infectioncontrol/guidelines/environmental/background/animals.html

Chandler, C. (2017). *Animal-assisted therapy in counseling*. Routledge.

Chubak, J., Hawkes, R., Dudzik, C., Foose-Foster, J., Eaton, L., Johnson, R., & Macpherson, C. (2017). Pilot study of therapy dog visits for inpatient youth with cancer. *Journal of Pediatric Oncology Nursing, 34*(5), 331–341. https://doi.org/10.1177/1043454217712983

Clark, S., Martin, F., McGowan, R., Smidt, J., Anderson, R., Wang, L., Turpin, T., Langenfeld-McCoy, N., Bauer, B., & Mohabbat, A. (2020). The impact of a 20-minute animal-assisted activity session on the physiological and emotional states in patients with fibromyalgia. *Mayo Clinic Proceedings, 95*(11), 2442–2461. https://doi.org/10.1016/j.mayocp.2020.04.037

Cole, K., Gawlinski, A., Steers, N., & Kotlerman, J. (2007). Animal-assisted therapy in patients hospitalized with heart failure. *American Journal of Critical Care, 16*(6), 575–585. https://doi.org/10.4037/ajcc2007.16.6.575

Dalton, K., Waite, K., Ruble, K., Carroll, K., DeLone, A., Frankenfield, P., Serpell, J., Thorpe, R., Morris, D., Agnew, J., Rubenstein, R., & Davis, M. (2020). Risks associated with animal-assisted intervention programs: A literature review. *Complementary Therapies in Clinical Practice, 39*, 101145. https://doi.org/10.1016/j.ctcp.2020.101145

De Assis, G., Schlichting, T., Mateus, B., Lemos, A., & Santos, A. (2021). Physical therapy with hippotherapy compared to physical therapy alone in children with cerebral palsy: Systematic review and meta-analysis. *Developmental Medicine and Child Neurology, 64*(3). https://doi.org/10.1111/dmcn.15042

Delta Society. (1996). *Standards of practice for animal-assisted activities and animal-assisted therapy*.

Ein, N., Li, L., & Vickers, K. (2018). The effect of pet therapy on the physiological and subjective stress response: A meta-analysis. *Stress Health, 34*(4), 477–489. https://doi.org/10.1002/smi.2812

Epilepsy Foundation. (2019). *Facts about seizure and epilepsy*. https://www.epilepsy.com/learn/about-epilepsy-basics/facts-about-seizures-and-epilepsy

Erich, M., Quinlan-Colwell, A., & O'Conner-Von, S. (2021). Distraction and relaxation. In M. Cooney & A. Quinlan-Colwell (Eds.), *Assessment and multimodal management of pain* (pp. 586–612). Elsevier.

Feng, Y., Lin, Y., Zhang, N., Jiang, X., & Zhang, L. (2021). Effects of animal-assisted therapy on hospitalized children and teenagers: A systematic review and meta-analysis. *Journal of Pediatric Nursing, 60*, 11–23. https://doi.org/10.1016/j.pedn.2021.01.020

Fike, L., Najera, C., & Dougherty, D. (2012, April–June). Occupational therapists as dog handlers: The collective experience with animal-assisted therapy in Iraq. *Army Medical Department Journal, 2012*, 51–54. http://www.cs.amedd.army.mil/amedd_journal.aspx

Fine, A. (2019). *Handbook on animal-assisted therapy: Foundations and guidelines for animal-assisted interventions* (5th ed.). Academic Press.

Fine, A., & Beck, A. (2019). Understanding our kinship with animals: Input for health care professionals interested in the human-animal bond. In A. Fine (Ed.), *Handbook on animal-assisted therapy: Foundations and guidelines for animal-assisted interventions* (pp. 3–12). Academic Press.

Fontaine, K. (2015). *Complementary & alternative therapies for nursing practice*. Pearson.

Friedmann, E., Katcher, A., Lynch, J., & Thomas, S. (1980). Animal companions and one-year survival of patients after discharge from a coronary care unit. *Public Health Reports, 95*(4), 307–312. https://www.jstor.org/stable/4596316

Friedmann, E., & Thomas, S. (1995). Pet ownership, social support, and one-year survival after acute myocardial infarction in the Cardiac Arrhythmia Suppression Trial (CAST). *American Journal of Cardiology, 76*, 1213–1217. https://doi.org/10.1016/S0002-9149(99)80343-9

Gasalberti, D. (2006). Alternative therapies for children and youth with special health care needs. *Journal of Pediatric Health Care, 20*(2), 133–136. https://doi.org/10.1016/j.pedhc.2005.12.015

Grandin, T., Fine, A., O'Haire, M., Carlisle, G., & Gabriels, R. (2019). The roles of animals for individuals with Autism Spectrum Disorder. In A. Fine (Ed.), *Handbook on animal-assisted therapy: Foundations and guidelines for animal-assisted interventions* (pp. 285–298). Academic Press.

Havey, J., Vlasses, F., Vlasses, P., Ludwig-Beymer, P., & Hackbarth, D. (2014). The effect of animal-assisted therapy on pain management use after joint replacement. *Anthrozoos, 27*(3), 361–369. https://doi.org/10.2752/175303714X13903827487962

Hetland, B., Bailey, T., & Prince-Paul, M. (2017). Animal assisted interactions to alleviate psychological symptoms in patients on mechanical ventilation. *Journal of Hospice and Palliative Nursing, 19*(6), 516–523. https://doi.org/10.1097/NJH.0000000000000391

Hetland, B., Heusinkvelt, J., Rupp, M., Fey, P., Murphy, C., Gillett, G., Micheels, T., & Baker, M. (2019, October). *Effectiveness of cleaning protocols for therapeutic animal robot used in the intensive care unit* [Poster presentation]. The Nursing Research and EBP Conference Cyberspace: The Next Nursing Frontier, Sioux Falls, SD.

Hung, L., Liu, C, Woldum E., Au-Yeung, A., Berndt, A., Wallsworth, C., Horne, N., Gregorio, M., Mann, J., & Chaudhury, H. (2019). The benefits of and barriers to using a social robot PARO in care settings: A scoping review. *BMC Geriatrics, 19*(1), 232. https://doi.org/10.1186/s12877-019-1244-6

International Association of Human-Animal Interaction Organizations. (2018). *IAHAIO White paper: The IAHAIO definitions for animal-assisted intervention and guidelines for wellness of animals involved*. https://iahaio.org/best-practice/white-paper-on-animal-assisted-interventions/

Johnson, R., & Meadows, R. (2010). Dog walking: Motivation for adherence to a walking program. *Clinical Nursing Research, 19*(4), 387–402. https://doi.org/10.1177/1054773810373122

Kanamori, M., Suzuki, M., Yamamoto, K., Kanda, M., Matsui, Y., Kojima, E., Fukawa, H., Sugita, T., & Oshiro, H. (2001). A day care program and evaluation of animal-assisted therapy for the elderly with senile dementia. *American Journal of Alzheimer's Disease & Other Dementias, 16*(4), 234–239. https://doi.org/10.1177/153331750101600409

Kawamura, N., Niiyama, M., & Niiyama, H. (2009). Animal-assisted activity experiences of institutionalized Japanese older adults. *Journal of Psychosocial Nursing, 47*(1), 41–47. https://doi.org/10.3928/02793695-20090101-08

Kim, S., Nam, Y., Ham, M., Park, C., Moon, M., & Yoo, D. (2021). Neurological mechanisms of animal-assisted intervention in Alzheimer's Disease: A hypothetical review. *Frontiers in Aging Neuroscience, 13*, 682308. https://doi.org/10.3389/fnagi.2021.682308

Krause-Parello, C., & Kolassa, J. (2016). Pet therapy: Enhancing social and cardiovascular wellness in community dwelling older adults. *Journal of Community Health Nursing, 33*(1), 1–10. https://doi.org/10.1080/07370016.2016.1120587

Krishna, N. (2009). *Dr. Dog—A programme for children with autism*. http://www.autismindia.com

Lai, N., Chang, S., Ng, S., Tan, S., Chaiyakunapruk, N., & Stanaway, F. (2019). Animal-assisted therapy for dementia. *Cochrane Database of Systematic Reviews, 11*, CD013243. https://doi.org/10.1002/14651858.CD013243.pub.2

Lust, E., Ryan-Haddad, A., Coover, K., & Snell, J. (2007). Measuring clinical outcomes of animal-assisted therapy: Impact on resident medication usage. *Consultant Pharmacist, 22*(7), 580–585. https://doi.org/10.4140/TCP.n.2007.580

Macauley, B. (2006). Animal-assisted therapy for persons with aphasia: A pilot study. *Journal of Rehabilitation Research & Development, 43*(3), 357–366. https://doi.org/10.1682/JRRD.2005.01.0027

Mano, M., Uchizono, M., & Nishimura, T. (2003). A trial of dog-assisted therapy for elderly people with Alzheimer's disease. *Journal of Japanese Society for Dementia Care, 2*, 150–157. https://doi .org/10.3390/ijerph17165713

Martin, F., & Farnum, J. (2002). Animal-assisted therapy for children with pervasive developmental disorders. *Western Journal of Nursing Research, 24*(6), 657–670. https://doi .org/10.1177/0193945023205555403

Moretti, F., DeRonchi, D., Bernabel, V., Marchetti, L., Ferrari, B., Forlani, C., & Atti, A. (2011). Pet therapy in elderly patients with mental illness. *Psychogeriatrics, 11*, 125–129. https://doi .org/10.1111/j.1479-8301.2010.00329.x

Murthy, R., Bearman, G., Brown, S., Bryant, K., Chinn, R., Hewlett, A., George, B., Goldstein, E., Holzman-Pazgal, G., Rupp, M., Wiemker, T., Weese, J., & Weber, D. (2015). Animals in health-care facilities: Recommendations to minimize potential risks. *Infection Control & Hospital Epidemiology, 36*(5), 495–516. https://doi.org/10.1017/ice.2015.15

Ng, Z., Albright, J., Fine, A., & Peralta, J. (2019). Our ethical and moral responsibility: Ensuring the welfare of therapy animals. In A. Fine (Ed.), *Handbook on animal-assisted therapy: Foundations and guidelines for animal-assisted interventions* (pp. 175–198). Academic Press.

Nightingale, F. (1860). Chattering hopes and advices. In *Notes on nursing: What it is and what it is not*. D. Appleton and Company. [American First Edition]. https://digital.library.upenn.edu/ women/nightingale/nursing/nursing.html#XII

Odendaal, J. (2000). Animal-assisted therapy: Magic or medicine? *Journal of Psychosomatic Research, 49*, 275–280. https://doi.org/10.1016/S0022-3999(00)00183-5

Odendaal, J., & Meintjes, R. (2003). Neurophysiological correlates of affiliative behavior between humans and dogs. *Veterinary Journal, 165*(3), 296–301. https://doi.org/10.1016/ S1090-0233(02)00237-X

O'Haire, M. (2017). Research on animal-assisted intervention and autism spectrum disorder, 2012–2015. *Applied Developmental Science, 21*(3), 200–216. https://doi.org/10.1080/10888691.20 16.1243988

Olsen, C., Pedersen, I., Bergland, A., Enders-Slegers, M., Patil, G., & Ihlebaek, C. (2016). Effect of animal-assisted interventions on depression, agitation and quality of life in nursing home residents suffering from cognitive impairment or dementia: A cluster randomized controlled trial. *International Journal of Geriatric Psychiatry, 31*(12), 1312–1321. https://doi.org/10.1002/ gps.4436

Park, S., Bak, A., Kim, S., Nam, Y., Kim, H., Yoo, D., & Moon M. (2020). Animal-assisted and pet-robot interventions for ameliorating behavioral and psychological symptoms of dementia: A systematic review and meta-analysis. *Biomedicines, 8*(6), 150. https://doi.org/10.3390/ biomedicines8060150

Peluso, S., de Rosa, A., de Lucia, N., Antenora, A., Illario, M., Esposito, M., & de Michele, G. (2018). Animal-assisted therapy in elderly patients: Evidence and controversies in dementia and psychiatric disorders and future perspectives in other neurological diseases. *Journal of Geriatric Psychiatry and Neurology, 31*(3), 149–157. https://doi.org/10.1177/0891988718774634

Perez-Gomez, J., Amigo-Gamero, H., Collado-Mateo, D., Barrios-Fernandez, S., Munoz-Bermejo, L., Garcia-Gordillo, M., Carlos-Vivas, J., & Adsuar, J. (2020). Equine-assisted activities and therapies in children with attention-deficit/hyperactivity disorder: A systematic review. *Journal of Psychiatric and Mental Health Nursing, 28.* https://doi.org/10.1111/jpm.12710

Pet Partners. (2018). *Standards of practice in animal-assisted interventions.*

Porter-Wenzlaff, L. (2007). Finding their voice: Developing emotional, cognitive, and behavioral congruence in female abuse survivors through equine facilitated therapy. *Explore, 3*(5), 529– 534. https://doi.org/10.1016/j.explore.2007.07.016

Powell, L., Edwards, K., McGreevy, P., Bauman, A., Podberscek, A., Neilly, B., Sherrington, C., & Stamatakis, E. (2019). Companion dog acquisition and mental well-being: A com-munity-based three-arm controlled study. *BMC Public Health, 19*, 1428 https://doi.org/ 10.1186/s12889-019-7770-5

Pruskowski, K., Gurney, J., & Cancio, L. (2020). Impact of the implementation of a therapy dog program on burn center patients and staff. *Burns, 46*, 293–297. https://doi.org/10.1016/j .burns.2019.11.024

Reddekopp, J., Dell, C. A., Rohr, B., Fornssler, B., Gibson, M., Carey, B., & Stempien, J. (2020). Patient opinion on visiting therapy dogs in a hospital emergency department. *International Journal of Environmental Research and Public Health, 17*(8), 2968. https://doi.org/10.3390/ijerph17082968

Rivera, M. (2010). *On dogs and dying: Inspirational stories from hospice hounds.* Purdue University Press.

Rodrigo-Claverol, M., Casanova-Gonzalvo, C., Malla-Clua, B., Rodrigo-Claverol, E., Jove-Naval, J., & Ortega-Bravo, M. (2019). Animal-assisted intervention improves pain perception in polymedicated geriatric patients with chronic joint pain: A clinical trial. *International Journal of Environmental Research and Public Health, 16*, 2843. https://doi.org/10.3390/ijerph16162843

Rodriguez, K., Herzog, H., & Gee, N. (2021). Variability in human–animal interaction research. *Frontiers in Veterinary Science, 7*, 619600. https://doi.org/1033389/fvets.2020.619600

Serpell, J. (2019). Animal-assisted interventions in historical perspective. In A. Fine (Ed.), *Handbook on animal-assisted therapy: Foundations and guidelines for animal-assisted interventions* (pp. 13–22). Academic Press.

Sobo, E., Eng, B., & Kassity-Krich, N. (2006). Canine visitation (pet) therapy: Pilot data on decreases in child pain perception. *Journal of Holistic Nursing, 24*(1), 51–57. https://doi.org/10.1177/0898010105280112

Therapy Dogs International. (2021). *Mission statement and history.* http://www.tdi-dog.org

U. S. Department of Veterans Affairs. (2021). *How common is PTSD in veterans?* https://www.ptsd.va.gov/understand/common/common_veterans.asp

Veterans Moving Forward. (2020). *Mission and vision – Veterans Moving Forward.* vetsfwd.org

Vizek, V., Arambasic, L., Kerestes, G., Kuterovac, G., & Vlahovic-Stetic, V. (2001). Pet ownership in childhood and socio-emotional characteristics, work values and professional choices in early adulthood. *Anthrozoos, 14*(4), 224–231. https://doi.org/10.2752/089279301786999373

Wawers, A., Bach, C., Heusinkvelt, J., Moody, A., Kinsella, S., Haefner, H., Kupzyk, K., & Hetland, B. (2021, March). *Animal assisted interactions with an animal robot during physical and occupational therapy sessions in the pediatric ICU: A feasibility study* [Poster presentation]. Midwest Nursing Research Society Annual Conference, Kansas City, MO (Virtual).

Weil, A. (2021). *Animal assisted therapy.* https://www.drweil.com/health-wellness/balanced-living/wellness-therapies/animal-assisted-therapy/

Wesley, M., Minatrea, N., & Watson, J. (2009). Animal-assisted therapy in the treatment of substance dependence. *Anthrozoos, 22*(2), 137–148. https://doi.org/10.2752/175303709X434167

Wharton, T., Whitworth, J., Macauley, E., & Malone, E. (2019). Pilot testing a manualized equine-facilitated cognitive processing therapy (EF-CPT) intervention for PTSD in veterans. *Psychiatric Rehabilitation Journal, 42*(3), 268–276. https://doi.org/10.1037/prj0000359

Wolff, A., & Frishman, W. (2005). Animal-assisted therapy and cardiovascular disease. In W. Frishman, M. Weintraub, & M. Micozzi (Eds.), *Complementary and integrative therapies for cardiovascular disease* (pp. 362–368). Elsevier Mosby.

Wood, W., Fields, B., Rose, M., & McClure, M. (2017). Animal-assisted therapies and dementia: A systematic mapping review using the Lived Environment Life Quality (LELQ) Model. *American Journal of Occupational Therapy, 71*(5), 105190030p1–7105190030p10. https://doi.org/10.5014/ajot.2017.027219

World Health Organization. (2020). *Dementia.* https://www.who.int/news-room/fact-sheets/detail/dementia

Yakimicki, M., Edwards, N., Richards, E., & Beck, A. (2018). Animal-assisted intervention and dementia: A systematic review. *Clinical Nursing Research, 28*(1), 9–29. https://doi.org/10.3928/19404921-20210924-01

Yamamoto, M., & Hart, L. (2019). Living with assistance dogs and other animals: Their therapeutic roles and psychosocial health effects. In A. Fine (Ed.), *Handbook on animal-assisted therapy: Foundations and guidelines for animal-assisted interventions* (pp. 61–77). Academic Press.

Manipulative and Body-Based Therapies

KUEI-MIN CHEN

Manipulative and body-based therapies, as previously classified by the National Center for Complementary and Integrative Health (NCCIH), focus primarily on the structures and systems of the body, including the bones and joints, the soft tissues, and the circulatory and lymphatic systems. Massage (Chapter 15), tai chi (Chapter 16), and relaxation therapies (Chapter 17) are among the most commonly used manipulative and body-based practices in this category. Although not specifically included as a complementary therapy on the NCCIH website, exercise (Chapter 18) is a body-based practice (also shown to impact mood and cognition) that is often recommended by nurses to patients to include in their daily health regimens; hence, exercise is included in this section of the text. More recently, the NCCIH has classified complementary approaches by their primary therapeutic input pertaining to how a given therapy is delivered or how the therapy is taken in. According to the new classification, therapies in this section are categorized as psychological (relaxation therapies), physical (massage), and a combination of psychological and physical (tai chi; NCCIH, 2021). However, in this text, we have chosen to organize therapies in sections for the reader according to the 2018 NCCIH classification to better differentiate the sections and respective therapies, and in so doing, we highlight commonalities among the therapies within the categories of the 2018 classification.

Although a number of the manipulative and body-based therapies are administered by specially trained therapists such as chiropractors and massage therapists, a number of the procedures can be and are administered by nurses, particularly certain types of massage and relaxation therapies. Massage can range from simple hand or foot massage to back rubs or full-body massages, the latter provided by nurses who have been trained as massage therapists. Massage has had a long history in nursing and was included as a nursing intervention in many of the early nursing texts. A variety of massage techniques have been part of healthcare systems in many countries (e.g., Japan, China, Greece, Egypt, Italy). A large number of relaxation therapies exist, including progressive relaxation, guided imagery, and deep breathing exercises; nurses choose from among these to fit the needs and preferences of patients in managing various health problems.

Although tai chi could be classified as an energy therapy, it has been placed in this section because tai chi involves certain postures and gentle movements with mental focus, breathing, and relaxation. Tai chi classes are common in community settings and long-term care facilities. A growing body of scientific research has supported that practicing tai chi may help improve balance and stability in older adults and those with Parkinson's disease, reduce back pain and pain from knee osteoarthritis and fibromyalgia, and improve quality of life and mood in people with chronic illnesses. Exercise is a common nonpharmacological and nonsurgical method for health promotion and the relief of diseases and symptoms. Studies of exercise largely show positive physical and psychological responses such as reductions in depression, anxiety, and stress. Exercise as a manipulative and body-based therapy is a very important area of study since patients want to be self-empowered and want guidance on which form of exercise is the best. Nurses' knowledge of exercise and its application in multiple populations assists in the delivery of expert nursing care.

Nurses will find more uses and safety aspects for manipulative and body-based therapies as exploration grows and as these treatments are rigorously investigated with more conditions and populations, particularly children. Nurses need to improve their knowledge and skills regarding manipulative and body-based therapies so that they can become more confident in assisting patients to integrate conventional treatment and manipulative and body-based therapies for illness management. Nurses also need to be aware of therapies or nuances of these therapies that exist in other healthcare systems and cultures so that they can either include and accommodate preferences or use such practices in the plan of care. Additionally, nurses need to be aware of these therapies and well informed so that they can caution patients about their use if appropriate, because some may be contraindicated with specific illnesses or conditions.

REFERENCE

National Center for Complementary and Integrative Health. (2021). *Complementary, alternative, or integrative health: What's in a name?* https://www.nccih.nih.gov/health/complementary-alternative-or-integrative-health-whats-in-a-name

Massage

MELODEE HARRIS

Massage is a widely used complementary therapy that has been employed by nurses since the time of Florence Nightingale. Early nurse specialists in massage traced the history of massage in textbooks such as *The Theory and Practice of Massage* (Goodall-Copestake, 1919), *Massage: An Elementary Text-book for Nurses* (Macafee, 1917), *Fundamentals of Massage for Students of Nursing* (Jensen, 1932), and *A Textbook of Massage for Nurses and Beginners* (Rawlins, 1933). The authors devoted extensive histories of massage "to teach the student appreciation for the subject" (Jensen, 1932, p. v). Macafee (1917) wrote, "The history of massage is as old as that of man" (p. 5). Both Eastern and Western cultures are a part of the history of the traditional nursing practice of massage.

In 3000 BCE, the Chinese documented the use of massage in *Cong Fau of Tao-Tse*. There is evidence in *Sa-Tsai-Tou-Hoei*, written in 1000 BCE and published in the 16th century, that the Japanese also used massage (Calvert, 2002; Jensen, 1932). Goodall-Copestake (1919) records how massage is associated with ancient Hindu writings. The Japanese translated massage or shampooing as *amma*. Natives from the Sandwich Islands used *lomi-lomi*, the Maoris of New Zealand used the term *romi-romi*, and the natives of Tong Island used *toogi-toogi* to mean massage (Kellog, 1895, p. 12). The French word *masser*, or "to shampoo," was applied to massage (Goodall-Copestake, 1919, p. 1; Jensen, 1932, p. 20).

The Greeks and Romans influenced the use of massage in Western civilizations. Hippocrates, the Father of Medicine, incorporated massage into the practice of medicine. In 380 BCE, Hippocrates wrote, "A physician must be experienced in . . . rubbing" (Goodall-Copestake, 1919, p. 2). Galen used massage principles with gladiator students in Pergamos (Jensen, 1932; Rawlins, 1933). In 1813, Per Henrik Ling of Sweden developed Swedish massage movements at the Royal Central Institute of Stockholm. In 1860, Dr. Johan Mezger of Amsterdam used massage on King Frederick VII (then crown prince) of Denmark, and his success promoted the popularity of massage across Scandinavia, the Netherlands, and Germany (Jensen, 1932). Although throughout history it has been known as an art and a complementary/alternative therapy, the practice of massage continues to build on a robust foundation, and evidence-based practices related to massage are evolving. In the Western world, massage may be used to treat a disease or syndrome diagnosed by a healthcare provider. Eastern or Asian massage is recommended by Eastern medical providers to treat disharmony and imbalance in the human body (Massage Therapy Body of Knowledge [MTBOK Task Force], 2010; Wieting, 2020). Western massage may use effleurage, petrissage, tapotement, or deep friction (Wieting, 2020). Eastern massage practices include shiatsu and may combine several techniques (Wieting, 2020). Today, across all cultures, massage is a holistic intervention that uses the natural healing process to connect the body, mind, and spirit.

DEFINITION

Massage is a part of almost every civilization. The definition and meaning of *massage* are influenced and interpreted by culture and the healing philosophy of the predominant healthcare discipline.

The term *massage* is derived from the Greek word *massein*, which means "to knead" (Calvert, 2002). The Arabic word *mass* or *mash*, "to press softly," also means "massage" (Goodall-Copestake, 1919, p. 1). The definition of *massage* varies by discipline. Nursing was among the first disciplines to use massage. Physicians, physical therapists, massage therapists, and even cosmetologists use massage.

Physicians term *massage* as medical massage. The Greeks and Romans influenced physicians to use massage. Hippocrates used the word *friction* for massage in the treatment of sprains (Jensen, 1932). Norstroëm (1868/1896) claimed that the use of massage came from bonesetters. Today, massage is used widely by doctors of osteopathic medicine.

Massage is within the scope of practice of physical therapy, and therapists use it across many settings (American Physical Therapy Association [APTA], 2013). Physical therapists use massage in sports medicine to reduce pain, rehabilitate, and boost the physical performance of athletes (Brummitt, 2008).

According to the MTBOK Task Force (2010), massage therapists have a broad interpretation of massage. *Massage, body massage, body rub, somatic therapy,* and other similar terms are equivalent to massage therapy. The terms *massage therapy* and *bodywork* are often used interchangeably. The use of bodywork by massage therapists also includes a more holistic approach to enhance awareness of the mind–body–spirit connection. Clinical massage entails more extensive assessment and techniques focused on symptoms to mean treatment, orthopedic, and medical massage (MTBOK Task Force, 2010, p. 40).

Nurses may seek further education and eligibility requirements to become Board Certified in Therapeutic Massage and Bodywork (NCBTMB, 2021). Bedside nurses are taught to use effleurage or slow-stroke back massage that does not require a separate license or training beyond nursing school. More than any other healthcare discipline, nurses have adopted massage into their curricula. In 1932, the National League for Nursing Education recommended 15 hours of lecture and training in massage for a nursing curriculum (Ruffin, 2011). Today, the National Council of State Boards of Nursing (NCSBN) includes complementary and alternative therapies in the NCLEX-RN® examinations. The NCSBN specifically mentions massage therapy in the 2019 NCLEX-RN test plan (NCSBN, 2018). Swedish massage movements such as effleurage or slow-stroke back massage continue to be taught in schools of nursing.

Overall, *massage* is a broad term. Attempts to operationalize a definition that includes art and science and covers interpretations from culture and discipline are challenging. The American Massage Therapy Association (AMTA) defined *massage* as "manual soft tissue manipulation, and includes holding, causing movement, and/or applying pressure to the body" (Fletcher, 2009, p. 59). Simply put, "massage is a therapeutic manipulation of the soft tissues of the body with the goal of achieving normalization of those tissues" (Wieting, 2020, para. 10).

SCIENTIFIC BASIS

Although massage is both an art and a science, early nurse massage specialists recognized massage as a science. Rawlins (1933) stated, "Massage is a science, not a fad of the times" (p. 19). Jensen (1932) defined *massage* as "the scientific manipulation of body tissue as a therapeutic measure" (p. 2).

Florence Nightingale based the use of nonpharmacological interventions such as massage on the environmental adaptation theory. Nightingale believed that nurses should promote the best possible environment that would allow natural laws to improve the healing process (Dossey et al., 2005).

Today, perhaps because of the relative lack of its study by rigorous research methods, massage is often thought of as more of an art than a science. Nurse researcher Dr. Tiffany Field established the first center in the world devoted to the science of touch and massage. The Touch Research Institute was established in 1992 at the University of Miami School of Medicine (Touch Research Institute, n.d.). Field was one of the first to study the effects of massage on weight gain in preterm infants (Field, 2002) and build the capacity for nursing science on massage.

Massage is used by nurses to promote health and wellness (Westerman & Blaisdell, 2016). It is used to increase circulation, relieve pain, induce sleep, reduce anxiety or depression, and improve quality of life (Rose, 2020). Massage produces therapeutic effects on multiple body systems: integumentary, musculoskeletal, cardiovascular, lymph, and nervous. Manipulating the skin and underlying muscle makes the skin supple. Massage increases or enhances movement in the musculoskeletal system by reducing swelling, loosening and stretching contracted tendons, and aiding in the reduction of soft tissue adhesions. Friction to the cutaneous and subcutaneous tissues releases histamines that, in turn, produce vasodilation of vessels and enhance venous return (Snyder & Taniguki, 2010).

Massage is a proposed mechanism for relaxation to reduce psychological and physiological stress (Harris & Richards, 2010). Stress is also an individual subjective experience. When the body interprets a physiological or psychological response as stressful, the sympathetic nervous system stimulates the hypothalamic–pituitary–adrenal axis in the brain (Christensen, 2020; Godoy et al., 2018). There is a release of stress hormones, such as cortisol and epinephrine (Melmed & Jameson, 2019). Tactile stimulation in the body tissues causes neurohormonal responses throughout the nervous system. Mechanoreceptors cause impulses to travel from the peripheral nervous system, up the ascending spinal cord to the brain (Gadhvi & Waseem, 2021). The stimulus is then interpreted in the higher brain, resulting in a neurological or biochemical response (Field, 2014b). Massage activates the parasympathetic nervous system to decrease the heart rate, blood pressure, and respiration, resulting in relaxation (Field, 2014b).

Stress is a biological response (Yaribeygi et al., 2017). The foundation of stress research is built on the work of Hans Seyles and other stress researchers and explains the psychological and physiological responses (Godoy et al., 2018). Studies show the benefits of massage for physiological and psychological health

(Barreto & Bartista, 2017) for the very young and very old (Field, 2018; Schaub et al., 2018). Preterm infants benefit from the effects of massage on weight gain, sleep cycles, cognition, gastrointestinal function, and pain (Johnson, 2019). A randomized control trial ($N = 53$) showed that foot massage and cognitive behavioral therapy reduced stress in middle-aged women (Lee, 2017). Another example of stress research shows the beneficial effects of mechanical massage on variability in heart rate and cortisol levels (Barreto & Batista, 2017). The objective measures from this small, randomized sample of participants ($N = 93$) from five study groups removed bias due to unique differences in therapists.

A growing field of contemporary research is focused on psychophysiological protocols for relaxation (Meier et al., 2020). Studies show that massage produces physiological and psychological indicators for the relaxation response (Harris & Richards, 2010; Kirschner & Kirschner, 2019). The reduction of pain, a frequent desired outcome of massage, is closely related to the relaxation response. Through the relaxation response, massage relieves pain by stimulating the large-diameter nerve fibers that have an inhibitory input on T-cells (Furlan et al., 2008). According to Wang and Keck (2004), "massaging the hands and feet stimulates the mechanoreceptors that activate the nonpainful nerve fibers, preventing pain transmission from reaching consciousness" (p. 59).

A block, randomized controlled trial ($N = 63$) showed increased heart rate variability and decreased repeated subjective measures of relaxation and stress in response to standardized massage protocols. One randomized controlled trial ($N = 66$) in women with chronic or somatoform back pain hypothesized that neuropsycho-regulatory massage therapy reduces pain (Baumgart et al., 2020). In comparison to traditional massage protocol, neuropsycho-regulatory massage manipulates the superficial fascia and skin. Traditional massage involves all layers of the skin on the back extending from the neck to sacral areas. The proposed mechanism is that neuropsycho-regulatory massage activates C-tactile fibers by slow superficial strokes to relieve back, shoulder, neck, and limb pain and associated depression. The outcome of the study indicated that neuropsycho-regulatory massage that targets C-tactile fibers is more effective than traditional massage for relieving pain, improving mood, and increasing physical activity.

INTERVENTION

Various strokes are used to produce friction and pressure on cutaneous and subcutaneous tissues. The type of stroke and the amount of pressure chosen depend on the desired outcomes and the body part being massaged.

There are a number of types of massage: *Swedish* (a massage using long, flowing strokes), *Esalen* (a meditative massage using light touch), *deep tissue or neuromuscular* (an intense kneading of the body), *sports massage* (a vigorous massage to loosen and ease sore muscles), *shiatsu* (a Japanese pressure-point technique to relieve stress), and *reflexology* (a deep foot massage that relates to parts of the body). The different types of massage incorporate a variety of strokes, varying levels of pressure, and a multitude of procedures. Massage strokes can be administered to the entire body or to specific areas of the body, such as the back, feet, or hands.

The environment in which massage is administered is important. The room must be warm enough for the person to be comfortable because shivering could negate the effects of the massage. In addition, privacy needs to be ensured.

Adding music and aromatherapy to sessions has been thought to increase the effectiveness of massage. Before administering massage, the nurse should explain the intervention, obtain a history, and secure the permission of the patient.

MASSAGE STROKES IN NURSING

In 1895, Dr. J. H. Kellog from Battle Creek, Michigan, wrote *The Art of Massage* to teach nurses and other practitioners how to use massage techniques (Calvert, 2002; Kellog, 1895). Although massage was prescribed by physicians early in nursing history, nurses responded by showing leadership to specialize in massage. Commonly used strokes in administering massage include effleurage, friction, pressure, petrissage, vibration, and percussion.

Effleurage

Effleurage is a slow, rhythmic stroking, with light skin contact. Effleurage may be applied with varying degrees of pressure, depending on the part of the body being massaged and the outcome desired. The palmar surface of the hands is used for larger surfaces and the thumbs and fingers for smaller areas. On large surfaces, long, gliding strokes approximately 10 to 20 inches in length are applied.

Friction Movements

In *friction movements*, moderate, constant pressure to one area is made with the thumbs or fingers. The fingers may be held in one place or moved in a small circumscribed area.

Pressure Stroke

The *pressure stroke* is similar to the friction stroke. However, pressure strokes are made with the whole hand.

Petrissage

Petrissage, or kneading, involves lifting a large fold of skin and the underlying muscle and holding the tissue between the thumb and fingers. The tissues are pushed against the bone, then raised and squeezed in circular movements. The grasp on the tissues is alternately loosened and tightened. Tissues are supported by one hand while being kneaded with the other. Variations include pinching, rolling, wringing, and kneading with fists or fingers. Petrissage is limited to tissues having a significant muscle mass.

Vibration Strokes

Vibration strokes can be administered with either the entire hand or with the fingers. Rapid, continuous strokes are used. Because administering vibration strokes requires a significant amount of energy, mechanical vibrators are sometimes used.

Percussion Strokes

For *percussion strokes*, the wrist acts as a fulcrum for the hand, with the hand hitting the tissue. Strokes are made with a rapid tempo over a large body area. Tapping and clapping are variants of percussion strokes.

SLOW-STROKE BACK MASSAGE

Slow-stroke back massage, or *effleurage*, is a technique taught in nursing schools. See Exhibit 15.1 for a description of how to perform slow-stroke back massage.

Exhibit 15.1 *Technique for Slow-Stroke Back Massage*

1. Environment

- The room should be at a comfortable temperature.
- The lights should be dimmed.
- Noise should be eliminated.
- The nurse should keep talking at a minimum.

2. The Patient

- Ask the patient whether there is a need to use the bathroom or whether there is any way the nurse can assist to promote relaxation before beginning the massage.
- The patient should be assisted to a comfortable position.
- Clothing should be removed so the back is exposed.
- Modesty should be respected.

3. The Slow-Stroke Back Massage

- Palms of the hands and fingers are used (effleurage).
- The nurse warms their hands.
- The nurse applies nonallergenic lotion to their hands.
- Palms of the hands are placed in the sacral area on each side of the spine.
- Gentle pressure is applied.
- Long, slow, rhythmic, circular strokes are used to move upward on each side of the spine toward the base of the neck.
- Then long, slow, rhythmic, circular strokes are used to move downward on each side of the spine toward the sacral area.
- The masseur applies 12 to 15 strokes per minute to perform a rhythmic movement.
- The massage should continue until completion without removing the hands from the back.

4. Completion

- Remove hands from the spine.
- Replace clothing to the back.
- Replace bedcovers.
- Instruct the patient to rise slowly.
- Instruct the patient to stay hydrated.
- Quietly leave the room.

Source: Protocol adapted from Harris, M., Richards, K. C., & Grando, V. T. (2012). The effects of slow-stroke back massage on minutes of nighttime sleep on persons with dementia in the nursing home. *Journal of Holistic Nursing, 30*(4), 255–263. https://doi.org/10.1177/08980101112455948

HAND MASSAGE

Techniques for performing hand massage are outlined in Exhibit 15.2. One mixed-methods pilot study (Schaub et al., 2018) tested the effects of hand massage on stress biomarkers for salivary cortisol and salivary alpha-amylase on hospitalized persons with dementia ($N = 40$). There were larger decreases in salivary cortisol and alpha-amylase during the second and third week and clinically significant results based on nurses' notes for patients' verbal and physical responses. There are various techniques for hand massage that are easy to use with many populations,

---

Exhibit 15.2 *Techniques for Hand Massage*

Each hand is massaged for 2½ minutes. Do not massage if the hand is injured, reddened, or swollen. Protocols from 5 to 10 minutes for each hand have also been recommended (Kolcaba et al., 2006; Remington, 2002).

1. Back of hand

- Short, medium-length, straight strokes are done from the wrist to the fingertips; moderate pressure is used (effleurage).
- Large, half-circle, stretching strokes are made from the center to the side of the hand, using moderate pressure.
- Small, circular strokes are made over the entire hand, using light pressure (make small *O*s with the thumb).
- Featherlike, straight strokes are made from the wrist to the fingertips, using very light pressure.

2. Palm of hand

- Short, medium-length, straight strokes are made from the wrist to the fingertips, using moderate pressure (effleurage).
- Gentle milking and lifting of the tissue of the entire palm of the hand are done using moderate pressure.
- Small circular strokes are made over the entire palm, using moderate pressure (making little *O*s with index finger).
- Large, half-circle, stretching strokes are used from the center of the palm to the sides, using moderate pressure.

3. Fingers

- Each finger is gently squeezed from the base to the tip on both sides and the front and back, using light pressure.
- A gentle range of motion is performed on each finger.
- Gentle pressure is applied to each nail bed.

4. Completion

- The patient's hand is placed on yours and covered your other hand. The top hand is gently toward you several times. The patient's hand is turned over, and your other hand is gently drawn toward you several times.

including older adults (Kolcaba et al., 2006; Snyder et al., 1995) as well as infants and children (Field, 2002). A suggested period for administering massage is 2½ minutes per hand. The length of time is individualized for each patient, based on response.

MEASUREMENT OF OUTCOMES

Both physiological and psychological outcomes have been used to measure the effectiveness of massage. Indices of relaxation—heart rate, blood pressure, respiratory rate, skin temperature, cortisol level, and muscle tension—have been measured in many studies. Anxiety inventories and scales to determine pain level and quality of sleep, as well as quality-of-life indices, have been used to determine the efficacy of massage. Protocols for the duration of massage are needed. Typically, massage is dosed at 30- or 60-minute intervals because this is the duration of time used by massage therapists. The results of a randomized controlled trial ($N = 125$) used a 60-minute, once-weekly dose of massage in an 8-week protocol for osteoarthritis of the knee (Perlman et al., 2012). A follow-up randomized control trial (Perlman et al., 2019) showed overall similar results for efficacy and safety of 60-minute massage protocols once-weekly for osteoarthritis of the knee. Sherman et al. (2014) randomized 228 participants to five protocol groups and one control group to test the dosing of massage for neck pain. Results showed that a 60-minute protocol two to three times a week was more effective than shorter protocols. More research is needed to guide implementation and standardize massage protocols for other conditions. It is important that both short- and long-term effects of massage be measured.

PRECAUTIONS

Ernst (2003) reviewed the literature to determine adverse reactions to massage. Although a number of negative reactions were noted, the majority of these were associated with exotic types of massage and not with the Swedish massage technique. A review of the literature on Swedish massage (Baretto & Batista, 2017) indicates that although the incidence of adverse effects associated with massage is low, massage is not risk-free and should be performed by a trained provider. Herniated discs, spinal cord injury, soft tissue trauma, neurological impairment, and dissection of the vertebral artery are identified as some of the potential adverse effects associated with massage. Another review of the literature (Batavia, 2004) indicated the following contraindications to performing massage: arteritis, esophageal varices, unstable hypotension, advanced respiratory failure, postmyocardial infarction, aneurysm, emboli, arrhythmia, anticoagulant therapy/disease, heart failure, phlebitis, varicose veins, deep vein thrombosis, atherosclerosis, tumor, and cancer. Comfort touch is a type of massage that does not use massage techniques such gliding, kneading, or friction. Comfort touch is nurturing acupressure that is safe for older adults and those with a chronic illness. (Rose, 2020).

The patient's history of massage gathered by the nurse prior to the intervention provides information about past use of massage and any adverse responses. It is also important to determine a person's overall response to touch. Some people may be averse to being touched because of past negative experiences. Others may be hypersensitive to touch. One method for overcoming this sensitivity is beginning with light touch and slowly increasing the pressure. The area to be massaged is assessed for redness, bruises, edema, or rashes prior to performing massage.

Age-related changes are important considerations for massage. Older adults have more fragile skin and may take anticoagulants, which could cause bruising with massage. Osteoporosis and corticosteroids also place the older adult at risk for fracture. Arthritis, Parkinson's disease, and stroke may limit mobility. The nurse may need to modify massage techniques, positioning, and protocols when considering age-related changes and comorbidities (Rose, 2020).

Massage therapists and nurses have been reluctant to use massage with cancer patients (Gecsedi, 2002) because of the belief that the therapy may initiate or accelerate metastases. A physician's order is needed for body region and technique to be used. Factors considered are the location of the tumor, the stage of the cancer, and the location of any metastatic lesions. Pressure in the immediate area of the cancer is to be avoided. A pilot study ($N = 12$) comparing reflexology and Swedish massage to reduce physiological stress and pain and improve mood was conducted on nursing home residents with cancer (Hodgson & Lafferty, 2012). The results revealed that both techniques were feasible and produced measurable improvements in cortisol levels, pain, and mood. The study supports the need to develop guidelines for older adults with cancer in the nursing home.

Because blood pressure may be lowered during massage, monitoring for light-headedness is suggested after the initial massage sessions, particularly in older adults. If light-headedness does occur, allowing the person to remain recumbent for several minutes at the conclusion of the massage may help decrease the likelihood of hypotension and falls. Monitoring of blood pressure and pulse rate are required in patients with cardiac conditions to determine whether adverse effects are being experienced.

In patients with burns, relief from itching precedes evidence of a therapeutic effect on scar formation. However, skin breakdown can occur if massage is initiated too early. If there is fragile skin breakdown, massage should be temporarily discontinued. Simultaneous use of massage and creams should be monitored closely for skin irritation (Agency for Clinical Innovation [ACI], 2014).

USES

Exhibit 15.3 is a list of selected conditions for which massage is used. Evidence related to relaxation, pain, sleep, and other conditions is discussed in this section.

RELAXATION

Nurses use massage as an intervention to relieve physiological and psychological stress and promote relaxation (Harris & Richards, 2010). A national survey by the AMTA (2018), 29% of participants chose massage to decrease stress. Although stress research has included massage, the effects of massage on relaxation is a growing body of research (Meier et al., 2020).

COMFORT TOUCH

Comfort touch is a massage technique developed by Mary Katherine Rose (2020). Comfort touch is caring touch designed for chronically ill and older adults. Pain relief and relaxation are the primary goals of comfort touch.

Exhibit 15.3 *Uses of Massage*

- Behavioral abnormalities (Remington, 2002; Zhao et al., 2020).
- Comfort (Kolcaba et al., 2006; Rose, 2020).
- Decrease aggressive behaviors (Garner et al., 2008).
- Increase psychological well-being (Hattan et al., 2002).
- Increase weight in preterm infants (Field, 2018).
- Stress, pain, cognition, irritability in preterm infants (Johnson, 2019).
- Lessen neck pain (Sherman et al., 2014).
- Lessen fatigue (Currin & Meister, 2008).
- Lessen knee pain (Perlman et al., 2019).
- Promote relaxation/reduce stress (Harris & Richards, 2010; Meier et al., 2020).
- Promote sleep (Harris et al., 2012; Richards, 1998).
- Health promotion (Barreto & Battista, 2017).

DEPRESSION AND ANXIETY

A 20-minute effleurage with essential oils implemented three times a week for 2 weeks showed statistically significant reductions ($p < .001$) in State-Trait Anxiety Inventory scores and in heart and respiratory rates in patients ($N = 50$) in a psychiatric hospital (da Silva Domingos & Braga, 2015). In a quasi-experimental study ($N = 30$), there were statistically significant differences in anxiety ($p = .002$) and positive trending with a large effect size ($d = 1.3$) on the Hospital Anxiety and Depression Scale on patients in the intervention group after they received 5-minute hand massages (Prichard & Newcomb, 2015). Another study (Chen et al., 2013) revealed statistically significant decreases after back massage in systolic blood pressure ($p < .01$), diastolic blood pressure ($p < .01$), pulse ($p < .01$), and respiratory rate ($p < .01$), as well as a statistically significant difference in anxiety ($p = .02$) in participants ($N = 64$) with congestive heart failure.

BEHAVIORAL ABNORMALITIES

Several studies using hand massage reported a decrease in psychological indicators for stress (Hicks-Moore & Robinson, 2008; Kolcaba et al., 2006; Remington, 2002). Two randomized controlled trials on hand massage (Hicks-Moore & Robinson, 2008; Remington, 2002) used the Cohen Mansfield Agitation Index to test the effects of hand massage on reducing agitation. Hicks-Moore and Robinson (2008) and Remington (2002) reported statistically significant decreases in agitation 1 hour after hand massage in older participants. Kolcaba et al. (2006) showed statistically significant results for comfort using hand massage in the nursing home environment. One literature review (Zhao et al., 2020) of 23 studies on massage therapy and other nonpharmacological interventions showed that massage in combination with music or aromatherapy was beneficial for decreasing anxiety, stress, and other behavioral abnormalities in persons living with dementia.

BURNS

Massage is used in burn patients to control pain, anxiety, and scarring. There are physiotherapy and occupational therapy guidelines to break up collagen bundles, soften tissues, decrease itching, and prevent adhesions caused by burns (ACI, 2017). One randomized controlled trial (N = 90) with burn patients who received aromatherapy massage and inhalation massage showed statistically significant decreases in anxiety (p = .007) and pain (p < .001) compared with the control group (Seyyed-Rasodi et al., 2016). One systematic review showed moderate to strong effects on the management of scar tissue for hypertrophic burns (Deflorin et al., 2020), but there was poor quality of evidence and a lack of consistent measurement tools. One randomized controlled trial (Nedelec et al., 2018) in the review did not find evidence to support a long-term benefit from massage. Overall, more randomized controlled trials are needed.

HIV

One randomized controlled trial showed a 60-minute massage once weekly for 4 weeks had a positive impact on anxiety and hyperventilation, but not on depression and quality of life (Reychler et al., 2017). However, studies from an earlier Cochrane review (Hillier et al., 2010) showed improvements in CD4+ and killer cells as well as improved quality of life. A randomized controlled trial (Perez et al., 2015) in South Africa showed improved developmental outcomes, especially in hearing and speech for infants exposed to HIV. A literature review showed few studies on massage and HIV for full-term infants and more studies on preterm infants (Field, 2018). More research is needed across the life span.

PRETERM INFANTS

In a research review, Dr. Tiffany Field (2014a) outlined the benefits of massage on weight gain in preterm infants. Preterm infants experience significant stress. In one study in which preterm infants (N = 30) were randomly assigned to a massage therapy or exercise group, results suggested increased weight gain for the combination of tactile or kinesthetic stimulation (Diego et al., 2014). Two more recent literature reviews (Field, 2018; Johnson, 2019) show that massage has beneficial effects on the physical and mental health of preterm infants.

PAIN

Reduction of pain is another condition for which massage is often used. Numerous studies have found that massage does result in reduced pain (AMTA, 2018). According to a national survey (N = 1005) by the AMTA (2018), pain was the top reason for seeking massage services in 43% of adult participants. A Cochrane review (N = 13) revealed benefits for individuals with low back pain when massage was combined with exercise and education (Furlan et al., 2015). In a review of research on the use of massage and aromatherapy in patients with cancer, Wang and Keck (2004) reported a lessening of pain in postoperative patients, and Mok and Woo (2004) found that massage lessened pain in patients with strokes.

SLEEP

A randomized controlled trial of massage on participants ($N = 40$) after coronary artery bypass graft surgery showed decreased fatigue and more effective sleep (Nerbass et al., 2010). Two studies used objective measures for sleep to determine the effects of massage in older adults. Richards (1998) used polysomnography as an objective measure for sleep in hospitalized older men ($N = 69$) to compare a slow-stroke back massage intervention group between participants using relaxing music and a control group. Another randomized controlled pilot study (Harris et al., 2012) with patients with dementia in the nursing home ($N = 40$) used actigraphy to objectively measure sleep in participants receiving a 3-minute, slow-stroke back massage compared with a usual-care control condition. Although there were no statistically significant differences between participants in the intervention and control groups in either study, the results provided evidence for the clinical significance of using slow-stroke back massage for relaxation and sleep in the geriatric population.

CULTURAL APPLICATIONS

Shiatsu, a pressure-point type of massage, is popular in Japan and other Asian countries. Its underlying purpose is to rebalance the energy system in the body through pressure on specific points. Although shiatsu may not be comforting during administration, relaxation is often felt at the conclusion. Shiatsu may be used to help alleviate other conditions. Taniguki (2008) found shiatsu therapy to be highly efficacious in managing constipation in six older adult patients (from 81–93 years old) who were on bed rest and receiving home care.

In countries such as Japan, acupuncture and moxibustion are often used, in addition to massage, by massage therapists, who also often have a license to practice acupuncture and moxibustion. Therefore, in some research studies, because of the cultural implications, massage cannot be separated from acupuncture and moxibustion (Hirakawa et al., 2005).

In a multicultural qualitative study (Kilstoff & Chenoweth, 1998), hand massage was conducted on Chinese-, Italian-, Vietnamese-, Arab-, French-, and English-speaking participants ($N = 39$; 16 dyads of patients with dementia and caregivers; 7 day-care staff) in a dementia-care patient setting. The results showed a reduction in stress, decreased agitation, increased alertness, improved self-hygiene, and improved sleep. Family caregivers also reported less distress, improved sleep, and feelings of calm.

Massage is widely used around the world as illustrated in the accounts of nursing students (see Sidebars 15.1 and 15.2).

FUTURE RESEARCH

There is a lack of rigorous research on complementary therapies such as massage. Specific techniques, questions related to the person who should administer the massage, specific protocols, dose-finding studies, qualitative research, and studies to support the clinical significance of massage are all areas for further investigation to build nursing science in massage. One challenge in conducting research on massage is having a comparable control group. McNamara et al. (2003) compared massage and standard care in patients undergoing a diagnostic test.

Sidebar 15.1 *Massage: International Perspective From Thailand*

Thanchanok Wongvibul

Massage is one of the significant parts of Thai culture. Many people in Thailand may enjoy massage as a way to energize and relax their bodies; however, some people may recognize massage as part of healthcare. From various types of massage, Thai massage has been known as the most common therapeutic option among Thai people due to the distinct techniques involved in its provision of service. The traditional Thai massage is different from Western massages as it mainly focuses on circulation and pressure points, which help promote internal health and reduce muscle tension. In general, people can easily get Thai massage at massage shops or spas, and the price can range from $6 to $50 per hour depending on the place and the type of services performed. Moreover, people can also get Thai massage along with rehabilitation programs at clinics or alternative medicine hospitals. To perform Thai massage in Thailand, massage therapists are required to complete the training courses from the schools approved by the Thai Ministry of Public Health and have a professional license.

Sidebar 15.2 *Massage: International Perspective from China*

Sarah Walker

While living in Wuhan, China, for 3 years I had quite a few massages. The price was roughly 66 RMB, which came to US$11 at that time. The massage businesses with actual storefronts might make you pay a premium price. But the small ones located in apartments often had one or two blind staff members. It turns out that it is a common job for the blind community in China. Although these were fun and interesting, toward my last year in China, I discovered foot massages (zu bu anmo). These are much more popular and usually a little cheaper. Regular customers come in nearly every day after a hard day's work on their feet. Not only do they put flower petals in the water, but they will also give you a 5- to 10-minute back massage. After such a holistic pampering, they will trim your toenails and scrape off any dead skin. Many foreigners become regulars at these places and splurge on their budget for something that we know would be 3 to 5 times the price in Western countries.

Reflexology and Swedish massage (Hodgson & Lafferty, 2012) were compared on nursing home residents with cancer. A randomized controlled trial ($N = 401$) that compared structural and relaxation massage for low back pain used blinding to test the effectiveness of treatment for low back pain (Cherkin et al., 2012). More studies are needed that compare massage techniques for developing evidence-based practices. The results of a randomized controlled trial ($N = 125$; Perlman et al., 2019) showed that a 60-minute, once-weekly dose of massage was an optimal standard for future dose-finding studies in patients with osteoarthritis of the knee.

The following are suggestions for research that is needed so that practitioners may have more direction in using massage in clinical settings:

- Well-designed studies using blinding, randomization, and attention control groups with large sample sizes are needed.
- Few investigators have explored the impact that massage has on psychoneuroimmunological indices. Studies on the use of massage with patients with HIV infection and cancer would guide nurses in its use with these groups.
- Dose-finding studies for administering massage and the number of sessions that produce the best results need to be established. There is great variation in these two parameters in published studies. Because of time constraints in practice settings, this information would be very helpful to busy practitioners.
- Research studies on the benefits of massage using multimodal protocols, including exercise, aromatherapy, music, and other nonpharmacological interventions, are needed in the development of evidence-based practices.
- What, if any, is the effect of the gender of the therapist administering massage on the outcomes obtained? Few studies have reported on this factor.

REFERENCES

Agency for Clinical Innovation. (2014). *ACI statewide burn injury service: Physiotherapy and occupational therapy clinical practice.*

American Massage Therapy Association. (2018). *Massage therapy in integrative care and pain management.*

American Physical Therapy Association. (2013). *Minimum required skills of physical therapists graduates at entry-level.* http://www.apta.org/uploadedFiles/APTAorg/About_Us/Policies/Education/MinimumRequiredSkillsPTGrads.pdf

Barreto, D. M., & Batista, M. V. A. (2017). Swedish massage: A systematic review of its physical and psychological benefits. *Advances in Mind Body Medicine, 31*(2), 16–20.

Batavia, M. (2004). Contraindications for therapeutic massage: Do sources agree? *Journal of Bodywork and Movement Therapies, 8,* 48–57. https://doi.org/10.1016/S1360-8592(03)0008-6

Baumgart, S. B. E., Baumboch-Kraft, A., & Lorenz, J. (2020). Effect of psycho-regulatory massage therapy on pain and depression in women with chronic and/or somataform back pain: A randomized controlled trial. *Brain Science, 10,* 721. https://doi.org/10.3390/brainsci10100721

Brummitt, J. (2008). The role of massage in sports performance and rehabilitation: Current evidence and future direction. *North American Journal of Sports Physical Therapy, 3,* 7–21.

Calvert, R. N. (2002). *The history of massage.* Healing Arts Press.

Chen, W. L., Liu, G. J., Yeh, S. H., Chiang, M. C., Fu, M. Y., & Hsieh, Y. K. (2013). Effect of back massage intervention on anxiety, comfort, and physiologic responses in patients with congestive heart failure. *Journal of Alternative and Complementary Medicine, 19,* 464–470. https://doi.org/10.1089/acm.2011.0873

Cherkin, D. C., Sherman, K. J., Kahn, J., Wellman, R., Cook, A. J., Johnson, E., Erro, J., Delaney, K., & Deyo, R. A. (2012). A comparison of the effects of 2 types of massage and usual care on chronic low back pain. *Annals of Internal Medicine, 155*(1), 1–9. https://doi.org/10.7326/0003-4819-155-1-201107050-00002

Christensen, J. F. (2020). Stress & disease. In M. D. Feldman, J. F. Christensen, J. M. Satterfield, & R. Laponis (Eds.), *Behavioral medicine: A guide for clinical practice* (5th ed.). McGraw Hill.

Currin, J., & Meister, E. A. (2008). A hospital-based intervention using massage to reduce distress among oncology patients. *Cancer Nursing*, 3, 214–221. https://doi.org/10.1097/01.NCC.0000305725.65345.f3

da Silva Domingos, T., & Braga, E. M. (2015). Massage with aromatherapy: Effectiveness on anxiety of users with personality disorders in psychiatric hospitalization. *Journal of School of Nursing USP*, 49(3), 450–456. https://doi.org/10.1590/30080-6234201500003000013

Deflorin, C., Hohenauer, E., Stoop, R., van Daele, U., Cliisen, R., & Taeymans, J. (2020). Physical management of scar tissue: A systematic review and meta-analysis. *The Journal of Alternative and Complementary Medicine*, 26(10), 854–865. https://doi.org/10.1089/acm.2020.0109

Diego, M. A., Field, T., & Hernandez-Reif, M. (2014). Preterm infant weight gain is increased by massage therapy and exercise via different underlying mechanisms. *Early Human Development*, 90(3), 137–140. https://doi.org/10.1016/j.earlhumdev.2014.01.009

Dossey, B. M., Selanders, L. C., Beck, D., & Attewell, A. (2005). *Florence Nightingale today: Healing, leadership, global action*. American Nurses Association.

Ernst, E. (2003). The safety of massage therapy. *Rheumatology*, 42, 1101–1106. https://doi.org/10.1093/rheumatology/keg306

Field, T. (2002). Preterm infant massage therapy studies: An American approach. *Seminars in Neonatology*, 7, 487–494. https://doi.org/10.1053/siny.2002.0153

Field, T. (2014a). Massage therapy research review. *Complementary Therapies in Clinical Practice*, 20, 224–229.

Field, T. (2014b). *Touch* (2nd ed.). The MIT Press.

Field, T. (2018). Infant massage therapy research review. *Clinical Research in Pediatrics*, 1(2), 1–9.

Fletcher, B. (2009). A bridge between the mind and body: The effects of massage on body image state. *Undergraduate Review*, 5, 58–63. http://vc.bridgew.edu/undergrad_rev/vol5/iss1/13

Furlan, A.D., Giraldo, M., Baskwill, Irvin, E., Imamura, M. (2015). Massage for low-back pain. Cochrane Data-base of Systematic Reviews 2015, 9. Art. No.: CD001929. https://doi.org/10.1002/14651858.CD001929.pub3

Gadhvi, M., & Waseem, M. (2021). Physiology, sensory system. In *StatPearls*. StatPearls Publishing. https://www.ncbi.nlm.nih.gov/books/NBK547656/

Garner, B., Phillips, L. J., Schmidt, H. M., Markulev, C., O'Connor, J., Wood, S. J., Berger, G. E., Burnett, P., & McGorry, P. D. (2008). Pilot study evaluating the effect of massage therapy on stress, anxiety, and aggression in a young adult psychiatric inpatient unit. *Australian & New Zealand Journal of Psychiatry*, 42(5), 414–422. https://doi.org/10.1080/00048670801961131

Gecsedi, R. A. (2002). Massage therapy for patients with cancer. *Clinical Journal of Oncology Nursing*, 6, 52–54. https://doi.org/10.1188/02.CJON.52-54

Godoy, L. D., Ross, M. T., Delfino-Pereira, P., Garcia-Calrasco, N., & de leima Umeoka, E. H. (2018). A comprehensive overview on stress neurobiology: Basic concepts and clinical implications. *Frontiers in Behavioral Neuroscience*, 12, 127. https://doi.org/10.3389/fnbeh.2018.00127

Goodall-Copestake, B. M. (1919). *The theory and practice of massage* (2nd ed.). Paul B. Hoeber.

Harris, M., & Richards, K. C. (2010). The physiological and psychological effects of slow-stroke back massage and hand massage on relaxation in the elderly. *Journal of Clinical Nursing*, 19, 917–926. https://doi.org/10.1111/j.1365-2702.2009.03165.x

Harris, M., Richards, K. C., & Grando, V. T. (2012). The effects of slow-stroke back massage on minutes of nighttime sleep on persons with dementia in the nursing home. *Journal of Holistic Nursing*, 30(4), 255–263. https://doi.org/10.1177/08980101112455948

Hattan, J., King, L., & Griffiths, P. (2002). The impact of foot massage and guided relaxation following cardiac surgery: A randomized controlled trial. *Journal of Advanced Nursing*, 37, 199–207. https://doi.org/10.1046/j.1365-2648.2002.02083.x

Hicks-Moore, S., & Robinson, B. (2008). Favorite music and hand massage. *Dementia*, 7(1), 95–108. https://doi.org/10.1177/1471301207085369

Hillier, S. L., Louw, Q., Morris, L., Uwimana, J., & Statham, S. (2010). Massage therapy for people with HIV/AIDS. *Cochrane Database of Systematic Reviews*, (1), CD007502. https://doi.org/10.1002/14651858.CD007502.pub2

Hirakawa, Y., Masuda, Y., Kimata, T., Uemura, K., Kuzuya, M., & Iguchi, A. (2005). Effects of home massage rehabilitation for the bed-ridden elderly: A pilot trial with a three-month follow up. *Clinical Rehabilitation, 19*, 20–27. https://doi.org/10.1191/0269215505cr7950a

Hodgson, N. A., & Lafferty, D. (2012). Reflexology versus Swedish massage to reduce physiological stress and pain and improve mood in nursing home residents with cancer: A pilot study. *Evidence-Based Complementary & Alternative Medicine.* https://doi.org/10.1155/2012/456897

Johnson, S. (2019). "Helping babies: The mental and physical effects of massage therapy on preterm infants." *Intuition: The BYU Undergraduate Journal of Psychology, 14*(2), 14. https://scholarsarchive.byu.edu/intuition/vol14/iss2/14

Kellog, J. H. (1895). *The art of massage.* Good Health Publishing.

Kilstoff, K., & Chenoweth, L. (1998). New approaches to health and well-being for dementia day-care clients, family carers and day-care staff. *International Journal of Nursing Practice, 4*(2), 70–83. https://doi.org/10.1046/j.1440-172X.1998.00059.x

Kirschner, M., & Kirschner, R. (2019). Hand massage reduces perceived stress, anxiety and fatigue. *International Journal of Innovative Studies in Medical Sciences, 3*(4), 1–6.

Kolcaba, K., Schirm, V., & Steiner, R. (2006). Effects of hand massage on comfort of nursing home residents. *Geriatric Nursing, 27*, 85–91. https://doi.org/10.1016/j.gerinurse.2006.02.006

Lee, Y. M. (2017). Effects of combined foot massage and cognitive behavioral therapy on the stress response in middle-aged women. *Journal of Alternative and Complementary Medicine, 23*(6), 445. https://doi.org/10.1089/acm.2016.0421

Macafee, N. E. (1917). *Massage, an elementary text-book for nurses.* Reed & Witting.

Massage Therapy Body of Knowledge. (2010). *Massage therapy body of knowledge* (MTBOK) version 1.0.

McNamara, M. E., Burnham, D. C., Smith, C., & Carroll, D. L. (2003). The effects of back massage before diagnostic cardiac catheterization. *Alternative Therapies in Health and Medicine, 9*(1), 50–57. https://doi.org/10.4037/AJCC1998.7.4.288

Meier, M., Unternaehrer, E., Dimitroff, S. J., Benz, A., Bentele, U. U., Schorpp, S. M., Wenzel, M., & Pruessner, J. C. (2020). Standardized massage interventions as protocols for the induction of psychophysiological relaxation in the laboratory: A block randomized, controlled trial. *Scientific Reports, 10*(1), 14774. https://doi.org/10.1038/s41598-020-71173-w

Melmed, S., & Jameson, J. L. (2019). Physiology of anterior pituitary hormones. In J. L. Jameson, A. S. Fauci, D. L. Kasper, S. L. Hauser, D. L. Longo, & J. Loscalzo (Eds.), *Harrison's principles of internal medicine* (20th ed., pp. 2659–2663). McGraw Hill.

Mok, E., & Woo, C. P. (2004). The effects of slow-stroke massage on anxiety and shoulder pain in elderly stroke patients. *Complementary Therapies in Nursing & Midwifery, 10*, 209–216. https://doi.org/10.1016/j.ctnm.2004.05.006

National Certification Board for Therapeutic Massage and Bodywork. (2021). *Become certified: Earn the profession's highest credentials.* https://www.ncbtmb.org

National Council of State Boards of Nursing. (2018). *National Council of State Boards of Nursing: 2019 NCLEX-RN® detailed test plan: Item writer/item reviewer/nurse educator version.*

Nedelec, B., Couture, M. A., Calva, V., Poulin, C., Chouinard, A., Shashoua, D., Gauthier, N., Correa, J. A., de Oliveira, A., Mazer, B., & LaSalle, L. (2019). Randomized controlled trial of the immediate and long-term effect of massage on adult postburn scar. *Burns, 45*(1), 128–139. https://doi.org/10.1016/j.burns.2018.08.018

Nerbass, F. B., Feltrim, M. I. Z., de Souza, S. A., Ykeda, D. S., & Lorenzi-Filho, G. (2010). Effects of massage therapy on sleep quality after coronary artery bypass graft surgery. *Clinicals, 65*, 1105–1110. https://doi.org/10.1590/S1807-59322010001000100008

Norstroëm, G. M. (1896). *The handbook of massage.* Leland Stanford Junior University, reprinted in 1896 by the Lane Medical Library. (Original work published 1868)

Perez, E. M., Carrara, H., Bourne, L., Berg, A., Swanevelder, S., & Hendricks, M. K. (2015). Massage therapy improves the development of HIV-exposed infants living in a low socio-economic, peri-urban community of South Africa. *Infant Behavior & Development, 38*, 135–146. https://doi.org/10.1016/j.infbeh.2014.12.011

Perlman, A., Fogerite, S. G., Glass, O., Bechard, E., Ali, A., Njike, V. Y., Pieper, C., Dmitrieva, N. O., Luciano, A., Rosenberger, L., Keever, T., Milak, C., Finkelstein, E. A., Mahon, G., Campanile, G., Cotter, A., & Katz, D. L. (2019). Efficacy and safety of massage for osteoarthritis of the knee: A randomized clinical trial. *Journal of General Internal Medicine, 34,* 379–386. https://doi .org/10.1007/s11606-018-4763-5

Perlman, A. I., Ali, A., Njike, V. Y., Hom, D., Davidi, A., Gould-Fogeite, S., Milak, C., & Katz, D. L. (2012). Massage therapy for osteoarthritis of the knee: A randomized dose-finding trial. *PLoS ONE, 7*(2), e30248. https://doi.org/10.1371/journal.pone.0030248

Prichard, C., & Newcomb, P. (2015). Benefit to family members of delivering hand massage with essential oils to critically ill patients. *American Journal of Critical Care Nurses, 24*(5), 446–449. https://doi.org/10.4037/ajcc2015767

Rawlins, M. (1933). *A textbook of massage for nurses and beginners* (2nd ed.). Mosby.

Remington, R. (2002). Calming music and hand massage with agitated elderly. *Nursing Research, 51*(5), 317–323. https://doi.org/10.1097/00006199-200209000-00008

Reychler, G. Caty, G., Arcq, A., Lebrun, L., Belkhir, L., Yombi, J., & Marot, J. (2017). Effects of massage therapy on anxiety, depression, hyperventilation and quality of life in HIV infected patients: A randomized controlled trial. *Complementary Therapies in Medicine, 32,* 109–114. https://doi.org/10.1016/j.ctim.2017.05.002

Richards, K. C. (1998). Effect of a back massage and relaxation intervention on sleep in critically ill patients. *American Journal of Critical Care, 7,* 288–299.

Rose, M. K. (2020). *Comfort touch: Massage for the elderly and the ill.* Wolters Kluwer/Lippincott Williams & Wilkins.

Ruffin, P. T. (2011). A history of massage in nurse training school curricula (1860–1945). *Journal of Holistic Nursing, 29,* 61–67. https://doi.org/10.1177/0898010110377355

Schaub, C., Von Gunten, A., Morin, D., Wild, P., Gomez, P., & Popp, J. (2018). The effects of hand massage on stress and agitation among people with dementia in a hospital setting: A pilot study. *Applied Psychophysiology and Biofeedback, 43,* 319–332. https://doi.org/10.1007/ s10484-018-9416-2

Seyyed-Rasodi, A., Salehi, F., Mohammadpoorosi, A., Goljaryan, S., & Seyyedi, A. (2016). Comparing the effects of aromatherapy massage and inhalation aromatherapy on anxiety and pain in burn patients. *Burns, 42*(8), 1774–1780. https://doi.org/10.1016/j.burns.2016.06.014

Sherman, K. J., Cook, A. J., Wellman, R. D., Hawkes, R. J., Kahn, J. R., Deyo, R. A., & Cherkin, D. C. (2014). Five-week outcomes from a dosing trial of therapeutic massage for chronic neck pain. *The Annals of Family Medicine, 12*(2), 112–120. https://doi.org/10.1370/afm.1602

Snyder, M., Egan, E. C., & Burns, K. R. (1995). Efficacy of hand massage in decreasing agitation behaviors associated with care activities in persons with dementia. *Geriatric Nursing, 16*(2), 60–63. https://doi.org/10.1016/s0197-4572(05)80005-9

Snyder, M., & Taniguki, S. (2010). Massage. In M. Snyder & R. Lindquist (Eds.), *Complementary & alternative therapies in nursing* (6th ed., pp. 337–448). Springer Publishing Company.

Taniguki, S. (2008). *Use of Shiatsu with home care patients* (Unpublished manuscript).

Touch Research Institute. (n.d.). *Touch Research Institute.* http://www6.miami.edu/touch-research

Wang, H. L., & Keck, J. F. (2004). Foot and hand massage as an intervention for postoperative pain. *Pain Management Nursing, 5,* 59–65. https://doi.org/10.1016/j.pmn.2004.01.002

Westerman, K. F., & Blaisdell, C. (2016). Many benefits and little risk: The use of massage in nursing practice. *American Journal of Nursing, 116*(1), 35–39. https://doi.org/10.1097/01.NAJ .0000476164.97929.f2

Wieting, J.M. (2020). *Massage, traction, and manipulation.* Retrieved from https://emedicine .medscape.com/article/324-overview#showall

Yaribeygi, H., Panahi, Y., Sahraei, H., Johnston, T. P., & Sahebkar, A. (2017). The impact of stress on body function: A review. *EXCLI Journal, 16,* 1057–1072. https://doi.org/10.17179/excli2017-480

Zhao, H., Weiwei, G., & Zhang, M. (2020). Massage therapy in nursing as nonpharmacological interventions to control agitation and stress in patients with dementia. *Alternative Therapies, 16*(6), 29–33.

Tai Chi

KUEI-MIN CHEN

Time pressure is emerging as a contemporary malaise. A lack of time is the major barrier to exercising regularly. Failing to exercise may lead to mental strain, nervous breakdown, or inefficiency in daily work (Booth et al., 2017). Good health is essential; how to acquire and maintain a healthy mind and body are vital concerns. It is commonly recognized that exercise and other forms of physical activity have a wide range of health benefits, both physiological and psychological, for all age groups (Manferdelli et al., 2019). However, it is not easy to find an exercise that suits people of all ages.

Tai chi is one intervention that has received increasing attention among many professionals: nurses, physicians, occupational therapists, physical therapists, and recreational therapists. It is a manipulative and body-based therapy that can heighten individuals' awareness of their bodies and take advantage of their body structure for expressing feelings and ideas. Gradually, people become more aware of their total being, and harmony is enhanced.

DEFINITION

Tai chi, which means "supreme ultimate," is a traditional Chinese martial art (Koh, 1981) and a mind–body exercise. It involves a series of fluid, continuous, graceful, dance-like postures, and the performances of movements are known as *forms* (Yang, 2010). The graceful body movements engage in continuous body and trunk rotation, flexion/extension of the hips and knees, postural alignment, and coordination of the arms—integrated by mental concentration, the balanced shifting of body weight, muscle relaxation, and breath control. Movements are performed in a slow, rhythmic, and well-controlled manner (Clark, 2011).

Several styles of tai chi are practiced: *chen* (quick and slow large movements), *yang* (slow large movements), *wu* (mid-paced, compact movements), *sun* (quick, compact movements), and *wu hao* (small, subtle movements; Douglas & Douglas, 2012). Each style has a characteristic protocol that differs from the other styles in the postures or forms included, the order in which they appear, the pace at which movements are executed, and the level of difficulty; however, the basic principles are the same (Yang & Liang, 2016). For example, one significant difference between the *chen* and *yang* styles is that *yang* movements are relaxed, evenly paced, and graceful. The *yang* style is the most popular tai chi practiced by older adults (Liang & Wu, 2014). In comparison, the *chen* style is characterized by alternating slow, gentle movements with quick and vigorous ones as well as restrained and controlled actions, which reflects a more martial origin (Gu, 2011). Most tai chi movements were named after animals, such as "white crane spreads its wings" and "grasp the bird's tail" (Koh, 1981).

There are a few simplified forms of ancient tai chi. For example, the simplified tai chi exercise program (STEP), developed by Chen et al., (2006), encompasses three phases: warm-up, tai chi exercises, and cooldown. In the warm-up phase, nine exercises are designed to loosen the body from head to toe; the second phase includes 12 easy-to-learn and easy-to-perform tai chi movements; three activities in the cooldown phase help the body return to a preintervention state of rest. STEP differs from traditional tai chi styles in that it incorporates fewer leg movements, fewer knee bends, and less complicated hand gestures. It was specifically designed for older adults suffering from chronic illness (Chen et al., 2006).

SCIENTIFIC BASIS

Tai chi practice is closely linked to Chinese medicine theory, in which the vital life energy, chi (or *qi*), is thought to circulate throughout the body in discrete channels called meridians. Using correct postures and adequate relaxation, tai chi promotes the free flow of chi throughout the body, which improves the health of an individual. The movements of tai chi are regulated by the timing of deep breathing and the movement of the diaphragm. It offers a balanced exercise to the muscles and joints of various parts of the body (Clark, 2011). In addition, a peaceful state of mind and spiritual dedication to each movement during the exercise ensure that the central nervous system (CNS) is given sufficient training and is consequently toned up with time as the exercise continues. A strong CNS is essential for a healthy body, and various organs depend largely on its soundness (Clark, 2011).

INTERVENTION

In Asian countries such as Taiwan, it is common and popular for older adults to practice tai chi as a group, in the early morning, in parks, or on the athletic grounds of elementary schools. Tai chi practice groups are usually led by masters who are pleased to share the essence of tai chi with others. People who are interested in tai chi are welcome to join the groups and learn the movements from these masters. In Western countries such as the United States, there has been growing interest in the practice of tai chi. Various tai chi clubs are available to the public through community centers, health clinics, or private organizations. General information is widespread through websites, books, and videos. Tai chi is a convenient exercise that can be practiced in any place, at any time, and without any equipment.

TECHNIQUE

Although various styles of tai chi are practiced, the underlying practice principles are the same. The five essential principles of movement are (Hallisy, 2018)

- hand and leg movements should be synchronous;
- the emphasis should be on a soft, relaxed, rather than on a hard, tense position;
- moves should be practiced with a quiet and open mind;

▓ the soles of the feet should be rooted to the ground, with the knees bent in a low stance and the primary focus of awareness within the lower abdomen; and
▓ the physical force should be rooted in the feet, passed up through the legs as weight is shifted, and distributed by the pivoting of the waist.

In the physical performance, an individual must relax and think of nothing else before starting. The movements should be slow and rhythmic with natural breathing. Every action becomes easy and smooth, the waist turns freely, and the feelings of comfort and relaxation are gradually developed (Hallisy, 2018). In the spiritual aspect, tai chi is an exercise that produces harmony of the body and the mind. Each movement should be guided by thought instead of physical strength. For instance, to lift up the hands, an individual must first have the necessary mental concentration, and then the hands can be raised slowly in a proper manner. Hence, the breathing will become deeper, and the body will be strengthened (Hallisy, 2018).

GUIDELINES

The steps for performing the movement called "white crane spreads its wings" are presented in Exhibit 16.1.
Various videos on tai chi are also available. The following DVDs and/or books are useful for learning tai chi:

▓ *The Complete Illustrated Guide to Tai Chi: A Step-by-Step Approach to the Ancient Chinese Movement* (Clark, 2011) contains a complete introduction to the principles and practices of tai chi and is accompanied by clear and instructive photographs throughout. It includes sections on the basic principles of movement and the body, ways that tai chi can help heal, life energies, meridians, the seven major chakras, and step-by-step guides to the complete movement sequence.
▓ *Seated Tai Chi and Qigong: Guided Therapeutic Exercises to Manage Stress and Balance Mind, Body, and Spirit* (Quarta & Vallie, 2012) emphasizes that tai chi and qigong are the perfect antidote to the stresses of modern life and a great way to stay healthy. This illustrated guidebook provides an explanatory introduction

---

Exhibit 16.1 *Procedure for Performing "White Crane Spreads Its Wings"*

- Bring your right foot next to your left while your left palm circles clockwise up, palm down. At the same time, turn your body slightly to your left and rotate your right palm up.
- Bring your left foot a half step forward. Shift all your weight onto your right foot. At the same time, bring your right palm up past your left elbow and lift your left foot up slightly.
- Complete the movement by lowing your left palm down to waist level, palm down. Raise your right palm up to head level, palm facing inward, and touch down with your left foot into an empty stance.

Source: Adapted from Liang, S. Y., & Wu, W. C. (2014). *Simplified tai chi chuan: 24 postures with applications & standard 48 postures* (2nd ed.). Ymaa Publication Center.

to these forms of exercise and shows how to build up a program from easy to more challenging steps.

- *The Complete Idiot's Guide to T'ai Chi & Qigong Illustrated* (Douglas & Douglas, 2012) includes nearly 150 online videos that support the book and 300 richly detailed illustrations, giving it a highly effective how-to focus.
- *Simplified Tai Chi Chuan: 24 Postures with Applications & Standard 48 Postures* (Liang & Wu, 2014) is designed for self-study and can help people learn both the 24 simplified tai chi chuan 24 forms and the 48 simplified tai chi chuan 48 forms quickly and accurately.
- *Tai Chi Chuan Martial Applications: Advanced Yang Style* (Yang & Liang, 2016) includes a new, easy-to-follow layout. Each technique is presented in four to six large photographs with detailed instructions on how to perform the movements. Motion arrows are used on the photographs to help execute the movements correctly.
- *Learn the Basics of the Tai Chi Form in 10 Easy Steps: The Beginners Guide to the Tai Chi Form* (Read, 2018) includes video links and over 100 photos to guide people learn the basic moves of tai chi.
- *Tai Chi In 10 Weeks: A Beginner's Guide* (Kuhn, 2017) is designed to guide beginning students through the fundamentals of tai chi in ten weeks. It teaches readers 24 steps *yang*-style form and shares insight on warming up, healing, and avoiding injury.

MEASUREMENT OF OUTCOMES

Mind concentration and breathing control are two of the major tenets of tai chi practice (Yeung et al., 2018). When practicing tai chi with a peaceful, focused mind and incorporating smooth breathing into each movement, a person experiences physical and psychological relaxation, which leads to enhanced well-being in both states (Yeung et al., 2018). With this conceptual framework in mind, the measurement of the effects of tai chi should include both physical and psychological well-being. More studies have been done to measure the physical outcomes of tai chi practice (such as cardiovascular functioning), with little emphasis on psychological well-being outcomes (such as mood states).

USES

Tai chi is especially appropriate for older adults or for patients with chronic diseases because of its low intensity, steady rhythm, and low physical and mental tension (Chewning et al., 2020; Zhu et al., 2020). It has been shown to enhance cardiovascular and respiratory functions, improve health-related fitness, and promote positive health status (Lee et al., 2020; Manferdelli et al., 2019; Wang et al., 2016a). In addition, practicing tai chi has been effective in lowering blood pressure (Leung et al., 2019; Ma et al., 2018; Wang et al., 2016a). Studies also have indicated that tai chi increases postural stability, enhances balance (Bubela et al., 2019; Ghandali et al., 2017), and improves muscle strength and endurance (Bubela et al., 2019; Ghandali et al., 2017; Hwang et al., 2016), which leads to a reduction in the risk of falls (Bubela et al., 2019; Gallant et al., 2019; Hwang et al., 2016; Li et al., 2018). Tai chi also plays an important role in symptom control of chronic illnesses such as osteoarthritis (Field, 2016; Ghandali et al., 2017; Wang et al., 2016b).

In addition, studies have indicated that tai chi practice may also provide psychological benefits, such as enhanced positive mood states (Huang et al., 2019; Hwang et al., 2016; Wang et al., 2016a) and quality of sleep (Chan et al., 2016; Huston & McFarlane, 2016; Lü et al., 2017; Zhu et al., 2020).

Researchers have suggested that tai chi could be incorporated into community programs or senior center activities to promote the well-being of community-dwelling older adults. It could also be included as one of the activities in nursing homes or in rehabilitation programs in hospital settings (Desrochers et al., 2016; Polkey et al., 2018). Furthermore, tai chi has been applied to other populations. For example, tai chi improves the pulmonary function of children with asthma (Liao et al., 2019; Lin et al., 2017), serves as a therapy for patients with attention-deficit/hyperactivity disorder (Converse et al., 2020), increases the functional capacity of people with myocardial infarction (Wu et al., 2020), and enhances balance, gait, and mobility of people with Parkinson disease (Li et al., 2020; Zhu et al., 2020). Tai chi has also been practiced in many countries, including the United States, the United Kingdom, Australia, Hong Kong, Singapore, and Taiwan. How tai chi is used in the United Kingdom, as an example, is illustrated in Sidebar 16.1.

Sidebar 16.1 *Use of Tai Chi in the United Kingdom*

Graeme D. Smith

Although part of traditional Chinese medicine (TCM), tai chi appears to be increasingly used in the United Kingdom for health-related benefits and stress relief. To date, there is little U.K.-based research to support the popularity of this activity. Anecdotally, tai chi seems to be used mostly by older people for physical and mental health benefits. The National Health Service (NHS) in the United Kingdom notes that appropriate use of tai chi may prevent falls and improve overall psychological well-being in older adults. The basis of these claims may come from the improved balance control and flexibility those who practice tai chi may achieve. However, as with other forms of complementary and alternative medicine, high-quality rigorous research is required to substantiate these claims. Unfortunately, to date, such research is lacking.

Private healthcare providers in the United Kingdom also promote tai chi as a very low-impact, feel-good form of exercise. There would appear to be no real safety issues associated with using tai chi, although people who are pregnant or have a hernia, back pain, or severe osteoporosis are encouraged to speak to their family doctor before they start. Also, from a safety perspective, individuals are encouraged to find out about a tai chi instructor's qualifications and experience before they enroll in a program. At present, there is no statutory regulation of tai chi in the United Kingdom. Several tai chi bodies do exist, including the Tai Chi Union for Great Britain. This is the largest collective of independent tai chi instructors in the United Kingdom. They aim to unite tai chi practitioners and promote tai chi in all its aspects—health, aesthetic meditation, self-defense, and general improvement of standards. Tai Chi UK is another existing organization that claims tai chi can be "the ultimate holistic experience." The development of such groups is a clear indication of tai chi's increasing popularity in the United Kingdom.

PRECAUTIONS

Tai chi is unique for its slow graceful movements with low-impact, low-velocity, and minimal orthopedic complications and is a suitable conditioning exercise for older adults (Kasim et al., 2020; Okuyan & Deveci, 2020). Although many research studies have shown the benefits of tai chi, there are some contraindications to its practice, such as an acute stage of angina, ventricular arrhythmia, or myocardial ischemia. The instructor and the student have to be aware of these contraindications, and an initial assessment is necessary to determine an individual's exercise tolerance and other limitations (Wang et al., 2016a). While learning tai chi, a novice should be periodically evaluated in terms of progress, program adherence, cognitive response, muscular strength, balance, and level of flexibility at fairly regular (e.g., every 4 weeks) intervals for the first 60 days to 90 days of participation in such a program. Progression is individualized and is based on the preference of the instructor (Hermanns et al., 2018). It is strongly suggested that one learn tai chi from an experienced master who is able to teach the movements based on individual needs and physical tolerance. Advice on choosing a class is provided in Exhibit 16.2.

FUTURE RESEARCH

Overall, practicing tai chi appropriately has various benefits, as evidenced in the literature, and it is highly recommended for the appropriate populations. More studies about the effects of tai chi from a nursing perspective are needed to provide guidance o its use with various populations to nurses. Some questions for further research include:

- Which populations can most benefit from practicing tai chi, and are there conditions that would preclude its use?
- What is the nature of change in the well-being status of older adults who practice tai chi?
- What are the differences between well-being outcomes of beginners (people who are just starting to learn tai chi movements), practitioners (people who have practiced tai chi regularly for more than a year), and masters (people who have practiced tai chi regularly for more than a decade and are licensed by the National Tai Chi Association to be instructors)?

Exhibit 16.2 *Selecting a Tai Chi Class*

- If possible, find a studio or organization that specializes in tai chi.
- Find an experienced teacher (6–10 years of experience) who demonstrates and verbally explains the movements. Ask to observe a class before joining.
- Find a class with fewer than 20 students.
- Avoid purchasing any special clothing or equipment.

WEBSITES

Additional information can be found through the following useful websites:

- www.scheele.org/lee/tcclinks.html provides links to more than 100 other websites on tai chi and related topics.
- www.itcca.it/peterlim/index.htm is a valuable site with complete historical and background information on tai chi.

REFERENCES

Booth, F. W., Roberts, C. K., Thyfault, J. P., Ruegsegger, G. N., & Toedebusch, R. G. (2017). Role of inactivity in chronic diseases: Evolutionary insight and pathophysiological mechanisms. *Physiological Reviews, 97*(4), 1351–1402. https://doi.org/10.1152/physrev.00019.2016

Bubela, D., Sacharko, L., Chan, J., & Brady, M. (2019). Balance and functional outcomes for older community-dwelling adults who practice tai chi and those who do not: A comparative study. *Journal of Geriatric Physical Therapy, 42*(4), 209–215. https://doi.org/10.1519/JPT.0000000000000153

Chan, A. W., Yu, D. S., Choi, K. C., Lee, D. T., Sit, J. W., & Chan, H. Y. (2016). Tai chi qigong as a means to improve night-time sleep quality among older adults with cognitive impairment: A pilot randomized controlled trial. *Clinical Interventions in Aging, 11*, 1277–1286. https://doi.org/10.2147/CIA.S111927

Chen, K. M., Chen, W. T., & Huang, M. F. (2006). Development of the simplified tai-chi exercise program (STEP) for frail older adults. *Complementary Therapies in Medicine, 14*, 200–206. https://doi.org/10.1016/j.ctim.2006.05.002

Chewning, B., Hallisy, K. M., Mahoney, J. E., Wilson, D., Sangasubana, N., & Gangnon, R. (2020). Disseminating tai chi in the community: Promoting home practice and improving balance. *Gerontologist, 60*(4), 765–775. https://doi.org/10.1093/geront/gnz006

Clark, A. (2011). *The complete illustrated guide to tai chi: A step-by-step approach to the ancient Chinese movement.* HarperCollins.

Converse, A. K., Barrett, B. P., Chewning, B. A., & Wayne, P. M. (2020). Tai chi training for attention deficit hyperactivity disorder: A feasibility trial in college students. *Complementary Therapies in Medicine, 53*, Article 102538. https://doi.org/10.1016/j.ctim.2020.102538

Desrochers, P., Kairy, D., Pan, S., Corriveau, H., & Tousignant, M. (2016). Tai chi for upper limb rehabilitation in stroke patients: The patient's perspective. *Disability and Rehabilitation, 39*, 1313–1319. https://doi.org/10.1080/09638288.2016.1194900

Douglas, B., & Douglas, A. W. (2012). *The complete idiot's guide to t'ai chi & qigong illustrated.* Alpha.

Field, T. (2016). Knee osteoarthritis pain in the elderly can be reduced by massage therapy, yoga and tai chi: A review. *Complementary Therapies in Clinical Practice, 22*, 87–92. https://doi.org/10.1016/j.ctcp.2016.01.001

Gallant, M. P., Tartaglia, M., Hardman, S., & Burke, K. (2019). Using tai chi to reduce fall risk factors among older adults: An evaluation of a community-based implementation. *Journal of Applied Gerontology, 38*(7), 983–998. https://doi.org/10.1177/0733464817703004

Ghandali, E., Moghadam, S. T., Hadian, M. R., Olyaei, G., Jalaie, S., & Sajjadi, E. (2017). The effect of tai chi exercises on postural stability and control in older patients with knee osteoarthritis. *Journal of Bodywork and Movement Therapies, 21*(3), 594–598. https://doi.org/10.1016/j.jbmt.2016.09.001

Gu, Q. (2011). *Chen style taijiquan 56 form for competition.* Hong Kong Study Society.

Hallisy, K. M. (2018). Health benefits of tai chi: Potential mechanisms of action. *International Journal of Family & Community Medicine, 2*(5), 261–264. https://doi.org/10.15406/ijfcm.2018.02.00091

Hermanns, M., Haas, B. K., Rath, L., Murley, B., Arce-Esquivel, A. A., Ballard, J. E., & Wang, Y. T. (2018). Impact of tai chi on peripheral neuropathy revisited: A mixed-methods study. *Gerontology and Geriatric Medicine, 4*, Article 2333721418819532. https://doi.org/10.1177/2333721418819532

Huang, N., Li, W., Rong, X., Champ, M., Wei, L., Li, M., Mu, H., Hu, Y., Ma, Z., & Lyu, J. (2019). Effects of a modified tai chi program on older people with mild dementia: A randomized controlled trial. *Journal of Alzheimer's Disease, 72*(3), 947–956. https://doi.org/10.3233/JAD-190487

Huston, P., & McFarlane, B. (2016). Health benefits of tai chi: What is the evidence? *Canadian Family Physician, 62*(11), 881–890. https://www.cfp.ca/content/cfp/62/11/881.full.pdf

Hwang, H. F., Chen, S. J., Lee-Hsieh, J., Chien, D. K., Chen, C. Y., & Lin, M. R. (2016). Effects of home-based tai chi and lower extremity training and self-practice on falls and functional outcomes in older fallers from the emergency department: A randomized controlled trial. *Journal of the American Geriatrics Society, 64*(3), 518–525. https://doi.org/10.1111/jgs.13952

Kasim, N. F., van Zanten, J. V., & Aldred, S. (2020). Tai chi is an effective form of exercise to reduce markers of frailty in older age. *Experimental Gerontology, 135*(1), 110925. https://doi.org/10.1016/j.exger.2020.110925

Koh, T. C. (1981). Tai chi chuan. *American Journal of Chinese Medicine, 9*, 15–22. https://doi.org/10.1142/s0192415x81000032

Kuhn, A. (2017). *Tai chi in 10 weeks: A beginner's guide.* YMAA Publication Center.

Lee, T. L., Sherman, K. J., Hawkes, R. J., Phelan, E. A., & Turner, J. A. (2020). The benefits of T'ai Chi for older adults with chronic back pain: A qualitative study. *The Journal of Alternative and Complementary Medicine, 26*(6), 456–462. https://doi.org/10.1089/acm.2019.0455

Leung, L. Y., Chan, A. W., Sit, J. W., Liu, T., & Taylor-Piliae, R. E. (2019). Tai chi in Chinese adults with metabolic syndrome: A pilot randomized controlled trial. *Complementary Therapies in Medicine, 46*, 54–61. https://doi.org/10.1016/j.ctim.2019.07.008

Li, F., Harmer, P., Fitzgerald, K., Eckstrom, E., Akers, L., Chou, L. S., Pidgeon, D., Voit, J., & Winters-Stone, K. (2018). Effectiveness of a therapeutic Tai Ji Quan intervention vs a multimodal exercise intervention to prevent falls among older adults at high risk of falling: A randomized clinical trial. *JAMA Internal Medicine, 178*(10), 1301–1310. https://doi.org/10.1001/jamainternmed.2018.3915

Li, Q., Liu, J., Dai, F., & Dai, F. (2020). Tai chi versus routine exercise in patients with early- or mild-stage Parkinson's disease: A retrospective cohort analysis. *Brazilian Journal of Medical and Biological Research, 53*(2), Article e9171. http://dx.doi.org/10.1590/1414-431X20199171

Liang, S. Y., & Wu, W. C. (2014). *Simplified Tai Chi Chuan: 24 postures with applications & standard 48 postures* (2nd ed.). YMAA Publication Center.

Liao, P. C., Lin, H. H., Chiang, B. L., Lee, J. H., Yu, H. H., Lin, Y. T., Yang, Y. H., Li, P. Y., Wang, L. C., & Sun, W. Z. (2019). Tai chi chuan exercise improves lung function and asthma control through immune regulation in childhood asthma. *Evidence-Based Complementary and Alternative Medicine, 2019*, Article 9146827. https://doi.org/10.1155/2019/9146827

Lin, H. C., Lin, H. P., Yu, H. H., Wang, L. C., Lee, J. H., Lin, Y. T., Yang, Y. H., Li, P. Y., Sun, W. Z., & Chiang, B. L. (2017). Tai-chi-chuan exercise improves pulmonary function and decreases exhaled nitric oxide level in both asthmatic and nonasthmatic children and improves quality of life in children with asthma. *Evidence-Based Complementary and Alternative Medicine, 2017*, Article 6287642. https://doi.org/10.1155/2017/6287642

Lü, J., Huang, L., Wu, X., Fu, W., & Liu, Y. (2017). Effect of Tai Ji Quan training on self-reported sleep quality in elderly Chinese women with knee osteoarthritis: A randomized controlled trial. *Sleep Medicine, 33*, 70–75. https://doi.org/10.1016/j.sleep.2016.12.024

Ma, C., Zhou, W., Tang, Q., & Huang, S. (2018). The impact of group-based tai chi on health-status outcomes among community-dwelling older adults with hypertension. *Heart & Lung, 47*(4), 337–344. https://doi.org/10.1016/j.hrtlng.2018.04.007

Manferdelli, G., La Torre, A., & Codella, R. (2019). Outdoor physical activity bears multiple benefits to health and society. *The Journal of Sports Medicine and Physical Fitness, 59*(5), 868–879. https://doi.org/10.23736/S0022-4707.18.08771-6

Okuyan, C. B., & Deveci, E. (2020). The effectiveness of tai chi chuan on fear of movement, prevention of falls, physical activity, and cognitive status in older adults with mild cognitive impairment: A randomized controlled trial. *Perspectives in Psychiatric Care.* Advanced online publication.. https://doi.org/10.1111/ppc.12684

Polkey, M. I., Qiu, Z. H., Zhou, L., Zhu, M. D., Wu, Y. X., Chen, Y. Y., Ye, S. P., He, Y. S., Jiang, M., He, B. T., Mehta, B., Zhong, N. S., & Luo, Y. M. (2018). Tai chi and pulmonary rehabilitation compared for treatment-naive patients with COPD: A randomized controlled trial. *Chest*, *153*(5), 1116–1124. https://doi.org/10.1016/j.chest.2018.01.053

Quarta, C. W., & Vallie, M. M. (2012). *Seated tai chi and qigong: Guided therapeutic exercises to manage stress and balance mind, body and spirit*. Singing Dragon.

Read, P. (2018). *The beginners guide to the tai chi form*. Blurb.

Wang, C., Schmid, C. H., Iversen, M. D., Harvey, W. F., Fielding, R. A., Driban, J. B., Price, L. L., Wong, J. B., Reid, K. F., Rones, R., & McAlindon, T. (2016a). Comparative effectiveness of tai chi versus physical therapy for knee osteoarthritis. *Annals of Internal Medicine*, *165*(2), 77–86. https://doi.org/10.7326/M15-2143

Wang, Y. T., Li, Z., Yang, Y., Zhong, Y., Lee, S. Y., Chen, S., & Chen, Y. P. (2016b). Effects of wheelchair tai chi on physical and mental health among elderly with disability. *Research in Sports Medicine*, *24*(3), 157–170. https://doi.org/10.1080/15438627.2016.1191487

Wu, B., Ding, Y., Zhong, B., Jin, X., Cao, Y., & Xu, D. (2020). Intervention treatment for myocardial infarction with tai chi: A systematic review and meta-analysis. *Archives of Physical Medicine and Rehabilitation*, *101*(12), 2206–2218. https://doi.org/10.1016/j.apmr.2020.02.012

Yang, J. M. (2010). *Tai chi chuan classical yang style: The complete form qigong*. Yang's Martial Arts Association.

Yang, J. M., & Liang, T. T. (2016). *Tai chi chuan martial applications: Advanced yang style* (3rd ed.). Ymaa Publication Center.

Yeung, A., Chan, J. S. M., Cheung, J. C., & Zou, L. (2018). Qigong and tai-chi for mood regulation. *Focus*, *16*(1), 40–47. https://doi.org/10.1176/appi.focus.20170042

Zhu, M., Zhang, Y., Pan, J., Fu, C., & Wang, Y. (2020). Effect of simplified Tai Chi exercise on relieving symptoms of patients with mild to moderate Parkinson's disease. *The Journal of Sports Medicine and Physical Fitness*, *60*(2), 282–288. https://doi.org/10.23736/S0022-4707.19.10104-1

Relaxation Therapies

MICHELE M. EVANS AND SUSAN M. BEE

During the past decade, stress was recognized as a global problem by the World Health Organization (WHO, 2013), and the recent COVID-19 pandemic has amplified these concerns. The cost of stress, measured in health impacts to clients and providers, is growing. Given this persistent level of global stress, it has become increasingly important that both clinicians and clients develop stress-reducing techniques. Relaxation therapies can be used to decrease stress by reducing muscle tension in the body. Many relaxation therapies exist and have been shown to help manage stress, offer pain relief, and promote health. The ones discussed in this chapter range from simple and easily implemented diaphragmatic breathing (DB) to more complex methods, such as progressive muscle relaxation (PMR) and autogenic training (AT). Using a combination of these therapies is common because they provide variety in terms of time to learn and to use. Evidence supporting the use of these strategies continues to grow, making them good options for health symptom management and promotion of wellness.

DEFINITION

Relaxation therapies help reduce the tension that exists in muscles, which often generalizes to other areas of the body, including the mind. Effective relaxation can reduce the destructive impacts and symptoms of stress-induced illnesses and improve a person's quality of life. Relaxation is a form of self-care that can benefit clients, students, and healthcare providers themselves. Teaching clients relaxation techniques allows them to become more active partners in their healthcare.

Relaxed DB uses the diaphragm when a breath is taken. The purpose of relaxed breathing is to slow breathing and to reduce the use of shoulder, neck, and upper chest muscles to breathe more efficiently, which improves oxygenation to the entire body.

PMR is the tensing and releasing of successive muscle groups. This technique was introduced by Jacobson (1938) and is still used widely today. A person's attention is drawn to discriminating between the feelings experienced when a muscle group is relaxed and when it is tensed; eventually, with practice, the person is able to relax the muscles just by focusing on them.

AT is a relaxation method that uses both imagery and body awareness to reduce stress and muscle tension. This technique was developed and published by the German neurologist Schultz (Schultz & Luthe, 1959) and addresses autonomic sensations that lead to muscle relaxation.

SCIENTIFIC BASIS

The aim of relaxation therapies is to reduce stress and the accompanying effects that stress has on the body. Real and perceived events and thoughts can create stress that activates the sympathetic nervous system. This begins a cascade of physical and chemical reactions. The heart pounds and blood pressure rises, respirations become shallow, pupils dilate, and the muscles tense as the body prepares to cope with the stressor. This is often called the *fight-or-flight* response. The parasympathetic nervous system is known as the rest-and-digest or rest-and-restore response. When one response is activated, the other is quiet. Prolonged activation of the sympathetic nervous system over time can have deleterious effects on the body. The desired outcome of relaxation strategies is the mitigation of persisting high levels of stress and activation of the parasympathetic nervous system (Jacobson, 1938).

When a person breathes, the body takes in oxygen and releases carbon dioxide. If the body detects an imbalance in these two gases, it signals for changes in breathing that may lead to fast, shallow breathing called *hyperventilation*, often in response to stressful events or pain. DB is a relaxation technique that uses the diaphragm to breathe deeply and improve oxygenation to the entire body. It is a learned skill, and practice is required for optimal benefit. Evidence from a comprehensive review by Hopper (2019) suggests that diaphragmatic breathing as an isolated intervention may decrease both physiologic biomarkers and psychological measures of stress. Research from Schmidt et al., (2012) provides evidence that using DB for 10 minutes three times per day significantly reduces the self-rating of anxiety, depression, fatigue, sleep quality, and pain.

Jacobson (1938) reported that PMR decreased the body's oxygen consumption, metabolic rate, respiratory rate, muscle tension, premature ventricular contractions, and systolic and diastolic blood pressure and increased alpha brain waves. Subsequent studies, including that of Izgu (2020), have validated Jacobson's findings, additionally finding that PMR resulted in an improvement in pain, fatigue, and quality of life in patients with Type 2 diabetes. Also pertinent are timely findings that PMR training can reduce anxiety, depression, and sleep quality in COVID-19 patients during isolation (Xiao et al., 2020).

AT reduces excessive autonomic arousal, and it is effective in raising dysfunctionally low levels of autonomic functions such as a low heart rate. It is known as a self-regulatory model. AT may not only affect sympathetic tone but may also activate the parasympathetic system. The increase in parasympathetic dominance results in peripheral vasodilation and increased feelings of warmth and heaviness in the body. A meta-analysis regarding the effectiveness of autogenic training on the stress response found that AT decreased anxiety and depression and increased high-frequency heart rate variability (Seo, 2019).

INTERVENTION

Relaxation means more than simply having peace of mind or resting. It means eliminating tension from the body and mind. Learning relaxation skills requires the person to focus on the mind–body connection, such as when muscles are tensed, and practice ways to relax the muscles to improve overall health and wellness.

TECHNIQUES

DB TECHNIQUE

DB can be used before and during stressful situations, such as a painful procedure, or for overall health enhancement as part of routine self-care. It is a relatively simple relaxation technique that can be taught and used in virtually any healthcare setting and does not require extensive training of the instructor or the client. The instructions for DB are found in Exhibit 17.1. Emphasis needs to be placed on the person practicing DB throughout the day until it becomes a natural way of breathing. For the best effect, an individual should practice this technique frequently when not anxious or short of breath. A recent investigation by Russell and colleagues (2017) found that including a "post exhalation rest break" in diaphragmatic breathing improved high-frequency heart rate variability (which is positively associated with self-regulatory control). Access naturalhealthperspective.com/resilience/deep-breathing.html for succinct information on DB.

PMR TECHNIQUE

Numerous techniques for muscle relaxation have been developed since Jacobson published his technique in 1938. Often, the procedures include attention to breathing (Schaffer & Yucha, 2004). The instructor assists the individual in identifying a place that is quiet and restful in which to practice relaxation. A comfortable chair that provides support for the body is recommended. Clothing should be loose and not restrictive; shoes, glasses, and contact lenses should be removed. The person may wish to use the bathroom before practicing muscle relaxation.

The PMR therapy or variations of it, developed by Bernstein and Borkovec (1973) is widely used. They combined the 108 muscles and muscle groups of

---

Exhibit 17.1 *Instructions for Diaphragmatic (Deep) Breathing*

1. Sit comfortably with feet flat on the floor.
2. Loosen tight clothing around the abdomen and waist.
3. Place hands in the lap or at the sides.
4. Breathe in slowly (through the nose if possible), allowing the abdomen to expand with inhalation.
5. Exhale at the normal rate.
6. Use pursed-lip breathing—which creates a very small opening between lips through which to breathe out—if desired.

Exhibit 17.2 *Guidelines for Progressive Muscle Relaxation for 14 Muscle Groups*

General Information

Instruct clients to tense a specific muscle group when they hear "tense" and to release the tension when they hear "relax." Tension is held for 7 seconds. Draw attention to the feeling of tension and relaxation. When muscles are relaxed, attention is drawn to the differences between the two states.

Tensing Specific Muscle Groups

- Dominant hand and forearm: Make a tight fist and hold it.
- Dominant upper arm: Push elbow down against the arm of the chair.
- Repeat instructions for the nondominant arm.
- Forehead: Lift eyebrows as high as possible.
- Central face (cheeks, nose, eyes): Squint eyes and wrinkle nose.
- Lower face and jaw: Clench teeth and widen mouth.
- Neck: Pull chin down toward chest but do not touch chest.
- Chest, shoulders, and upper back: Take a deep breath and hold it; pull shoulder blades back.
- Abdomen: Pull stomach in and try to protect it.
- Dominant thigh: Lift leg and hold it straight out.
- Dominant calf: Point toes toward the ceiling.

Repeat instructions for the nondominant side.

Source: Adapted from Bernstein, D., & Borkovec, T. (1973). *Progressive relaxation training.* Research Press.

Jacobson's original technique into the initial tensing and relaxing of 14 muscle groups. Subsequently, the number of groups was reduced to seven and then four (Exhibit 17.2). Although Bernstein and Borkovec included instructions for tensing muscles of the feet, those are not included in Exhibit 17.2 because spasms in the foot may result when tensing these muscles. The ultimate goal is to achieve muscle relaxation throughout the body without initially having to tense the muscles. Through practice, the individual acquires a mental image of how the muscles feel when they are relaxed and is able to relax them using this image.

Education on the scientific basis for the use of PMR is provided during the first session. Stressors, the impact of stress on the body, and the signs and symptoms of high levels of stress are discussed. Descriptions and demonstrations for achieving tension of each muscle group are given, and participants then practice tensing each of the muscle groups.

After progressing through all the muscle groups, the instructor asks the client to identify whether tension remains in any of them. The instructor observes the client to assess general relaxation, focusing on slowed, deeper breathing; arms relaxed and shoulders forward; and feet apart with toes pointing out. At the conclusion of the session, 2 or 3 minutes are provided for the client to enjoy the feelings associated with relaxation. Terminating relaxation is done gradually.

The instructor counts backward from four to one. The individual is given the opportunity to ask questions or discuss the feelings experienced.

Bernstein and Borkovec (1973) proposed using 10 sessions to teach PMR. However, in many studies, instruction has been limited to fewer sessions with positive results obtained. A critical factor in determining the number of teaching sessions needed is ensuring that people have mastered relaxing the muscle groups and have integrated PMR into their lifestyles.

An essential factor in the effectiveness of PMR and other relaxation techniques is daily practice. At least one 15-minute practice session a day is recommended. Schaffer and Yucha (2004) suggest two 10-minute practice sessions daily. Helping clients find a time of day to practice relaxation is an important component of instruction. Often, an audiotape of the instructions is provided for home practice. Clients are also instructed to use the relaxation technique anytime they feel tense or before an event that may cause them to become anxious and tense. Refer to www.guidetopsychology.com/pmr.htm for comprehensive instructions on PMR.

AT TECHNIQUE

AT is a relaxation method that is self-generated or self-guided using relaxation phases. A healthcare provider familiar with the therapy can help in learning the method. AT is gaining worldwide use and is intended to create a feeling of warmth and heaviness throughout the body while a profound state of physical relaxation, bodily health, and mental health is experienced. AT is most effective when done in a quiet place while wearing loose clothing and not wearing shoes. Practice should be done at a time when the individual has not recently eaten a large meal. The person focuses intently on inner experiences and excludes external events. When the session finishes, people relax with their eyes closed for a few seconds and then get up slowly. To maintain proficiency, practicing at least once a day is recommended. Instructions for self-guided AT are given in Exhibit 17.3. Refer to www.guidetopsychology.com/autogen.htm for an example of in-depth instructions on phases to be used for relaxation.

Exhibit 17.3 *Instructions for Self-Guided AT*

AT consists of a warm-up period of breathing and progressively learning six phases of relaxation that all together may take several months to fully master. On completion, a person will progress through and include the following:

- *Warm-up:* focused breathing on slow exhalation
- *Phase 1:* heaviness—arms and legs are heavy
- *Phase 2:* warmth—arms and legs are warm
- *Phase 3:* a calm heart—heartbeat is calm
- *Phase 4:* breathing—breathing is steady
- *Phase 5:* stomach—stomach is soft and warm
- *Phase 6:* cool forehead—forehead is cool
- *Completion:* feel supremely calm

MEASUREMENT OF OUTCOMES

Although findings from many studies have shown positive outcomes from the use of relaxation techniques, positive results have not been reported in all the research in which these therapies were explored. Reasons for the differences in outcomes may relate to the wide variation in the types of relaxation techniques, the length and type of instruction, the degree of mastery of the therapy, and irregular or sporadic practice of the procedures.

A variety of outcomes have been used to measure the efficacy of relaxation techniques. Physiological measurements that are often used include respiratory rate, heart rate, and blood pressure. Electromyogram readings are occasionally taken to determine the degree of tension in the specific muscle groups. Practitioners need to be alert to underlying pathology or medications that may interfere with a reduction in physiological parameters.

Anxiety is the most frequently used subjective measure. The State-Trait Anxiety Inventory (STAI) Scale by Spielberger et al. (1983) has been widely used. People's self-reports about feelings of relaxation have been included in many studies because satisfaction is a good indicator of whether an individual will continue to use an intervention. Reports of reduction of pain, symptoms of depression, increases in comfort, and improved sleep are other results that have been used to measure the effects of these techniques.

PRECAUTIONS

Although muscle-relaxation techniques have been used with multiple populations and have been demonstrated to be an effective therapy for nurses to use, some cautions should be observed. It is important for practitioners to know whether clients practice the relaxation techniques on a regular basis because this may affect the pharmacokinetics of medications. Adjustment in doses of medication for hypertension, diabetes, and seizures may be indicated.

The relaxation of muscles may produce a hypotensive state. People are instructed to remain seated for a few minutes after practice. Movement in place and the gradual resumption of activities help raise the blood pressure. Taking a person's blood pressure at the conclusion of teaching sessions helps identify those who are prone to hypotensive states after muscle relaxation and AT because the relaxation therapy may have caused hypotension.

Some individuals with chronic pain have reported a heightened awareness of pain following the tensing and relaxing of muscles. Concentrating on tensing and relaxing muscles may draw attention to the pain rather than to the muscle sensation. A good assessment of clients is needed to determine whether negative outcomes are occurring.

Children younger than school age lack the discipline to do AT. Also, those with limited mental ability, acute central nervous system disorders, or uncontrolled psychosis may be unable to process the in-depth instructions (Linden, 2007). In some clients, AT may produce the side effects of anxiety, sadness, resurfaced memories and suppressed thoughts, or reawakened pain sensation from old illnesses or injuries. These effects may stem from the disinhibition of various cortical processes due to the autogenic formulas and the focus on body sensations (Lehrer, 2009).

USES

Promoting an understanding of the anticipated positive benefits of the therapies is critical. Relaxation therapies have been used to achieve a variety of outcomes in diverse populations. Exhibit 17.4 lists conditions and populations, including the country in which the research was conducted, showing the widespread use of these therapies. The use of DB, PMR, and AT to reduce anxiety and stress, relieve pain, and promote health is discussed. As noted in the list of uses, studies have been carried out worldwide.

Exhibit 17.4 *Selected Studies Supporting Use of Therapies*

THERAPY	HEALTH CONDITION	STUDY AUTHORS	COUNTRY OF STUDY
DB	Chronic pain and fibromyalgia (pain tolerance, self-efficacy, heart rate variability, functional impact on daily life)	Schmidt et al. (2012) Tomas-Carus (2018)	United States Portugal
DB	Anxiety, depression, and prenatal attachment in gestational diabetes	Fiskin (2018)	Turkey
DB	Type 2 diabetes mellitus	Hedge et al. (2012)	India
DB	Pain and anxiety during burn care	Park et al. (2013)	South Korea
DB	Coronary heart disease	Chung et al. (2010)	Taiwan
DB	Chronic obstructive pulmonary disease	Yamaguti et al. (2012)	Brazil
DB	Gastroesophageal reflux disease	Halland (2021)	United States
DB and PMR	Asthma	Georga (2019)	Greece
DB and PMR	Hypertension during pregnancy	Aalami et al. (2016)	Iran
PMR	Anxiety and self-efficacy in patients undergoing extremity fracture surgery	Xie (2016)	China
PMR	Cancer (decreasing nausea and vomiting)	Zhang (2017)	China
PMR	Chronic obstructive pulmonary disease	Chegeni (2018); Yilmaz (2017)	Iran Turkey
PMR	Night eating syndrome	Vander Wal et al. (2015)	United States

THERAPY	HEALTH CONDITION	STUDY AUTHORS	COUNTRY OF STUDY
PMR	COVID 19 patients (negative emotions and sleep quality)	Xiao et al. (2020)	China
PMR	Migraine headaches	Meyer et al. (2016)	Germany
PMR	Pain, fatigue, and quality of life in diabetes	Izgu (2020)	Turkey
PMR	Chemotherapy-inducednausea	Tian (2020)	China
PMR	Postcesarean pain, sleep, and physical activities	Ismail (2018)	Egypt
PMR	Schizophrenia	Melo-Dias et al. (2014)	Portugal
PMR and AT	Reduced benzodiazepine use in patients with medically unexplained symptoms	Hashimoto (2020)	Japan
AT	Anxiety, depression, distress in hemodialysis patients	Cavallaro & Alibrandi (2020)	Italy
AT	Poststroke anxiety	Golding et al. (2016)	United Kingdom
AT	Anxiety disorder	Miu et al. (2009)	Netherlands
AT	Insomnia	Bowden et al. (2012)	United Kingdom
AT	Chronic fatigue syndrome	Kutsenko (2018)	Ukraine
AT	Breastfeeding self-efficacy	Rahayu & Yunarsih (2018)	Indonesia
AT	Sexual arousal	Stanton & Meston (2017)	United States

Exhibit 17.4 *Selected Studies Supporting Use of Therapies (continued)*

AT = autogenic training; DB = diaphragmatic breathing; PMR = progressive muscle relaxation.

REDUCTION OF ANXIETY AND STRESS

As noted in Exhibit 17.4, these therapies have been effective in reducing the stress associated with a number of conditions. DB training significantly improved anxiety and depression in women with gestational diabetes (Fiskin & Sahin, 2018). Golding et al. (2016) reported a reduction in anxiety scores using AT with poststroke patients. Miu et al. (2009) found that AT increased heart rate variability and facilitated vagal control of the heart, reducing symptoms of anxiety. Relaxation techniques can be used to both decrease and prevent stress, which is a risk factor for many health conditions.

PAIN

Relaxation therapies have been used extensively in the management of many types of pain. Muscle tension increases the perception of pain, so lessening anxiety and tension may help in reducing it. Research by Schmidt et al. (2012) with patients with fibromyalgia found that the use of three 10-minute daily DB sessions showed significant improvements in pain severity, fatigue, pain self-efficacy, cold pressor tolerance, and heart rate variability in measurements 2 weeks apart. Similarly, Tomas-Carus (2018) found that 12 weeks of daily DB practice resulted in a significant improvement in pain threshold and functional capacity in a study of patients with fibromyalgia. A significant reduction in pain levels was found in patients with burns using DB (Park et al., 2013). In a 6-week PMR program, migraine headache frequency was significantly decreased. PMR was suggested to operate by enhancing self-efficacy in managing headaches and reducing associated pain episodes (Meyer et al., 2016).

COVID-19

The sudden and rapid expansion of COVID-19 illness provided an additional need for stress reduction across the globe and several researchers have investigated how relaxation strategies could be helpful to both patients and providers. Liu et al. (2021) utilized DB to improve sleep quality and relieve anxiety among first-line nurses in China during the pandemic. Additionally, in separate studies, researchers found that PMR training reduced anxiety, depression, and/or sleep quality in hospitalized COVID-19 patients during isolation when compared to that of controls (Liu et al., 2020; Xiao et al., 2020).

CULTURAL APPLICATIONS

Almost every culture has therapies for reducing stress. These include the use of various herbal preparations or potions, use of muscle exercises such as yoga, or spiritual practices. The three relaxation therapies described in this chapter or variations of them are commonly used in a number of cultures. Sidebar 17.1 describes therapies used in the Republic of Singapore.

Sidebar 17.1 *Use of Relaxation Therapies in the Republic of Singapore*

Siok-Bee Tan

In Singapore, relaxation techniques may be taught by nurses, psychologists, therapists, or other health professionals. The number of practitioners using these strategies is not substantial. At present, most nurses working in Singapore hospitals who use relaxation techniques employ deep diaphragmatic breathing. Fewer nurses use progressive muscle relaxation and autogenic training because a minority has been trained in these techniques and because these therapies are not suited to a fast-paced hospital environment. Nevertheless, in mental health institutions, relaxation techniques are more widely used. In outpatient areas, relaxation techniques can also be better utilized. For example, nurses who attend

Sidebar 17.1 *Use of Relaxation Therapies in the Republic of Singapore (continued)*

the Chronic Disease Management Workshop teach both deep diaphragmatic breathing and progressive muscle relaxation.

As an advanced practice nurse in Singapore, I use a combination of medical, nursing, and therapy models in clinical care. I specialize in helping patients who have intractable pain and chronic neurological conditions by utilizing various relaxation techniques. Techniques are important, but it is also crucial to ensure that a rapport is established first for the success of relaxation therapies. For example, in the practice of autogenic training, the key is to access the subconscious mind with relaxation. This requires considerable time and discipline to learn. In a culture in which patients mostly prescribe to medication and surgery, it is a challenge to get patients to adopt the technique for relaxation. With rapport, patients have the trust to commit their time to practice and, in turn, be able to bypass the critical factor of the conscious mind to access the subconscious mind to install the positive suggestions. I have successfully empowered many patients in using the healing powers of the mind as they get into a trance state during autogenic training.

It would be prudent to enable a greater number of nurses in Singapore to complete training in relaxation therapies, not only for the financial savings it may provide by shortening hospital stays but also for the benefits it provides to patients by equipping them with tools to manage anxiety and concerns at home. However, there is a need to have a shift in the hospital culture for relaxation techniques to be fully used. Relaxation techniques must be viewed as an advancement in pain and anxiety care and must be given an opportunity to be implemented by health professionals. The hospital culture in Singapore is focused on medication or surgery. However, there is some hope because mind–body interventions are slowly gaining entry into mainly medically dominated treatment. Patient care will be optimal if more healthcare professionals are willing to use complementary techniques as part of the recovery regimen.

Work-related demands result in poor health and well-being for a substantial number of nurses, which leads to increased absenteeism, high attrition, and reduced performance. Their stress also affects their working relationship with fellow nursing staff, their interactions with patients, and, therefore, their delivery of care. Thus, nursing management in Singapore has explored ways to enable nurses to embrace tools of self-care that will promote resiliency in their work environment, such as mindfulness and deep breathing practices and strategies. Mindfulness is increasingly gaining recognition as a tool for improving care, competence, and compassion among healthcare practitioners and, as a result, their patients. The practice of mindfulness cultivates the ability to purposefully focus one's attention on internal experiences, as well as interaction with the external environment, and to view these experiences more objectively, accepting them without judgment.

Nursing management in one Singapore hospital engaged a psychologist to conduct an introductory mindfulness and deep-breathing program for nurse leaders. This psychologist also supports new nurses and leaders during orientation programs. The psychologist has also facilitated a 5-week mindfulness and deep-breathing course, 2 hours each session, with a group of 16 nurses. This course

(continued)

Sidebar 17.1 *Use of Relaxation Therapies in the Republic of Singapore (continued)*

aimed to prepare nurse trainers, who will then facilitate courses for other nurses within their clinical areas.

Nurses who attended the program reported a positive impact of mindfulness and its benefits applied to the context of their daily lives at home and at work. They were motivated to continue their practice after the end of the program. The hospital in Singapore hopes to form a culture that will promote the ongoing practice of mindfulness and deep breathing. This is consistent with their vision of creating a culture shift to an environment full of empathy, compassion, and kindness.

Although relaxation strategies are helpful in reducing stress and anxiety in many conditions, it is important to note that these interventions alone may not be the most effective treatment for generalized anxiety disorder or major depression. According to the National Center for Complementary and Integrative Health (2016) website, a more comprehensive cognitive behavioral approach that includes relaxation has been found to be the most helpful for these conditions.

HEALTH PROMOTION IN VARIOUS POPULATIONS

Nursing has been at the forefront of teaching clients about health-promotion practices. Reducing and managing stress is an important preventive health strategy, and these therapies can be used for reducing risks for numerous conditions. Although relaxation therapies may not reduce heart rate and blood pressure in those who have readings within the normal range, using these techniques on a regular basis by healthy people may help prevent the development of hypertension. PMR and DB were found to decrease both systolic and diastolic blood pressure in pregnant women (Aalami et al., 2016). In healthy adults, DB was found to not only improve attention and negative affect but to also improve cortisol levels (Ma, 2017). Relaxation training can improve health in additional ways. AT was found to improve sexual arousal in sexually functional women (Stanton & Meston, 2017) and to have positive impacts on breastfeeding self-efficacy (Rahayu & Yunarsih, 2018). Sleep is essential for overall health; Bowden et al. (2012) found that the use of AT resulted in significant improvement in sleep-onset latency and stated that study participants ($N = 153$) with insomnia reported feeling more refreshed and energized. Those with Type 2 diabetes mellitus responded positively to DB, with significant reductions in fasting and postprandial plasma glucose and glycated hemoglobin levels (Hedge et al., 2012). This therapy may have the potential to be a preventive measure for a condition that is increasing in the United States.

TECHNOLOGY-BASED DELIVERY OF RELAXATION STRATEGIES

There is considerable interest in promoting more independence for individuals to maintain their health and wellness. As interest in relaxation methods has grown, the number of electronic applications and resources to instruct and support their use has also expanded. A number of researchers have recently investigated outcomes of using electronically delivered relaxation strategies, that is, online-based or smartphone application–based relaxation. A recent study in Spain found a reduction in COVID-19 anxiety levels in students by using combined PMR, autogenic, and abdominal breathing delivered via a telematic workshop (Ozamiz-Etxebarria, 2020). Several research projects have looked at the use of PMR with headaches utilizing a smartphone-based relaxation treatment and found that application use was associated with a reduction in the number of headache days (Minen et al., 2019; Usmani et al., 2021).

Practical examples of these technologies are available for various portable devices, although there is no specific research supporting their effectiveness. Breathe2Relax is an app created by National Center for Telehealth and Technology that helps users relax and relieve stress through exercises such as diaphragmatic breathing. It is completely free and available on the Apple App Store or Google Play. The Apple Watch includes a free app called Breathe that uses an animated flower to guide breath rate. Breathe creates a visual cue to breathe in as the flower slowly expands and to breathe out as the flower contracts. For those interested in PMR, there are several platforms available for purchase, such as the Progressive Muscle Relaxation, PMR Pro, and Superchill PMR, at Google Play or the Apple App Store. Free internet-based instruction for various relaxations are readily searchable; the interested reader may try a guided diaphragmatic breathing meditation from Mayo Clinic at www.mayoclinic.org/healthy-lifestyle/stress-management/multimedia/meditation/vid-2008474.

Electronically delivered relaxation strategies could be promising options in the future due to overall accessibility, less need for provider face-to-face availability, and the low cost of these resources. These resources have the potential to reach individuals with less healthcare access related to location or expense. The limitations of research to date have been small sample sizes, less robust methodologies, and reliance on subjective measures. While individuals may search out various independent resources on the internet and mobile devices, healthcare providers will need to ensure the scientific integrity of the sources before making recommendations.

FUTURE RESEARCH

Relaxation therapies discussed in this chapter have been used singly and in combination with other therapies to reduce and prevent stress. A scientific body of knowledge is emerging to guide the use of these techniques in practice, but more research is necessary. The following are several areas in which studies are needed:

- Although the number of randomized experimental studies on relaxation methods has grown, many of the studies have been completed with relatively small samples. Replication with larger sample sizes will provide greater support for these interventions.
- Clinical evidence for the feasibility and effectiveness of mobile device applications and internet-based sites for learning and using relaxation therapies will continue to present an important research opportunity.
- As the focus of healthcare becomes more individualized, it is important to identify relaxation therapies most likely to be effective for people based on their genetic information, cultural background, and lifestyle preferences. Studies connecting phenotype with genotype will be informative.

■ More research concentrating on using these therapies for health promotion and disease prevention in primary care settings may help improve the delivery of healthcare. Studies focusing on healthcare cost savings related to the use of relaxation strategies will be beneficial.

REFERENCES

Aalami, M., Jafarnejad, F., & ModarresGharavi, M. (2016). The effects of progressive muscular relaxation and breathing control technique on blood pressure during pregnancy. *Iranian Journal of Nursing and Midwifery Research, 21*(3), 331–336. https://doi.org/10.4103/1735-9066.180382

Bernstein, D., & Borkovec, T. (1973). *Progressive relaxation training*. Research Press.

Bowden, A., Lorenc, A., & Robinson, N. (2012). Autogenic training as a behavioural approach to insomnia: A prospective cohort study. *Primary Health Care Research & Development, 13*(2), 175–185. https://doi.org/10.1017/S1463423611000181

Cavallaro, M. F., & Alibrandi, A. (2020). The autogenic training on dialysis as a mental place of serenity and well-being. *Journal of Clinical and Developmental Psychology, 2*(2), 12–23. https://doi.org/10.6092/2612-4033/0110-2335

Chegeni, P. S, Gholami, M, Azargoon, A, Hossein, P. A. H., Birjandi, M, & Norollahi, H. (2018). The effect of progressive muscle relaxation on the management of fatigue and quality of sleep in patients with chronic obstructive pulmonary disease: A randomized controlled clinical trial. *Complementary Therapies in Clinical Practice, 31*, 64–70. https://doi.org/10.1016/j.ctcp.2018.01.010

Chung, L., Tsai, P., Liu, B., Chou, K., Lin, W., Shyu, Y., & Wang, M. (2010). Home-based deep breathing for depression in patients with coronary heart disease: A randomized controlled trial. *International Journal of Nursing Studies, 47*, 1346–1353. https://doi.org/10.1016/j.ijnurstu.2010.03.007

Fiskin, G., & Sahin, N. (2018). Effect of diaphragmatic breathing exercise on psychological parameters in gestational diabetes: A randomized controlled trial. *European Journal of Integrative Medicine, 23*, 50–56. https://doi.org/10.1016/j.eujim.2018.09.006

Georga, G., Chrousos, C., Artemiadis, A., Panagiotis, P. P., Bakakos, P., & Darviri, C. (2019). The effect of stress management incorporating progressive muscle relaxation and biofeedback-assisted relaxation breathing on patients with asthma: A randomized controlled trial. *Advances in Integrative Medicine, 6*(2), 73–77. https://doi.org/10.1016/j.aimed.2018.09.001

Golding, K., Kneebone, I., & Fife-Schaw, C. (2016). Self-help relaxation for post-stroke anxiety: A randomized, controlled pilot study. *Clinical Rehabilitation, 30*(2), 174–180. https://doi.org/10.1177/0269215515575746

Halland, M., Bharucha, A. E., Crowell, M. D., Ravi, K., & Katzka, D. A. (2021). Effects of diaphragmatic breathing on the pathophysiology and treatment of upright gastroesophageal reflux: A Randomized controlled trial. *The American Journal of Gastroenterology, 116*, 86–94. https://doi.org/10.14309/ajg.0000000000000913

Hashimoto, K., Takeuchi, T., Koyama, A., Hiiragi, M., Suka, S., & Hashizume, M. (2020). Effect of relaxation therapy on benzodiazepine use in patients with medically unexplained symptoms. *BioPsychoSocial Medicine, 14*, 13. https://doi.org/10.1186/s13030-020-00187-7

Hedge, S., Adhikari, P., Subbalakshmi, N., Nandini, M., Rao, G., & D'Souza, V. (2012). Diaphragmatic breathing exercise as a therapeutic intervention for control of oxidative stress in type 2 diabetes mellitus. *Complementary Therapies in Clinical Practice, 18*, 151–153. https://doi.org/10.1016/j.ctcp.2012.04.002

Hopper, S., Murray, S. L., Ferrara, L. R., & Singleton, J. K. (2019). Effectiveness of diaphragmatic breathing for reducing physiological and psychological stress in adults: A quantitative systematic review. *JBI Database of Systematic Reviews and Implementation Report, 17*, 1855–1876. https://doi.org/10.11124/JBISRIR-2017-003848

Ismail, N., & Elgzar, W. T. (2018). The effect of progressive muscle relaxation on post caesarean section pain, quality of sleep and physical activities limitation. *International Journal of Security and Networks, 3,* 14. https://doi.org/10.20849/ijsn.v3i3.461

Izgu, N., Metin, Z. G., Karadas, C., Ozdemir, L., Metinarikan, N., & Corapcioglu, D. (2020). Progressive muscle relaxation and mindfulness meditation on neuropathic pain, fatigue, and quality of life in patients with type 2 diabetes: A randomized clinical trial. *Journal of Nursing Scholarship, 52*(5), 476–487. https://doi.org/10.1111/jnu.12580

Jacobson, E. (1938). *Progressive relaxation.* University of Chicago Press.

Kutsenko, V. (2018). Application of autogenetic training technique in integrated rehabilitation of patients with chronic fatigue syndrome. *Sports Medicine and Physical Rehabilitation, 1,* 82–86.

Lehrer, P. (2009). Relaxation therapies. In L. Freeman (Ed.), *Mosby's complementary and alternative medicine: A research-based approach* (3rd ed., pp. 148–150). Mosby Elsevier.

Linden, W. (2007). *Autogenic training.* Guilford Press.

Liu, K., Chen, Y., Wu, D., Lin, R., Wang, Z., & Pan, L. (2020). Effects of progressive muscle relaxation on anxiety and sleep quality in patients with COVID-19. *Complementary Therapies in Clinical Practice, 39,* 101132. https://doi.org/10.1016/j.ctcp.2020.101132.

Liu, Y., Jiang, Y., Shi, T., Liu, Y. N., Liu, X., Xu, G., Li, F., Wang, Y. L., & Wu, X. Y. (2021). The effectiveness of diaphragmatic breathing relaxation training for improving sleep quality among nursing staff during the COVID-19 outbreak: A before and after study. *Sleep Medicine, 78,* 8–14. https://doi.org/10.1016%2Fj.sleep.2020.12.003

Ma, X., Yue, Z. Q., Gong, Z. Q., Zhang, H, Duan, N. Y., Shi, Y. T., Wei, G. X., & Li, Y. F. (2017). The effect of diaphragmatic breathing on attention, negative affect and stress in healthy adults. *Frontiers in Psychology, 8,* 874. https://doi.org/10.3389/fpsyg.2017.00874

Melo-Dias, C., Apostolo, J., & Cardoso, D. (2014). Effectiveness of progressive muscle relaxation training for adults diagnosed with schizophrenia: A systematic review protocol. *JBI Database of Systematic Reviews & Implementation Reports, 12*(10), 85–97. https://doi.org/10.11124/jbisrir-2014-1639

Meyer, B., Keller, A., Wohlbier, H., Overath, C., Muller, B., & Krupp, P. (2016). Progressive muscle relaxation reduces migraine frequency and normalizes amplitudes of contingent negative variation (CNV). *Journal of Headache and Pain, 17,* 37. https://doi.org/10.1186/s10194-016-0630-0

Minen, M., Adhikari, S., Seng, E. K., Berk, T., Jinich, S., Powers, S., & Lipton, R. B. (2019). Smartphone-based migraine behavioral therapy: A single-arm study with assessment of mental health predictors. *Nature Partner Journals Digital Medicine, 2,* 46. https://doi.org/10.1038/s41746-019-0116-y

Miu, A. C., Heilman, R. M., & Miclea, M. (2009). Reduced heart rate variability and vagal tone in anxiety, trait versus state, and the effects of autogenic training. *Autonomic Neuroscience-Basic & Clinical, 145*(1/2), 99–103. https://doi.org/10.1016/j.autneu.2008.11.010

National Center for Complementary and Integrative Health. (2016). *Relaxation techniques for health.* https://nccih.nih.gov/health/stress/relaxation.htm

Ozamiz-Etxebarria, N., Santa María, M. D., Munitis, A. E., & Gorrotxategi, M. P. (2020). Reduction of COVID-19 anxiety levels through relaxation techniques: A study carried out in northern Spain on a sample of young university students. *Frontiers in Psychology, 11,* 2038. https://doi.org/10.3389/fpsyg.2020.02038

Park, E., Oh, H., & Kim, T. (2013). The effects of relaxation breathing on procedural pain and anxiety during burn care. *Burns, 39,* 1101–1106. http://www.elsevier.com/locate/burns

Rahayu, D., & Yunarsih, Y. (2018). Improving breast feeding self efficacy with autogenic training relaxation. *The 2nd Joint International Conferences, 2,* 64–68.

Russell, E. B., Scott, A. B., Boggero, I. A., & Carlson, C. R. (2017). Inclusion of a rest period in diaphragmatic breathing increases high frequency heart rate variability: Implications for behavioral therapy. *Psychophysiology, 54*(3), 358–365. https://doi.org/10.1111/psyp.12791

Schaffer, S. D., & Yucha, C. B. (2004). Relaxation & pain management: The relaxation response can play a role in managing chronic and acute pain. *American Journal of Nursing, 104*(8), 75–82. https://doi.org/10.1097/00000446-200408000-00044

Schmidt, J., Joyner, M., Tonyan, H., Reid, K., & Hooten, W. (2012). Psychological and physiological correlates of a brief intervention to enhance self-regulation in patients with fibromyalgia. *Journal of Musculoskeletal Pain, 20*(3), 211–221. https://doi.org/10.3109/10582452.2012.704142

Schultz, J. H., & Luthe, W. (1959). *Autogenic training: A psycho-physiological approach in psychotherapy.* Grune & Stratton.

Seo, E., & Kim, S. (2019). Effect of autogenic training for stress response: A systematic review and meta-analysis. *Journal of Korean Academy Nursing, 49*(4), 361–374. https://doi.org/10.4040/jkan.2019.49.4.361

Spielberger, C., Gorsuch, R., Luschene, R., Vagg, P., & Jacobs, G. (1983). *Manual for STAI.* Consulting Psychological Press.

Stanton, A., & Meston, C. A. (2017). Single session of autogenic training increases acute subjective and physiological sexual arousal in sexually functional women. *Journal of Sex & Marital Therapy, 43*(7), 601–617. https://doi.org/10.1080/0092623x.2016.1211206

Tian, X., Tang, R. Y., Xu, L., Xie, W., Chen, H., Pi, Y. P., & Chen, W. Q. (2020). Progressive muscle relaxation is effective in preventing and alleviating of chemotherapy-induced nausea and vomiting among cancer patients: A systematic review of six randomized controlled trials. *Support Care Cancer, 28*(9), 4051–4058. https://doi.org/10.1007/s00520-020-05481-2

Tomas-Carus, P., Branco, J. C., Raimundo, A., Parraca, J. A., Batalha, N., & Biehl-Printes, C. (2018). Breathing exercises must be a real and affective intervention to consider in women with fibromyalgia: A pilot randomized controlled trial. *The Journal of Alternative and Complementary Medicine, 24,* 825–832. https://doi.org/10.1089/acm.2017.0335

Usmani, S., Balcer, L., Galetta, S., & Minen, M. (2021). Feasibility of smartphone-delivered progressive muscle relaxation in persistent post-traumatic headache patients. *Journal of Neurotrauma, 38*(1), 94–101. https://doi.org/10.1089/neu.2019.6601

Vander Wal, J., Maraldo, T., Vercellone, A., & Gagne, D. (2015). Education, progressive muscle relaxation therapy, and exercise for the treatment of night eating syndrome: A pilot study. *Appetite, 89,* 136–144. https://doi.org/10.1016/j.appet.2015.01.024

World Health Organization. (2013). *Guidelines for the management of conditions specifically related to stress.*

Xiao, C. X., Lin, Y. J., Lin, R. Q., Liu, A. N., Zhong, G. Q., & Lan, C. F. (2020). Effects of progressive muscle relaxation training on negative emotions and sleep quality in COVID-19 patients: A clinical observational study. *Medicine, 99*(47), e23185. https://doi.org/10.1097%2FMD.000000000002318

Xie, L., Deng, Y., Zhang, J., Richmond, C.J., Tang, Y., & Zhou, J. (2016). Effects of progressive muscle relaxation intervention in extremity fracture surgery patients. *Western Journal of Nursing Research, 38,* 155–168. https://doi.org/10.1177/0193945914551509

Yamaguti, W., Claudino, R., Neto, A., Chammas, M., Gomes, A., Salge, J., & Carvalho, C. (2012). Diaphragmatic breathing training program improves abdominal motion during natural breathing in patients with chronic obstructive pulmonary disease: A randomized controlled trial. *Archives of Physical Medicine and Rehabilitation, 93,* 571–577. https://doi.org/10.1016/j.apmr.2011.11.026

Yilmaz, C. K., & Kapucu, S. (2017). The effect of progressive relaxation exercises on fatigue and sleep quality in individuals with COPD. *Holistic Nursing Practice, 31*(6), 369–377. https://doi.org/10.1097/hnp.0000000000000234

Zhang, L. J., Cai, S., Zhao, H., Liang, Y. T., Ye, M. L., & Chen, C. (2017). Study on effects of progressive muscle relaxation training on nausea and vomiting, cancer related fatigue and negative emotion of patients with lung cancer undergoing chemotherapy. *Chinese General Practice Nursing, 15*(27), 3338–3341.

18

Exercise

DERECK L. SALISBURY, ERICA N. SCHORR, ULF G. BRONÄS,
AND DIANE TREAT-JACOBSON

Exercise is well recognized as a lifelong endeavor essential for energetic, active, and healthy living. In large, longitudinal studies, it has been established that morbidity and mortality are reduced in physically fit individuals compared with sedentary individuals (Blair et al., 1989, 1996; Mandsager et al., 2018). Although the research supporting the benefits of exercise is substantial, (a) it is often overlooked in the practice of conventional Western medicine, and (b) compliance to current physical activity and exercise guidelines is poor as only one in four adults and one in five adolescents currently meet the physical activity guidelines for aerobic and muscular strengthening activities (Centers for Disease Control and Prevention, U.S. Department of Health and Human Services, 2018).

In 1996, the U.S. Surgeon General (U.S. Department of Health and Human Services, 1996) issued a report identifying millions of inactive Americans as being at risk for a wide range of chronic diseases and ailments, including coronary heart disease (CHD), Type 2 diabetes mellitus (T2DM), colon cancer, hip fractures, hypertension, and obesity. Since this landmark document, several updates and position statements have been made by governing associations in 2007 (Haskell et al., 2007), 2008 (U.S. Department of Health and Human Services, Office of Disease Prevention and Health Promotion, 2008), 2011 (Garber et al., 2011), and 2018 (U.S. Department of Health and Human Services, Office of Disease Prevention and Health Promotion, 2018).

The most recent guidelines, the U.S. Department of Health and Human Services publications including the 2018 Physical Activity Guidelines for Americans (U.S. Department of Health and Human Services, 2018) and *Healthy People 2030* (Office of Disease Prevention and Health Promotion, U.S. Department of Health and Human Services, 2020) continue to specify several objectives for improving health, including physical activity and exercise. These publications provide more evidence, justifications, and strategies behind the previous publication recommendations (U.S. Department of Health and Human Services, Office of Disease Prevention and Health Promotion, 2008) for reducing the percentage of adults who do not participate in any physical activity and increasing the percentage of persons, regardless of age or health status, who engage in moderate-intensity physical activity on most days of the week. In addition, these updates now provide objectives and strategies to enhance adherence to physical activity guidelines that are specific to schools and workplaces, including increasing the number of students who participate in daily physical education classes and increasing the proportion of work sites that offer physical activity and exercise programs, respectively (Office of Disease Prevention and Health Promotion, U.S. Department of Health and Human Services, 2020).

It is important to recognize the role of exercise as a component of good health. Exercise, either alone or as an alternative or complementary therapy, has been linked to many positive physiological and psychological responses, from a reduction in the stress response to an increased sense of well-being (Pedersen, 2019). Exercise *must* be an integral part of one's personal lifestyle if it is to have optimal effects. Maintaining physical fitness should be enjoyable and rewarding for people of all ages and can contribute significantly to extending longevity and improving quality of life (Bermejo-Cantarero et al., 2021; Kodama et al., 2009). Nurses' knowledge of exercise and its application in multiple populations assists in the delivery of expert nursing care. This chapter discusses the definition, physiological basis, application, and promotion of exercise as a nursing intervention in a variety of populations, and specific cultural applications.

DEFINITION

Physical activity is defined as "any bodily movement produced by skeletal muscles that results in caloric expenditure" (Caspersen et al., 1985; Dasso, 2019). Definitions of *exercise* are complex and vary according to the scientific discipline; however, they all incorporate physical activity into their descriptions. Exercise is commonly defined as a voluntary physical activity that is planned, structured, repetitive, and undertaken to sustain or improve health and any aspect of physical fitness (i.e., cardiorespiratory fitness, muscle strength, body composition, balance, or flexibility; Dasso, 2019).

Exercise is commonly classified according to the rate of energy expenditure, which is expressed either in relative terms according to the percentage of peak oxygen consumption (VO_2) or in absolute terms such as metabolic equivalents of task (METs). Exercise can also be classified as aerobic or anaerobic. Exercise is aerobic when the energy demand by the working muscles is supplied by aerobic adenosine triphosphate (ATP) production as allowed by inspired oxygen and mitochondrial enzymatic capacity (American College of Sports Medicine [ACSM], 2018). In general, aerobic exercise increases demand on the respiratory, cardiovascular, and musculoskeletal systems. Sustained periods of work require aerobic metabolism at a level compatible with the body's oxygen supply capabilities (i.e., oxygen uptake equals oxygen requirements of the tissues). *Anaerobic exercise* is the term used when energy demand exceeds what the body is able to produce through the aerobic process or when the body is performing short bursts of high-intensity exercise, such as in resistance and sprint training (ACSM, 2018).

SCIENTIFIC BASIS

Better understanding of exercise physiology and the body's response to various stages of physical activity assists in developing exercise programs appropriate for the individual and the goal of the exercise training session. The response of the body to exercise occurs in stages. The initial response to acute exercise is a withdrawal of parasympathetic stimulation of the heart through the vagus nerve. This results in a rapid increase in heart rate (HR) and cardiac output (Tipton, 2006). The sympathetic stimulation occurs more slowly and becomes a dominant factor once HR is above approximately 100 beats per minute. Sympathetic stimulation is fully completed after approximately 10 to 20 seconds, during which time a large sympathetic outburst occurs and the heart overshoots the rate needed but then returns to the rate required for increased activity.

The brain stimulates the initial cardiovascular response together with impulses from muscles being exercised, and these impulses are sent to the brain; an increase in HR is initiated, and the blood flow is shunted toward the exercising muscles (Astrand et al., 2004). During this phase, there is a slow adjustment of respiration and circulation, resulting in an oxygen deficit; the initial energy needed by the exercising tissue is fueled mainly by the anaerobic metabolism of creatine phosphate and anaerobic glycolysis (Jones & Poole, 2005).

As exercise continues, VO_2 increases in a linear fashion in relation to the intensity of exercise. The increase in VO_2 is caused by an increase in oxygen extraction by the working muscles and an increase in cardiac output. Oxygen extraction by the working muscle tissues is approximately 80% to 85%, or a threefold increase from rest, in sedentary and moderately active individuals. This is caused by an increase in the number of open capillaries, thereby reducing diffusion distances and increasing capillary blood volume (Fletcher et al., 2013). Cardiac output is increased to meet the increased oxygen demands of the working muscle. The increase in cardiac output is caused by increased stroke volume, which is due to an increase in ventricular filling pressure brought on by increased venous return and decreased peripheral resistance offered by the exercising muscles. Together with the withdrawal of parasympathetic stimulation and increases in sympathetic stimulation, the increase in HR further accentuates the increase in cardiac output, as well as increased myocardial contractility (from positive inotropic sympathetic impulses to the heart; Astrand et al., 2004). In normal individuals, cardiac output can increase four- to fivefold, allowing for increased delivery of oxygen to exercising muscle beds and facilitating the removal of lactate, carbon dioxide (CO_2), and heat. Ventilation increases to deliver oxygen and to allow for the elimination of CO_2. Blood pressure (BP) increases as a result of increased cardiac output and the sympathetic vasoconstriction of vessels in the nonexercising muscles, viscera, and skin. During this "steady state" exercise phase, oxygen uptake equals oxygen tissue requirement, aerobic metabolism of glucose and fatty acids occurs, and there is no accumulation of lactic acid (Tipton, 2006).

As exercise becomes more strenuous, there is a shift toward anaerobic metabolism, resulting in increased production of lactic acid (Tipton, 2006). The anaerobic threshold is a point during exercise at which ventilation abruptly increases despite linear increases in work rate (Beaver et al., 1986). As exercise goes beyond the steady state, the oxygen supply does not meet the oxygen requirement, and energy is provided through anaerobic glycolysis and creatine phosphate breakdown. This increases proton release and phosphate accumulation, increasing acidosis (Robergs et al., 2004; Westerblad et al., 2002). Shortly beyond the anaerobic threshold, fatigue and dyspnea ensue and work ceases, coinciding with a significant drop in blood glucose levels. Exercise at a level that allows for a greater contribution of energy via aerobic metabolism and less involvement of the anaerobic system (and hence glucose as the primary fuel) may delay the onset of these biochemical fatigue-inducing changes.

Following cessation of exercise, there is a period of rapid decline in oxygen uptake, followed by a slow decline toward resting levels. This slow phase of oxygen uptake return is called *excess postexercise oxygen consumption* (LaForgia et al., 2006). During this period, the body attempts to resynthesize used creatine phosphate, remove lactate, restore muscle and blood oxygen stores, decrease body temperature, return to resting levels of HR and BP, and lower circulating catecholamines (Astrand et al., 2004).

INTERVENTION

Healthy People 2030 is a continuing set of data-driven national objectives for the United States to achieve by 2030 to improve health (Office of Disease Prevention and Health Promotion, U.S. Department of Health and Human Services, 2020). Physical activity is emphasized as a health behavior objective and target within *Healthy People 2030*. The overarching goal is to improve health, fitness, and quality of life through the practice of habitual physical activity. Twenty-three specific objectives (and evidence-based resources) are further provided to promote adherence to physical activity guidelines for specific age groups and health status (Office of Disease Prevention and Health Promotion, U.S. Department of Health and Human Services, 2020). Furthermore, the ACSM (Garber et al., 2011), specifically states that exercise is an important way to achieve physical activity goals and is considered to be beneficial to health and reduces the risk of the following:

- dying prematurely
- dying prematurely from CHD
- acquiring T2DM
- incurring hypertension
- developing colon cancer

The updated reports have provided even more new evidence that adhering to the recommendations in the Physical Activity Guidelines for Americans (U.S. Department of Health and Human Services, 2018) consistently, over time, can lead to even more long-term health benefits across the life span than previously thought, including the following:

- prevention of eight types of cancer (bladder, breast, colon, endometrium, esophagus, kidney, stomach, lung) in adults
- reducing feelings of uneasiness and despair
- reducing the risk of dementia including from Alzheimer's disease
- for older adults, lowering the risk of falls and injuries from falls
- for pregnant women, reducing the risk of postpartum depression
- for youth, help improve cognition
- for all age groups, reducing the risk of excessive weight gain

Given that exercise can enhance health and well-being in all age groups, across a broad spectrum of health and disease, it is important for nurses to recognize opportunities to promote exercise as a nursing intervention. There are countless activities included under the umbrella of exercise. When prescribing an exercise intervention, it is important to consider the goals of the individual, health, medical, exercise, and physical activity histories, as well as the patient's personal exercise preference, to ensure both safety and compliance during the exercise training program (see the section on precautions). A complete, multimodal exercise training program should involve each of the following modalities: resistance, flexibility, neuromuscular (i.e., functional fitness training), and aerobic; specific exercise selections within each given modality should be prescribed based on the needs of the individual.

RESISTANCE TRAINING

Resistance training is any exercise that causes the muscles to contract against an external resistance with the expectation of increases in strength, mass, and/or endurance (ACSM, Chodzko-Zajko, et al., 2009). This external resistance can be provided through the use of a variety of equipment, including machines and lower cost alternatives, such as free weights and rubber exercise tubing or bands. Furthermore, external resistance can be provided by one's own body weight or even household items such as bricks or jugs of water. Resistance training has physiological and healthy aging–promoting effects, which include increasing bone, muscle, and connective tissue strength and improving insulin sensitivity, BP, mental health, and body composition. Because of this, the ACSM has included it in its recommendations since 1998 (ACSM, 1998). The current guidelines state that resistance training should be performed 2 to 3 days per week, with specific recommendations based on the goals and experience of the individual. Briefly, for the novice to improve muscular strength, resistance training should involve 8 to 10 of the major muscle groups with one set of 8 to 12 repetitions performed at a resistance that induces moderate fatigue (rating of perceived exertion [RPE] 12–13/20; ACSM, 2009; Garber et al., 2011).

FLEXIBILITY TRAINING

Flexibility training (stretching) is an important, but often neglected part of an exercise training program. Stretching is particularly important for older adults to attenuate aging-related declines in joint range of motion, loss of skeletal muscle elasticity, and functional mobility (Stathokostas et al., 2012). Furthermore, stretching is important in the maintenance of postural stability and the prevention and management of nonspecific low back pain (Gordon & Bloxham, 2016). Flexibility exercises should be performed 2 to 3 days per week and target major muscles of the shoulder girdle, chest, neck, trunk, lower back, hips, and legs. Each stretch should be moved slowly into a position that induces mild discomfort (but not sharp pain) and held (static) for 10 to 30 seconds (Garber et al., 2011).

NEUROMUSCULAR TRAINING

Neuromuscular exercise training focuses on the implementation of exercises designed to challenge balance and proprioception. During the past few decades, there has been an increase in the popularity of non-Western styles of exercise that fall under the category of neuromuscular exercise, including qigong and related movements in yoga and tai chi (Humberstone & Stuart, 2016). These forms of exercise build on meditative movement and, as such, may provide a more enjoyable form of exercise (Humberstone & Stuart, 2016). Furthermore, the dynamic movements and isometric muscle contractions performed in these exercises have been shown to increase muscular strength, physical fitness, and joint range of motion, particularly in novices, deconditioned people, and older adults (Sivaramakrishnan et al., 2019; Solloway et al., 2016; Youkhana et al., 2016). Of note, neuromuscular exercise can be incorporated in select resistance training exercises such as step-ups, lunges, or exercises (such as a dumbbell shoulder press) while standing on one leg. The optimal effectiveness and dose of neuromuscular exercise training have yet to be established; however, performing 60 minutes weekly (i.e., 20-minute sessions 3 days a week) has been shown to improve measures of neuromotor performance (Garber et al., 2011).

AEROBIC EXERCISE TRAINING

The focus of the exercise intervention and prescription hereafter is devoted to aerobic exercise training. An exercise session, particularly one focused on aerobic exercise, should involve three phases: warm-up, aerobic exercise, and cooldown. These phases are designed to allow the body an opportunity to sustain internal equilibrium by gradually adjusting physiological processes to the stress of exercise and thus maintaining homeostasis.

WARM-UP PHASE

The goal of the warm-up is to allow the body time to adapt to the rigors of aerobic exercise. Warming up results in an increase in muscle temperature, a higher need for oxygen to meet the increased metabolic demands of the exercising muscles, dilation of capillaries to increase circulation, adjustments within the neural respiratory center to the demands of exercise, and a shunting of blood flow from the splanchnic beds to the exercising muscles, resulting in increased venous return (ACSM, 2018). A good warm-up also increases flexibility and decreases the risk for developing arrhythmias and adverse myocardial ischemic events during the exercise session (ACSM, 2018). The warm-up, 5 to 10 minutes of low- to moderate-intensity aerobic exercise, should achieve an HR within 20 beats per minute of the target HR for the subsequent aerobic exercise portion of the training session. In addition, a warm-up may incorporate stretching exercises. If stretching is incorporated in the warm-up, it should be performed after the low-intensity aerobic activity. Specific recommendations for performing flexibility exercises were discussed previously.

AEROBIC EXERCISE PHASE

The aerobic phase of exercise is also known as the *conditioning phase*. The aerobic phase, which is typically the focus of aerobic exercise prescription, consists of four essential components—frequency, intensity (which is usually measured as a relative percentage of maximal aerobic capacity), time (session duration), and type (mode of exercise)—that are often collectively referred to in the literature as *FITT* (ACSM, 2018). The combination of these components determines the effectiveness of the exercise and is known as the *training volume* or *dose*. The mode of exercise should involve rhythmic, continuous movement of large muscle groups—walking, jogging, cycling, swimming, or cross-country skiing (Garber et al., 2011). In general, the frequency should be 5 days per week, with a duration of at least 30 minutes for health benefits (Garber et al., 2011).

Because most people are not meeting the current key guidelines, and knowing the significant health benefits associated with exercise, guidance for adults no longer requires physical activity (including exercise) to occur in bouts of at least 10 minutes. The current guidelines now state that the duration of exercise is cumulative, and any amount of exercise is better than none (Piercy et al., 2018). Pertaining to the intensity of exercise, it can be either moderate or vigorous. For moderate-intensity exercise, 150 minutes or more per week is the target, and if the exercise performed is vigorous, the duration can be shortened to 75 minutes per week (ACSM, 2018). Moreover, moderate and vigorous exercise can be combined to achieve the recommended activity dose per week (Garber et al., 2011). For individual determination of intensity, target HRs and RPE should be used (Table 18.1). For most people, physical fitness improvements may be gained with moderate-intensity exercise.

As physical fitness improves, it may be necessary to increase one of the FITT components (i.e., frequency, intensity, or duration) to gain additional benefits. The accumulated amount of daily moderate to vigorous physical activity and exercise is what is important. Although those who perform at least 150 minutes per week of accumulated moderate physical activity show significant health benefits compared with sedentary individuals, additional health benefits are gained by doing physical activity beyond the equivalent of 300 minutes of moderate-intensity physical activity a week (Piercy et al., 2018). However, a balance still needs to be achieved to obtain maximal benefit with the least risk and discomfort. Adjustment of exercise volume, particularly the intensity component is important not only for safety reasons but also for comfort and enjoyment of the activity. As tolerance develops, any or all of the exercise components can be increased to meet the person's aerobic capacity. For example, if an individual is comfortable with the intensity of the exercise, the duration and frequency can be increased to further improve the training effect.

Table 18.1 Monitoring "Target" Levels of Exercise

Intensity	% HR Method	% HRR	RPE
Light	57–<64	30–<39	9–11
Moderate	64–<76	40–59	12–13
Vigorous	>76	≥60	14+

Note: HR = heart rate; HRR = heart rate reserve; RPE = rating of perceived exertion.
HR method: target HR, $HR_{max/peak}$ (intensity).
HRR method: target heart rate ($HR_{max/peak} - HR_{rest}$) × (% intensity) + HR_{rest}; HR_{rest} is determined after 5 minutes of seated, quiet rest; $HR_{max/peak}$ is determined directly from a graded exercise or physical fitness test (i.e., 10-m shuttle walk or 6-minute walk test), or it is estimated from taking 220 and subtracting it from one's age. RPE is based off the Borg 15 Category RPE scale.
Source: Adapted with permission from American College of Sports Medicine. (2018). Guidelines for exercise testing and prescription (10th ed.). Lippincott Williams & Wilkins/Wolters Kluwer.

COOLDOWN PHASE

Immediately following endurance exercise, the person should engage in a cooling-down period. The cooldown allows the body to return to its normal resting state. This allows the HR and BP to return to resting levels and attenuates postexercise hypotension by improving venous return. The cool-down also improves heat dissipation and elimination of blood lactate and provides a means to combat any potential postexercise rise in catecholamines (ACSM, 2018). Cooling-down exercises should last 5 to 10 minutes and may include walking slowly and deep breathing. It should be noted that the cool-down period is a great time to perform static flexibility exercises due to the increased compliance of the skeletal muscles induced by the aerobic exercise training session.

TOOLS FOR MONITORING THE INTENSITY OF THE INTERVENTION

Prior to a thorough description of the evidence-based recommendations in regard to the intervention, terminology commonly used in monitoring the intensity component of the intervention should be defined. Exercising individuals should monitor the response of their bodies to the activity to ensure that the intensity is appropriate (Table 18.1). This can be done in several ways, including monitoring target HR and RPE and applying the talk test.

MONITORING TARGET HR

The most common way to objectively monitor relative exercise intensity is through monitoring of HR. Two established methods are the HR max method (Shookster et al., 2020) and heart rate reserve (HRR) method (Karvonen & Vuorimaa, 1988) based on the peak HR achieved on a cardiopulmonary exercise or physical fitness test or an age-predicted maximum HR estimated from a prediction equation (Table 18.1). Regardless of the method used to calculate target HR zones, HR should be assessed a third of the way to halfway through the exercise session and immediately after stopping exercise. Exercise intensity can be increased or decreased based on this measurement.

RATING OF PERCEIVED EXERTION

RPE is the subjective intensity of effort, strain, discomfort, and/or fatigue that is experienced during exercise (Borg, 1998). The RPE can be quantified using a variety of scales, most notably the Borg 15 Category RPE scale (ranges from 6–20; Borg, 1998) and the OMNI Picture System of Perceived Exertion scales (ranges from 0–10; Utter et al., 2004). In addition, differentiated (overall body) and undifferentiated (legs; chest/breathing) RPE can be assessed by the individual during the exercise session. This concept is important because the exercise modality used may influence the perceptual response, particularly the differentiated perceptual signal arising from the activated anatomical region (Mays et al., 2014).

THE TALK TEST

The Talk Test is a well-validated tool to measure the intensity of day-to-day physical activities and can replace target HR monitoring when an individual is exercising at a moderate intensity (Foster et al., 2008; Reed & Pipe, 2014). While exercising, the intensity is evaluated by asking the patient if they can speak comfortably (Fletcher et al., 2013). If the exercise prevents the individual from talking comfortably, the intensity is considered to be greater than moderate (i.e., hard/vigorous). If talking is comfortable, the intensity is considered sub-moderate (i.e., light). Exercise between these thresholds is considered moderate. A variation of this technique is to whistle; if the individual is unable to whistle, the intensity is too great and should be decreased if the goal is to exercise at moderate intensity.

SPECIFIC TECHNIQUE: WALKING

One of the strategies identified by *Healthy People 2030* to improve health and quality of life through daily physical activity is promoting an increase in "the proportion of adults who walk or bike to get places" (Office of Disease Prevention and Health Promotion, U.S. Department of Health and Human Services, 2020). Walking is one of the simplest ways to get active and stay active and can have a significant impact on health. Moreover, it is an exercise in which most people of all age groups and varying levels of ability can use to improve endurance. A major advantage is that walking requires no special equipment, facilities, or new skills. It is also safer and easier to maintain than many other forms of exercise. Intensity, duration, and frequency are easily regulated and adjusted to accommodate a wide range of physical capabilities and limitations. The initial intensity should be outlined at the start of the program and is dependent on baseline levels of conditioning, physical or disease-related limitations or precautions, and outcome goals.

A walking program can be approached in two ways. The exercise can be completed in one or more daily sessions. For example, a previously sedentary individual may wish to begin an exercise program consisting of 10-minute walks and progressively increase the time or intensity as physical fitness increases. The more traditional alternative is to engage in one longer session (of at least 30 minutes in duration) at least five times per week. The American Heart Association (AHA, 2021b) contains many resources for individuals interested in starting a walking program. Additionally, the AHA provides a 6-week beginner walking plan for the beginner walker who wants to improve overall health and increase energy. Walks start at 10 minutes or less and gradually work up to 30-plus minutes (AHA, 2021a). Tips for fitness walking are presented in Exhibit 18.1.

MEASUREMENT OF OUTCOMES

The appropriate measure of the effectiveness of an exercise intervention depends on the specific exercise prescribed and the goals of the intervention. Changes in atherosclerotic risk factors (i.e., cholesterol levels, triglycerides, insulin sensitivity, waist circumference, BP, body mass index [BMI]) may be measured if cardiovascular health is the primary outcome of the exercise program. If cardiovascular fitness is the targeted outcome, an aerobic exercise program would be prescribed, and improvements in the cardiovascular system such as increased cardiac output, VO_2, and improved local circulation would be used to determine the effectiveness of the intervention (Balady et al., 2010; Fletcher et al., 2013). Cardiovascular response to submaximal exercise may provide further information and may be

> ### Exhibit 18.1 *Tips for Fitness Walking*
>
> - Warm up by performing a few stretches.
> - Think tall as you walk. Stand straight with your head level and your shoulders relaxed.
> - Your heel will hit the surface first. Use smooth movements rolling from heel to toe.
> - Keep your hands free and let your arms swing naturally in opposition to your legs.
> - When you are ready to pick up the pace, quicken your step and lengthen your stride, but do not compromise your upright posture or smooth, comfortable movements.
> - To increase your intensity, burn more calories, and tone your upper body, bend your arms at the elbows and pump your arms. Keep your elbows close to your body.
> - Breathe in and out naturally, rhythmically, and deeply.
> - Use the talk test to check your exercise intensity or take your pulse to see whether you are within your target heart rate.
> - Cool down during the last 3 to 5 minutes by gradually slowing your pace to a stroll.
>
> *Source:* Adapted from American Heart Association. (2013). *Start walking now.* https://www.heart.org/HEARTORG/HealthyLiving/PhysicalActivity/Walking_UCM_460870_SubHomePage.jsp

even more beneficial in assessing the impact on quality of life, as most activities of daily living (ADLs) are performed at submaximal intensity. Exercise prescribed to improve function may use parameters such as improved joint mobility, prevention or reduction of osteoporosis, and improved strength in determining exercise effectiveness.

Assessment may determine changes in physical functioning and disability (e.g., Short Physical Performance Battery (Guralnik et al., 1994), 6-Minute Walk Test (American Thoracic Society, 2002), Timed Up and Go Test (Podsiadlo & Richardson, 1991), ability to perform ADL, changes in symptoms and activity tolerance, and other variables that reflect an individual's ability to function in daily life. Lower-intensity programs, which may not demonstrate great changes in maximal exercise capacity, might produce sufficient changes in these outcome variables to make a difference in an individual's quality of life. Such programs would be especially appropriate in older and very sedentary individuals, for whom low-intensity exercise can produce a modest increase in fitness and more significant improvements in function. Development and implementation of programs designed to meet the specific needs of patients can help maximize functional and quality-of-life outcomes.

USES

Populations for whom exercise is particularly beneficial include, but are not limited to, children, older adults, and those with affective, cognitive, metabolic, cardiovascular, and pulmonary diseases. The application and demonstrated effects of exercise intervention (with a focus on aerobic exercise) in each of these populations are briefly discussed.

OVERWEIGHT CHILDREN AND ADOLESCENTS

The prevalence of overweight children and adolescents remains alarmingly high (Centers for Disease Control and Prevention, U.S. Department of Health and Human Services, 2021). Of particular concern are the increasing rates of T2DM and metabolic syndrome diagnosed in overweight children and adolescents (Centers for Disease Control and Prevention, U.S. Department of Health and Human Services, 2017), problems that used to be limited primarily to adults. A lack of physical activity and excess caloric intake cause central obesity, which, in turn, is believed to promote developing these conditions (Institute of Medicine, 2011). The current recommendations are essentially the same as for healthy adults, with a focus on greater training dose: 60 to 90 minutes of enjoyable, moderate physical activity 5 days a week (Donnelly et al., 2009). The current guidelines also explicitly state that achieving weight loss by exercise alone is difficult and therefore recommend that a weight-loss regimen should be a combination of calorie restriction and increased physical activity (Donnelly et al., 2009).

OLDER ADULTS

The fastest growing segment of the population in the United States is one with individuals older than the age of 65. Older adults are especially prone to the "hazards of immobility" that affect many of the body's systems, which contribute to attenuated quality of life and functional independence. The benefit of exercise as a therapy to prevent or delay functional decline and disease and improve quality of life is demonstrated by the numerous favorable changes occurring in response to exercise. Specifically, exercise promotes motor control through improved coordination, reaction time, and power, each being important for improving body functioning and performing ADLs.

It is particularly important to tailor or customize exercise programs for older adults, who may have specific limitations. Exercise needs to be initiated at lower levels and increased gradually. Previously sedentary older individuals may be more comfortable initiating an exercise program with some supervision, which allows them to become accustomed to this new level of activity in a safe environment. Group exercise may be especially appealing to older adults (ACSM, Chodzko-Zajko, et al., 2009). The current guidelines recommend—with the specific inclusion of resistance training 2 (or more) nonconsecutive days per week—using 8 to 10 major muscle groups and one set of 10 to 15 repetitions at a moderate intensity (12–13/20) based on the RPE scale (ACSM, Chodzko-Zajko, et al., 2009). Moreover, the guidelines recommend that older individuals should perform flexibility and balance (e.g., dancing) exercises a minimum of 10 minutes, two to three times per week, to prevent age-related reductions in range of motion and, hence, prevent falls (ACSM, Chodzko-Zajko, et al., 2009).

INDIVIDUALS WITH AFFECTIVE DISORDERS

Exercise is an effective, although underused, intervention for individuals with affective disorders. There is considerable evidence supporting the positive effects of exercise in combating depression and anxiety (Kazeminia et al., 2020; Miller et al., 2020; Rhyner & Watts, 2016). There are fewer, if any, side effects when compared with pharmacotherapy, and exercise is often more cost-effective than psychotherapy and pharmacotherapy. Although most studies have evaluated the effects of aerobic activity as an intervention, anaerobic activity has also been shown to be beneficial in alleviating depression (Gordon et al., 2018). This suggests that improvement in mood is associated with exercise in general, rather than increased aerobic capacity. Exercise prescription guidelines for persons with affective disorders will likely differ little from prescriptions used for healthy adults (ACSM, 2018). When prescribing exercise, it is important to consider two additional factors: (1) undertreated or untreated depression can negatively affect adherence to exercise programs, and (b) significant comorbidities exist between affective disorders and chronic diseases (i.e., cardiovascular disease [CVD] and its risk factors; Bonnet et al., 2005; Härter et al., 2003).

INDIVIDUALS WITH MILD COGNITIVE IMPAIRMENT OR ALZHEIMER'S DEMENTIA

Because of the mixed effectiveness of medications, exercise has been considered as a treatment for mild cognitive impairment (MCI) and late-stage Alzheimer's dementia (AD), and as a prevention strategy (Cass, 2017; Northey et al., 2018). Aerobic exercise appears to improve brain blood flow and stimulate the production and release of neurotrophic factors that collectively can enhance neurogenesis and increase hippocampal volume (Tari et al., 2019), all of which are important contributing factors to the preservation of brain function with aging. Both aerobic and resistance training have shown promise as a treatment modality for MCI and AD by attenuating declines in cognitive function, reducing neuropsychiatric symptoms, and increasing functional capacity (Huang et al., 2021; Panza et al., 2018; Yu et al., 2019). As with affective disorders, exercise training has been shown to have fewer side effects and better adherence compared with pharmacotherapy. Although no specific exercise recommendations have been established to date, it appears that exercise programs that focus on moderate- to vigorous-intensity aerobic exercise training performed 3 to 4 days per week for at least 45 minutes/ session over the course of 6 months holds the most promise in attenuating the cognitive decline seen in people with AD (Panza et al., 2018; Yu et al., 2019).

INDIVIDUALS WITH CARDIOVASCULAR DISEASE

Cardiac rehabilitation is an available, but underutilized, therapy that is prescribed for those with CHD or chronic heart failure (CHF), providing a safe environment for the initiation of an exercise program (Ades et al., 2017). Programs usually have several phases and are tailored to the specific needs, limitations, and characteristics of individuals, helping them resume active and productive lives (McMahon et al., 2017). There are multiple mechanisms by which exercise training can decrease the risk of cardiovascular events mediated by its anti-atherosclerotic, anti-arrhythmic, anti-ischemic, and antithrombotic effects (Barone Gibbs et al., 2021; Franklin et al., 2020). Exercise training has been shown to improve symptom-limited exercise capacity in patients with CHD or CHF, primarily as a result of peripheral hemodynamic adaptations. CHD or CHF patients have a low skeletal muscle oxidative capacity, which is significantly improved with training, despite relatively low workloads and exercise intensities (Piña et al., 2003; Tucker et al., 2018). Prior to training, patients are often unable to perform ADL without symptoms. Following cardiac rehabilitation, patients function further above the ischemic threshold in performing ADLs and thus require a lower percentage of maximal effort to perform activities. This increases stamina and endurance and helps maintain independence (Piña et al., 2003).

Peripheral artery disease (PAD), a prevalent atherosclerotic occlusive disease, limits functional capacity and is related to decreased quality of life (McDermott et al., 2004; Regensteiner et al., 2008). Individuals with PAD typically experience exercise-induced ischemic pain in the lower extremities, known as claudication (Hiatt et al., 2008). Exercise training is one of the most effective interventions available for the treatment of claudication caused by PAD (Treat-Jacobson, McDermott, Bronas, et al., 2019). Aerobic exercise training in the form of treadmill walking, the most commonly studied mode of exercise therapy, has been shown to improve peak walking distance up 180 m (Fakhry et al., 2012). Optimally, prior to program initiation, an exercise prescription should be generated based on a graded exercise test, and patients should start training at the intensity at which the onset of claudication occurs (Treat-Jacobson, McDermott, Beckman, et al., 2019). During a typical session, patients exercise at a moderate pace until they experience moderate to moderately severe claudication. At that point, they rest until the pain subsides. This exercise/rest pattern is repeated throughout the exercise session. The most effective exercise programs for the treatment of claudication include the following components: the patient should exercise to the point of moderate/moderately severe claudication (3–4 rating on a 5-point scale); the exercise session should be at least 30 minutes in length, with at least three sessions per week; and the exercise program should continue for at least 12 weeks with intermittent walking as the most effective mode of exercise (Treat-Jacobson, McDermott, Bronas, et al., 2019). In addition, a number of studies have shown that modalities of exercise that avoid claudication (i.e., upper body ergometry, total body recumbent stepping) or walking performed at intensities that are pain-free or produce only mild levels of claudication can achieve health benefits comparable to walking at moderate or higher levels of claudication and should be used by those for whom walking training is not suitable (Treat-Jacobson, McDermott, Beckman, et al., 2019; Treat-Jacobson, McDermott, Bronas, et al., 2019).

INDIVIDUALS WITH CARDIOVASCULAR DISEASE RISK FACTORS

HYPERTENSION

Hypertension (HTN) is the most common, costly, but modifiable major risk factor for the development of CVD and premature mortality, affecting nearly half (46%) of the U.S. adult population (Benjamin et al., 2019). Aerobic exercise training is well known for its anti-hypertensive effects, influencing BP at rest and at submaximal exercise/activity workloads. Emphasis should be placed on aerobic exercise training, as resting BP reductions of 5 to 7 mmHg are seen following aerobic exercise training in individuals with HTN (Cornelissen & Smart, 2013). This magnitude of BP reduction is associated with a 20% to 30% risk reduction for CVD (Whelton et al., 2002). Growing evidence suggests that resistance training is an efficacious strategy for the management of HTN and should be used as a supplement to aerobic exercise training (MacDonald et al., 2016). Special factors to consider when prescribing exercise in individuals with HTN are found in Table 18.2.

DIABETES MELLITUS

Regular exercise in people with impaired glucose tolerance (prediabetes) and T2DM commonly results in several positive physiological adaptations, including improved glucose tolerance, increased insulin sensitivity, and reduced

Table 18.2 *Evidence-Based, Population-Specific Aerobic Exercise Recommendations and Key References*

Condition	Frequency	Intensity	Duration (minutes)	Special Considerations
Healthy Adults (Garber et al., 2011)	5 d/wk (moderate) 3 d/wk (vigorous)	Moderate or vigorous	30–60 (moderate) 20–60 (vigorous)	Select modes that maximize interest and tolerability.
Older Adults (American College of Sports Medicine, Chodzko-Zajko, et al., 2009)	Same as healthy	RPE 12–13 (moderate) RPE 14–15 (vigorous)	Same as healthy	Select modes that minimize fall risk in frail individuals or those with a fall history.
Children (U.S. Department of Health and Human Services, 2018)	Daily	Moderate and vigorous	≥ 60	Moderate corresponds to noticeable increases in RR and HR; vigorous corresponds to substantial increases in RR and HR. Youth should avoid exercise in hot, humid environments and be properly hydrated.
Obese (Donnelly et al., 2009)	≥5 d/wk	40%–60% HRR (novice) ≥60% HRR (experienced)	Progress to 60	Maximize caloric expenditure, greater volume of exercise required. Target a minimal reduction in body weight of at least 5%–10% of initial body weight over 3–6 months. Incorporate concurrent dietary changes by reducing caloric intake by 500–1,000 kcal/day.

(continued)

Table 18.2 *Evidence-Based, Population-Specific Aerobic Exercise Recommendations and Key References (continued)*

Condition	Frequency	Intensity	Duration (minutes)	Special Considerations
Cognitive decline (MCI and AD; Huang et al., 2021; Yu et al., 2019)	3–4 d/wk	40%–60% HRR	45 +	Specific recommendations are not documented; the available evidence for aerobic exercise attenuating cognitive decline is limited to several randomized controlled trials. Aerobic fitness is correlated to cognitive function.
Attentive disorders (Hearing et al., 2016)	Same as healthy	Same as healthy	Same as healthy	Undertreated or untreated depression can negatively affect adherence to exercise.
HTN (Pescatello et al., 2015)	≥5 d/wk	40%–60% HRR	30–60	Medical consultation in people with uncontrolled hypertension is recommended prior to start. Maintain BP ≤220/105 mmHg while exercising. BP-lowering effects of aerobic exercise are immediate (postexercise hypotension). Medications such as beta-blockers can limit aerobic capacity.
DM (Colberg et al., 2016)	3–7 d/wk	40%–60% HRR (novice) ≥60% HRR (experienced)	20–60	Greater benefits observed with greater volume of exercise. Timing of exercise should be considered in individuals taking antiglycemic agents. Measure glucose prior to and after exercise and adjust CHO intake as necessary.
CAD (Fletcher et al., 2013; Squires et al., 2018)	3–5 d/wk	40%–80% HRR; 12–16 RPE	20–60	Exercise intensity should be prescribed 10 bpm under ischemic threshold if applicable. ECG monitoring is indicated based on risk stratification.

Condition	Frequency	Intensity	Duration (minutes)	Special Considerations
PAD (Treat-Jacobson, McDermott, Beckman, et al., 2019; Treat-Jacobson, McDermott, Bronas, et al., 2019)	3 d/wk	40%–60% peak workload on treadmill test—see Special Consideration	Accumulate 30+ minutes of exercise (preferably walking) per session	Exercise prescription is modality-specific For walking-based exercise, walk to moderate claudication (3–4/5 rating), followed by seated rest until ischemic pain subsides. For individuals with severe PAD, contraindications to or low treadmill exercise capacity, use nonwalking exercise modality.
COPD (Garvey et al., 2016)	3–5 d/wk	40%–60% HRR, progress to ≥60% HRR, titrate based on symptoms	Based on dyspnea, may be intermittent or continuous, accumulate 30+ minutes	Intensity should be further modified to promote 4–6 rating on Borg category (C) ratio (R) or CR 10 scale. SpO2 should be maintained above 88% to 90% during exercise. Supplemental O_2 may be utilized when necessary. Individuals suffering from acute exacerbations should limit exercise until symptoms have subsided.

Note: AD = Alzheimer's dementia; BP = blood pressure; bpm = beats per minute; CAD = coronary artery disease; CHO = carbohydrate; COPD = chronic obstructive pulmonary disease; DM = diabetes mellitus; HR = heart rate; HRR = heart rate reserve; HTN = hypertension; kcal = kilocalorie; MCI = mild cognitive impairment; PAD = peripheral artery disease; RPE = rating of perceived exertion; RR = respiratory rate; %SaO2 = percent oxygen saturation.
Borg CR 10 scale; scale used to determine the magnitude of perceived exertion.

hemoglobin A1c (HbA1c; Colberg et al., 2016). In people with insulin-dependent T2DM, exercise training has been shown to lower the requirement of exogenous insulin (ACSM, 2018). A growing body of evidence, which has focused on vascular function in T2DM, chronic microvascular adaptations seen in this population following exercise training included enhanced endothelial function and enhanced capillary perfusions and density (Olver & Laughlin, 2016). This is clinically relevant given the microvascular complications seen with T2DM (Chatterjee et al., 2017). Specific exercise prescriptions are based on healthy weight loss and maintenance because 90% of people with T2DM are obese. Studies suggest that weight loss can produce remission of T2DM in a dose-dependent manner; therefore, moderate to high volumes of aerobic exercise are recommended (Magkos et al., 2020). Additionally, resistance training is more important in the treatment of hyperglycemia and should be encouraged (Codella et al., 2018) because T2DM is an independent risk factor for an accelerated decline in functional status and muscle strength (Anton et al., 2013).

INDIVIDUALS WITH PULMONARY DISEASE

Chronic obstructive pulmonary disease (COPD) is a common, preventable and treatable disease that is characterized by persistent respiratory symptoms and airflow limitation that is due to airway and/or alveolar abnormalities, usually caused by significant exposure to noxious particles or gases (Mirza et al., 2018). The hypoxic and inflammatory state induced by COPD results in skeletal muscle dysfunction, a condition characterized by reduced Type I oxidative fibers and mitochondrial dysfunction (Jaitovich & Barreiro, 2018). Both the reduced capacity for alveolar gas diffusion and reduced oxidative capacity of the skeletal muscles attribute to the increasing breathlessness and muscular fatigue particularly seen on exertion. Upper body skeletal muscle fatigue is most commonly noted (McKeough et al., 2016) as activities such as changing a tire can become exceedingly difficult. The increased fatigue seen in the upper body skeletal muscles is most likely due to the increasee need to recruit this musculature to assist in ventilatory mechanics. As the disease progresses, an inability to perform ADLs and disability are often seen. The benefits to COPD patients from pulmonary rehabilitation are considerable, and rehabilitation has been shown to be the most effective therapeutic strategy to improve shortness of breath, health status, and exercise tolerance (Garvey et al., 2016; Mirza et al., 2018). The focus of pulmonary rehabilitation is aerobic exercise training, which most notably improves cardiovascular function and skeletal muscle oxidative capacity, thereby enhancing oxygen delivery, extraction, and utilization. In turn, these training effects can lower the demands and stress put on the pulmonary system during exertion. Light to moderate aerobic exercise is known to reduce fatigue, whereas high-intensity training of at least 60% to 80% of peak work rate is associated with maximal physiologic improvements in aerobic fitness, endurance, and ventilation at submaximal work rates (Garvey et al., 2016). Resistance training is also increasingly important for individuals with COPD to improve skeletal muscle strength and endurance in an attempt to attenuate the skeletal muscle dysfunction and disability and increase the performance of ventilatory accessory muscles (Liao et al., 2015).

PRECAUTIONS

Before an exercise program is initiated, preparticipation screening procedures are recommended. However, a possible barrier to becoming physically active is the requirement for exercise preparticipation health screening, which may involve a visit to a healthcare provider and/or diagnostic testing to potentially identify exercise contraindications (Franklin, 2014). Unnecessary referral to healthcare providers for screening may lead to a higher incidence of false-positive exercise test responses, necessitating medical follow-up and additional studies when they are not required. Such studies can place unnecessary financial and other burdens on the healthcare system and barriers to exercise participation for the patient (Franklin, 2014). The most recent preparticipation screening algorithm provided by the ACSM (Riebe et al., 2015) helps navigate this issue and further identifies (a) who should receive medical clearance before initiating an exercise, (c) patients with clinically significant disease(s) who may benefit from participating in a medically supervised exercise program, and (c) medical conditions that may require exclusion from exercise programs until those conditions are abated or better controlled. In general, previously sedentary individuals with or presenting with symptoms suggestive of cardiovascular, metabolic, or renal disease, should consult a physician prior to initiating an exercise program (Riebe et al., 2015).

To avoid injury, it is important to begin an exercise program slowly, follow safety guidelines, and exercise consistently. Potential exercise-related injuries include muscle and joint pain, cramps, blisters, shin splints, low back pain, tendinitis, and other sprains or muscle strains. The most commonly reported adverse event of exercise is musculoskeletal injury; approximately 25% of adults between 20 and 85 years of age reported an injury occurring at least once during 1 year (Hootman et al., 2002). It is possible that some of these are misclassified as injuries instead of muscle soreness due to a rapid increase in volume or intensity of training without proper knowledge of the principles of training.

When exercising, it is important to follow guidelines to help promote exercise safety. These include (a) stretching the muscles and tendons prior to beginning exercise, (b) wearing appropriate footwear and clothing, (c) choosing a modality that is appropriate for skill and fitness level, and (d) learning the exercise properly and continuing good form even with increased speed or intensity (AHA, 2021c; U.S. Department of Health and Human Services, 2018). If exercise-related injuries occur, they can usually be treated with one or a combination of therapies, including rest, ice, compression, and elevation (Järvinen et al., 2007).

ADHERENCE TO EXERCISE PROGRAMS

Maintaining the exercise program is key to the effectiveness of the intervention. Given the poor adherence to physical activity (and exercise) guidelines, it is important for nurses to understand and provide evidence-based strategies to maximize adherence if exercise is to be used as a form of preventative medicine or therapy. Adherence to exercise training is considered a multifactorial problem with several biosocial contributing factors. Biosocial factors associated with favorable exercise adherence include higher socioeconomic status and education levels, marital status; good health (fewer health conditions or better self-rated health) and better physical and cognitive function, fewer depressive symptoms, supervised exercise programs, and extrinsic motivators (wearable technologies, etc.; Rivera-Torres et al., 2019).

Exhibit 18.2 *Facilitating Adherence to Exercise*

Make exercise as enjoyable as possible:
- Exercise with friends (make exercise a social experience).
- Start low and progress slowly (trying too much too soon can result in sore muscles or injury).
- Choose an exercise modality that you enjoy (if running is not fun, perhaps swimming or biking is more appropriate).

Incorporate exercise into the lifestyle:
- Make exercise part of your daily routine.
- Choose an exercise mode that is convenient for your daily routine.
- Combine exercise with your family activities.

Set goals and monitor progress:
- Set (and achieve) realistic short- and long-term goals. This can provide a sense of accomplishment while enhancing intrinsic motivation and confidence.
- Create a record or graph. This supplies a visual of progress and may provide insight into adjustments to the exercise program that aid in achieving goals while enhancing motivation.

Source: Rivera-Torres, S., Fahey, T. D., & Rivera, M. A. (2019). Adherence to exercise programs in older adults: Informative report. *Gerontology & Geriatric Medicine, 5*, 2333721418823604. https://doi.org/10.1177/2333721418823604; Spiteri, K., Broom, D., Bekhet, A. H., de Caro, J. X., Laventure, B., & Grafton, K. (2019). Barriers and motivators of physical activity participation in middle-aged and older-adults - A systematic review. *Journal of Aging and Physical Activity, 27*(4), 929–944. https://doi.org/10.1123/japa.2018-0343.

When considering both the barriers and facilitators of exercise, important suggestions that can increase adherence to exercise programs that can be made include: making exercise enjoyable and part of a lifestyle and monitoring progress (Rivera-Torres et al., 2019; Spiteri et al., 2019) (Exhibit 18.2).

MOBILE HEALTH TECHNOLOGIES

Mobile health technologies (m-Health), which includes mobile applications, mobile devices, short messaging service, and voice calling, provide an opportunity to address low rates of adherence to both physical activity and exercise guidelines (Schorr et al., 2021). Over the last decade, m-Health technology, especially the wearable technology and mobile applications markets, have grown substantially and gained global popularity. Interventions using m-Health technologies have the potential to improve low rates of exercise adherence by providing individuals with continuous and individualized feedback, support, and guidance on lifestyle physical activity and encouraging self-care; both critical components of chronic disease management. While the Technology Acceptance Model and Post-Acceptance Model explain the basic factors that determine behavioral intention, and thus usage of m-Health technology, there exists a need for further study on the individualized factors that influence m-Health technology adoption and sustained usage, as well as the efficacy, cost, and scalability to successfully leverage m-Health technologies as a preventive measure to reduce the burden of advanced illness (i.e., CVD; Barone Gibbs et al., 2021; Burke et al., 2015; Schorr et al., 2021). Additionally, people are paying closer attention to what goes into and onto their bodies and how little or how much they are moving them. As a result, an entire industry has developed that has the potential to enhance adherence to both physical activity and exercise guidelines.

DETRAINING

Detraining refers to the partial or complete loss of training-induced fitness adaptations as a consequence of training cessation (Mujika & Padilla, 2000, 2001). Once participation in exercise has ceased, there is a rapid return to pre-exercise levels of physical fitness. The majority of the decline occurs during the first 5 weeks following exercise cessation and is usually complete within 12 weeks (Mujika & Padilla, 2000, 2001). In general, rates of detraining are similar for men and women and even among older adults. During detraining, blood volume (and stroke volume) decrease, which are large contributing factors in the loss of cardiorespiratory fitness. With disuse, the muscle tissues atrophy, which is a contributing factor to muscular strength losses. In addition, the decreased caloric expenditure leads to a positive energy balance, which can result in increased accumulation of adipose tissue and BMI.

CULTURAL APPLICATIONS

The benefits of exercise and physical activity appear to be equal across gender and race; however, this topic remains poorly studied and recommendations are based primarily on assumptions that findings in one population will carry over to another. It should be mentioned that there exist cultural preferences, including religious and ethnic preferences, in the use of exercise and physical activity. Although there has been little systematic investigation regarding these preferences, their potential influence should be considered when prescribing exercise and physical activity. For example, with certain ethnicities, it may be beneficial to make exercise modifications for garments that cover the body.

The use of alternate exercise techniques has gained popularity during the past few decades, especially among older adults. These forms of physical activity include meditative forms of movement in the practice of qigong and its specific forms such as tai chi and yoga (discussed in separate chapters in this book). Within these alternative forms of physical activity, numerous styles and movements have been reported, but the overarching theme remains the same. Although the evidence base for this type of exercise is less strenuous than for structured Western-style exercise (e.g., walking), it appears that these forms of physical activity may provide health benefits, especially in improving balance and lowering the fear of falling. However, most reported studies have been small and have used large variations of these techniques.

Other cultures have also been able to incorporate daily physical activity as part of their usual routine, either by necessity or by choice. For example, European countries have facilitated walking and cycling as modes of transportation by incorporating walkways and bicycle lanes in city planning. These forms of transportation are also culturally accepted as the primary modes of transportation in those countries, whereas in the United States, this is commonly not the case. Exercise in Sweden, as one example of activity incorporated into the European lifestyle, is presented in Sidebar 18.1. Sidebar 18.2 illustrates another country in which activity is incorporated into lifestyles; in Nigeria, the work life of farmers keeps them active and fit.

Sidebar 18.1 *Exercise in Sweden*

Ulf G. Bronäs

In Sweden (as in most of Europe), major cities are built to facilitate walking and cycling as the primary modes of transportation to and from work, school, day care, grocery shopping, and places of entertainment. Walkways and bicycle lanes are incorporated into city planning and allow for easy access for most people. It is common for parents to bring their children to day care by walking or using a specialized bicycle child seat assembled on the back of the bicycle. Once the child is older, the family bikes together to day care or school. Parents drop their children off at day care or school and continue biking either to work or to a mass-transit station. More than 60% of Swedes use public transportation to and from work, which facilitates both walking and bicycling. These modes of transportation are culturally accepted and used as primary methods of transportation in Sweden and throughout Europe. It is often said that to experience Europe, one must walk the cities. The cities are built to promote walking; it is the most convenient (and least expensive) form of transportation. The availability of multiple walkways and bicycle lanes is evident in the cities, allowing the population the option of incorporating daily physical activity into their lives.

Sidebar 18.2 *Exercise in Nigeria*

Gladys O. Igbo

As far as exercise is concerned, in my home country of Nigeria, people exercise at levels that are not all that different from the United States recommendations for exercise, and they use some elements of movement and exercise as part of their healing modalities. In considering exercise and activity, one must bear in mind that in Nigeria, most individuals exercise "naturally" as farmers; during cultivating seasons, there are a lot of vigorous movements involved in daily work activities. Likewise, exercise is commonly used as part of the recovery process when someone becomes ill. Growing up there, I witnessed a lot of early morning rising and walking out in nature, especially when someone was ill and was trying to recover fast and well. I continue to value exercise; I advocate exercise as part of health promotion as a nurse and in my role as a fitness trainer in a health club in the United States. In Nigeria, we may not have traditional "health clubs," so to speak, like most developed countries do, with required dues and memberships. However, most Nigerians do have the basic knowledge of how incorporating some activities of movement to help in their quest for good health and health enhancement.

There is a clear need for future city planning to incorporate safe, accessible, and enjoyable walkways and bicycle lanes so that the American population can incorporate daily physical activity into their lives and gain the health benefits associated with increased physical activity levels. This will help change the cultural perspective of physical activity in this country and support walking and/or bicycling as a preferred mode of transportation.

FUTURE RESEARCH

There are many gaps in our knowledge related to exercise, its measurement, the benefits, and methods for improving exercise adherence. Specific areas of needed research include

- investigations of cultural and ethnic differences in physical activity and response to exercise;
- investigations of the benefit of exercise in individuals with disabilities, including mental and physical disabilities;
- development of strategies to increase lifelong physical activity and exercise; and
- determine if electronic or social media can improve short- and long-term adherence.

WEBSITES

GENERAL GUIDELINES AND INFORMATION

- Centers for Disease Control and Prevention (CDC) (www.cdc.gov/physicalactivity)
- President's Council on Physical Fitness and Sports (www.fitness.gov)
- U.S. Department of Health and Human Services, Physical Activity Guidelines (https://health.gov/our-work/physical-activity)
- Healthy People 2030 (https://health.gov/healthypeople)

GUIDELINES AND INFORMATION PERTAINING TO FAMILIES AND COMMUNITIES

- CDC (www.cdc.gov/physicalactivity/index.html)
- National Institutes of Health—Exercise and Physical Activity (www.nia.nih.gov/health/exercise-physical-activity)
- Office of the Surgeon General (www.surgeongeneral.gov/obesityprevention/index.html)
- President's Council on Physical Fitness and Sports (www.presidentschallenge.org)

SCHOOLS

- CDC, Division of Adolescent and School Health (www.cdc.gov/healthyschools/physicalactivity/index.htm)

COMMUNITIES

- Federal Highway Administration (www.fhwa.dot.gov/environment/bicycle _pedestrian)
- National Institutes of Health (www.nhlbi.nih.gov/health/public/heart/obesity/ wecan)
- National Park Service (www.nps.gov/ncrc/programs/rtca/helpfultools/ht _publications.html)

WORKSITE

- CDC, Healthier Worksite Initiative (https://www.cdc.gov/physicalactivity/ worksite-pa/)

ACRONYMS

ACSM: American College of Sports Medicine
AD: Alzheimer's dementia
ADL: activities of daily living
AHA: American Heart Association
ATP: adenosine triphosphate
BMI: body mass index
BP: blood pressure
CDC: Centers for Disease Control
CHD: coronary heart disease
CHF: chronic heart failure
CVD: cardiovascular disease
COPD: chronic obstructive pulmonary disease
HR: heart rate
HRR: heart rate reserve
HTN: hypertension
MCI: mild cognitive impairment
METs: metabolic equivalents of task
PAD: peripheral artery disease
RPE: rating of perceived exertion
T2DM: type 2 diabetes mellitus
USDHHS: U.S. Department of Health and Human Services
VO2: peak oxygen consumption

REFERENCES

Ades, P. A., Keteyian, S. J., Wright, J. S., Hamm, L. F., Lui, K., Newlin, K., Shepard, D. S., & Thomas, R. J. (2017). Increasing cardiac rehabilitation participation from 20% to 70%: A road map from the Million Hearts Cardiac Rehabilitation Collaborative. *Mayo Clinical Proceedings, 92*(2), 234–242. https://doi.org/10.1016/j.mayocp.2016.10.014

American College of Sports Medicine. (1998). American College of Sports Medicine position stand. Exercise and physical activity for older adults. *Medicine and Science in Sports and Exercise, 30*(6), 992–1008. https://doi.org/10.1097/00005768-199806000-00032

American College of Sports Medicine. (2009). American College of Sports Medicine position stand. Progression models in resistance training for healthy adults. *Medicine & Science in Sports & Exercise, 41*(3), 687–708. https://doi.org/10.1249/MSS.0b013e3181915670

American College of Sports Medicine. (2018). *ACSM's Guidelines for Exercise Testing and Prescription* (10th ed.). Lippincott Williams & Wilkins/Wolters Kluwer.

American College of Sports Medicine, Chodzko-Zajko, W. J., Proctor, D. N., Fiatarone Singh, M. A., Minson, C. T., Nigg, C. R., Salem, G. J., & Skinner, J. S. (2009). American College of Sports Medicine position stand. Exercise and physical activity for older adults. *Medicine and Science in Sports and Exercise, 41*(7), 1510–1530. https://doi.org/10.1249/MSS.0b013e3181a0c95c

American Heart Association. (2021a). *Six week beginner walking plan.* https://www.heart.org/idc/groups/heart-public/@wcm/@fc/documents/downloadable/ucm_449261.pdf

American Heart Association. (2021b). *Walking.* https://www.heart.org/HEARTORG/HealthyLiving/PhysicalActivity/Walking_UCM_460870_SubHomePage.jsp

American Heart Association. (2021c). *Why is walking the most popular form of exercise?* https://www.heart.org/en/healthy-living/fitness/walking/why-is-walking-the-most-popular-form-of-exercise

American Thoracic Society. (2002). ATS statement: Guidelines for the six-minute walk test. *American Journal of Respiratory & Critical Care Medicine, 166*(1), 111–117. https://doi.org/10.1164/ajrccm.166.1.at1102

Anton, S. D., Karabetian, C., Naugle, K., & Buford, T. W. (2013). Obesity and diabetes as accelerators of functional decline: Can lifestyle interventions maintain functional status in high risk older adults? *Experimental Gerontology, 48*(9), 888–897. https://doi.org/10.1016/j.exger.2013.06.007

Astrand, P.-O., Kaare, R., Dahl, H., & Stromme, S. (2004). *Textbook of work physiology: Physiological bases of exercise* (Vol. 4). Human Kinetics.

Balady, G. J., Arena, R., Sietsema, K., Myers, J., Coke, L., Fletcher, G. F., Forman, D., Franklin, B., Guazzi, M., Gulati, M., Keteyian, S. J., Lavie, C. J., Macko, R., Mancini, D., Milani, R. V., & Council on Epidemiology and Prevention, and Council on Peripheral Vaascular Disease, and Interdisciplinary Council on Quality of Care and Outcomes Research, and on behalf of the American Heart Association Exercise, Cardiac Rehabilitation, and Prevention Committee of the Council on Clinical Cardiology. (2010). Clinician's Guide to cardiopulmonary exercise testing in adults: A scientific statement from the American Heart Association. *Circulation, 122*(2), 191–225. https://doi.org/10.1161/CIR.0b013e3181e52e69

Barone Gibbs, B., Hivert, M. F., Jerome, G. J., Kraus, W. E., Rosenkranz, S. K., Schorr, E. N., Spartano, N. L., & Lobelo, F. (2021). Physical activity as a critical component of first-line treatment for elevated blood pressure or cholesterol: Who, what, and how?: A scientific statement from the American Heart Association. *Hypertension, 78*, e26–e37. https://doi.org/10.1161/HYP.0000000000000196

Beaver, W. L., Wasserman, K., & Whipp, B. J. (1986). Bicarbonate buffering of lactic acid generated during exercise. *Journal of Applied Physiology, 60*(2), 472–478. https://doi.org/10.1152/jappl.1986.60.2.472

Benjamin, E. J., Muntner, P., Alonso, A., Bittencourt, M. S., Callaway, C. W., Carson, A. P., Chamberlain, A. M., Chang, A. R., Cheng, S., Das, S. R., Delling, F. N., Djousse, L., Elkind, M. S. V., Ferguson, J. F., Fornage, M., Jordan, L. C., Khan, S. S., Kissela, B. M., Knutson, K. L., . . . Virani, S. S. (2019). Heart disease and stroke statistics-2019 update: A report from the American Heart Association. *Circulation, 139*(10), e56–e528. https://doi.org/10.1161/cir.0000000000000659

Bermejo-Cantarero, A., Álvarez-Bueno, C., Martínez-Vizcaino, V., Redondo-Tébar, A., Pozuelo-Carrascosa, D. P., & Sánchez-López, M. (2021). Relationship between both cardiorespiratory and muscular fitness and health-related quality of life in children and adolescents: A systematic review and meta-analysis of observational studies. *Health and Quality of Life Outcomes, 19*(1), 127. https://doi.org/10.1186/s12955-021-01766-0

Blair, S. N., Kampert, J. B., Kohl, H. W., 3rd, Barlow, C. E., Macera, C. A., Paffenbarger, R. S., Jr., & Gibbons, L. W. (1996). Influences of cardiorespiratory fitness and other precursors on cardiovascular disease and all-cause mortality in men and women. *Journal of the American Medical Association, 276*(3), 205–210. https://doi.org/10.1001/jama.276.3.205

Blair, S. N., Kohl, H. W., 3rd, Paffenbarger, R. S., Jr., Clark, D. G., Cooper, K. H., & Gibbons, L. W. (1989). Physical fitness and all-cause mortality. A prospective study of healthy men and women. *Journal of the American Medical Association, 262*(17), 2395–2401. https://doi.org/10.1001/jama.262.17.2395

Bonnet, F., Irving, K., Terra, J. L., Nony, P., Berthezène, F., & Moulin, P. (2005). Anxiety and depression are associated with unhealthy lifestyle in patients at risk of cardiovascular disease. *Atherosclerosis, 178*(2), 339–344. https://doi.org/10.1016/j.atherosclerosis.2004.08.035

Borg, G. (1998). *Borg's Perceived Exertion and Pain Scales*. Human Kinetics.

Burke, L. E., Ma, J., Azar, K. M., Bennett, G. G., Peterson, E. D., Zheng, Y., Riley, W., Stephens, J., Shah, S. H., Suffoletto, B., Turan, T. N., Spring, B., Steinberger, J., & Quinn, C. C. (2015). Current science on consumer use of mobile health for cardiovascular disease prevention: A scientific statement from the American Heart Association. *Circulation, 132*(12), 1157–1213. https://doi.org/10.1161/cir.0000000000000232

Caspersen, C. J., Powell, K. E., & Christenson, G. M. (1985). Physical activity, exercise, and physical fitness: Definitions and distinctions for health-related research. *Public Health Reports, 100*(2), 126–131. https://doi.org/10.2307/20056429

Cass, S. P. (2017). Alzheimer's disease and exercise: A literature review. *Current Sports Medicine Reports, 16*(1), 19–22. https://doi.org/10.1249/jsr.0000000000000332

Centers for Disease Control and Prevention, U.S. Department of Health and Human Services. (2017). *New CDC report: More than 100 million Americans have diabetes or prediabetes*. https://www.cdc.gov/media/releases/2017/p0718-diabetes-report.html

Centers for Disease Control and Prevention, U.S. Department of Health and Human Services. (2018). *Trends in meeting the 2008 physical activity guidelines, 2008–2018*. https://www.cdc.gov/physicalactivity/downloads/trends-in-the-prevalence-of-physical-activity-508.pdf

Centers for Disease Control and Prevention, U.S. Department of Health and Human Services. (2021). *Obesity facts |Overweight and obesity*. https://www.cdc.gov/obesity/data/childhood.html

Chatterjee, S., Khunti, K., & Davies, M. J. (2017). Type 2 diabetes. *Lancet, 389*(10085), 2239–2251. https://doi.org/10.1016/s0140-6736(17)30058-2

Codella, R., Ialacqua, M., Terruzzi, I., & Luzi, L. (2018). May the force be with you: Why resistance training is essential for subjects with type 2 diabetes mellitus without complications. *Endocrine, 62*(1), 14–25. https://doi.org/10.1007/s12020-018-1603-7

Colberg, S. R., Sigal, R. J., Yardley, J. E., Riddell, M. C., Dunstan, D. W., Dempsey, P. C., Horton, E. S., Castorino, K., & Tate, D. F. (2016). Physical activity/exercise and diabetes: A position statement of the American Diabetes Association. *Diabetes Care, 39*(11), 2065–2079. https://doi.org/10.2337/dc16-1728

Cornelissen, V. A., & Smart, N. A. (2013). Exercise training for blood pressure: A systematic review and meta-analysis. *Journal of the American Heart Association, 2*(1), e004473. https://doi.org/10.1161/JAHA.112.004473

Dasso, N. A. (2019). How is exercise different from physical activity? A concept analysis. *Nursing Forum, 54*(1), 45–52. https://doi.org/10.1111/nuf.12296

Donnelly, J. E., Blair, S. N., Jakicic, J. M., Manore, M. M., Rankin, J. W., Smith, B. K., & American College of Sports, M. (2009). American College of Sports Medicine Position Stand. Appropriate physical activity intervention strategies for weight loss and prevention of weight regain for adults. *Medicine and Science in Sports and Exercise, 41*(2), 459–471. https://doi.org/10.1249/MSS.0b013e3181949333

Fakhry, F., van de Luijtgaarden, K. M., Bax, L., den Hoed, P. T., Hunink, M. G., Rouwet, E. V., & Spronk, S. (2012). Supervised walking therapy in patients with intermittent claudication. *Journal of Vascular Surgery, 56*(4), 1132–1142. https://doi.org/10.1016/j.jvs.2012.04.046

Fletcher, G. F., Ades, P. A., Kligfield, P., Arena, R., Balady, G. J., Bittner, V. A., Coke, L. A., Fleg, J. L., Forman, D. E., Gerber, T. C., Gulati, M., Madan, K., Rhodes, J., Thompson, P. D.,

Williams, M. A., & American Heart Association Exercise, on behalf of the American Heart Association Exercise, Cardiac Rehabilitation, and Prevention Committee of the Council on Clinical Cardiology, Council on Nutrition, Physical Activity and Metabolism, Council on Cardiovascular and Stroke Nursing, and Council on Epidemiology and Prevention. (2013). Exercise standards for testing and training: A scientific statement from the American Heart Association. *Circulation, 128*(8), 873–934. https://doi.org/10.1161/CIR.0b013e31829b5b44

Foster, C., Porcari, J. P., Anderson, J., Paulson, M., Smaczny, D., Webber, H., Doberstein, S. T., & Udermann, B. (2008). The talk test as a marker of exercise training intensity. *Journal of Cardiopulmonary Rehabilitaion and Prevention, 28*(1), 24–30; quiz 31–22. https://doi.org/10.1097/01.hcr.0000311504.41775.78

Franklin, B. A. (2014). Preventing exercise-related cardiovascular events: Is a medical examination more urgent for physical activity or inactivity? *Circulation, 129*(10), 1081–1084. https://doi.org/10.1161/circulationaha.114.007641

Franklin, B. A., Thompson, P. D., Al-Zaiti, S. S., Albert, C. M., Hivert, M. F., Levine, B. D., Lobelo, F., Madan, K., Sharrief, A. Z., & Eijsvogels, T. M. H. (2020). Exercise-related acute cardiovascular events and potential deleterious adaptations following long-term exercise training: Placing the risks into perspective—an update: A scientific statement from the American Heart Association. *Circulation, 141*(13), e705–e736. https://doi.org/10.1161/cir.0000000000000749

Garber, C. E., Blissmer, B., Deschenes, M. R., Franklin, B. A., Lamonte, M. J., Lee, I. M., Nieman, D. C., Swain, D. P., & American College of Sports Medicine. (2011). American College of Sports Medicine position stand. Quantity and quality of exercise for developing and maintaining cardiorespiratory, musculoskeletal, and neuromotor fitness in apparently healthy adults: Guidance for prescribing exercise. *Medicine and Science in Sports and Exercise, 43*(7), 1334–1359. https://doi.org/10.1249/MSS.0b013e318213fefb

Garvey, C., Bayles, M. P., Hamm, L. F., Hill, K., Holland, A., Limberg, T. M., & Spruit, M. A. (2016). Pulmonary rehabilitation exercise prescription in chronic obstructive pulmonary disease: Review of selected guidelines: An official statement from the American Association of Cardiovascular and Pulmonary Rehabilitation. *Journal of Cardiopulmonary Rehabilitation and Prevention, 36*(2), 75–83. https://doi.org/10.1097/hcr.0000000000000171

Gordon, B. R., McDowell, C. P., Hallgren, M., Meyer, J. D., Lyons, M., & Herring, M. P. (2018). Association of efficacy of resistance exercise training with depressive symptoms: Meta-analysis and meta-regression analysis of randomized clinical trials. *JAMA Psychiatry, 75*(6), 566–576. https://doi.org/10.1001/jamapsychiatry.2018.0572

Gordon, R., & Bloxham, S. (2016). A systematic review of the effects of exercise and physical activity on non-specific chronic low back pain. *Healthcare (Basel), 4*(2). https://doi.org/10.3390/healthcare4020022

Guralnik, J. M., Simonsick, E. M., Ferrucci, L., Glynn, R. J., Berkman, L. F., Blazer, D. G., Scherr, P. A., & Wallace, R. B. (1994). A short physical performance battery assessing lower extremity function: Association with self-reported disability and prediction of mortality and nursing home admission. *Journal of Gerontology, 49*(2), M85–M94. https://doi.org/10.1093/geronj/49.2.m85

Härter, M. C., Conway, K. P., & Merikangas, K. R. (2003). Associations between anxiety disorders and physical illness. *European Archives of Psychiatry and Clinical Neuroscience, 253*(6), 313–320. https://doi.org/10.1007/s00406-003-0449-y

Haskell, W. L., Lee, I. M., Pate, R. R., Powell, K. E., Blair, S. N., Franklin, B. A., Macera, C. A., Heath, G. W., Thompson, P. D., & Bauman, A. (2007). Physical activity and public health: Updated recommendation for adults from the American College of Sports Medicine and the American Heart Association. *Medicine and Science in Sports and Exercise, 39*(8), 1423–1434. https://doi.org/10.1249/mss.0b013e3180616b27

Hearing, C. M., Chang, W. C., Szuhany, K. L., Deckersbach, T., Nierenberg, A. A., & Sylvia, L. G. (2016) Physical exercise for the treatment of mood disorders: A critical review. *Curr Behav Neurosci Rep, 3*(4), 350–359. https://doi.org/1007s50473-016-0089-y

Hiatt, W. R., Goldstone, J., Smith, S. C., Jr., McDermott, M., Moneta, G., Oka, R., Newman, A. B., Pearce, W. H., & American Heart Association Writing Group. (2008). Atherosclerotic Peripheral Vascular Disease Symposium II: Nomenclature for vascular diseases. *Circulation, 118*(25), 2826–2829. https://doi.org/10.1161/circulationaha.108.191171

Hootman, J. M., Macera, C. A., Ainsworth, B. E., Addy, C. L., Martin, M., & Blair, S. N. (2002). Epidemiology of musculoskeletal injuries among sedentary and physically active adults. *Medicine & Science in Sports & Exercise, 34*(5), 838–844. https://doi.org/10.1097/00005768-200205000-00017

Huang, X., Zhao, X., Li, B., Cai, Y., Zhang, S., Wan, Q., & Yu, F. (2021). Comparative efficacy of different exercise interventions on cognitive function in patients with MCI or dementia: A systematic review and network meta-analysis. *Journal of Sport and Health Science.* https://doi.org/10.1016/j.jshs.2021.05.003

Humberstone, B., & Stuart, S. (2016). Older women, exercise to music, and yoga: Senses of pleasure? *Journal of Aging and Physical Activity, 24*(3), 412–418. https://doi.org/10.1123/japa.2015-0115

Institute of Medicine. (2011). *Early childhood obesity prevention policies.* The National Academics Press. https://doi.org/10.17226/13124

Jaitovich, A., & Barreiro, E. (2018). Skeletal muscle dysfunction in chronic obstructive pulmonary disease. What we know and can do for our patients. *American Journal of Respiratory Critical Care Medicine, 198*(2), 175–186. https://doi.org/10.1164/rccm.201710-2140CI

Järvinen, T. A., Järvinen, T. L., Kääriäinen, M., Aärimaa, V., Vaittinen, S., Kalimo, H., & Järvinen, M. (2007). Muscle injuries: Optimising recovery. *Best Practices and Research in Clinical Rheumatology, 21*(2), 317–331. https://doi.org/10.1016/j.berh.2006.12.004

Jones, A. M., & Poole, D. C. (2005). Oxygen uptake dynamics: From muscle to mouth--an introduction to the symposium. *Medicine & Science in Sports & Exercise, 37*(9), 1542–1550. https://doi.org/10.1249/01.mss.0000177466.01232.7e

Karvonen, J., & Vuorimaa, T. (1988). Heart rate and exercise intensity during sports activities. Practical application. *Sports Medicine, 5*(5), 303–311. https://doi.org/10.2165/00007256-198805050-00002

Kazeminia, M., Salari, N., Vaisi-Raygani, A., Jalali, R., Abdi, A., Mohammadi, M., Daneshkhah, A., Hosseinian-Far, M., & Shohaimi, S. (2020). The effect of exercise on anxiety in the elderly worldwide: A systematic review and meta-analysis. *Health and Quality of Life Outcomes, 18*(1), 363. https://doi.org/10.1186/s12955-020-01609-4

Kodama, S., Saito, K., Tanaka, S., Maki, M., Yachi, Y., Asumi, M., Sugawara, A., Totsuka, K., Shimano, H., Ohashi, Y., Yamada, N., & Sone, H. (2009). Cardiorespiratory fitness as a quantitative predictor of all-cause mortality and cardiovascular events in healthy men and women: A meta-analysis. *Journal of the American Medical Association, 301*(19), 2024–2035. https://doi.org/10.1001/jama.2009.681

LaForgia, J., Withers, R. T., & Gore, C. J. (2006). Effects of exercise intensity and duration on the excess post-exercise oxygen consumption. *Journal of Sports Sciences, 24*(12), 1247–1264. https://doi.org/10.1080/02640410600552064

Liao, W. H., Chen, J. W., Chen, X., Lin, L., Yan, H. Y., Zhou, Y. Q., & Chen, R. (2015). Impact of resistance training in subjects with COPD: A systematic review and meta-analysis. *Respiratory Care, 60*(8), 1130–1145. https://doi.org/10.4187/respcare.03598

MacDonald, H. V., Johnson, B. T., Huedo-Medina, T. B., Livingston, J., Forsyth, K. C., Kraemer, W. J., Farinatti, P. T., & Pescatello, L. S. (2016). Dynamic resistance training as stand-alone antihypertensive lifestyle therapy: A meta-analysis. *Journal of the American Heart Association, 5*(10). https://doi.org/10.1161/jaha.116.003231

Magkos, F., Hjorth, M. F., & Astrup, A. (2020). Diet and exercise in the prevention and treatment of type 2 diabetes mellitus. *Nature Reviews Endocrinology, 16*(10), 545–555. https://doi.org/10.1038/s41574-020-0381-5

Mandsager, K., Harb, S., Cremer, P., Phelan, D., Nissen, S. E., & Jaber, W. (2018). Association of cardiorespiratory fitness with long-term mortality among adults undergoing exercise treadmill testing. *JAMA Network Open, 1*(6), e183605. https://doi.org/10.1001/jamanetworkopen.2018.3605

Mays, R. J., Goss, F. L., Nagle, E. F., Gallagher, M., Schafer, M. A., Kim, K. H., & Robertson, R. J. (2014). Prediction of VO2 peak using OMNI Ratings of Perceived Exertion from a submaximal cycle exercise test. *Perceptual and Motor Skills, 118*(3), 863–881. https://doi.org/10.2466/27.29 .PMS.118k28w7

McDermott, M. M., Liu, K., Greenland, P., Guralnik, J. M., Criqui, M. H., Chan, C., Pearce, W. H., Schneider, J. R., Ferrucci, L., Celic, L., Taylor, L. M., Vonesh, E., Martin, G. J., & Clark, E. (2004). Functional decline in peripheral arterial disease: Associations with the ankle brachial index and leg symptoms. *Journal of the American Medical Association, 292*(4), 453–461. https://doi .org/10.1001/jama.292.4.453

McKeough, Z. J., Velloso, M., Lima, V. P., & Alison, J. A. (2016). Upper limb exercise training for COPD. *Cochrane Database Systematic Reviews, 11*(11), CD011434. https://doi .org/10.1002/14651858.CD011434.pub2

McMahon, S. R., Ades, P. A., & Thompson, P. D. (2017). The role of cardiac rehabilitation in patients with heart disease. *Trends in Cardiovascular Medicine, 27*(6), 420–425. https://doi .org/10.1016/j.tcm.2017.02.005

Miller, K. J., Gonçalves-Bradley, D. C., Areerob, P., Hennessy, D., Mesagno, C., & Grace, F. (2020). Comparative effectiveness of three exercise types to treat clinical depression in older adults: A systematic review and network meta-analysis of randomised controlled trials. *Ageing Research Reviews, 58*, 100999. https://doi.org/10.1016/j.arr.2019.100999

Mirza, S., Clay, R. D., Koslow, M. A., & Scanlon, P. D. (2018). COPD guidelines: A review of the 2018 GOLD report. *Mayo Clinic Proceedings, 93*(10), 1488–1502. https://doi.org/10.1016/j .mayocp.2018.05.026

Mujika, I., & Padilla, S. (2000). Detraining: Loss of training-induced physiological and performance adaptations. Part II: Long term insufficient training stimulus. *Sports Medicine, 30*(3), 145–154. https://doi.org/10.2165/00007256-200030030-00001

Mujika, I., & Padilla, S. (2001). Cardiorespiratory and metabolic characteristics of detraining in humans. *Medicine & Science in Sports & Exercise, 33*(3), 413–421. https://doi .org/10.1097/00005768-200103000-00013

Northey, J. M., Cherbuin, N., Pumpa, K. L., Smee, D. J., & Rattray, B. (2018). Exercise interventions for cognitive function in adults older than 50: A systematic review with meta-analysis. *British Journal of Sports Medicine, 52*(3), 154–160. https://doi.org/10.1136/bjsports-2016-096587

Office of Disease Prevention and Health Promotion, U.S. Department of Health and Human Services. (2020). *Healthy people 2030.* https://health.gov/healthypeople

Olver, T. D., & Laughlin, M. H. (2016). Endurance, interval sprint, and resistance exercise training: Impact on microvascular dysfunction in type 2 diabetes. *American Journal of Physiology-Heart and Circulatory Physiology, 310*(3), H337–H350. https://doi.org/10.1152/ajpheart.00440.2015

Panza, G. A., Taylor, B. A., MacDonald, H. V., Johnson, B. T., Zaleski, A. L., Livingston, J., Thompson, P. D., & Pescatello, L. S. (2018). Can exercise improve cognitive symptoms of Alzheimer's disease? *Journal of the American Geriatric Society, 66*(3), 487–495. https://doi .org/10.1111/jgs.15241

Pedersen, B.K. (2019). Physical activity and muscle-brain crosstalk. *National Review of Endocrinology, 15* (7), 383-392. https://doi.org/10.1038/s41574-019-0174-x

Pescatello, L. S., MacDonald, H. V., Lamberti, L., & Johnson, B. T. (2015). Exercise for hypertension: A prescription update integrating existing recommendations with emerging research. *Current Hypertension Reports, 17*(11), 87. https://doi.org/10.1007/s11906-015-0600-y

Piercy, K. L., Troiano, R. P., Ballard, R. M., Carlson, S. A., Fulton, J. E., Galuska, D. A., George, S. M., & Olson, R. D. (2018). The physical activity guidelines for Americans. *Journal of the American Medical Association, 320*(19), 2020–2028. https://doi.org/10.1001/jama.2018.14854

Piña, I. L., Apstein, C. S., Balady, G. J., Belardinelli, R., Chaitman, B. R., Duscha, B. D., Fletcher, B. J., Fleg, J. L., Myers, J. N., & Sullivan, M. J. (2003). Exercise and heart failure: A statement from the American Heart Association Committee on Exercise, Rehabilitation, and Prevention. *Circulation, 107*(8), 1210–1225. https://doi.org/10.1161/01.cir.0000055013.92097.40

Podsiadlo, D., & Richardson, S. (1991). The timed "Up & Go": A test of basic functional mobility for frail elderly persons. *Journal of the American Geriatric Society, 39*(2), 142–148. https://doi.org/10.1111/j.1532-5415.1991.tb01616.x

Reed, J. L., & Pipe, A. L. (2014). The talk test: A useful tool for prescribing and monitoring exercise intensity. *Current Opinion in Cardiology, 29*(5), 475–480. https://doi.org/10.1097/hco.0000000000000097

Regensteiner, J. G., Hiatt, W. R., Coll, J. R., Criqui, M. H., Treat-Jacobson, D., McDermott, M. M., & Hirsch, A. T. (2008). The impact of peripheral arterial disease on health-related quality of life in the peripheral arterial disease awareness, risk, and treatment: New resources for survival (PARTNERS) program. *Vascular Medicine, 13*(1), 15–24. https://doi.org/10.1177/1358863X07084911

Rhyner, K. T., & Watts, A. (2016). Exercise and depressive symptoms in older adults: A systematic meta-analytic review. *Journal of Aging and Physical Activity, 24*(2), 234–246. https://doi.org/10.1123/japa.2015-0146

Riebe, D., Franklin, B. A., Thompson, P. D., Garber, C. E., Whitfield, G. P., Magal, M., & Pescatello, L. S. (2015). Updating ACSM's recommendations for exercise preparticipation health screening. *Medicine & Science in Sports & Exercise, 47*(11), 2473–2479. https://doi.org/10.1249/mss.0000000000000664

Rivera-Torres, S., Fahey, T. D., & Rivera, M. A. (2019). Adherence to exercise programs in older adults: Informative report. *Gerontology & Geriatric Medicine, 5*, 2333721418823604. https://doi.org/10.1177/2333721418823604

Roberts, R. A., Ghiasvand, F., & Parker, D. (2004). Biochemistry of exercise-induced metabolic acidosis. *American Journal of Physiology Regulatory, Integrative and Comparative Physiology, 287*(3), R502–R516. https://doi.org/10.1152/ajpregu.00114.2004

Schorr, E. N., Gepner, A. D., Dolansky, M. A., Forman, D. E., Park, L. G., Petersen, K. S., Still, C. H., Wang, T. Y., & Wenger, N. K. (2021). Harnessing mobile health technology for secondary cardiovascular disease prevention in older adults: A scientific statement from the American Heart Association. *Circulation: Cardiovascular Quality and Outcomes, 14*(5), e000103. https://doi.org/10.1161/hcq.0000000000000103

Shookster, D., Lindsey, B., Cortes, N., & Martin, J. R. (2020). Accuracy of commonly used age-predicted maximal heart rate equations. *International Journal of Exercise Science, 13*(7), 1242–1250.

Sivaramakrishnan, D., Fitzsimons, C., Kelly, P., Ludwig, K., Mutrie, N., Saunders, D. H., & Baker, G. (2019). The effects of yoga compared to active and inactive controls on physical function and health related quality of life in older adults- systematic review and meta-analysis of randomised controlled trials. *International Journal of Behavioral Nutrition and Physical Activity, 16*(1), 33. https://doi.org/10.1186/s12966-019-0789-2

Solloway, M. R., Taylor, S. L., Shekelle, P. G., Miake-Lye, I. M., Beroes, J. M., Shanman, R. M., & Hempel, S. (2016). An evidence map of the effect of Tai Chi on health outcomes. *Systematic Reviews, 5*(1), 126. https://doi.org/10.1186/s13643-016-0300-y

Spiteri, K., Broom, D., Bekhet, A. H., de Caro, J. X., Laventure, B., & Grafton, K. (2019). Barriers and motivators of physical activity participation in middle-aged and older-adults—A systematic review. *Journal of Aging and Physical Activity, 27*(4), 929–944. https://doi.org/10.1123/japa.2018-0343

Squires, R. W., Kaminsky, L. A., Porcari, J. P., Ruff, J. E., Savage, P. D., & Williams, M. A. (2018). Progression of exercise training in early outpatient cardiac rehabilitation: An official statement from the American Association of Cardiovascular and Pulmonary Rehabilitation. *Journal of Cardiopulmonary Rehabililation and Prevention, 38*(3), 139–146. https://doi.org/10.1097/hcr.0000000000000337

Stathokostas, L., Little, R. M., Vandervoort, A. A., & Paterson, D. H. (2012). Flexibility training and functional ability in older adults: A systematic review. *Journal of Aging Research, 2012*, 306818. https://doi.org/10.1155/2012/306818

Tari, A. R., Norevik, C. S., Scrimgeour, N. R., Kobro-Flatmoen, A., Storm-Mathisen, J., Bergersen, L. H., Wrann, C. D., Selbæk, G., Kivipelto, M., Moreira, J. B. N., & Wisløff, U. (2019). Are the neuroprotective effects of exercise training systemically mediated? *Progress in Cardiovascular Diseases, 62*(2), 94–101. https://doi.org/10.1016/j.pcad.2019.02.003

Tipton, C. M. (2006). *ACSM's advanced exercise physiology*. Lippincott Williams & Wilkins.

Treat-Jacobson, D., McDermott, M. M., Beckman, J. A., Burt, M. A., Creager, M. A., Ehrman, J. K., Gardner, A. W., Mays, R. J., Regensteiner, J. G., Salisbury, D. L., Schorr, E. N., & Walsh, M. E. (2019). Implementation of supervised exercise therapy for patients with symptomatic peripheral artery disease: A science advisory from the American Heart Association. *Circulation, 140*(13), e700–e710. https://doi.org/10.1161/cir.0000000000000727

Treat-Jacobson, D., McDermott, M. M., Bronas, U. G., Campia, U., Collins, T. C., Criqui, M. H., Gardner, A. W., Hiatt, W. R., Regensteiner, J. G., & Rich, K. (2019). Optimal exercise programs for patients with peripheral artery disease: A scientific statement from the American Heart Association. *Circulation, 139*(4), e10–e33. https://doi.org/10.1161/cir.0000000000000623

Tucker, W. J., Lijauco, C. C., Hearon, C. M., Jr., Angadi, S. S., Nelson, M. D., Sarma, S., Nanayakkara, S., La Gerche, A., & Haykowsky, M. J. (2018). Mechanisms of the improvement in peak VO(2) with exercise training in heart failure with reduced or preserved ejection fraction. *Heart, Lung and Circulation, 27*(1), 9–21. https://doi.org/10.1016/j.hlc.2017.07.002

U.S. Department of Health and Human Services. (1996). *Physical activity and health: A report of the surgeon general*. U.S. Department of Health and Human Services, Centers for Disease Control and Prevention, National Center for Chronic Disease Prevention and Health Promotion.

U.S. Department of Health and Human Services. (2018). *Physical activity guidelines for Americans* (2nd ed). https://health.gov/sites/default/files/201909/Physical_Activity_Guidelines_2nd_edition.pdf

U.S. Department of Health and Human Services, Office of Disease Prevention and Health Promotion. (2008). *Physical activity guidelines for Americans*. https://health.gov/our-work/nutrition-physical-activity/physical-activity-guidelines

U.S. Department of Health and Human Services, Office of Disease Prevention and Health Promotion. (2018). *Physical Activity Guidelines for Americans*. healthysd.gov/physical-activity-guidelines-for-Americans-2nd-editon/

Utter, A. C., Robertson, R. J., Green, J. M., Suminski, R. R., McAnulty, S. R., & Nieman, D. C. (2004). Validation of the Adult OMNI Scale of perceived exertion for walking/running exercise. *Medicine and Science in Sports and Exercise, 36*(10), 1776–1780. https://doi.org/10.1249/01.mss.0000142310.97274.94

Westerblad, H., Allen, D. G., & Lännergren, J. (2002). Muscle fatigue: Lactic acid or inorganic phosphate the major cause? *News in Physiological Sciences, 17*, 17–21. https://doi.org/10.1152/physiologyonline.2002.17.1.17

Whelton, S. P., Chin, A., Xin, X., & He, J. (2002). Effect of aerobic exercise on blood pressure: A meta-analysis of randomized, controlled trials. *Annals of Internal Medicine, 136*(7), 493–503. https://doi.org/10.7326/0003-4819-136-7-200204020-00006

Youkhana, S., Dean, C. M., Wolff, M., Sherrington, C., & Tiedemann, A. (2016). Yoga-based exercise improves balance and mobility in people aged 60 and over: A systematic review and meta-analysis. *Age Ageing, 45*(1), 21–29. https://doi.org/10.1093/ageing/afv175

Yu, F., Salisbury, D. L., & Kelly, K. (2019). *The Alzheimer's rx: Aerobic exercise*. Cygnus Media, LLC.

IV

Biologically Based Therapies

MARGO HALM

Biologically based therapies comprise natural products now classified as *nutritional approaches* by the National Center for Complementary and Integrative Health (NCCIH, 2021a). These natural products include herbal preparations (also called *botanicals*), vitamins, minerals, dietary supplements or nutraceuticals, essential oils, and live microorganisms (usually bacteria). One therapy that is becoming more commonly used by nurses, as well as in consumer self-care, is aromatherapy (Chapter 19). The essential oils used in aromatherapy are natural products. The most common use of essential oils by nurses is in the administration of aromatherapy externally—either by application to the skin or by inhalation. The essential oils used in aromatherapy need to be differentiated from the artificial (synthetic) oils found in many popular bath-and-body shops.

Chapter 20 explores herbal preparations, whereas Chapter 21 focuses on functional foods and nutraceuticals. People from the earliest times have used herbal preparations to improve health or cure illnesses. Hildegard of Bingen, a Benedictine nun, wrote treatises in the 12th century detailing a large number of natural products, such as herbs that could be used in healing (Encyclopedia of World Biography, 2004). Herbal product compounds for traditional Chinese medicine were documented in the Chinese *Materia Medica* as early as 400 BCE (Beijing Digital Museum of Traditional Chinese Medicine, 2012).

Although the use of herbal preparations decreased in the 20th century as new medicines evolved, there has been a resurgence in the public's use of natural products. With marketing all around us, natural products are readily available. Consumers can purchase products from natural food, grocery, and big-box retail stores; provider offices; and internet websites. The 2012 National Health Interview Survey (NHIS) included questions about the use of natural products (NCCIH, 2016) and found 17.7% of those surveyed used one or more nonvitamin/nonmineral natural products. In the 2015 National Consumer Survey on Medication

Experience and Pharmacist Role, 35% of U.S. adults (N = 26,157) reported using at least one herbal medicine, with an average number of 2.6 per adult. The predictors of herbal medicine use were higher education, chronic health conditions, as well as the use of mail-order pharmacy and over-the-counter (OTC) products (Rashrash et al., 2017). In a German focus group study, young, middle-aged, and older adults cited the main reasons for using herbal products were to promote health and prevent chronic and acute illness but, most important, to treat mild to moderate illnesses, such as head and chest colds and musculoskeletal issues (Welz et al., 2018). The use of natural products continues to be a part of healing practices in many non-Western healthcare systems as well. For example, herbal preparations are a prominent part of Native American healing practices and traditional Chinese medicine. Preparations from natural products used in other parts of the world are illustrated in the international sidebars included within the chapters of this section.

On top of this regular use, many consumers rushed to stockpile natural products during the COVID-19 pandemic in order to have sufficient supply to buffer their risk. Consumer demand for herb remedies focused on products for respiratory and flu-like symptoms, such as Vitamin C and D, honey, garlic, honeysuckle, cinnamon twig, and peony root that could boost the immune system (Caspani, 2020; Khabour & Hassanein, 2021). In one study, the use of natural products was significantly associated with higher age (>50) and level of fear about the virus (Khabour & Hassanein, 2021). A dramatic rise in Google searches for *"immune boost"* and *"immune boosting"* were also observed as the pandemic began to unfold (Wagner et al., 2020). The social media platform Instagram featured commercial posts claiming products had beneficial "immune-boosting" qualities without any critique of validity, leading to the spread of inaccurate information (Wagner et al., 2020). Indeed, while the science is emerging on the effectiveness of herbs, vitamins, minerals, and other dietary recommendations against COVID-19 (Alagawany et al., 2021; Silveira et al., 2020), sufficient evidence is not yet available to guide clinical practice or self-care. If misused, some herbal preparations could actually boost the immune system and contribute to the deadly cytokine storm some patients with COVID-19 have experienced (Ries, 2020).

The majority of the products in the category of natural products (e.g., nonprescription supplements, food additives)—including nutraceuticals—are available OTC. Since natural products do not require a prescription, healthcare professionals are often not actively involved in conversations and decisions regarding their use. As noted, natural products are an integral part of health practices in many cultures across the globe. Natural products may interact with prescribed medications or other treatments. These interactions range from reduced absorption with lessened pharmaceutical effectiveness to potentiation of drug effects which may contribute to the mild to serious side effects (e.g., tachycardia, hypertension) or adverse events (e.g., hemorrhage, stroke) that may be associated with these products (Coxeter et al., 2004; Hussain, 2011; Tachjian et al., 2010; Wolf et al., 2021). Furthermore, the greater number of natural products used, the higher the probability the patient will experience interactions of any kind (Wolf et al., 2021). Thus, it is critical that the healthcare team be aware of a patient's use of natural products. Careful, specific inquiry about their use needs to be a part of all patient assessments. Healthcare professionals, including students, must understand the uses, contraindications, and precautions associated with various natural products. Becoming well informed will allow members of the healthcare team to be more effective in their roles to educate and counsel patients on the safe use of natural products and, thus, better understand that "natural" does not always mean the product is safer or a better option for health (NCCIH, 2021b). Such understanding will also serve students and healthcare professionals in their own personal use of natural products for self-care or management of diseases and conditions.

NCCIH launched an app *HerbList*™ to help consumers navigate information about popular herbs and herbal supplements (www.nih.gov/news-events/news-releases/nih-launches-herblist-mobile-app-herbal-products). Available on the Apple App and Google Play stores, *HerbList*™ includes research-based information on the safety and effectiveness of herbal products. *Mosby's Handbook of Herbs and Natural Supplements* is another app available on the Apple App Store. This app provides information on uses, doses, side effects/adverse reactions, interactions, client considerations, and patient teaching points related to many herbs and natural supplements. The Natural Standard database (https://natural medicines.therapeuticresearch.com/) also provides high-quality evidence-based information on natural products that are generally recognized as safe (GRAS) by the FDA.

Research on natural products, especially herbal preparations, has only recently begun in the United States. However, a considerable body of research has been developed in other countries such as Germany. The German *Commission E Monographs* (Klein et al., 1999) is akin to the *Physician's Desk Reference* (PDR) in the United States. Specific monographs containing reliable information related to herbal preparations are included on the American Botanical Council website (https://cms.herbalgram.org/commissione/index.html).

REFERENCES

Alagawany, M., Attia, Y. A., Farag, M. R., Elnesr, S. S., Nagadi, S. A., Shafi, M. E., Khafaga, A., Ohran, H., Alaqil, A., & Mohamed, E. (2021). The strategy of boosting the immune system under the COVID-19 pandemic. *Frontiers in Veterinary Science, 7,* 712. https://doi.org/10.3389/fvets.2020.570748

Beijing Digital Museum of Traditional Chinese Medicine. (2012). *Classic literature of traditional Chinese medicine.* http://en.tcm-china.info/culturehistory/literature/75830.shtml

Caspani, M. (2020, March 9). *U.S. coronavirus threat fuels demand for traditional herbal remedies.* https://www.reuters.com/article/us-health-coronavirus-usa-herbs/u-s-coronavirus-threat-fuels-demand-for-traditional-herbal-remedies-idUSKBN20W2GR

Coxeter, P. D., McLachlan, A. J., Duke, C. C., & Roufogalis, B. D. (2004). Herb-drug interactions: An evidence-based approach. *Current Medicinal Chemistry, 11*(11), 1513–1525. https://doi.org/10.2174/0929867043365198

Encyclopedia of World Biography. (2004). *Hildegard of Bingen.* http://www.encyclopedia.com/doc/1G2-3404708047.html

Hussain, S. (2011). Patient counseling about herbal-drug interactions. *African Journal of Traditional, Complementary and Alternative Medicines, 8*(5S), 152. https://doi.org/10.4314/ajtcam.v8i5S.8

Khabour, O. F., & Hassanein, S. F. (2021). Use of vitamin/zinc supplements, medicinal plants, and immune boosting drinks during COVID-19 pandemic: A pilot study from Benha city, Egypt. *Heliyon, 7*(3), e06538. https://doi.org/10.1016/j.heliyon.2021.e06538

Klein, S., Rister, R., & Riggins, C. (1999). *The complete German Commission E monographs: Therapeutic guide to herbal medicines.* American Botanical Council.

National Center for Complementary and Integrative Health. (2016). *NCCIH facts-at-a-glance and mission.* https://nccih.nih.gov/about/ataglance

National Center for Complementary and Integrative Health. (2021a). *Complementary, alternative, or integrative health: What's in a name?* https://www.nccih.nih.gov/health/complementary -alternative-or-integrative-health-whats-in-a-name?

National Center for Complementary and Integrative Health. (2021b). *Natural doesn't necessarily mean safer, or better.* https://www.nccih.nih.gov/health/know-science/natural-doesnt-mean-better

Rashrash, M., Schommer, J. C., & Brown, L. M. (2017). Prevalence and predictors of herbal medicine use among adults in the United States. *Journal of Patient Experience, 4*(3), 108–113. https://doi.org/10.1177/2374373517706612

Ries, J. (2020). *Herbal remedies and COVID-19: What to know.* https://www.healthline.com/health-news/herbal-remedies-covid-19-what-to-know

Silveira, D., Prieto-Garcia, J. M., Boylan, F., Estrada, O., Fonseca-Bazzo, Y. M., Jamal, C. M., Magalhães, P., Pereira, E., Tomczyk, M., & Heinrich, M. (2020). COVID-19: Is there evidence for the use of herbal medicines as adjuvant symptomatic therapy? *Frontiers in Pharmacology, 11*, 1479. https://doi.org/10.3389/fphar.2020.581840

Tachjian, A., Maria, V., & Jahangir, A. (2010). Use of herbal products and potential interactions in patients with cardiovascular diseases. *Journal of the American College of Cardiology, 55*(6), 515–525. https://doi.org/10.1016/j.jacc.2009.07.074

Wagner, D. N., Marcon, A. R., & Caulfield, T. (2020). "Immune boosting" in the time of COVID: Selling immunity on Instagram. *Allergy, Asthma & Clinical Immunology, 16*(1), 1–5. https://doi.org/10.1186/s13223-020-00474-6

Welz, A. N., Emberger-Klein, A., & Menrad, K. (2018). Why people use herbal medicine: Insights from a focus-group study in Germany. *BMC Complementary and Alternative Medicine, 18*(1), 92. https://doi.org/10.1186/s12906-018-2160-6

Wolf, C. P., Rachow, T., Ernst, T., Hochhaus, A., Zomorodbakhsch, B., Foller, S., Rengsberger, M., Hartmann, M., & Hübner, J. (2022). Interactions in cancer treatment considering cancer therapy, concomitant medications, food, herbal medicine and other supplements. *Journal of Cancer Research and Clinical Oncology, 148*(2), 461–473. https://doi.org/10.1007/s00432-021-03625-3

Aromatherapy

LINDA L. HALCÓN & JANET TOMAINO

Aromatherapy is a relatively recent addition to nursing care in the United States, although it is growing in popularity within healthcare settings worldwide. Aromatherapy is offered by nurses in many countries, including Switzerland, Germany, Australia, Canada, Japan, Korea, and the United Kingdom, and it has been a medical specialty in France for many years. This modality is particularly well suited to nursing because it incorporates the therapeutic value of sensory experience (i.e., smell) and often includes the use of touch in the delivery of care. It also builds on a rich heritage of botanical therapies within nursing practice (Libster, 2002, 2012).

Aromatherapy has been part of herbal or botanical medicine for millennia. There is evidence of plant distillation and the use of essential oils and other aromatic plant products dating back 5,000 years. In ancient Egypt and the Middle East, plant oils were used in embalming, incense, perfumery, and healing. Therapeutic applications of essential oils were recorded as part of Greek and Roman medicine, and essential oils have been used in Ayurvedic medicine and in traditional Chinese medicine for more than 1,000 years. With the expansion of trade and improvements in distillation methods, essential oils became common elements of herbal medicine and perfumery in Europe during the Middle Ages (Keville & Green, 2009). In the late 1800s, scientists noted the association between environmental exposure to plant essential oils and the prevention of disease, and microbiologists conducted studies showing the in vitro activity of certain plant oils against microorganisms (Battaglia, 2003). More recent studies confirm the antimicrobial properties of essential oils (Sakkas & Papadopoulou, 2017; Solorzano-Santos & Miranda-Novales, 2012).

The development of clinical aromatherapy within the context of modern Western health science began in France just prior to World War I when chemist René-Maurice Gattefossé was healed of a near-gangrenous wound with lavender essential oil. He subsequently championed its use for infections and battle wounds. Physician Jean Valnet and nurse Marguerite Maury followed Gattefossé in promoting the therapeutic value of essential oils in Europe, and, in the 1930s, interest in the anti-infective value of essential oils began to appear in the European and Australian medical literature (Price & Price, 2011). The use of essential oils continued sporadically as a nonconventional treatment modality in the West until the recent explosion of interest in botanical medicines when its use became more visible and widespread. In their groundbreaking survey research on the use of complementary and alternative therapies in the United States, Eisenberg et al. (1998) reported that 5.6% of 2,055 adults surveyed used aromatherapy. Some large surveys estimating the overall prevalence of complementary therapies have not included aromatherapy as a separate modality (Barnes et al., 2008; Tindle et al., 2005); surveys of special populations, however, suggest its continuing and sometimes increasing use by the public (Akilen et al., 2014; Bowe et al., 2015; Egan et al., 2012; Fisher et al., 2016; Posadzki et al., 2013).

DEFINITION

There are many operant definitions of *aromatherapy*, and some of them contribute to common misconceptions. The word *aromatherapy* can lead people to believe that it simply involves smelling scents, but this is incorrect. It is important to remember that the widespread use of synthetic scents in household and personal products is not considered aromatherapy. Styles (1997) defined aromatherapy as the use of essential oils for therapeutic purposes that encompass the mind, body, and spirit—a broad definition that is consistent with holistic nursing practice. The National Cancer Institute (NCI, 2021) defines aromatherapy as the "therapeutic use of essential oils (also known as volatile oils) from plants (flowers, herbs, or trees) for the improvement of physical, emotional, and spiritual well-being." (paragraph 5) Buckle (2000) defined clinical aromatherapy in nursing as the use of essential oils for expected and measurable health outcomes. We define aromatherapy as "the evidence-informed use of plant essential oils for preventive or therapeutic purposes." Although aromatherapy clinical research has increased markedly in recent years, the evidence for using aromatherapy in nursing practice sometimes may be difficult to establish. There are findings for and against the use of a number of essential oils, however, and it is important to evaluate the available scientific data for individual essential oils and for specific conditions or symptoms.

Essential oils are obtained from a variety of plants worldwide, but not all plants produce essential oils. For those that do, the essential oils may be found in plants' flowers, leaves, stems, bark, roots, seeds, resin, or peels. Most essential oils are obtained by steam distillation of specific plant material. Steam-distilled essential oils are concentrated substances made up of the oil-soluble, lower molecular-weight chemical constituents found in the source plant material. Essential oils from citrus fruit peels are usually obtained by expression (similar to grating or grinding), but they also may be distilled. Carbon dioxide (CO_2) extraction is increasingly accepted by scientists and practitioners as an acceptable method for obtaining certain essential oils; however, other types of solvent extraction generally are not preferred for clinical use. Expressed and CO_2-extracted essential oils contain a broader range of chemicals present in the plant material; thus, they may have different therapeutic properties than distilled essential oils. Essential oils do not necessarily have the same medicinal properties as the plants from which they are derived because they do not contain the whole spectrum of chemicals present in the whole plant.

Nurses have an important role in helping patients differentiate among the range of botanical products that are easily available. Misunderstanding the origin and makeup of these products can result in unnecessary risk. The most commonly used botanical products can be viewed as a continuum (Exhibit 19.1). On one end of the continuum are *whole herbs*, referring to unprocessed material from whole plants or parts of plants (Exhibit 19.1, far-right box). This is the oldest and most

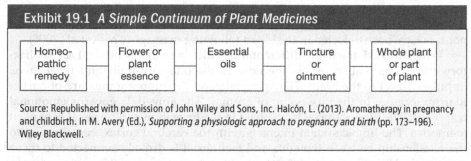

Exhibit 19.1 *A Simple Continuum of Plant Medicines*

Homeo-pathic remedy	Flower or plant essence	Essential oils	Tincture or ointment	Whole plant or part of plant

Source: Republished with permission of John Wiley and Sons, Inc. Halcón, L. (2013). Aromatherapy in pregnancy and childbirth. In M. Avery (Ed.), *Supporting a physiologic approach to pregnancy and birth* (pp. 173–196). Wiley Blackwell.

common form of botanical medicines worldwide. *Tinctures* and *ointments* are different from the whole plant and are also different from essential oils (Exhibit 19.1, second box from right). They are often confused with each other, and it is important that nurses understand the difference so that they can provide advice on their relative safety. Tinctures contain chemicals obtained from the plant material using alcohol as a solvent, and they include both water-soluble and oil-soluble chemicals. Tinctures are often taken orally or sublingually, with the dose and timing depending on the practitioner and the purpose. They are not as concentrated as essential oils. Ointments are made using vegetable oil (e.g., olive oil) rather than alcohol as the solvent. Plant-based tinctures and ointments are widely available. *Flower essences* (Exhibit 19.1, second box from left) also are often confused with essential oils. Essences contain some of the water-soluble chemicals present in the original plant material, and they also are thought to contain the vibrations or frequencies of the plants they are made from. *Homeopathy* (Exhibit 19.1, far-left box) was developed in Europe and was very popular in the United States in the late 1800s and early 1900s (Dooley, 2002). It declined in popularity as biomedicine became the dominant paradigm, although it is still an important healthcare paradigm in some European countries. Homeopathic remedies contain no molecules of the materials from which they are made. They are thought to work subtly on a vibrational level to promote balance and healing. Homeopathic remedies may be prescribed by a homeopathic physician or may be obtained over the counter. Homeopathy is becoming more popular in the United States once again; thus, nurses may benefit from understanding its basic concepts and differentiating it from other approaches.

SCIENTIFIC BASIS

Essential oils processed by any of the methods noted above are highly volatile, complex mixtures of organic chemicals consisting of terpenes and terpenic compounds. The chemistry of an essential oil largely determines its therapeutic properties. There are 60 to 300 separate chemicals in each essential oil, and the proportions of the constituents for a particular plant species vary depending on a host of genetic and environmental factors. Knowing the plant species, the chemotype, the part of the plant used, the country of origin, and the method of extraction can provide information about an essential oil's chemical constituents using readily available aromatherapy textbooks.

The pharmacological activity of essential oils begins on entry into the body through the olfactory, respiratory, gastrointestinal, or integumentary systems. All body systems can be affected once the chemical molecules making up essential oils reach the circulatory and nervous systems. A proportion of the compounds within an essential oil finds its way into the body, however applied (Tisserand &

Young, 2014), although the degree and rate of absorption vary depending on the route of administration. Inhaled aromas have the fastest effect, although compounds have been detected in the blood following massage (Cross et al., 2008).

When inhaled, the many different molecules in each essential oil act as olfactory stimulants that travel via the nose to the olfactory bulb, and from there, impulses travel to the brain. The amygdala and the hippocampus are of particular importance in the processing of aromas. The amygdala governs emotional responses. The hippocampus is involved in the formation and retrieval of explicit memories. The limbic system interacts with the cerebral cortex, contributing to the relationship between thoughts and feelings; it is directly connected to those parts of the brain that control heart rate, blood pressure, breathing, stress levels, and hormone levels (Kiecolt-Glaser et al., 2008). Although inhaling essential oils affects the mind and body through the process of olfaction, most molecules from any inhaled vapor travel to the lungs, where they may be absorbed into the circulatory system (Tisserand, 2016). Tisserand and Young (2014, p. 139) cited several essential oils, including *Lavandula angustifolia* (true lavender), *Lavandula x intermedia* (lavandin), and *Citrus bergamia* (bergamot), that are thought to reduce the effect of external emotional stimuli by increasing gamma-aminobutyric acid (GABA). GABA inhibits neurons in the amygdala, producing a sedative effect. The literature increasingly supports physiological and psychological bases for the neurological actions of essential oils (Bagetta et al., 2010; Bikmoradi et al., 2015; Chien et al., 2012; Igarashi et al., 2014; Lizarraga-Valderrama, 2020).

It is estimated that, at most, approximately 10% (5%–20%) of an essential oil may be absorbed through the skin on topical application (Cross et al., 2008; Tisserand, 2016), and there is controversy about skin penetration among essential oil researchers. Essential oils seem to be absorbed through the skin by working through the phospholipid bilayer via an intracellular route before the components of the essential oils reach the dermis and the bloodstream (Tisserand, 2016). In some instances, topically applied essential oil preparations have been used to enhance the dermal penetration of drugs (Nielsen, 2006; Valgimigli et al., 2012; Williams & Barry, 1989). There is some debate among essential oil experts about the rate and extent of penetration and absorption; however, there is evidence that penetration can vary depending on the condition of the skin, the age of the patient, the body part affected, and the carrier or vehicle for the essential oil. In addition, massage can enhance dermal penetration through heat and friction, and occlusion can enhance penetration. Essential oils are metabolized by the liver and excreted from the body mainly through the kidneys but also through respiration and insensate loss (Tisserand, 2016).

INTERVENTION

The choice of application method depends on patient characteristics and preferences, the symptom or condition being treated, the nurse's knowledge and practice parameters, the targeted outcome, and the properties and chemical components of the essential oil.

INHALATION DELIVERY METHOD

Essential oils are not always pleasant smelling, although inhalation is one of the simplest and most direct application procedures. Direct inhalation in a clinical setting can easily be delivered using cotton balls, patches, or inhaler sticks. Direct steam inhalation is not typically used in a clinical setting, but it can be a very effective method to use at home. Inhalation of essential oils also is facilitated by diffusers operated by heat, battery, or electricity. This method is best used at home or in a private setting and is not recommended in a public or clinical setting. There are several ways to receive the benefits of inhaled essential oils in clinical settings.

Cotton balls are the most simple to use.
Directions for use:

- Apply one to two drops of the selected essential oil or essential oil blend on a cotton ball.
- Place the cotton ball in a small plastic cup such as a med cup or souffle cup with lid or a small plastic bag.
- Advise the patient to hold the container approximately 6 inches from their nose while inhaling for 5 to 10 minutes.
- Close the container between uses.
- To use with patients who are unable to hold a container, tape the cotton ball to the upper part of their clothing within close range to their nose.
- For confused patients who may be at risk of placing the cotton ball in their mouth, tape it to the back of their clothing or place it inside the pillowcase.
- These directions can be repeated as needed every 30 minutes for symptom relief or three to four times per day for overall comfort.
- Replace or refresh the cotton ball every 8 hours.

Prefilled patches are convenient alternatives to taping a cotton ball to clothing.
Directions for use:

- Peel back the cover to expose the prefilled essential oil disk.
- Remove the backing, and then gently stick it to the patient's upper clothing.
- Patches are recommended to be changed every 8 hours.

Inhaler sticks with essential oil–filled inner wicks are used in a similar way as the cotton ball method. A number of essential oil companies sell premade inhaler sticks that are very convenient to use in a clinical setting. Empty tubes with wicks can be purchased to make your own if desired (Exhibit 19.2).
To create your own essential oil inhaler:

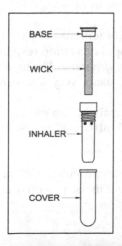

BASE

WICK

INHALER

COVER

Exhibit 19.2 *Inhaler Stick*

- Place the wick inside the inner tube.
- Drop 15 to 20 drops of an essential oil onto the wick.
- Snap the bottom cap in place and screw the outer cover in place.
- Apply a label if using it in a clinical setting or if using several different essential oils or mixtures.
- If choosing more than one essential oil per inhaler stick, keep the total drops at 15 to 20.
- Advise the patient to remove the outer cap and inhale from the inner tube while gently moving it back and forth approximately 6 inches from their nose.
- Replace the cap between uses. Inhaler sticks last for weeks to months depending on the essential oil and how frequently it is left open.

Direct steam inhalation can be effective for relieving sinus congestion and cold symptoms for self-care, but this method generally is not used in clinical settings. For home use:

- Place one to five drops of the selected essential oil or blend in a bowl filled with steamy hot water.
- Place a towel over your head and close your eyes as you inhale over the steamy essential oil water for 5 to 10 minutes.
- Be cautious to not get your face too close to the hot water and to keep your eyes closed throughout the treatment.

TOPICAL DELIVERY METHOD

Topical, or dermal, application combines the inhalation effects with local or systemic absorption effects. Diluted essential oils applied with massage and compresses or in a bath are common delivery methods that can be used for self-care and in some clinical settings.

Massage can facilitate the absorption of essential oils through the skin and can reduce the patient's perceived stress and pain, thus enhancing the healing process and possibly their communication.

- Simple 5-minute hand and/or foot massages with diluted essential oils are an excellent way to induce a rapid relaxation response.
- Mixtures for massage are generally 1% to 3% essential oil concentration (Tisserand & Young, 2014), using very low concentrations when massaging large areas of the body.
- To create an approximate 2% mixture for massage, add two drops of the selected essential oil to 1 teaspoon (5 ml) of cold-pressed vegetable oil, scent-free lotion, cream, or gel (Exhibit 19.3).

Some essential oil companies provide prediluted essential oil blends for massage. These can be more efficient to use in a busy clinical setting.

Exhibit 19.3 *Essential Oil Concentration Table*

Approximated essential oil per 30 ml of diluent	Concentration
6 drops	1%
12 drops	2%
18 drops	3%
24 drops	4%
30 drops	5%

Compresses can be a useful method for applying essential oils to treat skin conditions or minor injuries for self-care; however, they may not be acceptable in many clinical settings.

To prepare a compress:

■ Add four to six drops of essential oil to a bowl of warm or cool water depending on the treatment goal, soak a soft cotton cloth in the mixture, wring it out, and apply the cloth to the affected area, contusion, or abrasion.
■ Cover the compress with plastic wrap to retain moisture; then place a towel over the plastic wrap and keep it in place for as long as desired or comfortable (up to 4 hours; Buckle, 2003).

Essential oil therapeutic baths can be very useful for self-care and in some clinical settings, such as long-term care.

■ Consider using baths for relaxation or when experiencing sore muscles.
■ Five to 10 drops of the essential oil may be dissolved first in a dispersant, such as 1 tablespoon of a carrier oil, and then placed in the bathwater.
■ Because essential oils are not soluble in water, they float on top of the water if used without a dispersant (Tisserand Institute, n.d.-a) This could result in an uneven and too concentrated exposure.
■ An essential-oil bath should last approximately 10 to 15 minutes.
■ For additional benefits of soothing muscles and joints, the essential oil-carrier blend also may be dissolved in one cup of Epsom salts before adding to the bathwater.

GENERAL GUIDELINES FOR USE OF ESSENTIAL OILS

Nurses should be aware of general safety guidelines for patient education and in practice. These include the following:

■ Store essential oils away from open flames; they are volatile and highly flammable.

- Store essential oils in a cool place away from sunlight; use amber- or dark blue-colored glass containers. Close the container immediately after use. Essential oils can oxidize in the presence of heat, light, and air, changing their chemistry and thus their actions in unpredictable ways.
- Be aware that essential oils can stain clothing and textiles and that undiluted essential oils can degrade some plastics. Take appropriate precautions.
- Keep essential oils away from children and pets unless you are well versed in clinical aromatherapy. The literature contains cases of adverse reactions or deaths related to improper applications or accidental ingestion in young children and pets (Halicioglu et al., 2011).
- Use essential oils with care in pregnancy, especially in the first trimester (Conrad, 2019; Conrad & Adams, 2012; Halcón, 2013).
- Use essential oils from reputable suppliers. Seek the advice of a trained aromatherapist or the recommendation of a knowledgeable clinical provider. If using essential oils in clinical or research settings, test results verifying the chemical constituency should be obtained.
- Special care is needed when using essential oils with or around people who have a history of severe asthma or multiple allergies. Be sure to ask.
- Despite the relative safety of essential oils when used properly, sensitization and skin irritation can occur with topical application, especially when using them undiluted. In these cases, any residual essential oil solution should be removed with oil or lotion and rinsed with water, and its use should be discontinued. Most such reactions resolve without treatment; however, a healthcare provider should be consulted if discomfort/itching is severe or persists.
- If an essential oil gets into the eyes, rinse the eyes with copious amounts of sterile saline solution or cold tap water for 15 to 30 minutes (Tisserand Institute, n.d.-b).

MEASUREMENT OF OUTCOMES

The selection of suitable methods for assessing aromatherapy effects depends on the problem for which essential oils are used and the targeted outcomes of treatment. Using simple rating scales of pain, anxiety, or nausea to assess aromatherapy effects on patients' comfort in a clinical setting is efficient and can be easily documented. Using more complex types of measurements may be more suitable for measuring outcomes with aromatherapy research. For example, if lavender is used with a patient in a clinical setting to promote comfort, then pain and anxiety rating scores may be the most appropriate measures to use. If lavender is used to promote sleep, measures might include physiological markers, changes in sleep patterns, or a comparison of signs and symptoms of insomnia between a treated group and another group that is similar in all ways other than the treatment. For psychological conditions such as depression or anxiety, many reliable survey instruments are available and can be further validated by adding physiological measures such as cortisol levels or skin temperature and conductance. For infectious disease outcomes, standard laboratory tests can be used to measure the effect of treatment on microbial load. Other useful measures could include digital photography, quality-of-life scales, tests of cognitive performance, and electroencephalogram results. Using established measurement tools when possible is helpful in facilitating interpretation and comparing the effects of essential oils with those of other approaches.

CREDENTIALING

There is neither a recognized national certification examination for aromatherapists nor a governing body. The Aromatherapy Registration Council, a nonprofit entity established in 2000, administers a national examination and can provide the public with a list of registered aromatherapy practitioners. Nurses and health professionals wishing to use aromatherapy in their practice should check with their licensing bodies; nurses should check with their state board of nursing. In the United States, some nurse practice acts include language that specifically addresses the use of integrative therapies, including aromatherapy (Tomaino, 2020). Many states allow nurses to use aromatherapy in their practice if they have received specialized education.

Many courses are available, and health professionals should choose one relevant to their own clinical practice. There are no requirements in the United States at this time for a person administering aromatherapy to be certified or accredited; however, Canadian nurses have established criteria for practice. The length of training programs in aromatherapy may range from one weekend to several years. Generally, it is not necessary to be a health professional to enroll in these educational programs. Some of these educational programs are taught by nurses and include a clinical focus which would benefit nurses who want to use aromatherapy within their practice or clinical area. The National Association of Holistic Aromatherapy (www.naha.org) and the Alliance for International Aromatherapists (www.alliance-aromatherapists.org), two large aromatherapy professional organizations in the United States, list aromatherapy programs that meet specific education criteria.

Despite the lack of uniform credentialing, it is no longer unusual for hospitals and other clinical settings to include aromatherapy services, and nurses often have spearheaded these changes. To safely provide essential oils for patients, nurses must possess basic clinical aromatherapy education and insist that policies and procedures include good quality assurance and quality control. Sample aromatherapy policies and guidelines for developing a clinical program are available in an online course offered by the University of Minnesota on Coursera (Tomaino, 2019). The Alliance of International Aromatherapists (n.d.) has made policy and pediatric clinical guidelines developed by nurse aromatherapists available for its members.

PRECAUTIONS

Aromatherapy is a very safe complementary therapy if it is used with knowledge and within accepted guidelines. Many essential oils have been tested by the food and beverage industry for use as flavorings and preservatives, and much research has been carried out by the perfume and tobacco industries. Although most of the essential oils commonly used in clinical aromatherapy have been given generally-regarded-as-safe (GRAS) status, this only means that they are considered safe in minute amounts in foods and cosmetics. It does not give carte-blanche approval for all uses. Nurses should not administer essential oils orally, as this is outside a nurse's scope of practice and poisonings have been documented (Jacobs & Hornfeldt, 1994; Janes et al., 2005). Advanced practice nurses with prescriptive authority *and* specific training in the oral administration of essential oils are an exception, however. According to Tisserand and Young (2014), most poisonings involve ingestion accidents with young children; however, adults also have been known to ingest toxic amounts and types of essential oils. Most essential oils should not be used during the first trimester of pregnancy and should be used cautiously anytime during pregnancy (Conrad, 2019). Nurses need to be aware of essential oils that can cause photosensitivity, such as bergamot (*C. bergamia*) and other citrus oils (Keljova et al., 2010), and they should provide appropriate patient education and protection when these are used. Numerous cases of contact dermatitis following skin applications of essential oils have been reported (Brown & Browning, 2016; Fettig et al., 2014; Rudback et al., 2015), underscoring the importance of diluting essential oils for topical use and knowing which essential oils are most likely to be irritating or sensitizing.

Essential oils are very concentrated and potent compounds, and in most cases, they must be diluted in carrier oils for topical use. Tea tree (*Melaleuca alternifolia*) and lavender (*L. angustifolia*) are among the few exceptions to this rule. These essential oils can be used at full strength for immediate treatment of minor cuts, abrasions, and small burns; however, they should be diluted for follow-up treatment.

Some essential oils are known to be carcinogenic and others are contraindicated in people with specific conditions. Knowledge and common sense should guide nurses' thinking in this regard. For example, stimulant essential oils should not be used for patients with conditions for which stimulants are contraindicated. Essential oils can potentiate or decrease the effects of medications, often by increasing or decreasing metabolic enzymes (Tisserand, 2016). Extra care is needed when using essential oils with patients receiving chemotherapy because they may affect the absorption rate of cancer-treating and other drugs (Fox et al., 2011; Jain et al., 2008; Lim et al., 2009; Paduch et al., 2007; Williams & Barry, 1989). In short, it cannot be assumed that all essential oils are safe in all situations simply because they are *natural*.

Product identity confusion is another potential threat to safety. As noted, essential oils should not be confused with herbal extracts. They are completely different chemical mixtures, and they cannot be used interchangeably. Besides their chemical dissimilarities, herbal extracts and teas are usually taken internally, whereas essential oils generally are not. Nurses share responsibility for ensuring product integrity when essential oils are used in clinical practice. Chemical testing of essential oils used in patient care should be incorporated into ongoing aromatherapy quality assurance/quality control programs.

Nurses using essential oils regularly should protect themselves from unintended effects. Because essential oils are volatile, aerosolized molecules are inhaled by those applying them as well as by patients. It has been demonstrated that hand dermatitis may be associated with long-term unprotected use of lotions and other products containing essential oils (Crawford et al., 2004; Uter et al., 2010).

Perhaps one of the greatest risks in aromatherapy is using an incorrect essential oil for a particular health outcome. This could stem from a nurse's lack of knowledge of plant taxonomy. Many essential oils have familiar common names such as lavender, rose, and rosemary, but it is important to know the full botanical name. For example, "lavender" is a common name that refers to *three different kinds* of lavender *and* several hybrids. The genus of lavender is *Lavandula*, and all lavenders begin with this word. *L. angustifolia* is one of the most widely used and researched essential oils and is recognized as a relaxant and soporific. The other two species used in aromatherapy have very different properties. *Lavandula latifolia* (spike lavender) is a stimulant and expectorant; *Lavandula stoechas* is antimicrobial and not safe to use for long periods. The picture is further complicated by the hybrid *L. x intermedia* with its three chemotypes. Nurses who use aromatherapy clinically must know the full botanical name of each essential oil they intend to use. The botanical names of essential oils commonly used in clinical settings are found in Exhibit 19.4.

Exhibit 19.4 *Example of Essential Oils Used in a Clinical Setting*

ESSENTIAL OIL	BOTANICAL NAME	COMMON INDICATIONS FOR USE	CONSIDERATIONS
Bergamot	*Citrus bergamia*	Anxiety/stress, insomnia, overall comfort, pain,	Use caution for topical use- keep exposed areas from ultraviolet light for 18 hours after application; excellent choice for stressful situations
Black Pepper	*Piper nigrum*	Pain, smoking cessation	Consider blending with other essential oil(s) to use for smoking cessation via inhalation
Chamomile (Roman)	*Chamaemelum nobilis*	Anxiety/stress, calming, pain, sleep	Good choice for children; antispasmodic and antiinflammatory properties; consider blending with other essential oils
Frankincense	*Boswellia carterii* *Boswellia sacra*	Anxiety/stress, grief support, pain	Good choice for labor pain and end-of-life care; consider blending with other essential oil(s)
Ginger	*Zingiber officinales*	Fatigue, GI discomfort, nausea	Consider blending with other essential oils when using for chemo-induced nausea (due to potential negative smell memory)
Lavender	*Lavandula angustifolia*	Anxiety/stress, insomnia, pain	Good choice for overall comfort; good choice for children
Sweet Marjoram	*Origanum majorana*	Anxiety/stress, calming, insomnia, pain	Antispasmodic and sedating properties; consider blending with other essential oils
Sweet Orange	*Citrus sinensis*	Anxiety/stress, calming, GI discomfort, low mood,	Good choice for children
Peppermint	*Mentha x piperita*	Fatigue, GI discomfort, low mood, nausea, odor control, postsurgery & postdelivery urinary retention	Not for use with children less than 6 years of age; consider blending with other essential oils when using for chemo-induced nausea (due to potential negative smell memory)

(continued)

Exhibit 19.4 *Example of Essential Oils Used in a Clinical Setting (continued)*			
ESSENTIAL OIL	**BOTANICAL NAME**	**COMMON INDICATIONS FOR USE**	**CONSIDERATIONS**
Spearmint	*Mentha spicata*	GI discomfort/nausea, fatigue, low mood	Good choice for children; consider blending with other essential oils when using for chemo-induced nausea (due to potential negative smell memory)
Tea Tree	*Melaleuca alternifolia*	Bacterial and fungal infections; odor control	Topical use as antimicrobial; requires provider order

USES

Many health outcomes that fall within the domain of nursing practice can be addressed with essential oils, either alone or combined with other approaches. Essential oils can affect people psychologically and physically. They can increase or decrease sympathetic activity in individuals, affecting heart rate, blood pressure, plasma adrenaline, and plasma catecholamine levels (Chuang et al., 2014; Menezes et al., 2010; Watanabe et al., 2015). The effect of essential oil odors can be relaxing or stimulating, depending on a person's previous experiences, likes and dislikes, and the chemistry of the essential oil used; therefore, it is important to explore patient preference and the purpose for which the oil is being used when selecting essential oils for therapeutic purposes. Examples of essential oils used in clinical settings are shown in Exhibit 19.4.

Essential oils are used therapeutically to address a broad range of symptoms and body systems, and there are many aromatherapy texts describing their uses and recommending particular essential oils for specific conditions or symptoms. It is difficult to identify evidence other than case studies or historical anecdotes for some of these uses; however, with increased clinical use in recent years there is a more robust evidence base for a number of essential oils and clinical outcomes. The main applications of essential oils in conventional healthcare settings are to help address pain, symptoms of anxiety or depression, nausea, sleeplessness, or agitation and to prevent or treat infections. Nurse midwives have long incorporated essential oils into their practices, notably to reduce pain and aid relaxation during and after childbirth (Burns et al., 2000; Conrad & Adams, 2012; Einion, 2016; Ghiasi et al., 2019; Imura et al., 2006; Musil, 2013; Sheikhan et al., 2012). In long-term care and hospital settings, essential oils are used to help reduce anxiety and agitation in patients with or without dementia (Bowles et al., 2002; Goes et al., 2012; Kritsidima et al., 2009; Lin et al., 2007; Morris, 2008; O'Connor et al., 2013; Woelk & Schlafke, 2010; Yoshiyama et al., 2015), promote sleep and reduce night-time sedation (Dyer et al., 2016; Ko et al., 2021; Lillehei et al., 2015), and promote wound healing (Culliton & Halcón, 2011; Lusby et al., 2006). Aromatherapy can be a helpful intervention for palliative and end-of-life nursing care (Pounds, 2012; Tomaino, 2015).

Aromatherapy is used to address acute or chronic pain (Bagheri et al., 2020; de Sousa, 2011; Gedney et al., 2004; Ghelardini et al., 1999; Irmak et al., 2015; Kim et al., 2007; Noruzi et al., 2021), fatigue and nausea (Adib-Hajbaghery et al., 2015; Bagheri-Nesami et al., 2016; Lua et al., 2015; Lua & Zakaria, 2012; Pearson, 2015), infection (Bassol & Juliani, 2012; de Sousa et al., 2017; Gelmini et al., 2016; Paule, 2001; Thompson et al., 2011), and mood and cognition (Goes et al., 2015; Morris, 2008; Moss et al., 2010; Nagata et al., 2014). The literature also includes studies reporting the use of essential oils in the treatment of head lice and scabies (Barker & Altman, 2010; Choi et al., 2010; Greive & Barnes, 2018; Gutierrez et al., 2016; Thomas et al., 2016), postdelivery and postsurgical urinary retention (Fryatt & Bell, 2020; Mukurji et al., 2006; Phillips, 1998; Uvin et al., 2015), as an aid to smoking cessation (Cordell & Buckle, 2013; Rose & Behm, 1994), and drug withdrawal (Kunz et al., 2007; Lemme, 2009).

There is considerable and growing international literature on the use of plant essential oils against pathogenic microorganisms. The efficacy of essential oils in the treatment and prevention of infectious diseases has important implications for patient health as well as disinfection and hygiene (Edwards-Jones et al., 2004; Enshaieh et al., 2007; Muthaiyan et al., 2012), especially with the increase in resistance bacteria (Hammer et al., 2008). Methicillin-resistant *Staphylococcus aureus* and other microorganisms have been found to be sensitive to tea tree oil (*M. alternifolia*; Carson et al., 2005; Halcón & Milkus, 2004; Hammer et al., 2012). Preliminary work suggests that essential oils may also be effective in other difficult-to-treat infections and wounds (Culliton & Halcón, 2011; Sherry et al., 2003).

PEDIATRIC APPLICATIONS

Aromatherapy has been one of the integrative therapies most used for and by children, as evidenced by prevalence studies (Adams et al., 2013; Grossoehme et al., 2013; Simpson & Roman, 2001), the multitude of aromatherapy products advertised and sold for babies and children, and anecdotally by the increase in pediatric toxicity cases in emergency rooms and poison control centers. Knowledge and common sense are needed to guide nurses and parents in the safe application of essential oils in pediatrics. As an example, peppermint contains menthol and 1,8-cineole, and it has the potential of triggering a reflex known as pediatric hyper-reactivity (PHR) that could lead to an adverse respiratory response such as laryngoconstriction and reflex apnea in children younger than 2 years of age (Horváth & Ács, 2015). To be on the safe side, many clinical settings do not use peppermint for pediatric patients younger than 6 years of age. Hospital pediatric units generally limit aromatherapy to the safest essential oils and common symptoms such as pain (e.g., true lavender, Roman chamomile), nausea (e.g., ginger, spearmint, mandarin), and perceived anxiety (e.g., true lavender, sweet orange). Research suggests that essential oils may be quite helpful in addressing these symptoms (Kiberd et al., 2016; Malachowska et al., 2016; O'Flaherty et al., 2012). With vulnerable populations such as infants and small children, we recommend applying the precautionary principle (if a substance has not been proved safe, do not use it unless there is a compelling reason) and the integrative nursing principle that advises "moving from least intensive/invasive [therapies] to more, depending on need and context (Kreitzer & Koithan, 2014, p.12). For example, if a child has postoperative nausea and vomiting, imagery or acupressure (neither of which involve chemical substance exposure) could be tried first and then followed by offering an inhalation of spearmint if other approaches were not helpful. Extending this mode of thinking, if the aromatherapy is not helpful, the nurse could consider a pharmaceutical antiemetic.

Toxicity in children, as with others, is related to dose, meaning unsafe concentrations, inappropriate application methods, or unsafe essential oils. Essential oils are highly concentrated mixtures of many volatile chemicals, even though they are derived from plants. Chronic and acute reactions are usually caused by topical applications or ingestion. To avoid accidental ingestion of essential oils by small children, it is recommended that the oils be treated as medications and kept out of reach. They can be stored inside childproof medication containers at home. In addition, essential oils should be sold and stored in bottles with integral drop dispensers and clearly labeled with all ingredients (Fitzgerald & Halcón, 2010). Allergic contact dermatitis is not uncommon (Brown & Browning, 2016; Storan et al., 2016), and essential oil concentrations in skin or massage products should be lower for children than for adults. Tisserand and Young (2014) recommend concentrations of less than 0.2% for full-term infants up to 3 months, less than 0.5% up to 24 months, less than 2% up to 6 years, and no greater than 3% from 6 to 15 years. These guidelines assume that there is a good health rationale. Nurses who are knowledgeable about essential oils can introduce them in pediatric practice and remain within safety guidelines.

CULTURAL APPLICATIONS

There are regional, cultural, and religious traditions and preferences for the types of essential oils used therapeutically. For example, Ayurvedic practices include many essential oils that are produced in the Indian subcontinent, including those from sandalwood, jasmine, and other floral or spicy aromatic plants. Africa is the source of oils such as frankincense, myrrh, ylang-ylang, ravensara, and others. In Europe and much of the United States, essential oil production focuses on herbs or flowers that grow and thrive in temperate climates, such as peppermint, lavender, and basil. Citrus oils are produced in warmer regions. However, the lines are not as distinct as in earlier times when the procurement of essential oils was more limited to native and local plants. Plants are routinely transported and grown in nonnative areas, and the essential oils most commonly used for therapeutic purposes are now readily available throughout the world, obtainable through global trade and internet sales. For a description of the development of a clinical aromatherapy practice in a tertiary care center in the United Kingdom, see Sidebar 19.1.

Cultural plant-healing traditions often have been altered and adapted by newcomers. The case of Australian tea tree oil provides an example of the adaptation of cultural and regional health practices over time. *M. alternifolia* grows in one area of Australia as a native plant, and it was used as an herbal anti-infective medicine by Aboriginal peoples for centuries. More than 200 species of the genus *Melaleuca* are native to Australia and New Zealand, and only a few have been explored for modern medicinal uses as essential oils (Weiss, 1997). *M. alternifolia* is one of many plants referred to as "tea tree" in Australia and New Zealand, hence the importance of relying on Latin names for identification. The healing properties of this plant were noted by European explorers and settlers, and at some point, the foliage was distilled to produce a very concentrated antiseptic substance—tea tree oil. Since the early 1900s, there has been intermittent interest in tea tree oil on the

Sidebar 19.1 *Aromatherapy in a U.K. Tertiary Cancer Centre*

Jacqui Stringer

The Christie is a tertiary cancer center in the North West of England that specializes in the acute care of vulnerable cancer patients. The Christie has used aroma in the true sense of the word as an additional support to help relaxation since the 1990s. My nursing practice at the Christie began in the hematology unit where I took care of patients who were completely healthy until they attended their general practitioner with "fatigue" or a long-standing minor infection, only to be admitted with a life-threatening condition (leukemia). This was a terrifying experience for them as they were put in isolation, given potentially life-threatening treatments, and were allowed minimal, if ,any contact with their loved ones for support due to their vulnerability to infection. This experience shifted my focus from giving the treatment to giving support because it was quite clear that as nurses, we didn't have a lot of time to do this. I found that massage touch was a very powerful tool for reducing stress and calming anxiety; however, the potency of the relaxation appeared to be extended and deepened if anchored by using essential oils in the massage oil. This is now well validated and documented in the literature (e.g., work from Tiffany Field and her team), and I was able to add supporting data while working on my PhD. We know that the olfactory system is directly linked to our emotions and to the limbic system. We are joining the dots a lot better now, to understand the significant impact of aroma on our psychological well-being.

I have not only nursing training, but also a degree in psychology; that plus my role as a research nurse at the time meant that research was embedded in my brain, with safety and ethical use of essential oils being a fundamental consideration for me when I started the service. I buried myself in the research, ensured the relevant paperwork was in place, and then got consent from both my clinical director and the trust governance committee before we commenced the service. My practice of aromatherapy on the Christie's hematology unit grew as nurses contacted me to help them with particular situations, such as a skin reaction due to treatment, when steroids didn't work. They then began asking me to help them with topical infections in patients who had compromised immune systems. For several years, I worked in conjunction with a consultant microbiologist to select essential oils with relevant antimicrobial action to ensure they had activity against the microorganisms causing the infection and that worked in synergy with conventional antibacterial agents. As an example, there were times with challenging wounds when I would send the microbiologist a swab taken from the wound and he would culture the organisms in the presence of various oils. He would then advise me about which oils would be effective. I then added that information to my clinical knowledge in order to decide which oils were the safest most efficacious ones to use in that situation.

It is important to note that I started out in a slow, steady, and safe manner and gradually built my unique practice from there. I never used oils "first line" for example, only when it was clear that conventional products were not effective. I never work in isolation but always as part of the multidisciplinary team so that I

(continued)

Sidebar 19.1 *Aromatherapy in a U.K. Tertiary Cancer Centre (continued)*

have the understanding, opinions, and consent of other clinicians to use oils in any given situation. I think this is so critical; physicians have ultimate responsibility for the patients in their care and as such they need to have confidence in what I am doing, to know that I will always work in a safe and professional manner.

Currently there are no guidelines, policies, or insurance for nurses who are not also qualified aromatherapists to use aromatherapy at the Christie, other than when the product has been blended by an aromatherapist following a thorough assessment and with clear instructions for use. Personally, I would not be comfortable with any nurse using essential oils unless they have the relevant training, with such a vulnerable patient cohort. The Christie employs aromatherapists who have the level of aromatherapy training that meets the qualifications for carrying the required insurance for their practice. Most of the aromatherapists don't practice clinical aromatherapy; they primarily use aromasticks with the patients to facilitate enhanced well-being, especially during the pandemic when the use of touch has had to be severely curtailed. However, we may administer aromatherapy foot massages for those patients in very distressed states who find it difficult to engage with the therapist on a cognitive level due to, for example, extreme distress or pain. In these challenging times, we still try to give service users (patients and staff) as much of a sensory experience as possible while maintaining social distance. When we can't meet the patients face to face, we teach them techniques over the phone or send aromasticks to them based on the description of what they need and like. Then we go through a visualization over the phone with them while they're smelling their own aromasticks so they can start anchoring memories into that positivity.

I am humbled by the trust put in me to develop the aromatherapy practice we have at the Christie, and I would always encourage other healthcare organizations desiring to use aromatherapy to work with your colleagues to build up trust and "start small, safe, and simple."

part of the medical community. This interest has expanded in recent years, partly through partnerships between the Australian government and the private agricultural sector to expand tea tree oil's economic impact. Both public and private funding was provided for excellent scientific research on the antimicrobial properties of tea tree oil, subsequently added to by healthcare researchers and scientists around the world. Extensive information can be found on the website of the University of Western Australia (www.marshallcentre.uwa.edu.au and https://research-repository.uwa.edu.au/en/publications/). Tea tree is now an important plantation crop, and the antimicrobial properties of tea tree oil (*M. alternifolia*) are somewhat known in Western biomedical healthcare settings but more widely so by the public. Affordable, pure essential oil or health products with tea tree oil as a major ingredient are available worldwide, benefiting the Australian agricultural sector as well as healthcare. For a description of aromatherapy and issues relevant to its use in nursing practice in Australia, see Sidebar 19.2.

Sidebar 19.2 *Aromatherapy in Nursing Practice in Australia*

Trisha Dunning

Anecdotally, aromatherapy is one of the most popular complementary therapies Australian nurses use, often combined with massage. National population data about the use of complementary and alternative medicine (CAM) suggest approximately 70% of nurses use CAM, including aromatherapy; however, there are no national data about the number of nurses who are qualified aromatherapists, work as aromatherapists in private practice, or incorporate aromatherapy in their nursing practice. One reason for the lack of such data is that aromatherapy is a self-regulated practice, unlike nursing. Currently, traditional Chinese medicine (TCM) is the only CAM regulated by the Australian Health Practitioner Regulation Agency.

Most Australians who use aromatherapy do so on a self-selected basis, and many may not understand the risks and benefits of essential oils or how to use them appropriately. In addition, aromatherapy products are often purchased from pharmacies, health food shops, local community markets, and supermarkets, where expert advice is not available and there is no guarantee of quality. Significantly, the public often confuses fragrances and essential oils, largely due to the marketing of fragrance products in beauty and home care.

Many CAM professional groups—including the International Aromatherapy and Aromatic Medicine Association, the organization most aromatherapists in Australia (including nurses) belong to—have specific requirements for membership. Membership rules include completing accredited courses, ensuring knowledge is current, and holding professional indemnity. Aromatherapy training is delivered at certificate and diploma levels by various private education providers and can often be completed online. Many of these courses lead to qualifications in beauty therapy rather than clinical aromatherapy. Some university CAM courses include information about aromatherapy. The quality of these courses varies in course content, teaching quality, amount and quality of supervised clinical practice, and assessment criteria.

Aromatherapy is used in a variety of clinical settings in Australia; however, it may not always be truly integrated into care plans and the outcomes are not always monitored systematically. Key areas of practice in which aromatherapy is used include palliative and cardiovascular care to manage stress and pain, promote relaxation, and improve emotional well-being. Essential oils are mostly used externally in vaporizers and massage, applied to furnishings and clothing, or used in baths.

Until recently, aromatherapy was commonly used in older adult care facilities to address odor, reduce stress, promote sleep, and reduce the need for sedatives. One program, Creative Ways to Care, was developed to assist caregivers in home care for relatives with dementia. The program had been widely implemented in older care settings. However, CAM use (including aromatherapy) in such facilities has declined since the Aged Care Funding Instrument (ACFI) was introduced and residents now have to pay for CAM therapies. The introduction of the ACFI has also affected the enrollment in CAM courses.

(continued)

Sidebar 19.2 *Aromatherapy in Nursing Practice in Australia (continued)*

A number of factors affect aromatherapy safety and quality:
- the individual (reason for using essential oils knowledge, health status, concomitant use of other CAM, conventional medicines)
- the practitioner (knowledge, competence)
- essential oils and carrier substances (labels, quality, purity, storage conditions, manufacturing processes)
- application method (internal or external use)
- environment (where aromatherapy is delivered)
- an evidence base for use (articulated in policies and procedures or guidelines)
- the regulation of products and practitioners (Essential oils are regulated as medicines under the Therapeutic Goods Act [1989] and must meet a range of other regulations such as labeling and packaging.)

A growing interest in the discovery of new plant medicines with health applications or profit possibilities has fueled expanded research on essential oils. In addition to laboratory and human studies aimed at improving health, research also is aimed at improved food preservation and the resultant prevention of foodborne illness and the eradication or control of insect-borne and parasitic diseases such as malaria (Samarasekera et al., 2008; Singh et al., 2008, 2021). As new essential oils are produced and tested for health and environmental applications (Baik et al., 2008; Dongmo et al., 2008), their production can provide international trade opportunities and improved agricultural diversity, in addition to providing affordable natural medicines. The sustainability of plant sources of essential oils is a growing concern, however, especially with essential oils derived from slow-maturing trees such as sandalwood, frankincense, myrrh, and rosewood. Their future is threatened by agricultural and economic factors as well as climate change.

Nurses have a role in this discussion. We have a responsibility to learn more about the sustainability of the plants from which our recommended clinical essential oils are derived. It is sometimes difficult to obtain good information about the essential oils used, and nurses often are not aware of the sources of essential oils used in their facilities. We encourage nurses, as providers and consumers of aromatherapy, to ask questions that may lead to deeper discussions:

- Ask your suppliers or the purchasers of essential oils in your institution about fair-trade practices. Asking the question will prompt buyers to seek fair-trade products when possible. Many people would be willing to pay a little more for products that benefit rather than deplete source communities and the environment.
- Although threatened plants that produce essential oils are some of the most exquisite and have great health benefits, they can be used judiciously. Sometimes other essential oils or other varieties with no concerns about sustainability can be used instead, or smaller amounts can be used.

As nurses learn more about essential oils and their chemistries and properties, they will be able to assess each individual situation and contribute deeply to these conversations.

FUTURE RESEARCH

The future of clinical aromatherapy is promising. Although aromatherapy researchers continue to face challenges related to the products themselves, such as smell blinding, synergistic and antagonistic effects when different oils are combined, possible confounding with aromatherapy massage, and natural variation in products, many more studies are being conducted and published, both in integrative therapies journals and in specialty journals. Nurses and other health professionals need to be aware of these challenges and critical of aromatherapy research reports, as they are about all research, since publication bias can occur in any direction. More work is needed to test the efficacy of essential oils already in common use and to extend the practice of aromatherapy in clinical settings where, for some conditions and individuals, it can be a cost-effective alternative or adjunct therapy with fewer side effects than pharmaceuticals and other biomedical treatments.

If current trends continue, aromatherapy (inhalation and topical) will be a standard care measure for addressing nursing diagnoses in acute, long-term, and community-based care. In some cities, most hospitals and nursing homes already have an aromatherapy program included in nursing protocols. Integrative nursing is a paradigm to guide and ground the growth of programs in healthcare settings and allow nurses to remain informed by evidence and view aromatherapy interventions in a larger context. Expanded applications, such as wound care and dermatological or oral preparations to address medical diagnoses, are very promising and will require multidisciplinary collaboration. Nursing perspectives will be important to ensure that essential oils are used to support health holistically.

WEBSITES

The following are websites that nurses may find helpful in identifying more information about essential oils:

- Alliance of International Aromatherapists: (www.alliance-aromatherapists .org)
- Aromatherapy Registration Council: (www.aromatherapycouncil.org)
- National Association of Holistic Aromatherapists: (www.naha.org)

SUSTAINABILITY RESOURCES

The following are websites that nurses may find helpful in identifying more information about the sustainability of essential oil plants:

- Airmid Institute
  https://airmidinstitute.org/
- Convention on International Trade in Endangered Species of Wild Fauna and Flora (CITIES)
  https://cites.org/eng/disc/what.php

https://cites.org/sites/default/files/eng/cop/18/inf/E-CoP18-Inf-053.pdf
▦ United Plant Savers
https://unitedplantsavers.org/learning-to-define-sustainability-lessons-for
-essential-oil-consumers/

REFERENCES

Adams, D., Dagenais, S., Clifford, T., Baydala, L., King, W., Hervas-Malo, M., Moher, D., & Vohra, S. (2013). Complementary and alternative medicine use by pediatric specialty outpatients. *Pediatrics, 131*(2), 225–232. https://doi.org/10.1542/peds.2012-1220

Adib-Hajbaghery, M., & Hosseini, F. (2015). Investigating the effects of inhaling ginger essence on post-nephrectomy nausea and vomiting. *Complementary Therapies in Medicine, 23*(6), 827–831. https://doi.org/10.1016/j.ctim.2015.10.002

Akilen, R., Pimlott, Z., Tsiami, A., & Robinson, N. (2014). The use of complementary and alternative medicine by individuals with features of metabolic syndrome. *Journal of Integrative Medicine, 12*(3), 171–174. https://doi.org/10.1016/S2095-4964(14)60012-1

Alliance of International Aromatherapists. (n.d.). Membership. https://www.alliance-aroma therapists.org/

Bagetta, G., Morrone, L., Rombola, L., Amantea, D., Russo, R., Berliocchi, L., Sakurada, S., Sakurada, T., Rotiroti, D., & Corasaniti, M. (2010). Neuropharmacology of the essential oil bergamot. *Fitoterapia, 81*(6), 453–461. https://doi.org/10.1016/j.fitote.2010.01.013

Bagheri, H., Salmani, T., Nourian, J., Mirrezaie, S. M., Abbasi, A, Mardani, A., & Vlaisavljevic, Z. (2020). The effects of inhalation aromatherapy using lavender essential oil on postoperative pain of inguinal hernia: A randomized controlled trial. *Journal of PeriAnesthesia Nursing, 35*(6), 642–648. https://doi.org/10.1016/j.jopan.2020.03.003

Bagheri-Nesami, M., Shorofi, S., Nikkhah, A., Espahbodi, F., & Ghaderi Koolaee, F. (2016). The effects of aromatherapy with lavender essential oil on fatigue levels in haemodialysis patients: A randomized clinical trial. *Complementary Therapies in Clinical Practice, 22*, 33–37. https://doi.org/10.1016/j.ctcp.2015.12.002

Baik, J., Kim, S., Lee, J., Oh, T., Kim J., Lee, N., & Hyun, C. (2008). Chemical composition and biological activities of essential oils extracted from Korean endemic citrus species. *Journal of Microbiology and Biotechnology, 18*(1), 74–79. https://www.jmb.or.kr/submission/Journal/018/JMB018-01-12.pdf

Barker, S. C., & Altman, P. M. (2010). A randomised, assessor blind, parallel group comparative efficacy trial of three products for the treatment of head lice in children—Melaleuca oil and lavender oil, pyrethrins and piperonyl butoxide, and a "suffocation" product. *BMC Dermatology, 10*(1), 6. https://doi.org/10.1186/1471-5945-10-6

Barnes, P. M., Bloom, B., & Nahin, R. (2008). Complementary and alternative medicine use among adults and children: United States 2007. *National Health Statistics Report,* (12), 1–23. https://www.cdc.gov/nchs/data/nhsr/nhsr012.pdf

Bassol, I. H. N., & Juliani, H. R. (2012). Essential oils in combination and their antimicrobial properties. *Molecules, 17*(4), 3989–4006. https://doi.org/10.3390/molecules17043989

Battaglia, S. (2003). *The complete guide to aromatherapy* (2nd ed.). International Centre of Holistic Aromatherapy.

Bikmoradi, A., Seifi, Z., Poorolajal, J., Araghchian, M., Safiaryan, R., & Oshvandi, K. (2015). Effect of inhalation aromatherapy with lavender essential oil on stress and vital signs in patients undergoing coronary artery bypass surgery: A single-blinded randomized clinical trial. *Complementary Therapies in Medicine, 23*(3), 331–338. https://doi.org/10.1016/j.ctim.2014.12.001

Bowe, S., Adams, J., Lui, C. W., & Sibbritt, D. (2015). A longitudinal analysis of self-prescribed complementary and alternative medicine use by a nationally representative sample of 19,783 Australian women, 2006–2010. *Complementary Therapies in Medicine, 23*(5), 699–704. https://doi.org/10.1016/j.ctim.2015.06.011

Bowles, E. J., Griffiths, M., Quirk, L., & Croot, K. (2002). Effects of essential oils and touch on resistance to nursing care procedures and other dementia-related behaviours in a residential care facility. *International Journal of Aromatherapy, 12*(1), 22–29. https://doi.org/10.1054/ijar.2001.0128

Brown, M., & Browning, J. (2016). A case of psoriasis replaced by allergic contact dermatitis in a 12-year-old boy. *Pediatric Dermatology, 33*(2), e125–e126. https://doi.org/10.1111/pde.12737

Buckle, J. (2000). The 'M' technique: physical hypnotherapy for the critically ill. *Massage & Bodywork, 15*(1), 52–5, 58–9, 64. http://www.positivehealth.com/article/touch/the-m-technique-touch-for-the-critically-ill-or-actively-dying

Buckle, J. (2003). *Clinical aromatherapy: Essential oils in practice* (2nd ed.). Churchill Livingstone.

Burns, E. E., Blamey, C., Ersser, S. J., Barnetson, L., & Lloyd, A. J. (2000). An investigation into the use of aromatherapy in intrapartum midwifery practice. *Journal of Alternative and Complementary Therapies, 6*(2), 141–147. https://doi.org/10.1089/acm.2000.6.141

Carson, C., Hammer, K., Messager, S., & Riley, T. (2005). Tea tree oil: A potential alternative for the management of methicillin-resistant *Staphylococcus aureus* (MRSA). *Australian Infection Control, 10*(1), 32–34. https://doi.org/10.1016/S0195-6701(98)90267-5

Chien, L-W., Cheng, S., & Liu, C. (2012). The effect of lavender aromatherapy on autonomic nervous system in midlife women with insomnia. *Evidence-Based Complementary & Alternative Medicine, 2012*, 1–8. https://doi.org/10.1155/2012/740813

Choi, H.-Y., Yang, Y.-C., Lee, S. H., Clark, J. M., & Ahn, Y.-J. (2010). Efficacy of spray formulations containing binary mixtures of clove and eucalyptus oils against susceptible and pyrethroid/malathion-resistant head lice (Anoplura: Pediculidae). *Journal of Medical Entomology, 47*(3), 387–391. https://doi.org/10.1603/ME09119

Chuang, K. J., Chen, H. W., Liu, I. J., Chuang, H. C., & Lin, L. Y. (2014). The effect of essential oil on heart rate and blood pressure among solus por aqua workers. *European Journal of Preventive Cardiology, 21*(7), 823–828. https://doi.org/10.1177/2047487312469474

Conrad, P. (2019). *Women's health aromatherapy*. Singing Dragon.

Conrad, P., & Adams, C. (2012). The effects of clinical aromatherapy for anxiety and depression in the high risk postpartum woman—A pilot study. *Complementary Therapies in Clinical Practice, 18*(3), 164–168. https://doi.org/10.1016/j.ctcp.2012.05.002

Cordell, B., & Buckle, J. (2013). The effects of aromatherapy on nicotine craving on a U. S. campus: A small comparison study. *The Journal of Alternative and Complementary Medicine, 19*(8), 709–713. https://doi.org/10.1089/acm.2012.0537

Crawford, G., Katz, K., Ellis, E., & James, W. (2004). Use of aromatherapy products and increased risk of hand dermatitis in massage therapists. *Archives of Dermatology, 140*(8), 991–996. https://doi.org/10.1001/archderm.140.8.991

Cross, S., Russell, M., Southwell, I., & Roberts, M. (2008). Human skin penetration of the major components of Australian tea tree oil applied in its pure form and as a 20% solution *in vitro*. *European Journal of Pharmaceutics & Biopharmaceutics, 69*(1), 214–222. https://doi.org/10.1016/j.ejpb.2007.10.002

Culliton, P., & Halcón, L. (2011). Chronic wound treatment with topical tea tree oil. *Alternative Therapies in Health and Medicine, 17*(2), 46–47.

de Sousa, D. (2011). Analgesic-like activity of essential oils constituents. *Molecules, 16*(3), 2233–2252. https://doi.org/10.3390/molecules16032233

de Sousa, D., Silva, R. H. N., Silva, E. F. D., & Gavioli, E. C. (2017). Essential oils and their constituents: An alternative source for novel antidepressants. *Molecules, 22*(8), 1290. https://doi.org/10.3390/molecules22081290

Dongmo, P., Tchoumbougnang, F., Sonwa, E., Kenfack, S., Zollo, P., & Menut, C. (2008). Antioxidant and anti-inflammatory potential of essential oils of some *Zanthoxylum* (Rutaceae) of Cameroon. *International Journal of Essential Oil Therapeutics, 2*(2), 82–88. https://hal.archives-ouvertes.fr/hal-00460458

Dooley, T. R. (2002). *Homeopathy: Beyond flat earth medicine* (2nd ed.). Timing Publications.

Dyer, J., Cleary, L., McNeill, S., Ragsdale-Lowe, M., & Osland, C. (2016). The use of aromasticks to help with sleep problems: A patient experience survey. *Complementary Therapies in Clinical Practice, 22,* 51–58. https://doi.org/10.1016/j.ctcp.2015.12.006

Edwards-Jones, V., Buck, R., Shawcross, S., Dawson, M., & Dunn, K. (2004). The effect of essential oils on methicillin-resistant *Staphylococcus aureus* using a dressing model. *Burns, 30*(8), 772–777. https://doi.org/10.1016/j.burns.2004.06.006

Egan, B., Gage, H., Hood, J., Poole, K., McDowell, C., Maguire, G., & Storey, L. (2012). Availability of complementary and alternative medicine for people with cancer in the British National Health Service: Results of a national survey. *Complementary Therapies in Clinical Practice, 18*(2), 75–80. https://doi.org/10.1016/j.ctcp.2011.11.003

Einion, A. (2016). Aromatherapy in midwifery practice. *Practising Midwife, 19*(5), 12, 14–15.

Eisenberg, D. M., Davis, R. B., Ettner, S. L., Appel, S., Wilken, S., Van Rompay, M. I., & Kessler, R. C. (1998). Trends in alternative medicine in the USA, 1990–1997: Results of a follow-up national survey. *Journal of the American Medical Association, 280*(18), 1569–1575. https://doi.org/10.1001/jama.280.18.1569

Enshaieh, S., Jooya, A., Siadat, A., & Iraji, F. (2007). The efficacy of 5% topical tea tree oil gel in mild to moderate acne vulgaris: A randomized, double-blind placebo-controlled study. *Indian Journal of Dermatology, Venereology and Leprology, 73*(1), 22–25. https://doi.org/10.4103/0378-6323.30646

Fettig, J., Taylor, J., & Sood, A. (2014). Post-surgical allergic contact dermatitis to compound tincture of benzoin and association with reactions to fragrances and essential oils. *Dermatitis, 25*(4), 211–212. https://doi.org/10.1097/DER.0000000000000057

Fisher, C., Adams, J., Hickman, L., & Sibbritt, D. (2016). The use of complementary and alternative medicine by 7427 Australian women with cyclic perimenstrual pain and discomfort: A cross-sectional study. *BMC Complementary & Alternative Medicine, 16,* 129. https://doi.org/10.1186/s12906-016-1119-8

Fitzgerald, M., & Halcón, L. (2010). A pediatric perspective on aromatherapy. In T. Culbert & K. Olness (Eds.), *Integrative pediatrics* (pp. 123–145). Oxford University Press.

Fox, L. T., Gerber, M., DuPlessis, J., & Hamman, J. H. (2011). Transdermal drug delivery enhancement by compounds of natural origin. *Molecules, 16*(12), 10507–10540. https://doi.org/10.3390/molecules161210507

Fryatt, J., & Bell, P. (2020). Effect of peppermint oil on postoperative urinary retention. *Journal of Pediatric Nursing, 51,* 116–118. https://doi.org/10.1016/j.pedn.2020.01.001

Gedney, J., Glover, T., & Fillingim, R. (2004). Sensory and affective pain discrimination after inhalation of essential oils. *Psychosomatic Medicine, 66*(4), 599–606. https://doi.org/10.1097/01.psy.0000132875.01986.47

Gelmini, F., Belotti, L., Vecchi, S., Testa, C., & Beretta, G. (2016). Air dispersed essential oils combined with standard sanitization procedures for environmental microbiota control in nosocomial hospitalization rooms. *Complementary Therapies in Medicine, 25,* 113–119. https://doi.org/10.1016/j.ctim.2016.02.004

Ghelardini, C., Galeotti, N., Salvatore, G., & Mazzanti, G. (1999). Local anaesthetic activity of the essential oil of *Lavandula angustifolia*. *Planta Medica, 65*(8), 700–703. https://doi.org/10.1055/s-1999-14045

Ghiasi, A., Bagheri, L., & Haseli, A. (2019). A systematic review on the anxiolytic effect of aromatherapy during the first stage of labor. *Journal of Caring Sciences, 8*(1), 51–60. https://doi.org/10.15171/jcs.2019.008

Goes, T., Antunes, F., Alves, P., & Teixeira-Silva, F. (2012). Effect of sweet orange aroma on experimental anxiety in humans. *Journal of Alternative & Complementary Medicine, 18*(8), 798–804. https://doi.org/10.1089/acm.2011.0551

Goes, T., Ursulino, F., Almeida-Souza, T., Alves, P., & Teixeira-Silva, F. (2015). Effect of lemongrass aroma on experimental anxiety in humans. *Journal of Alternative & Complementary Medicine, 21*(12), 766–773. https://doi.org/10.1089/acm.2015.0099

Greive, K., & Barnes, T. (2018). The efficacy of Australian essential oils for the treatment of head lice infestation in children: A randomized controlled trial. *The Australasian Journal of Dermatology, 59*(2), e99–e105. https://doi.org/10.1111/ajd.12626

Grossoehme, D., Cotton, S., & McPhail, G. (2013). Use and sanctification of complementary and alternative medicine by parents of children with cystic fibrosis. *Journal of Health Care Chaplaincy, 19*(1), 22–32. https://doi.org/10.1080/08854726.2013.761007

Gutierrez, M., Werdin-Gonzalez, J., Stefanazzi, N., Bras, C., & Ferrero, A. (2016). The potential application of plant essential oils to control *Pediculus humanus capitis* (Anoplura: Pediculidae). *Parasitology Research, 115*(2), 633–641. https://doi.org/10.1007/s00436-015-4781-8

Halcón, L. (2013). Aromatherapy in pregnancy and childbirth. In M. Avery (Ed.), *Supporting a physiologic approach to pregnancy and birth* (pp. 173–195). Wiley Blackwell.

Halcón, L., & Milkus, K. (2004). *Staphylococcus aureus* and wounds: A review of tea tree oil (*Melaleuca alternifolia*) as a promising antibiotic. *American Journal of Infection Control, 32*(7), 402–408. https://doi.org/10.1016/S0196655304003657

Halicioglu, O., Astarcioglu, G., Yaprak, I., & Aydinlioglu, H. (2011). Toxicity of *Salvia officinalis* in a newborn and a child: An alarming report. *Pediatric Neurology, 45*(4), 259–260. https://doi.org/10.1016/j.pediatrneurol.2011.05.012

Hammer, K., Carson, C., & Riley, T. (2012). Effects of *Melaleuca alternifolia* (tea tree) essential oil and the major monoterpene component terpinen-4-ol on the development of single- and multistep antibiotic resistance and antimicrobial susceptibility. *Antimicrobial Agents & Chemotherapy, 56*(2), 909–915. https://doi.org/10.1128/AAC.05741-11

Hammer, K. A., Carson, C. F., & Riley, T. V. (2008). Frequencies of resistance to *Melaleuca alternifolia* (tea tree) oil and rifampicin in *Staphylococcus aureus, Staphylococcus epidermidis* and *Enterococcus faecalis. International Journal of Antimicrobial Agents, 32*(2), 170–173. https://doi.org/10.1016/j.ijantimicag.2008.03.013

Horváth, G., & Ács, K. (2015). Essential oils in the treatment of respiratory tract diseases highlighting their role in bacterial infections and their anti-inflammatory action: A review. *Flavour and Fragrance Journal, 30,* 331–341. https://doi.org/10.1002/ffj.3252

Igarashi, M., Ikei, H., Song, C., & Miyazaki, Y. (2014). Effects of olfactory stimulation with rose and orange oil on prefrontal cortex activity. *Complementary Therapies in Medicine, 22*(6), 1027–1031. https://doi.org/10.1016/j.ctim.2014.09.003

Imura, M., Misao, H., & Ushijima, H. (2006). The psychological effects of aromatherapy-massage in healthy postpartum mothers. *Journal of Midwifery & Women's Health, 51*(2), e21–e27. https://doi.org/10.1016/j.jmwh.2005.08.009

Irmak, S., Uysal, M., Tas, U., Esen, M., Barut, M., Somuk, B., Alatli, T., & Ayan, S. (2015). The effect of lavender oil in patients with renal colic: A prospective controlled study using objective and subjective outcome measurements. *Journal of Alternative & Complementary Medicine, 21*(10), 617–622. https://doi.org/10.1089/acm.2015.0112

Jacobs, M., & Hornfeldt, C. (1994). Melaleuca oil poisoning. *Clinical Toxicology, 32*(4), 461–464. https://doi.org/10.3109/15563659409011050

Jain, R., Aqil, M., Ahad, A., Ali, A., & Khar, R. K. (2008). Basil oil is a promising skin penetration enhancer for transdermal delivery of labetolol hydrochloride. *Drug Development and Industrial Pharmacy, 34*(4), 384–389. https://doi.org/10.1080/03639040701657958

Janes, S. E. J., Price, C. S. G., & Th‚mas, D. (2005). Essential oil poisoning: N-acetylcysteine for eugenol-induced hepatic failure and analysis of a national database. *European Journal of Pediatrics, 164*(8), 520–522. https://doi.org/10.1007/s00431-005-1692-1

Keljova, K., Jirova, D., Bendova, H., Gajdos, P., & Kolarova, H. (2010). Phototoxicity of essential oils intended for cosmetic use. *Toxicology In Vitro, 24*(8), 2084–2089. https://doi.org/10.1016/j.tiv.2010.07.025

Keville, K., & Green, M. (2009). *Aromatherapy: A complete guide to the healing art* (2nd ed.). Crossing Press.

Kiberd, M., Clarke, S., Chorney, J., d'Eon, B., & Wright, S. (2016). Aromatherapy for the treatment of PONV in children: A pilot RCT. *BMC Complementary & Alternative Medicine, 16* (1), 450. https://doi.org/10.1186/s12906-016-1441-1

Kiecolt-Glaser, J., Graham, J., Malarkey, W., Porter, K., Lemeshow, S., & Glaser, R. (2008). Olfactory influences on mood and autonomic, endocrine, and immune function. *Psychoneuroendocrinology, 33*(3), 328–339. https://doi.org/10.1016/j.psyneuen.2008.06.011

Kim, J. T., Ren, C. J., Fielding, G. A., Pitti, A., Kasumi, T., Wajda, M., Lebovits, A., & Bekker, A. (2007). Treatment with lavender aromatherapy in the post-anesthesia care unit reduces opioid requirements of morbidly obese patients undergoing laparoscopic adjustable gastric banding. *Obesity Surgery, 17*(7), 920–925. https://doi.org/10.1007/s11695-007-9170-7

Ko, L., Su, C., Yang, M., Liu, S., & Su, T. (2021). A pilot study on essential oil aroma stimulation for enhancing slow-wave EEG in sleeping brain. *Scientific Reports, 11*(1), 1078. https://doi.org/10.1038/s41598-020-80171-x

Kreitzer, M., & Koithan, M. (2014). *Integrative nursing.* Oxford University Press.

Kritsidima, M., Newton, T., & Asimakopoulou, K. (2009). The effects of lavender scent on dental patient anxiety levels: A cluster randomised-controlled trial. *Community Dentistry and Oral Epidemiology, 38*(1), 83–87. https://doi.org/10.1111/j.1600-0528.2009.00511.x

Kunz, S., Schultz, M., Lewitzky, M., Driessen, M., & Rau, H. (2007). Ear acupuncture for alcohol withdrawal in comparison with aromatherapy: A randomized-controlled trial. *Alcoholism: Clinical and Experimental Research, 31*(3), 436–442. https://doi.org/10.1111/j.1530-0277.2006.00333.x

Lemme, P. (2009). The use of essential oils in psychiatric medication withdrawal. *International Journal of Clinical Aromatherapy, 6*(2), 15–23. https://shop.ijca.net/43-2009

Libster, M. (2002). *Delmar's integrative herb guide for nurses.* Delmar Thompson Learning.

Libster, M. (2012). *The nurse herbalist: Integrative insights for holistic practice.* Golden Apple Publications.

Lillehei, A., Halcón, L., Savik, K., & Reis, R. (2015). Effect of inhaled lavender and sleep hygiene on self-reported sleep issues: A randomized controlled trial. *Journal of Alternative & Complementary Medicine, 21*(7), 430–438. https://doi.org/10.1089/acm.2014.0327

Lim, P. F. C., Liu, X. Y., & Chan, S. Y. (2009). A review on terpenes as skin penetration enhancers in transdermal drug delivery. *Journal of Essential Oil Research, 21*(5), 423–428. https://doi.org/10.1080/10412905.2009.9700208

Lin, P., Chan, W., Ng, B., & Lam, L. (2007). Efficacy of aromatherapy (*Lavender angustifolia*) as an intervention for agitated behaviours in Chinese older persons with dementia: A crossover randomized trial. *International Journal of Geriatric Psychiatry, 22*(5), 205–210. https://doi.org/10.1002/gps.1688

Lizarraga-Valderrama, L. R. (2020). Effects of essential oils on central nervous system: Focus on mental health. *Phytotherapy Research, 35*, 657–679. https://doi.org/10.1002/ptr.6854

Lua, P., Salihah, N., & Mazlan, N. (2015). Effects of inhaled ginger aromatherapy on chemotherapy-induced nausea and vomiting and health-related quality of life in women with breast cancer. *Complementary Therapies in Medicine, 23*(3), 396–404. https://doi.org/10.1016/j.ctim.2015.03.009

Lua, P. L., & Zakaria, N. S. (2012). A brief review of current scientific evidence involving aromatherapy use for nausea and vomiting. *Journal of Alternative & Complementary Medicine, 18*(6), 534–540. https://doi.org/10.1089/acm.2010.0862

Lusby, P. E., Coombes, A. L., & Wilkinson, J. M. (2006). A comparison of wound healing following treatment with *Lavandula x allardii* honey or essential oil. *Phytotherapy Research, 20*(9), 755–757. https://doi.org/10.1002/ptr.1949

Malachowska, B., Fendler, W., Pomykala, A., Suwala, S., & Mlynarski, W. (2016). Essential oils reduce autonomic response to pain sensation during self-monitoring of blood glucose among children with diabetes. *Journal of Pediatric Endocrinology & Metabolism, 29*(1), 47–53. https://doi.org/10.1515/jpem-2014-0361

Menezes, I. A., Barreto, C. M., Antoniolli, A. R., Santos, M. R., & de Sousa, D. P. (2010). Hypotensive activity of terpenes found in essential oils. *Zeitschrift für Naturforschung C: A Journal of Biosciences, 65*(9), 562–566. https://doi.org/10.1515/znc-2010-9-1005

Morris, N. (2008). The effects of lavender (*Lavandula angustifolia*) essential oil baths on stress and anxiety. *International Journal of Clinical Aromatherapy*, 5(1), 3–7.

Moss, L., Rouse, M., Wesnes, K. A., & Moss, M. (2010). Differential effects of the aromas of *Salvia* species on memory and mood. *Human Psychopharmacology: Clinical & Experimental*, 25(5), 388–396. https://doi.org/10.1002/hup.1129

Mukurji, G., Yiangou, Y., Corcoran, S. L., Selmer, I. S., Smith, G. D., Benham, C. D., Bountra, C., Agarwal, S. K., & Anand, P. (2006). Cool and menthol receptor TRPM8 in human urinary bladder disorders and clinical correlations. *BMC Urology*, 6, 1–11. https://doi.org/10.1186/1471-2490-6-6

Musil, A. (2013). Labor encouragement with essential oils. *Midwifery Today with International Midwife*, 113(Autumn), 57–58.

Muthaiyan, A., Biswas, D., Crandall, P., Wilkinson, B., & Ricke, S. (2012). Application of orange essential oil as an antistaphylococcal agent in a dressing model. *BMC Complementary & Alternative Medicine*, 12, 125. https://doi.org/10.1186/1472-6882-12-125

Nagata, K., Iida, N., Kanazawa, H., Fujiwara, M., Mogi, T., Mitsushima, T., Lefor, A. T., & Suqimoto, H. (2014). Effect of listening to music and essential oil inhalation on patients undergoing screening CT colonography: A randomized controlled trial. *European Journal of Radiology*, 83(12), 2172–2176. https://doi.org/10.1016/j.ejrad.2014.09.016

National Cancer Institute (NCI), National Institutes of Health. (2021). *Aromatherapy and essential oils*. https://www.cancer.gov/about-cancer/treatment/cam/hp/aromatherapy-pdq#:~:text=Aromatherapy%20is%20the%20therapeutic%20use%20of%20essential%20oils,cancer%20primarily%20as%20supportive%20care%20for%20general%20well-being

Nielsen, J. (2006). Natural oils affect the human skin integrity and the percutaneous penetration of benzoic acid-dose dependency. *Basic & Clinical Pharmacology & Toxicology*, 98(6), 575–581. https://doi.org/10.1111/j.1742-7843.2006.pto_388.x

Noruzi, M., Farmahini, M., Amirmohseni, L., Pourandish, Y., Shamsikhani, S., Heydari, A., & Hararani, M. (2021). The effects of inhalation aromatherapy on postoperative abdominal pain: A three-arm randomized controlled trial. *Journal of PeriAnesthesia Nursing*, 36(2), 147–152. https://doi.org/10.1016/j.jopan.2020.07.001

O'Connor, D., Eppingstall, B., Taffe, J., & van der Ploeg, E. (2013). A randomized, controlled cross-over trial of dermally-applied lavender (*Lavandula angustifolia*) oil as a treatment of agitated behaviour in dementia. *BMC Complementary & Alternative Medicine*, 13, 315. https://doi.org/10.1186/1472-6882-13-315

O'Flaherty, L., van Dijk, M., Albertyn, R., Millar, A., & Rode, H. (2012). Aromatherapy massage seems to enhance relaxation in children with burns: An observational pilot study. *Burns*, 38 (6), 840–845. https://doi.org/10.1016/j.burns.2012.01.007

Paduch, R., Kandefer-Szerszen, M., Trytek, M., & Fiedurek, J. (2007). Terpenes: Substances useful in human healthcare. *Archivum Immunologiae et Therapaie Experimentalis*, 55(5), 315–327. https://doi.org/10.1007/s00005-007-0039-1

Paule, A. (2001). Antimicrobial properties of essential oil constituents. *International Journal of Aromatherapy*, 11(3), 126–133. https://doi.org/10.1016/S0962-4562(01)80048-5

Pearson. S. (2015). Essential oils for prenatal nausea and digestion. *Midwifery Today with International Midwife*, 116, 44–46.

Phillips, S. A. (1998). *Use of peppermint oil to promote urination in women experiencing postoperative urinary retention* [Unpublished master's thesis]. University of Kansas.

Posadzki, P., Watson, L., Alotaibi, A., & Ernst, E. (2013). Prevalence of use of complementary and alternative medicine (CAM) by patients/consumers in the UK: Systematic review of surveys [Review]. *Clinical Medicine*, 13(2), 126–131.

Pounds, L. (2012). Art of aromatherapy for end-of-life care. *Beginnings*, 32(4), 20–23.

Price, S., & Price, L. (2011). *Aromatherapy for health professionals* (4th ed.). Churchill Livingstone.

Rose, J., & Behm, F. (1994). Inhalation of vapor from black pepper extract reduces smoking withdrawal symptoms. *Drug and Alcohol Dependence*, 34(3), 225–229. https://doi.org/10.1016/0376-8716(94)90160-0

Rudback, J., Islam, M., Borje, A., Nilsson, U., & Karlberg, A. (2015). Essential oils can contain allergenic hydroperoxides at eliciting levels, regardless of handling and storage. *Contact Dermatitis, 73*(4), 253–254. https://doi.org/10.1111/cod.12427

Sakkas, H., & Papadopoulou, C. (2017). Antimicrobial activity of basil, oregano, and thyme essential oils. *Journal of Microbiology and Biotechnology, 27*(3), 429–438. https://doi.org/10.4014/jmb.1608.08024

Samarasekera, R., Weerasinghe, I., & Hemalal, K. (2008). Insecticidal activity of menthol derivatives against mosquitoes. *Pest Management Science, 64*(3), 290–295. https://doi.org/10.1002/ps.1516

Sheikhan, F., Jahdi, F., Khoei, E. M., Shamsalizadeh, N., Sheikhan, M., & Haghani, H. (2012). Episiotomy pain relief: Use of lavender oil essence in primiparous Iranian women. *Complementary Therapies in Clinical Practice, 18*(1), 66–70. https://doi.org/10.1016/j.ctcp.2011.02.003

Sherry, E., Sivananthan, S., Warnke, P., & Eslick, G. (2003). Topical phytochemicals used to salvage the gangrenous lower limbs of type 1 diabetic patients. *Diabetes Research and Clinical Practice, 62*(1), 65–66. https://doi.org/10.1016/j.diabres.2003.07.001

Simpson, N., & Roman, K. (2001). Complementary medicine use in children: Extent and reasons. A population based study. *British Journal of General Practice, 51*(472), 914–916.

Singh, B, Tiwari, S., & Dubey, N. (2021). Essential oils and their nanoformulations as green preservatives to boost food safety against mycotoxin contamination of food commodities: A review. *Journal of the Science of Food and Agriculture, 101*(12), 4879–4890. https://doi.org/10.1002/jsfa.11255

Singh, G., Kiran, S., Marimuthu, P., de Lampasona, M., de Heluani, C., & Catalan, C. (2008). Chemistry, biocidal and antioxidant activities of essential oil and oleoresins from *Piper cubeba* (seed). *International Journal of Essential Oil Therapeutics, 2*(2), 50–59. https://www.researchgate.net/publication/233677516_Chemistry_biocidal_and_antioxidant_activities_of_essential_oil_and_oleoresins_from_Piper_cubeba_seed

Solorzano-Santos, F., & Miranda-Novales, M. (2012). Essential oils from aromatic herbs as antimicrobial agents. *Current Opinion in Biotechnology, 23*(2), 136–141. https://doi.org/10.1016/j.copbio.2011.08.005

Storan, E., Nolan, U., & Kirby, B. (2016). Allergic contact dermatitis caused by the tea tree oil-containing hydrogel Burnshield. *Contact Dermatitis, 74*(5), 309–310. https://doi.org/10.1111/cod.12531

Styles, J. (1997). The use of aromatherapy in hospitalized children with HIV. *Complementary Therapies in Nursing and Midwifery, 3*(1), 16–20. https://doi.org/10.1016/s1353-6117(97)80029-7

Thomas, J., Carson, C. F., Peterson, G. M., Walton, S. F., Hammer, K. A., Naunton, M., Davey, R. C., Spelman, T., Dettwiller, P., Kyle, G., Cooper, G. M., & Baby, K. E. (2016). Therapeutic potential of tea tree oil for scabies [Review]. *American Journal of Tropical Medicine & Hygiene, 94*(2), 258–66. https://doi.org/10.4269/ajtmh.14-0515

Thompson, P., Jensen, T., Hammer, K., Carson, C., Molgaard, P., & Riley, T. (2011). Survey of the antimicrobial activity of commercially available Australian tea tree (*Melaleuca alternifolia*) essential oil products in vitro. *Journal of Alternative & Complementary Medicine, 17*(9), 835–841. https://doi.org/10.1089/acm.2010.0508

Tindle, H., Davis, R., Phillips, R., & Eisenberg, D. (2005). Trends in the use of complementary and alternative medicine by U.S. adults: 1997–2002. *Alternative Therapies in Health and Medicine, 11*(1), 42–49.

Tisserand Institute. (n.d.-a). *Bath safety.* https://tisserandinstitute.org/safety/bath-safety/

Tisserand Institute. (n.d.-b). *What to do when experiencing an adverse reaction.* https://tisserandinstitute.org/safety/what-to-do-when-experiencing-an-adverse-reaction/

Tisserand, R. (2016). *Essential oil chemistry and pharmacology: The actions of aromatic compounds in the body.* Seminar. http://enhancementsaromatherapyllc.vpweb.com/upload/Tisserand%20flyer_2pg.pdf

Tisserand, R., & Young, R. (2014). *Essential oil safety* (2nd ed.). Churchill Livingstone.

Tomaino, J. (2015). *Aromatherapy for end-of-life care: Successes and challenges of a DNP project.* [Paper presentation]. International Integrative Nursing Symposium.

Tomaino, J. (2019). *Aromatherapy: Clinical use of essential oils.* [MOOC]. Coursera. https://www .coursera.org/learn/aromatherapy-clinical-use-essential-oils?specialization=integrative -health-and-medicine

Tomaino, J. (2020). Aromatherapy and your nurse practice act. *American Holistic Nurses Association Beginnings, 40*(4), 14–15. https://www.ahna.org/Home/Publications

Uter, W., Schmidt, E., Geier, J., Lessmann, H., Schnuch, A., & Frosch, P. (2010). Contact allergy to essential oils: Current patch test results (2000–2008) from the Information Network of Departments of Dermatology (IVDK). *Contact Dermatitis, 63*(5), 277–283. https://doi .org/10.1111/j.1600-0536.2010.01768.x

Uvin, P., Franken, J., Pinto, S., Rietjens, R., Grammet, L., Deruyver, Y., Alpizar, Y. A., Talavera, K., VEnnekens, R., Everaerts, W., De Ridder, D., & Voets, T. (2015). Essential role of transient receptor potential M8 (TRPM8) in a model of acute cold-induced urinary urgency. *European Urology, 68*(4), 655–661. https://doi.org/10.1016/j.eururo.2015.03.037

Valgimigli, L., Gabbanini, S., Berlini, E., Lucchi, E., Beltramini, C., & Bertarelli, Y. L. (2012). Lemon (*Citrus limon,* Burm. f.) essential oil enhances the trans-epidermal release of lipid-(A, E) and water-(B6, C) soluble vitamins from topical emulsions in reconstructed human epidermis. *International Journal of Cosmetic Science, 34*(4), 347–356. https://doi.org/ 10.1111/j.1468-2494.2012.00725.x

Watanabe, E., Kuchta, K., Kimura, M., Rauwald, H., Kamei, T., & Imanishi, J. (2015). Effects of bergamot (*Citrus bergamia* (Risso) Wright & Arn.) essential oil aromatherapy on mood states, parasympathetic nervous system activity, and salivary cortisol levels in 41 healthy females. *Forschende Komplementarmedizin, 22*(1), 43–49. https://doi.org/10.1159/000380989

Weiss, E. (1997). *Essential oil crops.* CAB International.

Williams, A., & Barry, B. (1989). Essential oils as novel skin penetration enhancers. *International Journal of Pharmaceutics, 57*(2), R7–R9. https://doi.org/10.1016/0378-5173(89)90310-4

Woelk, H., & Schlafke, S. (2010). A multi-center, double-blind, randomised study of the lavender oil preparation silexan in comparison to lorazepam for generalized anxiety disorder. *Phytomedicine, 17*(2), 94–99. https://doi.org/10.1016/j.phymed.2009.10.006

Yoshiyama, K., Arita, H., & Suzuki, J. (2015). The effect of aroma hand massage therapy for people with dementia. *Journal of Alternative & Complementary Medicine, 21*(12), 759–765. https:// doi.org/10.1089/acm.2015.0158

Herbal Medicines

GREGORY A. PLOTNIKOFF AND ANGELA S. LILLEHEI

Herbs and related natural products such as spices are the oldest and most widely used form of medicine in the world. The use of herbs for the treatment of disease and the promotion of well-being can be traced back in many cultures at least 2,500 years. In the 5th century BCE, Hippocrates recommended the leaves and bark of the willow tree (genus *Salix*) for pain and inflammation. In the more recent past, in the 1850s, Florence Nightingale's medicine box that she brought to the Crimean War contained quinine and powdered rhubarb, as well as other medicines, to administer to the wounded and sick soldiers (Florence Nightingale Museum of London, 2016). However, herbal medicines are not restricted to historical use. Today, in addition to the well-known examples of aspirin from the willow tree, digoxin from the foxglove plant *Digitalis purpurea*, and paclitaxel from the pacific yew tree *Taxus brevifolia*, both over-the-counter and prescription plant-derived medications are frequently used. These include anticholinergic agents, anticoagulants, antihypertensives, and antineoplastic agents. Just a small percentage of the world's plant species provide medicines. There are likely many more waiting to be discovered. The most recently celebrated example is that of a potent antimalarial medication. Chinese scientists, led by Dr. Tu Youyou, discovered and isolated artemisinin from sweet wormwood (*Artemesia annua* L), a plant used for medicinal purposes in China for more than 2,000 years. For her work, Dr. Tu was honored with the very prestigious Lasker-DeBakey Clinical Research Award in 2011 (Miller & Su, 2011).

The most comprehensive and reliable data on the use of herbal medicine in the United States come from the National Health Interview Survey (NHIS). Looking at combined data from 88,962 adults, nonvitamin, nonmineral dietary supplements were the most commonly used complementary health therapy in 2002 (17.7%), 2007 (17.7%), and most recently measured in 2012 (18.9%). For the purpose of this survey, complementary health included a variety of therapies and products with a history of use or origins outside of conventional Western medicine (Clarke et al., 2015).

The high prevalence of use in all regions of the United States and across all ages, genders, ethnicities, and medical diagnoses means that health professionals must address herbal medicine use in all patient encounters (Arcury et al., 2006; Cherniack et al., 2008). In the 2012 NHIS study, 33.2% of adults reported the use of complementary and alternative medicines (CAM) in the previous year (Clarke et al., 2015). Most would support complementary approaches when used in combination with conventional medical treatments (Barnes et al., 2004). This is significant. The use of herbal medicines often is not disclosed unless specifically requested by the nurse, pharmacist, or physician. Even in 2008, as many as 62.5% of regular herbal medicine users also used prescription medicines; however, only 33% routinely reported their use to their care provider (Archer & Boyle, 2008). The 2004 Council for Responsible Nutrition's survey of 1,000 randomly selected U.S. adults documented that 90% looked to healthcare professionals, including nurses, for guidance in herbal medicine use (Ward & Blumenthal, 2005). Thus, herbal medicine warrants significant attention by all nurses as a complementary, holistic therapy and as a potential risk for interaction with other conventional approaches.

DEFINITION

Herbal medicines, or plant-based therapies, continue to occupy a place of central importance in the world's many healing traditions. These include the use of single herbs in many Western traditions and multiple-herb combinations in traditional Asian medical systems. Frequently, herbs are part of an overarching belief system that may involve spiritual or metaphysical components. Herbal medicines are often included in the work of shamans and other traditional healers who serve as intermediaries with the spirit world. Herbal medicines are also a tool in traditional Asian medicine and are used, like acupuncture, to open blocked channels (meridians) for the free flow of *qi* (life spirit or force). And in Ayurveda, an Indian medical system, herbal medicines are used to balance energies or doshas (Jansen et al., 2021).

Herbal medicines, also known as *botanicals* or *phytotherapies*, are one component of the range of natural products sold in the United States as dietary supplements. Plant therapies for medicinal or health purposes include herbs from the whole plant or a part of the plant, plant extracts or tinctures, essential oils, flower essences, and homeopathic remedies. A variety of plant therapy types may be included in dietary supplements. In addition to herbal products, other dietary supplements include fungi-based products (mycotherapies) and vitamin, mineral, and nutritional therapies (nutraceuticals). Since the passage of the Dietary Supplement Health and Education Act of 1994 (DSHEA; U.S. Congress, 1994), these biological modifiers have been available over the counter as dietary supplements. Although neither food nor drug, these substances are still regulated by the Food and Drug Administration (FDA) but with less stringent requirements. Unlike foods and drugs, dietary supplements can be sold based on evidence of safety in the possession of the manufacturer and can only be removed from the market if the FDA can prove them unsafe under ordinary conditions of use.

Under the DSHEA, herbal medicines can be sold for "stimulating, maintaining, supporting, regulating, and promoting health" rather than for treating disease. As dietary supplements rather than drugs, herbal medicines cannot claim to restore normal (or correct abnormal) function. In addition, herbs cannot claim to "diagnose, treat, prevent, cure, or mitigate" (U.S. Congress, 1994). Herbal medicine companies can assert that their product supports cardiovascular health but not that it lowers cholesterol. To do so would suggest that the product is intended for treating a disease (hypercholesterolemia) and is therefore subject to FDA pharmaceutical regulations.

This has raised questions about what constitutes a disease. The FDA originally defined *disease* as any deviation, impairment, or interruption of the normal structure or function of any part, organ, or system of the body that is manifested by a characteristic set of one or more signs and symptoms. This definition generated many concerns. "Normal structure" appeared to be normed to a 30-year-old man and therefore did not account for gender or aging. For example, are menopause and menstrual cramps diseases? With no signs or symptoms, is hypercholesterolemia a disease or a risk factor? After significant public outcry, the FDA adopted the definition of *disease* found in the Nutrition Labeling and Health Act of 1990. Disease is considered damage to an organ, part, structure, or system of the body such that it does not function properly (e.g., cardiovascular disease) or a state of health leading to such (e.g., hypertension).

SCIENTIFIC BASIS

Significant research has been done on numerous single herbal agents using Western biomedical/scientific models. Beginning in 1978, the German government's Bundesgesunheitsamt (Federal Health Agency) began evaluating the safety and efficacy of phytomedicines. The health professionals charged with doing so, known as the Commission E, met until 1994 and evaluated 300 herbal medicines, of which they recognized 190 as suitable for medicinal use. The complete reports have been translated and are available from the American Botanical Council (2000).

Beginning in 1996, significant meta-analyses and review articles of single-herb products began appearing on a regular basis in leading Western medical journals. These are readily accessible via the National Library of Medicine's PubMed website (www.ncbi.nlm.nih.gov/PubMed). Compiling data from similar studies for analysis (meta-analysis) is complicated by the fact that many studies published to date have left out important information, including naming the specific plant species studied (e.g., echinacea versus *Echinacea purpurea*, *E. pallida*, or *E. angustifolia*), the parts used (stems, leaves, or roots), the chemical constituents, the form (pressed juice, powdered whole extract, aqueous extract, ethanol extract, or aqueous-ethanol extract), the formulation (stated proportions of water to alcohol or specifically extracted fractions and concentrations) and dosage.

The standardization of herbal medicines is crucial both for scientific study and consumer protection. Standardization is equated with reproducibility, guaranteed potency, quality of active ingredients, and documentable effectiveness. However, with herbal medicines, standardization presents several problems. First, the active ingredient may not be known. Second, there may be more than one active ingredient. Third, both the content and the activity of a herbal medicine may be related to the means of the herb's growth conditions, extraction, and processing. In addition, there is a lack of quality assurance along the distribution chain from growing and harvesting conditions to the end consumer product (Heinrich, 2015). This significantly complicates both research and counseling for health professionals and consumers.

A growing number of healthcare professionals are studying the effects of these substances. With an increase in the FDA's involvement, we can look forward to a more reliable herb market. Expanded knowledge of herbal indications may augment the safety and efficacy of herbal therapies for patients.

INTERVENTION

Herbal medicines and dietary supplements need to be addressed in clinical settings in the same manner one addresses pharmaceutical agents. Every health professional needs to be aware of the wide use of herbal medicines and other dietary supplements.

TECHNIQUE

Efficient and effective patient advocacy means including questions on alternative therapies as a standard part of each patient interview. Reasonable questions include "Are you using any herbs? Vitamins? Dietary supplements?" Follow-up questions could cover "What dose? What source? What directions are you following? Why are you taking it?" Asking about the source of information can be quite helpful, as in, "Are you working with any other health professionals?" As with all good interviewing, listening for understanding rather than agreement or disagreement enhances the therapeutic alliance. In addition to knowing the type of herb used, the dose of each herb, and the intended purpose of each herb, gathering information regarding the duration of herb use is also helpful in assessing patients and providing the best possible care.

Unfortunately, professionals often do not ask such questions, and up to 69% of CAM-using patients do not volunteer such information (Graham et al., 2005). This "don't ask, don't tell" policy makes no sense in patient care. All health professionals need to create a safe environment that is conducive to patients' open sharing of important information, such as herbal use or use of other complementary/ alternative therapies without fear of ridicule or other negative responses. "Ask, then ask again" is a practice policy foundational to safe and effective patient care.

PRECAUTIONS

A common misconception regarding herbal medicines is that herbs have no side effects because they are natural. However, herbs do indeed have side effects and may be toxic or poisonous if not used appropriately. Consider the toxicity of widely used natural products such as coffee, cocaine, and tobacco. Another dilemma is patients using herbs in lieu of their prescribed medications. Although herbs may be a good option in particular cases and conditions, the decision to decline medications should be based on fully informed judgments in partnership with a health professional.

Interviewing for herbal medicine use is crucial for identifying patients at risk for interactions with prescription medications or for excessive bleeding in surgery. Patients with special risks of drug interactions and drug–herb interactions include those taking the following pharmaceutical agents: anticoagulants, hypoglycemics, antidepressants, sedative-hypnotics, antihypertensives, and medications with narrow therapeutic windows such as digoxin and theophylline. The significance of having knowledge of the ingestion of herbal medicines is illustrated in the list of known interactions of St. John's wort with commonly prescribed agents (see Exhibit 20.1).

Pregnancy, lactation, breastfeeding, and childcare are special topics in herbal medicine use. For these situations, the most authoritative references are cited in Exhibit 20.2. In the absence of clinical trial data, use is guided by historical experience or breast milk analysis. Herbs that increase breast milk production, such as

Exhibit 20.1 *Effect of St. John's Wort on Bioavailability of Selected Medications*

St. John's wort decreases the bioavailability of the following:
- calcium channel blockers
- coumadin
- cyclosporine
- digoxin
- irinotecan
- oral contraceptives
- protease inhibitors
- simvastatin
- tacrolimus
- theophylline

Note: The effect can remain strong for weeks after stopping ingestion.

Source: Di, Y. M., Li, C. G., Xue, C. C., & Zhou, S. F. (2008). Clinical drugs that interact with St. John's wort and implication in drug development. *Current Pharmacology Design, 14*, 1723–1742. https://doi.org/10.2174/138161208784746798; Zhou, S. F., & Lai, X. (2008). An update on clinical drug interactions with the herbal antidepressant St. John's wort. *Current Drug Metabolism, 9*(5), 394–409. https://doi.org/10.2174/138920008784746391

fenugreek, are frequently recommended by the International Board of Certified Lactation Consultants Examiners (IBLCE).

Nursing can play a critical role in patient assessment regarding the use of herbal medicines and in the education of patients on the safety and use of medicinal herbs. Exhibit 20.3 lists key teaching points regarding herbal medicines. Herbal therapies are safe only if herbs are prepared in the right way and used for the precise indication, in the correct amounts, for the exact duration, and with appropriate monitoring. Potential herb–herb and herb–drug interactions should be considered when patients are using herbal products. The lack of national standards in the collection and preparation of herbal products complicates this field in the United States. Because many herbs have potential or actual risks that need to be recognized, it is important for health providers to have reliable and accessible sources of information to prevent adverse herb-related reactions and to identify and manage complications of herbal therapies; selected reputable herbal references are provided at the end of this chapter (see Exhibit 20.2 and other resources at the end of this chapter).

All serious adverse reactions should be reported to the FDA through the MedWatch program at 1-800-332-1088 or at www.fda.gov/Safety/MedWatch/

Exhibit 20.2 *Suggested Additional Reading for Pregnancy, Breastfeeding, Lactation, and Childcare*

Hale, T. W. (2004). *Medications and mother's milk: A manual of lactational pharmacology* (11th ed.). Pharmasoft Medical Publishers.
Humphrey, S. (2004). *The nursing mother's herbal*. Fairview Press.
Kemper, K. J. (2002). *The holistic pediatrician* (2nd ed.). Perennial Currents.
Romm, A. J. (2003). *The natural pregnancy book*. Ten Speed Press.

Exhibit 20.3 *Five Key Patient Teaching Points*
1. Just because it is natural does not mean it is safe.
2. Just because it is safe does not mean it is effective.
3. Labels may not equal contents.
4. Self-diagnosis and self-treatment can result in self-malpractice.
5. Herbs are never a replacement for an emergency department.

HowToReport/ucm167733.htm. An example of a complication associated with herbal therapy is illustrated in the case of the use of *Ma huang* (Ephedra), which was marketed in the United States as a major ingredient in formulations for weight reduction. The use of this herb had been linked to numerous adverse cardiovascular events, including stroke, myocardial infarction, and sudden death (Haller & Benowitz, 2000), and the FDA banned sales of this herb in April 2004.

USES

Given the volume and variety of products, herbal medicine knowledge relevant to nursing practice cannot be summarized quickly. According to the most recent NHIS to examine herbal medicine use, the most commonly used herbal medicines were echinacea, cranberry, garlic, ginseng, and ginkgo (Clarke et al., 2015). This chapter explores these common herbal medicines along with other important herbs from an evidence-based perspective (Table 20.1). Additionally, Table 20.2 identifies the use from a symptom perspective based on the reporting of the National Institutes of Health, National Center for Complementary and Integrative Health (NCCIH), Herbs at a Glance. There is a significant range of scientific data available on each, and the theoretical risks should be acknowledged and carefully considered both by patients and health professionals. Furthermore, the clinical knowledge related to combining herbal products with prescription and nonprescription drugs is only in the developmental stages; much remains to be known about interactions and side effects.

Chronic illness (such as cancer or autoimmune disease or chronic pain), surgery, and the use of prescription medications are three situations in which herbal medicine reviews by nurses are important. Echinacea does stimulate the immune system, but this is not necessarily a positive effect. Ginkgo biloba's pharmacological activity places people at risk in surgery. St. John's wort is effective for depression but can render many prescription medications ineffective or even toxic. Many herbs have a sufficient evidence base and potential as alternatives to Western medicine. However, herbal medicine in the United States is a very broad and multicultural phenomenon; it is difficult to know all products used by or all products of potential benefit to patients. Readers should be aware that there are reputable clinical resources readily accessible for assistance in informed decision-making (e.g., see Exhibit 20.2 and other resources at the end of this chapter).

The recent legalization of marijuana (*Cannabis sativa*) for distribution through approved dispensaries in 36 states and the District of Columbia deserves special attention. Medicinal marijuana is the first herbal medicine to require a prescription in the United States. Even before such changes in state laws, several prescription forms of cannabinoids existed in the United States and Canada. Dronabinol and nabilone were used for treating nausea and vomiting associated

Table 20.1 *Selected Commonly Used Herbal Medicines*

Herbal Medicine	Uses	Strength of Evidence	Safety (General: Avoid herbal medicine when pregnant or breastfeeding and for long-term use. Side effects are dose-specific.)
Asian Ginseng	Increase resistance to environmental stress, general tonic, improve physical stamina, memory, concentration, stimulate immune function, antiaging, and other health problems.	Many studies but most are of low quality	Adverse Effects: Can cause insomnia, menstrual problems, breast pain, increased heart rate, digestive problems, and high or low blood pressure Interactions: May interact with high blood pressure medications, statins, and antidepressants, along with other medications
Chamomile	Generalized anxiety disorder May improve sleep quality for noninsomniacs	Preliminary studies included in a review	General: Generally safe when used in similar doses of teas Adverse Effects: Possible allergic reactions Interactions: May interact with cyclosporin, warfarin, and other medications
Cranberry	UTI prevention for those who are at increased risk	Limited and inconsistent	Interactions: May interact with warfarin
Echinacea	Common cold and other infections—may slightly reduce chances of getting a common cold	Many studies on affect on common cold	Adverse Effects: Nausea, stomach pain, allergic reactions
Elderberry	Colds, flu and other conditions-may relieve symptoms	Preliminary research on flu and common cold	General: Raw unripe berries and leaves and stems contain toxins
Garlic	High blood pressure and high blood cholesterol	Limited	Adverse Effects: Breath and body odor, heartburn, stomach upset. Interactions: May interact with Warfarin and HIV drugs

(continued)

Table 20.1 *Selected Commonly Used Herbal Medicines (continued)*

Herbal Medicine	Uses	Strength of Evidence	Safety (General: Avoid herbal medicine when pregnant or breastfeeding and for long-term use. Side effects are dose-specific.)
Gingko or Gingko biloba	Anxiety, diabetic retinopathy, glaucoma, peripheral artery disease, PMS, schizophrenia, and vertigo	Small amount of evidence available	General: Raw or tasted ginkgo seeds and the leaves may contain toxins Adverse Effects: Headache, GI issues, palpitations, dizziness, and allergic skin reactions Interactions: May interact with anticoagulants
Passionflower	Anxiety and sleep problems. Pain, heart rhythm problems, menopausal issues, and attention-deficit/hyperactivity disorder	Small amount of evidence for use with anxiety Not enough evidence for other uses	General: Found to be safe for short-term use
St. John's Wort	Depression, menopausal issues, ADHD, OCD. Topically for wounds and muscle pain	Evidence that it is helpful for mild depression Limited evidence on other uses	Adverse Effects: Sensitivity to light, insomnia, anxiety, dizziness, GI issues, fatigue, headache, and sexual issues Interactions: May interact with many conventional medications: antidepressants, BCP, some statins, some heart medications, some cancer medications, and many others.
Tumeric	Arthritis, digestive disorders, respiratory infections, allergies, liver disease, depression	Much research done but little available on health effects	General: Has bioavailability issues

Based on the National Center for Complementary and Integrative Health. *Herbs at a Glance.* https://www.nccih.nih.gov/health/herbsataglance.

Note: UTI = urinary tract infection; PMS = premenstrual syndrome; HIV = human immunodeficiency virus; ADHD = attention deficit hyperactivity disorder; OCD = obsessive compulsive disorder; BCP = birth control pills; GI = gastrointestinal.

Table 20.2 *Herbal Medicines With Some Evidence for Identified Symptoms*

Symptoms/Uses	Herbal Medicines	Evidence
Support antidepression	St. John's Wort	Helpful for mild depression
Support antianxiety	Chamomille Passionflower Gingko biloba	Preliminary studies Small amount Small amount
Promote sleep	Chamomille	Limited for improved sleep quality for noninsomniacs
General tonic	Asian Ginseng	Limited
Promote urological immune support	Cranberry	Limited for prevention for those who have frequent UTIs
Promote immune support	Echinacea Elderberry	May slightly reduce chance of getting the common cold, Preliminary
Promote cardiovascular health	Garlic	Limited for high BP and high cholesterol

Based on the National Center for Complementary and Integrative Health. *Herbs at a Glance.* https://www.nccih.nih.gov/health/herbsataglance. Refer to Table 20.1 for safety information.

Note: UTI = urinary tract infection; BP = blood pressure.

with chemotherapy or anorexia with weight loss in patients with AIDS. However, since 1970, marijuana as an herbal medicine has been considered a Schedule 1 substance and therefore illegal and without medical value. This understanding has been challenged by the discovery of what has been termed the endocannabinoid system. The presence of cannabinoid receptors CB1 and CB2 in the central nervous system (CNS) and elsewhere suggests the possibility of many promising pharmaceutical applications (Bostwick, 2012; Bostwick et al., 2013).

The most frequent medical use of the leaves and flowering tops of the marijuana plant is for pain and muscle spasticity (Borgelt et al., 2013). Safety concerns for all patients include dizziness, impaired memory and cognition, increased risk of schizophrenia in adolescents, and accidental ingestions by children and pets. A cannabis withdrawal syndrome has also been described (Crippa et al., 2013). Cannabis use disorders (CUDs) exist, especially among patients with a diagnosis of substance abuse and bipolar illness personality disorders. Nurses and all health professionals increasingly need to screen patients for appropriate medical use (Lev-Ran et al., 2013) and monitor for both positive and negative effects (Cohen et al., 2019).

RECENT NURSING RESEARCH IN MEDICINAL HERBS

Research on the use of herbs for healing is an important area for nursing. Examples of nursing research in the use of medicinal herbs include the effectiveness of Indian turmeric powder and honey for oral mucositis in cancer patients, with findings of a significantly positive difference between groups (Francis &

Williams, 2014); the effects of flaxseed on menopausal symptoms and quality of life, with findings of decreased menopausal symptoms and increased quality of life among women who used flaxseed for 3 months (Cetisli et al., 2015); and the effect of saw palmetto for symptom management during radiation therapy for men with prostate cancer, with results demonstrating safety at dosages up to 960 mg daily (but no statistically significant results between groups for lower urinary tract symptoms, although results trended in a positive direction; Wyatt et al., 2015). More recent research includes systematic reviews on herbal medicine for insomnia, demonstrating insufficient evidence (Leach & Page, 2014); ginseng as a treatment for fatigue, demonstrating modest evidence for efficacy (Arring et al., 2018); chamomile in the treatment of PMS, with findings showing that chamomille is effective for PMS (Khalesi et al., 2019); and the efficacy and safety of herbal medicine (*Lianhuaqingwen*) for treating COVID-19, which found Lianhuaqingwen appeared to be effective when combined with conventional treatment for patients with mild COVID-19 (Liu et al., 2021).

MEDICINAL MUSHROOMS

In addition to a variety of medicinal herbs being used, a plant dietary supplement gaining ground in medicinal use, although outside the range of herbal therapy, is medicinal mushrooms. Many mushrooms contain biologically active polysaccharides in fruit bodies, cultured mycelium, and cultured broth. The chemical structure of the polysaccharides, specifically that of the glucans and specific proteins, is thought to be associated with enhancing innate and cell-mediated immune responses and to exhibit antitumor properties (Motta et al., 2021). Additional properties that medicinal mushrooms and fungi are thought to have include antioxidant, radical scavenging, cardiovascular, anti-hypercholesterolemic, detoxification, and antiviral, antibacterial, antiparasitic, and antifungal (Wasser, 2014). There is still controversy on the use of mushrooms in Western medicine, with claims frequently outweighing the evidence (Money, 2016). Authors of a narrative review concluded that there is possible potential when used as a complementary therapy for cancer, but there is not enough clinical evidence to support the routine use of medicinal mushrooms with cancer at this time (Jeitler et al., 2020).

The NHIS survey found a significant increase in the use of fish oil, probiotics or prebiotics, and melatonin from 2007 to 2012. Conversely, a decrease in the use of herbs such as echinacea, garlic, ginseng, *Ginkgo biloba*, and saw palmetto was found from 2007 to 2012 (Clarke et al., 2015). As new plant therapies are promoted and researched, the medicinal herbs used by patients and consumers will continue to shift, which makes it challenging to stay abreast of what evidence and research is available. Ongoing herbal therapy research by scientists, nurses, and other healthcare professionals will be imperative.

CULTURAL APPLICATIONS

The practice of Western herbalism in medicine parallels that of Western pharmaceutical interventions. One herb with a defined pharmacological activity can be applied to a given patient with a given medical diagnosis. Successful treatment is understood as relief or eradication of the offending symptoms. Herbal medicines differ from pharmaceuticals in that—unlike plant-derived medications such as digoxin—single active agents are not identified, isolated, purified, and concentrated for human use. There is a presumed synergy of multiple bioactive components. Also, dosing is not as clearly identified. Rigorous scientific studies are thus much more difficult to conduct than are pharmaceuticals.

In sharp contrast to the North American experience, Asian herbal traditions use formulas containing multiple herbs that are customized for the patient and often for unmeasurable constitutional states and unquantifiable outcomes. Up to 12 ingredients can exist in these formulas. Ingredients can include plants, mushrooms, and minerals. In Chinese formulas, animal parts are often included.

Of particular interest may be Japan's Kampo tradition, as described in Sidebar 20.1. Today, in Japan, medical students are routinely taught to prescribe 148 ancient, multiherb formulas that are approved by Japan's equivalent of the

Sidebar 20.1 *Kampo, Japan's Traditional Medicine*

Kenji Watanabe

Kampo, Japan's traditional medicine, is widely practiced, approved by the government's regulatory agencies, and covered by the national health plan. Unlike North American medical schools, Japanese medical students are taught to prescribe ancient, multiherb formulas. Both physicians and nurses are expected to know the common uses and common side effects of these formulas.

Kampo literally means "way of the Han dynasty," the governmental period of ancient China from 220 BCE to 200 CE. During this time, many key medical texts were prepared. Japanese healers reinterpreted these to fit Japanese culture and historical experience. For this reason, Kampo today has many similarities to traditional Chinese medicine (TCM). However, there are several key points of differentiation. First, the Kampo physical examination focuses on the abdomen. Tongue and pulse diagnoses are considered, but the abdominal examination, termed *fukushin*, is prioritized. Second, although many formulas are shared, Kampo uses may be quite different. Third, Kampo diagnostic and therapeutic approaches are standardized and easily work with Western diagnoses and treatment plans. There is robust scientific literature, especially in the basic sciences, to support the prescription of rational herbal medicine.

Kampo herbal formulas are widely prescribed in both university and community hospitals across Japan. The Japanese Society of Oriental Medicine (JSOM) has annual meetings that attract many thousands of practitioners. Kampo is well understood in Japan.

Kampo's popularity and documented safety have promoted increasing international interest. As a result, the JSOM has produced an introductory text in English. An excellent English translation of the works of revered Kampo master Keisetsu Otsuka has recently been published, and the International Society for Japanese Kampo Medicine (ISJKM) now holds international meetings in English (www.isjkm.com). Furthermore, in 2013, the journal *Evidence-Based*

Sidebar 20.1 *Kampo, Japan's Traditional Medicine (continued)*

Complementary & Alternative Medicine hosted a special issue on the collaboration of Japanese Kampo medicine and Western medicine. In addition, the World Health Organization (WHO) is developing a common platform for Western medicine and traditional medicine via the *International Classification of Diseases* (*ICD*). Under the revision from *ICD-10* to *ICD-11* (currently, the *ICD-11* beta is on the web at https://icd.who.int/dev11/l-m/en), traditional Asian medicine, including Kampo, will be incorporated. This will enhance mutual communication between Western medicine and Kampo internationally.

Related Articles of Interest to English-Speaking Audiences

Cameron, S., Reissenweber, H., & Watanabe, K. (2012). Asian medicine: Japan's paradigm [letter]. *Nature, 482*(7835), 35. https://www.nature.com/articles/482035a.pdf

Gepshtein, Y., Plotnikiff, G. A., & Watanabe, K. (2008). Kampo in women's health: Japan's traditional approach to premenstrual symptoms. *Journal of Alternative Complementary Medicine, 14*(4), 427–435. https://doi.org/10.1089/acm.2007.7064

Hirose, T., Shinoda, Y., Yoshida, A., Kurimoto, M., Mori, K., Kawachi, Y., Tanaka, K., Takeda, A., Yoshimura, T., & Sugiyama, T. (2016). Efficacy of daiokanzoto in chronic constipation refractory to first-line laxatives. *Biomedical Reports, 5*(4), 497–500. https://doi.org/10.3892/br.2016.754

Ilto, A., Munakata, K., Imazu, Y., & Watanabe, K. (2012). First nationwide attitude survey of Japanese physicians on the use of traditional Japanese medicine (Kampo) in cancer treatment. *Evidence-Based Complementary & Alternative Medicine, 2012*(2012), 1–8. Article ID 957082.

Iwase, S., Yamaguchi, T., Miyajo, T., Terawaki, K., Inui, Q., & Uesono, Y. (2012). The clinical use of Kampo medicines (traditional Japanese herbal treatments) for controlling cancer patients' symptoms in Japan: A national cross-sectional survey. *BMC Complementary and Alternative Medicine, 12*, 222. https://doi.org/10.1186/1472-6882-12-222

Kimata, Y., Ogawa, K., Okamoto, H., Chino, A., & Namiki, T. (2016). Efficacy of traditional (Kampo) medicine for treating chemotherapy-induced peripheral neuropathy: A retrospective case series study. *World Journal Clinical Cases, 4*(10), 310–317. https://doi.org/10.12998/wjcc.v4.i10.310

Kowago, K., Shindo, S., Inoue, H., Akasaka, J., Motohashi, S., Urabe, G., Sato, M., Uchiyama, H., & Ogino, H. (2016). The effect of hachimi-jio-gan (Ba-wei-di-huang-wan) on the quality of life of patients with peripheral arterial disease—A prospective study using Kampo medicine. *Annals of Vascular Diseases, 9*(4), 288–294. https://doi.org/10.3400/avd.oa.15-00133

Mizoguchi, K., & Ikarashi, Y. (2017). Multiple psychopharmacological effects of the traditional Japanese Kampo medicine Yokukansan, and the brain regions it effects. *Frontiers in Pharmacology, 21*(8), 149. https://doi.org/10.3389/fphar.2017.00149

Watanabe, K., Matsuura, K., Gao, P., Hottenbacher, L., Tokunaga, H., Nishimura, K., Imazu, Y., Reissenweber, H., & Witt, C. M. (2011). Traditional Japanese Kampo medicine: Clinical research between modernity and traditional medicine—The state of research and methodological suggestions for the future. *Evidence-Based Complementary & Alternative Medicine, 8*(1), 1–19.

FDA and covered by their national health plan. Approximately 70% of all physicians prescribe these multiherb formulas, including nearly 100% of Japanese gynecologists. Diagnosis is made by physical examination of the tongue, pulse, and abdomen. Diagnoses can be very subjective, such as *katakori* (literally frozen shoulder, but patients have full range of motion) and *hiesho* (cold condition with normal body temperatures). There is no one-to-one correlation between a condition such as *hiesho* and a formula. Several formulas exist and are used for multiple conditions. The correct formula is based on the patient's history, physical examination, and response to initial treatment (Plotnikoff et al., 2008). A recent study explored the efficacy and safety of *keishibukuryogan*, a traditional Japanese Kampo medicine, for hot flashes in prostate cancer patients receiving androgen deprivation therapy. It was found to be helpful (Shigehara et al., 2020). Another study looked at another Kampo medicine, hangeshashinto, and oral mucositis from chemotherapy. This Kampo medicine was found to reduce the duration of the oral mucositis (Taira et al., 2020). And in a review of Kampo with symptoms related to aging (geriatric syndrome), it appears that Kampo can be helpful in a variety of symptoms related to aging. The value of the multifaceted Kampo is proposed to be helpful in addressing multifactorial age-related issues (Takayama et al., 2020).

FUTURE RESEARCH

Before even Western single-herb medicines can be more widely accepted by the conventional allopathic medical system, more randomized, double-blind, placebo-controlled trials are needed in the United States. The NCCIH has funded and will likely continue to fund promising clinical trials of herbal therapies. Understudied areas of research for herbal therapies include the following:

- premenstrual and perimenopausal symptom management
- prevention of chemotherapy side effects, including peripheral neuropathy
- chronic pain
- disabling fatigue
- refractory insomnia

In addition, significant efforts are needed to identify the most promising herbal supports for radiation therapy, irritable bowel and inflammatory bowel, and gastroparesis, as well as asthma and heart disease.

Western medicine has yet to explore the potential benefits of the world's many healing traditions that use customized combinations of herbs. The Kampo traditional medicines of Japan may be the best place to start, given the rigorous approach to safety, the strength of the published preclinical data, and the extent of use by mainstream health professionals. This study requires a new paradigm, one that accounts for potential synergy and counterbalancing activities of multiple ingredients. Although intriguing preliminary data exist for many dietary supplements, the historic paucity of funding mechanisms in these areas has meant that scientific support for the use of many commercial products lags significantly behind consumer marketing efforts.

The key message is this: Medicinal herbs for symptom management and well-being can be used by nursing for patients using evidenced-based literature and a holistic framework. Nursing has the opportunity and challenge to play a key role in the research, practice, and clinical use of plant therapies for symptom management and overall well-being.

WEBSITES AND OTHER RESOURCES

- American Botanical Council (www.herbalgram.org)
- American Nutraceutical Association (www.americanutra.com)
- Blumenthal, M., Goldberg, A., & Brinckmann, J. (Eds.). (2000). *Herbal medicine— The expanded Commission E Monographs*. American Botanical Council.
- FDA Center for Food Safety and Applied Nutrition—a link to report adverse events (www.fda.gov/AboutFDA/CentersOffices/OfficeofFoods/CFSAN/Con tactCFSAN/default.htm)
- *HerbalGram magazine*—published quarterly by the American Botanical Council and the Herb Research Foundation (www.herbalgram.org)
- Herb Research Foundation (www.herbs.org)
- Micromedex Alternative Medicine Database—an authoritative, full-text drug-information resource; includes alternative medicine and is one of the most comprehensive resources for herbal medicine. (www.library.ucsf.edu/db/ micromedex.html)
- HerbList™--- is a mobile app on herbal products launched in 2018 by the National Institutes of Health to help consumers with information about popular herbs and herbal supplements. It can be downloaded from the Apple App Store or Google Play. (www.nccih.nih.gov/health/herblist-app)

REFERENCES

American Botanical Council. (2000). *Herbal medicine: Expanded Commission E monographs*.

Archer, E. L., & Boyle, D. K. (2008). Herb and supplement use among the retail population of an independent, urban herb store. *Journal of Holistic Nursing, 26*, 27–35. https://doi .org/10.1177/0898010107305326

Arcury, T. A., Suerken, C. K., Grzywacz, J. G., Bell, R. A., Lang, W., & Quandt, S. A. (2006). Complementary and alternative medicine use among older adults: Ethnic variation. *Ethnic Diseases, 16*, 723–731. https://ethndis.org/priorarchives/ethn-16-03-723.pdf

Arring, N. M., Millstine, D., Marks, L. A., & Nail, L. M. (2018). Ginseng as a treatment for fatigue: A systematic review. *Journal of Alternative and Complementary Medicine, 24*(7), 624–633. https:// doi.org/10.1089/acm.2017.0361

Barnes, P. M., Powell-Griner, E., McFann, K., & Nahin, R. L. (2004). Complementary and alternative medicine use among adults: United States, 2002. *Advance Data, 343*, 1–19. https://doi .org/10.1016/j.sigm.2004.07.003

Borgelt, L. M., Franson, K. L., Nussbaum, A. M., & Wang, G. S. (2013). The pharmacologic and clinical effects of medical cannabis. *Pharmacotherapy, 33*(2), 195–209. https://doi.org/10.1002/ phar.1187

Bostwick, J. M. (2012). Blurred boundaries: The therapeutics and politics of medical marijuana. *Mayo Clinic Proceedings, 87*(2), 172–186. https://doi.org/10.1016/j.mayocp.2011.10.003

Bostwick, J. M., Reisfield, G. M., & DuPont, R. L. (2013). Clinical decisions. Medicinal use of marijuana. *New England Journal of Medicine, 368*(9), 866–868. https://doi.org/10.1056/ NEJMclde1300970

Cetisli, N. E., Saruhan, A., & Kivcak, B. (2015). The effects of flaxseed on menopausal symptoms and quality of life. *Holistic Nursing Practice, 29*(3), 151–157. https://doi.org/10.1097/ HNP.0000000000000085

Cherniack, E. P., Ceron-Fuentes, J., Florez, H., Sandals, L., Rodriguez, O., & Palacios, J. C. (2008). Influence of race and ethnicity on alternative medicine as a self-treatment for common medical conditions in a population of multi-ethnic urban elderly. *Complementary Therapies in Clinical Practice, 14*, 116–123. https://doi.org/10.1016/j.ctcp.2007.11.002

Clarke, T. C., Black, L. I., Stussman, B. J., Barnes, P. M., & Nahin, R. L. (2015). Trends in the use of complementary health approaches among adults: United States, 2002–2012. *National Health Statistics Reports, 79*, 1–16. https://www.ncbi.nlm.nih.gov/pmc/articles/PMC4573565/

Cohen, K., Weizman, A., & Weinstein, A. (2019). Positive and negative effects of cannabis and cannabinoids on health. *Clinical Pharmacology & Therapeutics, 105*(5), 1139–1147. https://doi .org/10.1002/cpt.1381

Crippa, J. A., Hallak, J. E., Machado-de-Sousa, J. P., Queiroz, R. H., Bergamaschi, M., Chagas, M. H., & Zuardi, A. W. (2013). Canabidiol for the treatment of cannabis withdrawal syndrome: A case report. *Journal of Clinical Pharmacology and Therapeutics, 38*(2), 162–164. https://doi .org/10.1111/jcpt.12018

Di, Y. M., Li, C. G., Xue, C. C., & Zhou, S. F. (2008). Clinical drugs that interact with St. John's wort and implication in drug development. *Current Pharmacology Design, 14*, 1723–1742. https:// doi.org/10.2174/138161208784746798

Florence Nightingale Museum of London. (2016). *Medicines & chest.* http://florence-nightingale -collections.co.uk/view/objects/asitem/items$0040:227

Francis, M., & Williams, S. (2014). Effectiveness of Indian turmeric powder with honey on complementary therapy in oral mucositis: A nursing perspective among cancer patients in Mysore. *Nursing Journal of India, 105*(6), 258–260. https://pubmed.ncbi.nlm.nih.gov/26182820/

Freeman, M. P., Fava, M., Lake, J., Trivedi, M. H., Wisner, K. L., & Mischoulon, D. (2010). Complementary and alternative medicine in major depressive disorder: The American Psychiatric Association Task Force Report. *Journal of Clinical Psychiatry, 71*(6), 669–681. https://doi.org/10.4088/JCP.10cs05959blu

Graham, R. E., Ahn, A. C., Davis, R. B., O'Connor, B. B., Eisenberg, D. M., & Phillips, R. S. (2005). Use of complementary and alternative medical therapies among racial and ethnic minor-ity adults: Results from the 2002 National Health Interview Survey. *Journal of the National Medical Association, 97*, 535–545. https://www.ncbi.nlm.nih.gov/pmc/articles/PMC2568705/ pdf/jnma00185-0093.pdf

Haller, C. A., & Benowitz, N. L. (2000). Adverse cardiovascular and central nervous system events associated with dietary supplements containing ephedra alkaloids. *New England Journal of Medicine, 343*(25), 1833–1838. https://doi.org/10.1056/NEJM200012213432502

Heinrich, M. (2015). Quality and safety of herbal medical products: Regulation and the need for quality assurance along the value chains. *British Journal of Clinical Pharmacology, 80*(1), 62–66. https://doi.org/10.1111/bcp.12586

Jansen, C., Baker, J. D., Kodaira, E., Ang, L., Bacani, A. J., Aldan, J. T., Shimoda, L. M. N., Salameh, M., Small-Howard, A. L., Stokes, A. J., Turner, H., & Adra, C. N. (2021). Medicine in motion: Opportunities, challenges and data analytics-based solutions for traditional medicine inte-gration into western medical practice. *Journal of Ethnopharmacology, 267*, 113477. https://doi .org/10.1016/j.jep.2020.113477

Jeitler, M., Michalsen, A., Frings, D., Hübner, M., Fischer, M., Koppold-Liebscher, D. A, Murthy, V., & Kessler, C. S. (2020). Significance of medicinal mushrooms in integrative oncology: A nar-rative review. *Frontiers in Pharmacology, 11*, 580656. https://doi.org/10.3389/fphar.2020.580656

Khalesi, Z. B., Beiranvand, S. P., & Bokaie, M. (2019). Efficacy of Chamomile in the treatment of premenstrual syndrome: A systematic review. *Journal of Pharmacopuncture, 22*(4), 204–209. https://doi.org/10.3831/KPI.2019.22.028.

Leach, M. J., & Page, A. T. (2015). Herbal Medicine for insomnia: A systematic review and meta-analysis. *Sleep Medicine Reviews, 24*, 1–12. https://doi.org/10.1016/j.smrv.2014.12.003

Lev-Ran, S., Le Foll, B., McKenzie, K., George, T. P., & Rehm, J. (2013). Cannabis use and cannabis use disorders among individuals with mental illness. *Comprehensive Psychiatry, 54*(6), 589–598. https://www.sciencedirect.com/science/article/pii/S0010440X13000187?via%3Dihub

Liu, M.,Gao, Y., Yuan, Y., Yang, K., Shi, S., Tian, J., & Zhang, J. (2021). Efficacy and safety of herbal medicine (Lianhuaqingwen) for treating COVID-19: A systematic review and meta-analysis. *Integrative Medicine Research, 10*, 100644. https://doi.org/10.1016/j.imr.2020.100644.

Miller, L. H., & Su, X. (2011). Artemisinin: Discovery from the Chinese herbal garden. *Cell, 146*(6), 855–858. https://doi.org/10.1016/j.cell.2011.08.024

Money, N. (2016). Are mushrooms medicinal? *Fungal Biology, 120,* 449–453. https://doi.org/10.1016/j.funbio.2016.01.006

Motta, F., Gershwin, M. E., & Selmi, C. (2021). Mushrooms and immunity. *Journal of Autoimmunity, 117,* 102576. https://doi.org/10.1016/j.jaut.2020.102576

Plotnikoff, G. A, Watanabe, K., & Yashiro, F. (2008). Kampo: From old wisdom comes new knowledge. *HerbalGram, 78,* 46–56. https://www.herbalgram.org/media/12021/issue78.pdf

Shigehara, K., Isumi, K., Nakashima, K., Kawaguchi, S. Nohara, T., Kadono, Y., & Mizokami, A. (2020). Efficacy and safety of keishibukuryogan, a traditional Japanese Camp medicine, for hot flashes in prostate cancer patients receiving androgen deprivation therapy. *Translational Andrology and Urology, 9*(6), 2533–2540. https://doi.org/10.21037/tau-20-901

Taira, K., Fujiwara, K., Fukuhara, T., Koyama, S., Takeuchi, H. (2020). The effect of Hangeshashinto on oral mucositis caused by induction chemotherapy in patients with head and neck cancer. *Yonago Acta Medica, 63*(3), 183–187. https://doi.org/10.33160/yam.2020.08007

Takayama, S., Tomita, N., Arita, R., Ono, R., Kikuchi, A., & Ishii, T. (2020). Kampo medicine for various aging-related symptoms: A review of geriatric syndrome. *Frontiers in Nutrition, 7*(86). https://doi.org/10.3389/fnut.2020.0086

U.S. Congress. (1994). *103rd Congress. Dietary Supplement Health and Education Act of 1994.* Pub. L. 103–417. 108 Stat/4325-4335. Library of Congress.

Ward, E., & Blumenthal, M. (2005). Americans confident in dietary supplements according to CRN survey. *HerbalGram, 66,* 64–65. https://www.herbalgram.org/resources/herbalgram/issues/66/table-of-contents/article2829/

Wasser, S. P. (2014). Medicinal mushrooms science: Current perspectives, advances, evidences, and challenges. *Biomedical Journal, 37*(6), 345–356. https://doi.org/10.4103/2319-4170.138318

Wyatt, G. K., Sikorskii, A., Safikhani, A., McVary, K. T., & Herman, J. (2015). Saw palmetto for symptom management during radiation therapy for prostate cancer. *Journal of Pain and Symptom Management, 51*(6), 1046–1054. https://doi.org/10.1016/j.jpainsymman.2015.12.315

Zhou, S. F., & Lai, X. (2008). An update on clinical drug interactions with the herbal antidepressant St. John's wort. *Current Drug Metabolism, 9*(5), 394–409. https://doi.org/10.2174/138920008784746391

21

Functional Foods and Nutraceuticals

MELISSA H. FRISVOLD

In the 21st century, the focus of the relationship between eating habits and health is changing from an emphasis on health maintenance through recommended dietary allowances of nutrients, vitamins, and minerals to an emphasis on the use of foods to provide better health, increase vitality, and aid in preventing disease and many chronic illnesses. The connection between food and health is not new. Indeed, the adage "Let food be your medicine and medicine your food" was adopted long ago by Hippocrates (1932). The interest and consumer demand for functional foods and nutraceuticals continue to grow, which drives progressive research into the identification of applications for nutraceutical substances (Wildman, 2020).

Nutraceuticals, because of their safety and potential nutritive and therapeutic effects, have received considerable attention (Shende et al., 2016). They provide a viable alternative to modern medicines and may be a useful tool in healthy living. Prescription drugs often have adverse effects that for some patients are difficult to tolerate. Nutraceuticals have the potential for various therapeutic effects such as antilipid, anti-inflammatory, anticancer, and antioxidant activity (AlAli et al., 2021). In addition, nutraceuticals may also be effective in the treatment of diabetes, obesity, and hypertension (Bergamin et al., 2019).

It is predicted that by 2027, the global nutraceutical market will reach USD 722.49 billion (Businesswire, 2020). Part of this industry growth is attributed to a greater interest in weight loss and caloric reduction in countries such as the United States, India, and China (Businesswire, 2020). In 2019, functional foods generated a revenue of USD 187.51 billion (Businesswire, 2020). Higher per capita income, increased consumer awareness regarding health and wellness, and a high urbanization rate are suggested reasons for the higher consumption in North America of dietary supplements (Research and Markets, 2021). Functional food, dietary supplements, prebiotics, probiotics, dietary fiber, and medical food are all different types of nutraceuticals (Maurya et al., 2021). Leading vendors in the nutraceutical product industry are Kraft Heinz Company (U.S.), Conagra (U.S.), General Mills (U.S.), Nestle (Switzerland), Amway (U.S.), Nature's Bounty (U.S.), Freedom Food Group Limited (Australia), The Hain Celestial Group (U.S.), and Pfizer Inc. (U.S.)

(Intrado GlobeNewswire, 2021). Examples of nutraceutical products made by these companies include health drinks, energy drinks, dietary supplements, juices, dairy beverages, infant nutrition, snacks, and bakery products. These products may be enhanced with prebiotics, vitamins, fiber, omega-3 fatty acid, probiotics, proteins, and amino acids (this list is not exhaustive; Intrado GlobeNewswire, 2021).

Coverage of all nutraceuticals is beyond the scope of this chapter. A plethora of functional foods and nutraceuticals exist. In the interest of brevity, several selected products are covered in depth in this chapter. As discussed previously, the sales of nutraceuticals and functional foods are consumer-driven. To this end, a few of the topics that are of high interest to the American consumer are discussed in this chapter. A survey conducted in 2016 by the International Food Information Council Foundation (IFIC) found that nearly half of consumers were interested in weight loss/management and that about one third of Americans listed increased energy, cardiovascular health, healthy aging, or digestive health to be topics of interest to them (Food Insight, 2017). Because the use of nutraceuticals is so prevalent and because their use may impact health and wellness, it is important that nurses and other healthcare professionals know about them and their potential benefits and risks.

DEFINITION

According to Stephen DeFelice (1994), the Foundation for Innovation in Medicine coined the term *nutraceutical* in 1989 to give an identity to an area of health and medicine that held great promise. According to the foundation, a nutraceutical is any substance that may be considered a food or part of a food and provides health benefits. These products may range from dietary supplements, isolated nutrients, and herbal products to genetically engineered designer foods. The number and variety of nutraceuticals available in the United States are staggering; for example, many grocery stores carry cereals fortified with omega-3 fatty acids, ginseng-enriched sports drinks, dairy products with various strains of probiotics, and orange juice that contains added calcium. The intent of the Dietary Supplement Health and Education Act (DSHEA), passed in 1994, was to protect the rights of consumers to have access to dietary supplements (and thus nutraceuticals and functional foods) to promote good health (Food and Drug Administration [FDA], 2012). Under the provisions of the law, dietary supplement ingredients are exempt from drug regulations; thus, premarketing approval, including demonstration of benefit and safety, is not required (Haller, 2010).

Until recently, a formal definition in the United States did not exist for the term *functional foods*, which created a challenge for researchers and developers of these foods that wanted to sell them or educate the public about their products (Martirosyan & Singh, 2015). The following definition was accepted at a 2014 conference attended by representatives from the U.S. Department of Agriculture (USDA), the Functional Food Center (FFC), the Academic Society for Functional Foods and Bioactive Compounds (ASFFBC), and the Agricultural Research Service (ARS), to facilitate better communication among scientists, government officials, the public, and food experts. The accepted definition of functional foods is "natural or processed foods that contain known or unknown biologically-active compounds; which, in defined, effective non-toxic amounts, provide a clinically proven and documented health benefit for the prevention, management, or treatment of chronic disease" (Martirosyan & Singh, 2015, p. 215). The definition identifies the following key points about functional foods:

- Functional foods can be processed or natural.
- Functional foods contain known or unknown biologically active compounds.
- Functional foods must provide a clinically proven and documented health benefit.
- Functional foods that contain bioactive compounds must be consumed in effective nontoxic amounts (Martirosyan & Singh, 2015).

The Japanese, who were among the first to use functional foods, have highlighted three conditions that define a functional food:

- It is a food (not a capsule, tablet, or powder) derived from naturally occurring ingredients.
- It can and should be consumed as part of a daily diet.
- It has a particular function when ingested, serving to regulate a particular body process: enhancement of the biological defense mechanism, prevention of a specific disease, recovery from a specific disease, control of physical and mental conditions, and slowing of the aging process (PA Consulting Group, 1990).

According to these definitions, unmodified whole foods such as fruits and vegetables represent the simplest form of a functional food. For example, broccoli, carrots, or tomatoes would be considered functional foods because they contain high levels of physiologically active components such as beta-carotene, lycopene, and sulforaphane. Modified foods, including those that have been fortified with nutrients or enhanced with phytochemicals, are also within the realm of functional foods.

SCIENTIFIC BASIS

During the past century, there have been many changes in the types of foods people eat, reflecting the application of scientific findings and technological innovations in the food industry. Although much research has been conducted on nutrition and health and disease, scientific exploration of the use of nutraceuticals has been more limited.

Interest in foodstuffs has generated investigation to link nutrient and food intake with improvements in health or the prevention of disease. Studies in the epidemiological literature have been reviewed and suggest a possible association between a low consumption of fruits and vegetables and the incidence of certain diseases such as heart disease (He et al., 2006, 2007; Wang et al., 2014). A 2019 meta-analysis suggested that turmeric and curcuminoids could significantly decrease triglycerides and low-density lipoprotein (LDL) cholesterol and increase high-density lipoprotein (HDL) cholesterol (Yuan et al., 2019). A recent analyses of the Women's Health Initiative (WHI) Dietary Modification (DM) Clinical Trial suggests that the adoption of increased vegetable, fruit and grain intake was associated with a reduction in death from cancer in postmenopausal women (Chlebowski et al., 2020).

Much scientific study has been conducted on the role of the various products added to normal foods to enhance their ability to inhibit or prevent diseases. Many researchers regard dietary intake as the best means of acquiring necessary nutrients (Kottke, 1998). For example, the World Cancer Research Fund International/ American Institute for Cancer Research (2017) recommends the consumption of foods mostly of plant origin, which may protect against certain types of cancers. It is important to point out that these foods contain various micronutrients; therefore, it is difficult to tease out whether a certain element of the food alone is responsible for an identified protective effect. However, supplementation of nutrients is common.

DIETARY PLANT STANOLS AND STEROLS

The cholesterol-lowering potential of dietary plant stanols and sterols has been known for many years (Jones et al., 2018; Plat et al., 2012). Natural sources of plant sterols and stanols do not have enough plant sterols to markedly decrease the LDL-C cholesterol; therefore, foods supplemented with plant sterols and stanols are a better option to lower cholesterol (National Lipid Association, 2021). The use of plant stanols at doses of 2 to 3 g daily is reported to be effective in lowering LDL cholesterol by 9% to 12% (Ras et al., 2014; Ruuth et al., 2020; Trautwein et al., 2018). The modification of plant stanols and sterols structurally enables them to be easily incorporated into fat-containing foods without losing their effectiveness in lowering cholesterol (Cater & Grundy, 1998). Dietary plant stanols and sterols inhibit the absorption of cholesterol in the small intestine, which, in turn, can lower LDL blood cholesterol (Cabral & Klein, 2017; de Jong et al., 2003).

Historically, plant stanols have been added to margarine-like products or yogurt drinks. Plant sterols are also available in the form of a tablet or a pill (Cleveland Clinic, 2019). A chewable plant stanol ester food supplement was evaluated in a randomized, double-blind, controlled 4-week intervention. A dose of 2g/day lowered LDL cholesterol by 7.6%, providing a convenient dietary tool to regulate cholesterol levels (Laitinen et al., 2017). It has been suggested that lifestyle modification, which includes dietary changes such as the inclusion of plant stanols and sterols, should be the primary treatment for lowering cholesterol (Turpeinen et al., 2012). Thus, functional foods might offer a safe and easily attainable method for decreasing heart disease risk (Turpeinen et al., 2012). The European Society of Cardiology (2016) has the following recommendations for health professionals to help make patient care decisions in their practice—plant stanols/sterols of at least 2g/day with the main meal may be considered: In adults and children older than age 6 with familial hypercholesterolemia, as an adjunct to pharmacological therapy in high-risk patients who fail to achieve LDL-C goals on statins (or cannot tolerate a statin) and for individuals with high cholesterol who do not qualify for statin therapy.

Plant sterols and their esters are generally recognized as safe (GRAS) food-grade substances, a designation indicating that there has been a history of safe intake of these products with no demonstrated harmful health effects found in the research (Cleveland Clinic, 2019; Wrick, 2005).

Collagen

Collagen is an important protein produced by the human body: it aids in wound and tissue healing and the repair of the scalp, gums, and cornea and helps repair bone and blood vessels (León-López et al., 2019). Aging is a complex process that involves the loss of collagen and elastin (Lupu et al., 2020). After age 40, the human body begins to lose collagen at the rate of 1% per year and by age 80, production in the body can decrease by about 75% compared to young adults (León-López et al., 2019).

Supplementation with oral collagen may have health and wellness benefits. For example, a pilot study on oral supplementation with collagen peptides concluded that collagen peptides, along with a calf-strengthening program, may benefit Achilles tendinopathy patients (Praet et al., 2019). Clinical trials have demonstrated that the use of daily collagen peptides improved skin hydration and elasticity and reduced signs of aging (Asserin et al., 2015). Nutraceutical collagen peptides may promote cutaneous wound closure. A small pilot study using nutraceutical collagen peptides demonstrated significant wound closure (Mistry et al., 2021).

Currently sources of collagen are bovine, porcine, poultry, and marine. It is sold as pills, gummies, powder, and liquid/drinks (alliedmarketresearch/collagen, 2021). Collagen hydrolysate, a bioactive peptide, is used the most in the development of nutraceuticals (León-López et al., 2019).

Cinnamon

The common spice cinnamon is obtained from the inner bark of the genus *Cinnamomum*, a tropical evergreen tree. In Ayurvedic medicine, cinnamon is considered a remedy for digestive, respiratory, and gynecologic ailments (Ranasinghe & Galappaththy, 2016). The German Commission E recognizes *Cinnamomum verum* and *Cinnamomum aromaticum* to treat dyspeptic complaints, bloating, flatulence, and loss of appetite (Deros & Maffioli, 2020). In vitro and in vivo studies have demonstrated numerous medicinal benefits of *Cinnamomum zeylanicum* (Ranasinghe et al., 2013). Cinnamon demonstrates antihyperglycemic properties (Hayward et al., 2019; Ranasinghe, & Galappaththy, 2016; Ranasinghe et al., 2013), may reduce LDL cholesterol (Jamali et al., 2020; Ranasinghe, & Galappaththy, 2016), increase HDL cholesterol (Ranasinghe, & Galappaththy, 2016), reduce trigylcerides (Jamali et al., 2020; Maierean et al., 2017), have antioxidant properties (Ranasinghe, & Galappaththy, 2016; Zhu et al., 2020), provides bactericidal and fungicidal activity (Ranasinghe et al., 2013), and lower blood pressure (Ghavami et al., 2021; Hadi et al., 2020; Jamali et al., 2020; Ranasinghe, & Galappaththy, 2016). In a study of women with polycystic ovarian syndrome, cinnamon supplementation improved serum glycemic indices and the lipid profile as well (Borzoei et al., 2018).

A meta-analysis and systematic review of the effects of cinnamon (*Cinnamomum Zeylanicum*) supplementation on C-reactive protein (CRP) suggests that cinnamon may improve levels of serum CRP (Vallianou et al., 2019). A systematic review and meta-analysis found that cinnamon supplementation significantly reduced body weight, body mass index, and waist-to-hip ratio (Yazdanpanah et al., 2020). In addition, cinnamon supplementation at a dose of greater than 2 grams per day for more than 12 weeks has been found to significantly impact obesity (Mousavi et al., 2020). Cinnamon supplementation may improve liver enzymes in patients with Type II diabetes (Mousavi et al., 2021). Patients with metabolic diseases may benefit from cinnamon supplementation because of its beneficial effects on various cardiometabolic risk factors (Kutbi et al., 2021). It has been hypothesized that cinnamon's medicinal benefits may arise from multiple mechanisms of action, such as increased glucose transporter-4 receptor synthesis, the inhibition of pancreatic amylase, and increased glycogen synthesis in the liver, which, in turn, improves insulin sensitivity, improves lipid levels, and ultimately provides improved glycemic control (Beejmohun et al., 2014).

Cinnamon supplements appear to be safe when consumed in foods as a spice. It is important to remember that there are several different types of cinnamon and to know which type the consumer is using. The U.S. Food and Drug Administration has listed cinnamon as safe (GRAS) to consume (USFDA, 2020). However, use in larger amounts may have side effects such as gastrointestinal problems. Cassia cinnamon contains coumarin, which may be harmful to the liver. Little is known about the safety of cinnamon in pregnancy or in breastfeeding in amounts greater than commonly found in foods. Ultimately, cinnamon should not be used in place of conventional medical care (National Center for Complementary and Integrative Health, 2021).

INTERVENTION

Many people are using nutraceuticals. Hence, it is important that nurses include assessing nutraceutical use when obtaining the health history of a patient. Exhibit 21.1 presents guidelines for nurses to use in assessing patients. Reputable websites for information about foods and nutraceuticals appear at the end of this chapter. Patients should be encouraged to be open about their use of nutraceuticals as part of communicating their preferences and efforts toward good health. Likewise, the response of health providers should be open and nonjudgmental, despite the potential need to counsel changes or discontinuance of a nutraceutical based on the evidence or knowledge of the provider. The expertise of professionals of other disciplines may be called on as well, through referral or consultation, to ensure that the patient receives up-to-date information from the latest evidence regarding the safety and efficacy of any foods or products used.

Exhibit 21.1 *Guidelines: Nutraceutical Assessment Guide for Nurses*

- Screen for nutraceutical use as a routine part of the health assessment interview process. Because surgical complications can arise from nutritional supplement use, their dosage is often discontinued a few weeks before surgery.
- Acquire a working knowledge of functional foods and nutraceuticals that includes benefits/risks, costs, and possible drug interactions.
- Develop effective communication strategies to ensure that all members of a patient's healthcare team are aware of any nutraceutical use.
- Explore the reasons for the use of nutritional supplements and functional foods. Can the same benefits be achieved by using another product that is safer or less expensive?
- Consider the unique healthcare needs of various populations. It is important that pregnant women, children, older adults, and populations with certain medical conditions discuss any nutritional supplementation use with their healthcare provider prior to initiation.
- Provide educational resources for patients that are easy to access, timely, evidence-based, and easy to understand.
- Remember to consult with and refer patients to nutritionists—knowledgeable and accessible resources in this promising and rapidly changing area of health and wellness.

MEASUREMENT OF OUTCOMES

Outcomes of therapy can be assessed in a number of ways, depending on the nutraceutical and the intent of the therapy. For example, blood levels of the nutrient or effect on the target organ (e.g., bone density, with the use of calcium) could be monitored over time. Also, it is important that potential side effects of the therapy be evaluated in periodic physical assessments and comprehensive histories. Positive or negative changes in subjective health, energy, and symptoms, or those subsequent to changes in nutraceutical use, can also be assessed in individuals as data for tolerance as part of cost–benefit evaluation. Effective teaching of nutraceutical principles, intended purpose, and doses and effects of functional foods will result in informed use by clients and greater awareness of intended and adverse effects.

PRECAUTIONS

It is of paramount importance that nutraceutical use be assessed as part of the health history and nutritional assessment. Safe use, including safe dosage, drug interactions, and side effects, must be carefully considered. MEDLINE offers a system for checking interactions among commonly used nutraceuticals and prescription drugs (MEDLINE, 2021).

A consistent concern cited in the literature is the lack of regulation of nutraceuticals. Nutraceuticals are classified as dietary supplements and are required to register their facility with the FDA. Like the food industry, manufacturers of nutraceuticals are expected to comply with Current Good Manufacturing Practices (see the Electronic Code of Federal Regulations, 2021). The labeling standards for dietary supplements are similar to the food industry. There are, however, standards for what health claims can be made and how supplements are marketed (FDA Reader, 2019).

One safety mechanism in place to ensure the production of quality products for consumers is a voluntary dietary supplement verification program through the U.S. Pharmacopeial Convention (USP). If a product contains the USP-verified mark on its label, it demonstrates that the item has been tested and audited as a supplement that meets certain criteria for declared potency and amount, that it does not contain harmful levels of contaminants, and that it meets the FDA's good manufacturing practices (U.S. Pharmacopeial Convention, 2021).

USES

Nutraceuticals and functional foods have been used to promote health and prevent and treat illness. Functional foods and nutraceuticals can be used to target deficiencies, establish optimal nutritional balance, or treat diseases. Because heart disease, cancer, and stroke are leading causes of death in the United States, greater access to nutraceuticals that have been shown to improve risk-factor profiles is desirable. Furthermore, people in the United States and worldwide could benefit from nutraceuticals when deficiencies of specific nutrients are noted.

CHILDREN AND ADOLESCENTS

Nutraceuticals and functional foods may also play an important role in the health of children and adolescents. A study by Mintel in 2018, found that 25% of teens aged 15 to 17 years said they worry about staying healthy. Many of the nutraceuticals or functional food products come from the food manufacturing industry. For example, Cargill (2018) has been building better snacks for kids through the supplementation of nutritional products, such as chicory root fiber and prebiotic fibers; the use of alternative grains, such as chia and sorghum; and adding turmeric, beetroot, and sweet potato to substitute for artificial colors. Cargill has also found ways to hide healthfulness into their food products, such as using cauliflower pizza crust, macaroni and cheese with chickpea pasta, and adding vegetable servings to smoothies, desserts, and shakes.

Probiotics may be useful in preventing antibiotic-associated diarrhea (AAD) in children. Antibiotics are often prescribed to children; however, these agents alter the microbial balance within the gastrointestinal tract and may cause diarrhea. The Cochrane IBD Group concluded that there is moderate evidence to support the use of probiotics in the treatment of AAD (Guo et al., 2019).

Heart disease, once thought to be a disease of aging, is now recognized as starting in childhood (Brothers, 2017). One recommended approach to this problem is through dietary interventions that treat dyslipidemia with a low-fat diet supplemented with water-soluble fiber, plant stanols, and plant sterols in children older than age 6 with familial hypercholesterolemia (Gylling et al., 2014; Kwiterovich, 2008).

In 2001, the American Academy of Pediatrics (AAP) published a landmark survey of its members that looked at the beliefs and use of complementary and alternative therapies (CAM) in their respective practices. Based on the findings of this survey, in 2002, the AAP developed a task force to educate families, patients, and physicians about complementary therapies. One outcome of this task force was the recommendation to research the use of CAM therapies in the pediatric population. It is important to recognize that many families are using nutraceuticals such as nutritional supplements or functional foods with their children. Approximately one third of children and adolescents in the United State use dietary supplements (Stierman et al., 2020). The most frequently used supplements were multivitamin-mineral, single-ingredient vitamin D, single-ingredient vitamin C, a probiotic, melatonin, omega-3 fatty acid, botanical, and a multivitamin (Stierman et al., 2020).

WOMEN'S HEALTH AND NUTRITIONAL NEEDS

Throughout the life span, women have unique nutritional needs that place them at risk for nutrition-related diseases and conditions. Nutrition has been shown to have a significant influence on the risk of chronic disease and on the maintenance of optimal health status. A balanced diet is a key component of women's health. Foods such as iron-fortified cereals and calcium-fortified cereals and juices may be necessary to meet daily requirements. Although food should be the first choice in meeting such needs, nutritional supplementation may be necessary. Following are some examples of increased nutritional needs across the life span of women (Academy of Nutrition and Dietetics, 2021):

■ An increase in calcium during pregnancy and menopause is necessary.
■ Vitamin D needs increase as women age.
■ Folate and folic acid requirements increase during pregnancy to prevent birth defects.

■ Iron needs increase during menstruation and pregnancy and are lower after menopause.

It is also important to remember that intake of certain nutrients above a certain level can be teratogenic (e.g., too much vitamin A in the first trimester of pregnancy), and because many foods are often enriched with vitamins and minerals, it is possible to consume too much.

CULTURAL APPLICATIONS

The influence of culture on both the use and acceptance of functional foods is an important consideration. Food choices can be influenced by cultural identity in many societies (Reddy & van Dam, 2020). Food culture is defined as the practices, attitudes, and beliefs surrounding food and incorporates heritage and ethnicity. Since food culture can greatly impact health, understanding the culture of food is important for healthcare providers in order to monitor and evaluate changes and help develop interventions that are consistent with each person's culture (Kanter & Gittelsohn, 2020).

According to Kanter and Gittelsohn (2020), food culture is a ubiquitous aspect of all societies. A functional food or nutraceutical is more likely to be accepted if it is consistent with culture. A study by Mullie et al. (2009) found a correlation

Sidebar 21.1 *Nutraceuticals in Uganda*

Faith Sebuliba, Mukono, Uganda

Uganda is a country of oral traditions, therefore, most information about functional medicine and nutraceuticals is not written down. Information is passed down from generation to generation directly through verbal communication. I gathered information for this chapter by talking to a traditional herbalist and faculty from the Mukono Diocese School of Nursing & Midwifery.

The use of "nutraceuticals" is not common in Uganda. The reasons for this are thought to be related to cost. In addition, information about nutraceutical products is not well known.

Pineapple, lemon, ginger, avocado leaves, hibiscus leaves, and tea leaves are some of the foods that have medicinal use in Uganda. For example, it is not uncommon to brew leaves from avocado or hibiscus leaves to make tea. The tea made from avocado leaves is used to strengthen the blood and decrease anemia. Clay is mixed with herbs to make a poultice or make it into a drink or dry it for chewing. The poultice is used in pregnancy to soften bones to allow the baby to fit more easily through the birth canal. The dry clay is chewed to prevent nausea. These foods and herbs are readily available in the yards or gardens of many people in Uganda. Clay is sold on the streets of Uganda. These natural remedies are passed through oral traditions and the use of an herbalist is reserved for unusual cases. Most herbalists are known in the villages and do not charge a fee; however, those who advertise are the ones who do it as a business (processing, packaging, selling).

between culture and the intake of functional foods. For example, soy is widely used in Asian cultures and is considered to be a traditional food source, with customary soy intake being estimated at 30 to 50 g per day (Cornwell et al., 2004). Hence, the use of soy as a nutraceutical may be more widely and easily accepted by someone in an Asian culture because this food is already so widely used. In addition, how food itself is viewed within the context of culture may have a strong influence on the use of nutraceuticals and functional foods. The use of nutraceuticals in Uganda is described in Sidebar 21.1.

FUTURE RESEARCH

Although nutraceuticals have a long-standing historical use, increased interest in these substances to promote health, prevent disease, and treat specific medical conditions is reflected in heightened attention to nutritional science and growing consumption. A consistent theme throughout this chapter (and in this chapter published in previous editions of this book) has been the need for more research in this area. A review of the literature for this chapter consistently demonstrated that many of the articles were older than five years and reaffirmed the need for updated studies on nutraceuticals and functional foods. The book *Complementary and Alternative Medicine in the United States* (Institute of Medicine, 2005) summarizes succinctly what the goal for research in this arena should be: "In terms of medical therapies, a commitment to public welfare is the obligation to generate and provide to healthcare practitioners, policy makers, and the public access to the best information available on the efficacy of CAM therapies" (p. 169). Consistent with this sentiment, and because there is so much interest and hope in this area, interdisciplinary research teams may explore the following questions:

- Which of the current nutraceuticals should be incorporated into a normal diet on a regular basis to promote health?
- Are nutraceuticals cost-effective?
- What are the side effects associated with short- and long-term use of specific nutraceuticals?
- Can we increase research on the use of nutraceuticals in pediatric populations?
- What are innovative ways to educate healthcare providers about nutraceuticals?
- Can we discover more effective methods to educate the U.S. healthcare consumer and consumers around the globe about the benefits and risks of nutraceuticals?
- How does culture affect the use of functional foods?

WEBSITES

Reputable websites for information about foods and nutraceuticals include the following:

- Academy of Nutrition and Dietetics (www.eatright.org)
- American Nutraceutical Association (https://ancorpusa.com)
- International Food Information Council (https://ific.org)
- Food Insight (www.foodinsight.org)
- Journal of Nutraceuticals and Food Science (https://nutraceuticals.imedpub .com)

- Mayo Clinic (www.mayoclinic.org)
- National Institutes of Health—National Center for Complementary and Integrative Health (https://nccih.nih.gov)
- National Institutes of Health—National Library of Medicine (www.nlm.nih.gov)
- National Institutes of Health—Office of Dietary Supplements (https://ods.od.nih.gov)
- Natural Medicines Comprehensive Database (https://naturalmedicines.therapeuticresearch.com)
- U.S. Department of Agriculture—Food and Nutrition Information Center (www.nal.usda.gov/fnic)
- U.S. Department of Health and Human Services—Office of Disease Prevention and Health Promotion (https://health.gov)
- U.S. Food and Drug Administration—Center for Food Safety and Applied Nutrition (www.fda.gov/aboutfda/centersoffices/officeoffoods/cfsan)

REFERENCES

Academy of Nutrition and Dietetics. (2021). *Healthy eating for women.* http://www.eatright.org/resource/food/nutrition/dietary-guidelines-and-myplate/healthy-eating-for-women

AlAli, M., Alqubaisy, M., Aljaafari, M. N., AlAli, A. O., Baqais, L., Molouki, A., Abushelaibi, A., Lai, K.-S., & Lim, S.-H. E. (2021). Nutraceuticals: transformation of conventional foods into health promoters/disease preventers and safety considerations. *Molecules, 26,* 2540. https://doi.org/10.3390/molecules26092540

American Academy of Pediatrics. (2001). *Periodic Survey #49: Complementary and alternative medicine (CAM) therapies in pediatric practices.* http://www.aap.org/research/periodicsurvey/ps49bex.htm

Asserin, J., Lati, E., Shioya, T., & Prawitt, J. (2015). The effect of oral collagen peptide supplementation on skin moisture and the dermal collagen network: Evidence from an ex vivo model and randomized, placebo-controlled clinical trials. *Journal of Cosmetic Dermatology, 14*(4), 291–301. https://doi.org/10.1111/jocd.12174

Beejmohun, V., Peytavy-Izard, M., Mignon, C., Muscente-Paque, D., Deplanque, X., Ripoll, C., & Chapal, N. (2014). Acute effect of Ceylon cinnamon extract on postprandial glycemia: Alpha-amylase inhibition, starch tolerance test in rats, and randomized crossover clinical trial in healthy volunteers. *BMC Complementary and Alternative Medicine, 14,* 351. https://doi.org/10.1186/1472-6882-14-351

Bergamin. A., Mantzioris, E., Cross, G., Deo, P., Garg, S., & Hill, J. A. M. (2019). Nutraceuticals: reviewing their role in chronic disease prevention and management. *Pharmaceutical Medicine, 33*(4), 291–309. https://doi.org/10.1007/s40290-019-00289-w

Borzoei, A., Rafraf, M., & Asghari-Jafarabadi, A. (2018). Cinnamon improves metabolic factors without detectable effects on adiponectin in women with polycystic ovary syndrome. *Asia Pacific Journal of Clinical Nutrition, 27*(3), 556–563. https://doi.org/10.6133/apjcn.062017.13

Brothers, J. (2017, September 6). High cholesterol can be a danger for kids, too. *Children's Hospital of Philadelphia Health Tip of the Week Newsletter.* https://www.chop.edu/news/high-cholesterol-can-be-danger-kids-too

Businesswire. (2020). *$722+ billion nutraceutical market size and share breakdown by product and region – ResearchandMarkets.com.* https://www.businesswire.com/news/home/20200520005477/en/722-Billion-Nutraceutical-Market-Size-and-Share-Breakdown-by-Product-and-Region---ResearchAndMarkets.com

Cabral, E. E., & Klein, M. R. (2017). Phytosterols in the treatment of hypercholesterolemia and prevention of cardiovascular diseases. *Arquivos Brasileiros de Cardiologia, 109*(5). https://doi.org/10.5935/abc.20170158

Cargill. (2018). *What kids want: Exploring the changing world of kids' food products.* https://www.cargill.com/doc/1432133870774/kids-food-products.pdf

Cater, N. B., & Grundy, S. M. (1998). Lowering serum cholesterol with plant sterols and stanols: Historical perspectives. In T. T. Nguyen (Ed.), *New developments in the dietary management of high cholesterol* (Postgraduate Medicine Special Report, pp. 6–14). McGraw Hill.

Chlebowski, R. T., Aragaki, A. K., Anderson, G. L., Pan, K., Neuhouser, M. L., Manson, J. E., Thomson, C. A., Mossavar-Rahmani, Y., Lane, D. S., Johnson, K. C., Wactawski-Wende, J., Snetselaar, L., Rohan, T. E., Luo, J., & Barac, A. (2020). Dietary modification and breast cancer mortality: Long term follow up of the women's health initiative randomized trial. *Journal Clinical Oncology, 38*, 1419–1428. https://doi.org/10.1200/JCO.19.00435

Cleveland Clinic. (2019). *Boost your cholesterol-lowering potential with phytosterols*. https://my.clevelandclinic.org/health/articles/17368-phytosterols-sterols--stanols

Cornwell, T., Cohick, W., & Raskin, I. (2004). Dietary phytoestrogens and health. *Phytochemistry, 65*, 995–1016. https://doi.org/10.1016/j.phytochem.2004.03.005

DeFelice, S. L. (1994). *What is a true nutraceutical and what is the nature & size of the U.S. nutraceutical market?* The Foundation for Innovation in Medicine. http://www.fimdefelice.org/p2462.html

de Jong, A., Plat, J., & Mensink, R. P. (2003). Metabolic effects of plant sterols and stanols [review]. *Journal of Nutritional Biochemistry, 14*(7), 362–369. https://doi.org/10.1016/S0955-2863(03)00002-0

Deros, G., & Maffioli, P. (2020). Nutraceutical herbs and insulin resistance. In R. Wildman & R. Bruno (Eds.), *Handbook of nutraceuticals and functional foods* (3rd ed., pp. 232). TCRC Press.

Electronic Code of Federal Regulations. (2021). Title 21, Chapter 1, Subchapter B, Part 111. *Current good manufacturing practice in manufacturing, packaging, labeling or holding operations for dietary supplements*. https://www.ecfr.gov/cgi-bin/retrieveECFR?gp=&SID=afbc29dec95942418f63bc6d27f5a895&mc=true&n=pt21.2.111&r=PART&ty=HTML#sp21.2.111.e

European Society of Cardiology/European Atherosclerosis Society. (2016). *EAS/EAS Guidelines for the management of dyslipidaemias*. https://ora.ox.ac.uk/objects/uuid:b66cfed8-126f-4ed3-ac5a-cc6225b0e141/download_file?file_format=pdf&safe_filename=ESC_EAS_20dyslipidaemia_GL_document_third_revision_FINAL.pdf&type_of_work=Journal+article

FDA Reader. (2019). *How the FDA regulates nutraceuticals*. https://www.fdareader.com/blog/how-the-fda-regulates-nutraceuticalsgo

Food and Drug Administration. (2012). *Dietary supplements*. http://www.fda.gov/food/dietarysupplements

Food Insights. (2017). *Functional foods, sustainability, protein, CRISPR and what's "healthy" among top U.S. food and nutrition trends in 2017*. https://foodinsight.org/functional-foods-sustainability-protein-crispr-and-whats-healthy-among-top-u-s-food-and-nutrition-trends-in-2017/

Ghavami, A., Haghighian, H. K., Roshanravan, N., Ziaei, R., Ghaedi, E., Moravejolahkami, A. R., & Askari, G. (2021). What is the impact of cinnamon supplementation on blood pressure? A systematic review and meta-analysis. *Endocrine, Metabolic & Immune Disorders Drug Targets, 21*, 956–965. https://doi.org/10.2174/1871530320666200729143614

Globenewswire. (2021). *Nutraceutical products market size to reach USD 461.70 Bn by 2027/growing demand for fortified food owing to the increasing health consciousness amongst consumers will be the major factor driving the industry growth, says reports and data*. https://www.globenewswire.com/en/news-release/2021/01/28/2166007/0/en/Nutraceutical-Products-Market-Size-To-Reach-USD-461-70-Bn-By-2027-Growing-Demand-for-Fortified-Food-Owing-to-the-Increasing-Health-Consciousness-Amongst-Consumers-will-be-the-Major.html

Guo, Q., Goldenberg, J. Z., Humphrey, C., El Dib, R., & Johnston, B. C. (2019). Probiotics for the prevention of antibiotic-associated diarrhea. *Cochrane Database of Systematic Reviews*, (4), CD004827. https://doi.org/10.1111/jocd.12174

Gylling, H., Plat, J., Turley, S., Ginsberg, H. N., Ellegard, L., Jessup, W., Jones, P. J., Lutjohann, D., Maerz, W., Masana, L., Silbernagel, G., Staels, B., Boren, J., Catapano, A. L., De Backer, G., Deanfield, J., Descamps, O. S., Kovanen, P. T., Riccardi, G., Tokgozoglu, L., & Chapman, M. J. (2014). Plant sterols and plant stanols in the management of dyslipidaemia and

prevention of cardiovascular disease. *Atherosclerosis, 232*(2), 346–360. https://doi.org/10.1016/j
.atherosclerosis.2013.11.043

Hadi, A., Campbell, M. S., Hassani, B., Pourmasoumi, M., Salehi-Sahlabadi, A., & Hosseini, S.
A. (2020). The effect of cinnamon supplementation on blood pressure in adults: A systematic review and meta-analysis of randomized controlled trials. *Clinical Nutrition ESPEN, 36,*
10–16. https://doi.org/10.1016/j.clnesp.2020.01.002

Haller, C. A. (2010). Nutraceuticals: Has there been any progress? *Clinical Pharmacology &
Therapeutics, 87*(2), 137–141. https://doi.org/10.1038/clpt.2009.250

Hayward, N. J., McDougall, G. J., Farag, S., Allwood, J. W., Austin, C., Campbell, F., Horgan, G.,
& Ranawana, V. (2019). Cinnamon shows antidiabetic properties that are species-specific:
Effects on enzyme activity inhibition and starch digestion. *Plant Foods for Human Nutrition,
74,* 544–522. https://doi.org/10/1007/s11130-019-00760-8

He, F. J., Nowson, C. A., Lucas, M., & MacGregor, G. A. (2007). Increased consumption of fruit
and vegetables is related to a reduced risk of coronary heart disease: Meta-analysis of cohort
studies. *Journal of Hypertension, 21*(9), 717–728. https://doi.org/10.1038/sj.jhh.1002212

He, F. J., Nowson, C. A., & MacGregor, G. A. (2006). Fruit and vegetable consumption and
stroke: Meta-analysis of cohort studies. *Lancet, 367,* 320–326. https://doi.org/10.1016/S0140
-6736(06)68069-0

Hippocrates. (1932). *Hippocrates* (W. H. S. Jones, Trans.). Harvard University Press.

Institute of Medicine. (2005). *Complementary and alternative medicine in the United States.* National
Academies Press.

Jamali, N., Jalali, M., Saffari-Chaleshtori, J., Samare-Najaf, M., & Samareh, A. (2020). Effect of cinnamon supplementation on blood pressure and anthropometric parameters in patients with
type 2 diabetes: A systematic review and meta-analysis of clinical trials. *Diabetes & Metabolic
Syndrome, 14,* 119–125. https://doi.org/10.1016/j.dsx.2020.01.009

Jones, P. J. H., Shamloo, M., MacKay, D. S., Rideout, T. C., Myrie, S. B., Plat, J., Roullet, J. B., Baer, D.
J., Calkins, K. L., Davis, H. R., Duell, P. B., Ginsberg, H., Gylling, H., Jenkins, D., Lutjohann,
D., Moghadasian, M., Moreau, R. A., Mymin, D., Ostlund, Jr, R. E., . . . , Weingartner, O. (2018).
Progress and perspectives in plant sterol and plant stanol research. *Nutrition Reviews, 76*(10),
725–746. https://doi.org/10.1093/nutrit/nuy032

Kanter, R., & Gittelsohn, J. (2020). Measuring food culture: a tool for public health practice.
Current Obesity Reports, 9, 480–492. https://doi.org/10.1007/s13679-020-00414-w

Kottke, M. K. (1998). Scientific and regulatory aspects of nutraceutical products in the United
States. *Drug Development and Industrial Pharmacy, 24*(12), 1177–1195. https://doi.org/
10.3109/03639049809108576

Kutbi, E. H., Sohouli, M. H., Fatahi, S., Lari, A., Shidfar, F., Aljhdali, M. M., Alhoshan, F. M.,
Elahi, S. S., Almusa, H. A., & Abu-Zaid, A. (2021). The beneficial effects of cinnamon among
patients with metabolic diseases: a systematic review and dose-response meta-analysis of
randomized-controlled trials. *Critical Reviews in Food Science & Nutrition,* 1–19. https://doi
.org/10.1080/10408398.2021.1896473

Kwiterovich, P. (2008). Recognition and management of dyslipidemia in children and adolescents. *Journal of Clinical Endocrinology & Metabolism, 93*(11), 4200–4209. https://doi.org/10.1210/
jc.2008-1270

Laitinen, K., Gylling, H., Kaipiainen, L., Nissinen, M. J., & Simonen, P. (2017). Cholesterol lowering efficacy of plant stanol ester in a new type of product matrix, a chewable dietary supplement. *Journal of Functional Foods, 30,* 119–124. https://doi.org/10.1016/j.jff.2017.01.012

León-López, A., Morales-Peñaloza, A., Martinez-Juárez, V. M., Vargas-Torres, A., Zeugolis, D.
I., & Aguirre-Álvarez, G. (2019). Hydrolyzed collagen---sources and applications. *Molecules,
24*(22), 4031. https://doi.org/10.3390/molecules24224031

Lupu, M-A., Pircalabioru, G. G., Chifiriuc, M-C., Albulescu, R., & Tanase, C. (2020). Beneficial
effects of food supplements based on hydrolyzed collagen for skin care (review). *Experimental
and Therapeutic Medicine, 20*(1), 12–17. https://doi.org/10.3892/etm.2019.8342

Maierean, S. M., Serban, M. C., Sahebkar, A., Penson, P., & Banach, M. (2017). The effects of cinnamon supplementation on blood lipid concentrations: A systematic review and meta-analysis. *Journal of Clinical Lipidology, 11*(6), 1393–1406. https://doi.org/10/1016/j.jacl .2017.08.004

Martirosyan, D. M., & Singh, J. (2015). A new definition of functional food by FFC: What makes a new definition unique? *Functional Foods in Health and Disease, 5*(6), 209–223.

Maurya, A. P., Chauhan, J., Yadav, D. K., Gangwar, R., & Maurya, V. K. (2021). Nutraceuticals and their impact on human health. In C. Egbuna, A. P. Mishra, & M. R. Goyal (Eds.), *Preparation of phytopharmaceuticals for the management of disorders, the development of nutraceuticals and traditional medicine* (pp. 229–254). Elsevier. https://doi.org/10.1016/B978-0-12-820284-5.00011-3

MEDLINE. (2021). *Drugs, herbs and supplements.* https://medlineplus.gov/druginformation.html

Mintel. (2018). *IFT18: Generation Z set to impact the future of food and drink innovation.* https:// www.mintel.com/press-centre/food-and-drink/generation-z-set-to-impact-the-future -of-food-and-drink-innovation

Mistry, K., van derSteen, B., Clifford, T., vanHolthoon, F., Kleinnijenhuis, A., Prawwitt, J., Labus, M., Vanhoecke, B., Lovat, P. E., & McConnell, A. (2021). Potentiating cutaneous wound healing in young and aged skin with nutraceutical collagen peptides. *Clinical and Experimental Dermatology, 46,* 109–117. https://doi.org/10.1111/ced.14392

Mousavi, S. M., Jayedi, A., Bagheri, A., Zargarzadeh, N., Wong, A., Persad, E., Akhgarjand, C., & Koohdani, F. (2021). What is the influence of cinnamon supplementation on liver enzymes? A systematic review and meta-analysis of randomized controlled trials. *Phytotherapy Research, 35,* 5634. https://doi.org/10.1002/ptr.7200

Mousavi, S. M., Rahmani, J., Kord-Varkaneh, H., Sheikhi, A., Larijani, B., & Esmaillzadeh, A. (2020). Cinnamon supplementation positively affects obesity: A systematic review and dose-response meta-analysis of randomized controlled trials. *Clinical Nutrition, 39,* 123–133. https://doi.org/10.1016/j.clnu.2019.02.017

Mullie, P., Guelinckx, I., Clarys, P., Degrave, E., Hulens, M., & Vansant, G. (2009). Cultural, socioeconomic and nutritional determinants of functional food consumption patterns. *European Journal of Clinical Nutrition, 63,* 1290–1296. https://doi.org/10.1038/ejcn.2009.89

National Center for Complementary and Integrative Health. (2021). *Cinnamon.* https://www .nccih.nih.gov/health/cinnamon

National Lipid Association. (2021). *Plant sterols and stanols in foods and supplement.* https://www .lipid.org/sites/default/files/plant_sterols_im_food_sterol_supplements.pdf

PA Consulting Group. (1990). *Functional foods: A new global added value market?*

Plat, J., Mackay, D., Baumgartner, S., Clifton, P. M., Gylling, H., & Jones, P. J. J. (2012). Progress and prospective of plant sterol and plant stanol research: Report of the Maastricht meeting. *Atherosclerosis, 225,* 521–533. https://doi.org/10.1016/j.atherosclerosis.2012.09.018

Praet, S. F. E., Purdam, C. R., Welvaert, M., Vlahovich, N., Lovell, G., Burke, L. M., Gaida, J. E., Manzanero, S., Hughes, D., & Waddington, G. (2019). Oral supplementation of specific collagen peptides combined with calf-strengthening exercises enhances function and reduces pain in Achilles tendinopathy patients. *Nutrients, 11*(1), 76. https://doi.org/10.3390/ nu11010076

Ranasinghe, P., & Galappaththy, P. (2016). Health benefits of Ceylon cinnamon (Cinnamomum zeylanicum): A summary of the current evidence. *The Ceylon Medical Journal, 61*(1), 1–5. https://doi.org/10.4038/cmj.v61i1.8251

Ranasinghe, P., Pigera, S., Premakumara, G. A., Galappaththy, P., Constantine, G. R., & Katulanda, P. (2013). Medicinal properties of 'true' cinnamon (Cinnamomum zeylanicum): A systematic review. *BMC Complementary and Alternative Medicine, 12,* 275. https://doi .org/10.1186/1472-6882/13/275

Ras, R. T., Geleijnse, J. M., & Trautwein, E. A. (2014). LDL-cholesterol-lowering effect of plant sterols and stanols across different dose ranges: A meta-analysis of randomised controlled studies. *British Journal of Nutrition, 112,* 214–219. https://doi.org/10.1017/S0007114514000750

Reddy, G., & van Dam, R. M. (2020). Food, culture, and identity in multicultural societies: Insights from Singapore. *Appetite, 149,* 104633. https://doi.org/10.1016/j.appet.2020.104633

Research and Markets. (2021). *Global $272.4 billion dietary supplements market to 2028 – shift from pharmaceutical to nutraceutical products.* https://www.globenewswire.com/news-rele ase/2021/03/19/2196106/28124/en/Global-272-4-Billion-Dietary-Supplements-Market-to -2028-Shift-From-Pharmaceutical-To-Nutraceutical-Products.html

Ruuth, M., Aikas, L., Tigistu-Sahle, F., Lindholm, H., Simonen, P., Kovanen, P. T., Gylling, H., & Oorni, K. (2020). Plant stanol esters reduce LDL (Low-density lipoprotein) aggregation by altering LDL surface lipids. *Atherosclerosis, Thrombosis and Vascular Biology, 40*(9), 2310–2321. https://doi.org/10.1161/ATVBAHA.120.314329

Shende, P., Desai, D., & Gaud, R. S. (2016). Nutraceuticals: An imperative to wellness. *Research and Reviews: Journal of Pharmacy and Pharmaceutical Sciences, 5,* 69–74. https://www.rroij.com/ open-access/nutraceuticals-an-imperative-to-wellness-.pdf

Stierman, G., Mishra, S., Gahche, J. J., Potischman, G., & Hales, C. M. (2020). Dietary supple-ment use in children and adolescents aged < 19 years – United States, 2017–2018. *MMWR Morbidity, Mortality Weekly, 69,* 1557–1562. https://doi.org/10.15585/mmwr.mm6943a1

Trautwein, D. A., Koppenol, W. P., de Jong, A., Hiemstra, H., Vermeer, M. A., Noakes, M., & Luscombe-Marsh, D. D. (2018). Plant sterols lower LDL-cholesterol and triglycerides in dyslipidemic individuals with or at risk of developing type 2 diabetes; a randomized, double-blind, placebo-controlled study. *Nutrition & Diabetes, 8,* 30. https://doi.org/10.1038/ s41387-018-0039-8

Turpeinen, A. M., Ikonen, M., Kivimäki, A. S., Kautiainen, H., Vapaatalo, H., & Korpela, R. (2012). A spread containing bioactive milk peptides Ile–Pro–Pro and Val–Pro–Pro, and plant sterols has antihypertensive and cholesterol-lowering effects. *Food and Function, 3,* 621–627. https:// doi.org/10.1039/c2fo10286b

U.S. Department of Health and Human Services. (2020). USFDA. Department of Health and Human services. CFR- Code of Federal Regulations [Title-21, volume-3] revised on April 1, 2019; part-182- *Substances generally recognized as safe.* https://www.ecfr.gov/current/title-21/ chapter-I/subchapter-B/part-182

U.S. Pharmacopeial Convention. (2021). *USP verified dietary supplements.* https://www.quality -supplements.org/

Vallianou, N., Tsang, C., Taghizadeh, M., Davoodvandi, A., & Jafarnejad, S. (2019). Effect of cin-namon (Cinnamomum Zeylanidum) supplementation on serum C-reactive protein concen-trations: A meta-analysis and systematic review. *Complementary Therapies in Medicine, 42,* 271–278. https://doi.org/10.1016/j.ctim.2018.12.005

Wang, X., Ouyang, Y., Liu, J., Zhu, M., Zhao, G., Bao, W., & Hu, F. B. (2014). Fruit and vegetable consumption and mortality from all causes, cardiovascular disease, and cancer: Systematic review and dose-response meta-analysis of prospective cohort studies. *British Medical Journal, 349,* g4490. https://doi.org/10.1136/bmj.g4490

Wildman, R. E. C. (2020). Overview of nutraceuticals and functional foods. In R. Wildman & R. Bruno (Eds.), *Handbook of nutraceuticals and functional foods* (3rd ed., p. 3). TCRC Press.

World Cancer Research Fund International. (2017). *Our cancer prevention recommendation— Plant foods.* http://www.wcrf.org/int/research-we-fund/cancer-prevention-recommenda tions/plant-foods

Wrick, K. L. (2005). The impact of regulations in the business of nutraceuticals in the United States: Yesterday, today and tomorrow. In C. M. Hasler (Ed.), *Regulation of functional foods & nutraceuticals: A global perspective* (pp. 3–36). Wiley-Blackwell.

Yazdanpanah, Z., Azadi-Yazdi, M., Hooshmandi, H., Ramezani-Jolfaie, N., & Salehi-Abargouei, A. (2020). Effects of cinnamon supplementation on body weight and composition in adults: A systematic review and meta-analysis of controlled clinical trials. *Phytotherapy Research, 34,* 448–463. https://doi.org/10.1002/ptr.6539

Yuan, F., Dong, H., Gong, J., Wang, D., Hu, Meilin, Huang, Wenya, Fang, K., Qin, X., Qui, A., Yang, X., & Lu, F. (2019). A systematic review and meta-analysis of randomized controlled trials on the effects of turmeric and curcuminoids on blood lipids in adults with metabolic diseases. *Advances in Nutrition, 10*(5), 791–802. https://doi.org/10.1093/advances/nmz021

Zhu, C., Yan, H., Zheng, Y., Santos, H. O., Macit, M. S., & Zhao, K. (2020). Impact of cinnamon supplementation on cardiometabolic biomarkers of inflammation and oxidative stress: A systematic review and meta-analysis of randomized controlled trials. *Complementary Therapies in Medicine, 53*, 102517. https://doi.org/10.1016/j.ctim.2020 02517

V

Energy-Healing Therapies

CORJENA CHEUNG

According to the National Center for Complementary and Integrative Health (NCCIH, 2021), energy healing therapies are techniques that involve channeling healing energy through the hands of a practitioner into the client's body to restore a normal energy balance and, therefore, health. These therapies are based on the belief that the human body has a subtle energy system that interpenetrates the physical anatomy and extends outward beyond it. Energy healing offers the potential for a shift in physiological state and present moment awareness that may be a first step in altering the perspectives that sustain symptom burden (Rao et al., 2016). These therapies are often used with other complementary therapies and conventional medical treatments to treat a wide variety of ailments and health problems.

The concept of energy and its use is universal. Most cultures have a word to describe energy: *Qi* (pronounced *chee*) is a basic element of traditional Chinese medicine (TCM); *ki* is the Japanese word for energy; in India, it is *prana*; the Dakota Indian word for energy is *ton*; and the Sioux Indian word is *waken*. Scientists and consumers express some skepticism about the efficacy of energy-healing therapies because of the difficulty in determining how energy works and how the effects can be measured. As technology evolves, new ways to detect what has previously seemed invisible are being discovered.

Persons sometimes refer to two types of energy: veritable (measurable) and putative (yet to be measured). Hot and cold therapy (Chapter 22) is a veritable type. Putative therapies include healing touch (Chapter 23) and Reiki (Chapter 24). Much of TCM is based on the flow of energy throughout the body on meridians. Acupressure (Chapter 25) and reflexology (Chapter 26) are based on the flow of energy through meridians identified in TCM.

Healing touch encompasses a group of therapies used by nurses around the world. These techniques may or may not involve actual physical touching of the body. The nurse (or another therapist) seeks to bring energy into the patient or to balance energy within the person. Reiki, an energy-healing therapy originating in Japan, is becoming more widely used in the United States.

The body of research on energy healing therapies continues to grow; however, high-level evidence consistently demonstrating efficacy remains a challenge. Although difficulties are encountered in the measurement of outcomes from many energy-healing therapies, many people intuitively recognize the existence of energy forces and their impact on health promotion and healing. As can be noted in Part V of this book, nurses are interested in using energy healing therapies in their clinical practices as well as for self-care despite weak evidence. In the absence of harmful side effects of energy-healing therapies and the minimal time that is required for training patients, they can be safely employed by nurses and healers in efforts to provide relief and healing (Rogers et al., 2021).

REFERENCES

National Center for Complementary and Integrative Health. (2021). *Terms related to complementary and integrative health.* https://www.nccih.nih.gov/health/providers/terms-related-to-complementary-and-integrative-health

Rao, A., Hickman, L. D., Sibbritt, D., Newton, P. J., & Phillips, J. L. (2016). Is energy healing an effective non-pharmacological therapy for improving symptom management of chronic illnesses? A systematic review. *Complementary Therapies in Clinical Practice, 25,* 26–41. https://doi.org/10.1016/j.ctcp.2016.07.003

Rogers, L., Phillips, K., & Cooper, N. (2021). *Energy healing therapies: A systematic review and critical appraisal.* https://www.researchgate.net/publication/349039163_Energy_Healing_Therapies_A_Systematic_Review_and_Critical_Appraisal

Heat and Cold Therapies

MARGO HALM AND RUTH LINDQUIST

The picture of a nurse applying a cool cloth to a patient forehead is iconic. Such a picture is commonly used to portray the caring nature of the nurse and the nursing profession. The application of cool or cold therapies has been used throughout time as a therapeutic mode, including comfort and pain relief. Historically, Hippocrates prescribed cold drinks to reduce fevers, and Savonarola treated constipation by having people walk on cold, wet marble floors (Lehmann & de Lateur, 1982). The use of heat dates back to ancient Greeks and Egyptians as well. The application of heat and cold for therapeutic purposes is a very simple and effective therapeutic tool. To this day, innovative new uses for the application of heat and cold continue to be explored, tested, and utilized in patient care and for self-care. Indeed, a wide range of heat and cold applications are used for therapeutic purposes around the world.

The application of heat and cold enjoy a long tradition in nursing. Early records written by Florence Nightingale (1859/1992) document that she advocated the use of hot water bottles, warm bricks, and warm flannels to prevent patient chilling. Likewise, early textbooks on nursing fundamentals included procedures for therapeutic applications of heat and cold (Hampton, 1893; Vannier & Thompson, 1929), and subsequently, heat or cold applications were determined to be one of five cutaneous stimulation interventions used by advanced practice nurses for pain management (Mobily et al., 1994). As nonpharmacological interventions, heat and cold may be used when pharmacological approaches cannot be used or applied instead to boost the effectiveness of pharmacologic agents (Demirel & Cakir, 2020).

Heat and cold therapy may be applied to local tissues or to the whole body. When properly used, heat and/or cold therapy can have very favorable effects; it can relieve pain, reduce swelling, speed tissue healing, and increase or decrease the body's temperature. The therapeutic use of heat and cold as treatment modalities is not unique to nursing. Heat and cold are used, for example, in physical therapy, sports medicine, emergency medicine, the operating room, and dermatology.

This chapter provides an overview of the therapeutic applications of heat and cold by nurses for self-care and in healthcare settings. Intervention techniques for heat and cold applications in nursing are also illustrated. Research studies related to the selected use of these therapies are summarized, with areas for further research suggested.

HEAT

The application of heat as a therapeutic modality is commonly done by nurses for a wide array of patient conditions. The use of heat can range from the use of a warm compress on a superficial wound or the application of a warming blanket following surgery to the application of ultrasonic heat to promote comfort and tissue healing. The focus of this section is the therapeutic use of heat in topical applications.

DEFINITION

Heat is energy associated with the increased motion of atoms or molecules. It can be transmitted to tissues by conduction, convection, radiation, and conversion. Solids (e.g., heating pads), liquids (e.g., water and wax), and gases (e.g., steam) applied at temperatures between 40 °C and 45 °C (104 °F–113 °F) for 5 to 30 minutes can produce therapeutic effects in tissues (Lehmann, 1990). Therapeutic heating modalities used superficially include hot packs, forced-air warming blankets, or circulating water devices.

SCIENTIFIC BASIS

Heat therapy stimulates vasodilation which increases blood flow to targeted tissues. This increased blood flow brings an influx of oxygen, nutrients, antibodies, proteins, and leukocytes to promote better healing. Heat also increases the tissue elasticity of connective tissues and produces smooth muscle relaxation. When applied to a joint, heat induces smooth muscle relaxation, leading to increased joint flexibility. Newer evidence suggests heat influences overall host defense and physiological resilience, impacting the virulence of viral loads (Cohen, 2020).

INTERVENTION

The use of heat can reduce inflammation and edema and thus ease pain. Heat may be used to alleviate discomfort associated with joint stiffness, low back pain, muscle spasms, myalgia, perimenstrual pain, fibromyalgia, contractures, and bursitis. Heat is easy to use and may be applied in many ways, including a hot wet towel (compress), heat pack/patch, or heating pad. A hot bath or shower may also be effective in relieving pain, and moist heat may be used to drain abscesses. As pain in joints is common and often chronic, heat therapy is often used to provide relief. For the application of heat for arthritic pain, see Exhibit 22.1.

Exhibit 22.1 *Technique for Application of Heat for Chronic Arthritic Pain*

- Assess arthritic joint and subjective pain experienced.
- Obtain heat source—a heating pad with a digital dial to set the temperature and time as a reliable source of heat.
- Place a thin cloth barrier between the source heat pack and the tissue to prevent irritation.
- Apply the pad to the site of the injury.
- Limit heat application sessions to 20 minutes as a good general rule.
- If pain persists or worsens, seek medical attention to discuss plan for relief.

USES

Heat therapy can be beneficial to healing or for comfort in conditions such as arthritis, stiff muscles, and injuries to deeper tissues of the skin. Heat is an accessible and effective self-care treatment for conditions such as rheumatoid arthritis and premenstrual symptoms and in many rehabilitation applications. Heat has been used to treat headaches, migraines, tight muscles, and low back pain, as well as relieve labor and episiotomy pain. A recent meta-analysis examining the use of heat therapy for primary dysmenorrhea found favorable results for heat therapy on pain relief and quality of life, although there were few studies and small sample sizes (Jo & Lee, 2018). See Exhibit 22.2 for recent evidence on the effects of thermotherapy in other various patient populations, including orthopedic and obstetric/gynecologic.

Exhibit 22.2 *Effects of Heat Applications in Various Populations*

POPULATION	INTERVENTION	OUTCOMES	LEVEL OF EVIDENCE
ORTHOPEDIC			
Osteoarthritis knee Yildirim et al. (2010)	Digital moist heating pad at 40.6°C–46.1 °C (105°F–115°F) wrapped over affected knee for 20 minutes every other day for 4 weeks	• ↓ pain • Improved physical function • Improved general health perception • Improved social functioning	II
Neck/back sprain Garra et al. (2010)	Heating pad to strained area for 30 minutes	• ↓ pain	I
Low back pain French et al. (2006)	Heated wrap therapy applied to low back for 8 hours, or heated electric blankets at 42.2 °C (108 °F) for average therapy time of 25 minutes	• ↓ pain	I
OBSTETRIC/ GYNECOLOGIC			
Dysmenorrhea Potur and Kömürcü (2014)	Topical heat patch at 38.0 °C (102 °F) to lower abdomen for 8 hours	• ↓ pain at 4 and 8 hours	I
Labor Türkmen and Oran (2021)	Thermoforming (dry heat application method at 37.8 °C to 40 °C (100 °F–104 °F) to sacral area for 20 minutes at various stages of cervical dilatation	• ↓ pain at 4–5 cm & 6–7 cm dilatation interval • ↑ comfort at 8–9 cm dilatation interval • Less ↓ in comfort as labor progresses	II

OUTCOME MEASURES

The application of heat induces vasodilation bringing greater blood flow to affected tissues. Such vasodilation is associated with increases in tissue temperature and elasticity, relaxation of muscles, and reductions in pain. Other measures may include mobility, flexibility, and decreased stiffness; quality of life; health perceptions; relaxation; comfort; pain reduction; and physical, social, or role functioning.

PRECAUTIONS

When using heat, it is important to gain its benefit while avoiding the risks. In healthcare and in self-care, harm is still a risk and unfortunately still often experienced when heat is used therapeutically, especially when used with persons within vulnerable populations. Therefore, utmost caution must be used when applying heat therapies. Risks include thermal injury, skin irritation/damage, hyperthermia, and equipment injury.

Heat can be dangerous for younger and older individuals. It is also dangerous for individuals with acute injuries, bleeding disorders (due to vasodilation), and inadequate blood supplies; those with sensory/perceptual deficits who are unable to respond appropriately to burning sensations (such as diabetes, peripheral vascular disease, multiple sclerosis); and those who have disordered or immature temperature regulation. Frequent and close monitoring is essential to prevent harm. Staying hydrated is important to prevent dehydration. Due to vasodilation, care must be taken when changing position such as from a sitting or lying position to a standing position to avoid hypotension and fainting. Avoid using heat for extended amounts of time as excessive exposure may result in skin irritation, blisters, burns, and even more inflammation. Individuals should also never sleep with a therapeutic heating application of any sort.

CULTURAL APPLICATIONS

Many applications of heat are universally used around the world. The equipment or tools used may vary by region, reflecting materials common to geographic areas. However, the principles for indication, application, and precaution/safety remain virtually the same.

Certain applications of heat have more cultural roots. Native sweat lodges (Garrett et al., 2011), or "sweat therapy," is an example. In some healing traditions, cupping is performed with heat added to the cups to promote health. Assessment of heat and cold patterns is part of treatment approaches in traditional Chinese medicine. A number of cultures around the world, especially those in cold climates, use heat through sauna bathing, warm/hot tubs, and hot springs for therapeutic effects of relaxation or to relieve muscle tightness or soreness, as well as prevent or treat viral respiratory infections for self-care. Emerging evidence suggests regular sauna bathing improves respiratory, cardiovascular, and immune function, as well as boosts mood and quality of life (Cohen, 2020).

Indeed, sauna enthusiasts have long touted its benefits. Saunas may use heat external from the body (i.e., from warm air by electric or wood-burning heaters) or infrared light to heat the body from the inside without warming the air). Recently, researchers have been studying the effects of sauna baths on human health. In one recent study, researchers found 12 sessions of high-temperature sauna baths led to statistically significant changes in body composition among 23 healthy young men, including right leg muscle mass, bone mineral content, and bone mineral density (Toro et al., 2021).

Sauna baths and hot tubs are common throughout the world. Saunas are a common form of detoxification and cleansing in Finland. In Iceland, there are natural hot springs with natural minerals and milky waters perfect for bathing. For example, the Blue Lagoon is one of the most famous and popular hot springs in Iceland, comprised entirely of natural minerals, with temperatures of 38 °C to 29°C (110 °F–102 °F). Around the world, locations without such natural formations can emulate warm baths with man-made hot tubs, which are popular in spas, and even hotels, often pool-side. Intentions for health benefits and self-care are often interwoven with recreational and social pastimes; the use of saunas and hot springs are good examples (**Sidebars 22.1 and 22.2**).

Sidebar 22.1 *Personal Account of the Use of the Sauna in Finland for Self-Care*

Reino Lindqvist

Everyday sauna: In my family, we have a sauna bath regularly, twice a week. A typical sauna session takes 45 minutes or an hour at the most. Getting washed and having a shower is an essential part of going to the sauna, of course. But the most important thing is the actual time in the "steam room."

The stove, or *kiuas* as we call it, is heated to the temperature of about 60 °C to 70°C (no less but not much hotter either). You have to feel that the temperature is comfortable to your body. While sitting on the sauna bench, you have to take it easy; there is no hurry. To add heat and moisture in the sauna room, you throw a cup of water on the stones in the stove. Again carefully, since you don't want to burn yourself with the hot steam. Feeling the heat rise up and then gradually disappear gives you a very relaxating experience. You can repeat this as many times as you feel comfortable. In contrast to the steam and heat, you can have a cooling shower every now and then.

There is a saying in Finland: *Have your sauna as if you were in a church: Don't worry, don't hurry, be quiet, enjoy yourself.* A sauna is like a sanctuary to Finns. Following these simple rules, you'll feel like a new person after your sauna.

I don't know if the heat of a sauna really does clean out waste products inside you, but at least your skin is a lot cleaner after sauna.

Traditionally, Finns have their sauna at least on Saturday night. It means that the week's work is done and you are ready for a weekly holiday rest.

Savusauna, smoke sauna: We have also a log cabin about 10 miles from our home. There we have a special sauna called *savusauna*. It does not have a chimney at all. There is a fireplace built of stones in the corner of the sauna room but no bathroom, no shower, or other modern facilities. The fireplace is heated by burning wood under the stones. Smoke pours straight through the stones into the sauna room and out of the door and special valves into the open air.

(continued)

Sidebar 22.1 *Personal Account of the Use of the Sauna in Finland for Self-Care* *(continued)*

Heating up the sauna takes several hours, maybe half a day. So you have to be patient and not in a hurry when you decide to have a smoke sauna. After all, the wood has been burned down and the room has been properly ventilated; welcome to the SAUNA! This is not for busy business nerds.

Now, when the saavusauna is ready, you have all the time you want to enjoy the softest, gentlest heat that you have ever experienced while sitting on the sauna bench and listening to the silence and the sizzle of water on the hot stones. If you have a lake or a pond, even a pool outside, you can go out to swim or at least dip yourself in the refreshing water and relax.

Is it suitable to drink something during a sauna? Of course it is. Water, soda, juice. or beer but not, in my mind, wine or hard liquor. They may be even dangerous to you.

And once again, take your time to enjoy the experience. At night, after your sauna, you'll sleep like a baby and wake up in the morning feeling like a totally new person. This is my therapy and medicine for most troubles.

Sidebar 22.2 *Use of Hot Tubs and Hot Springs in Iceland*

Thora Jenny Gunnarsdottir

I live in Reykjavik, Iceland. Going to the swimming pool and diving into the hot tub or sitting in the warm healing waters of a hot spring increases my quality of life. If I go in the morning, it helps ease the stiffness of the body, and I can begin the day feeling rested and focused. If I go in the evening after a stressful day, then after a while, I start to witness how the stress and the tension gradually disappear, and I unwind—not to mention how it later improves my sleep. I try to engage in this experience at least two or three times a week to improve my general well-being. Another good reason to go to the hot tub is to catch up on gossip and other key talking points from the locals or just bring a friend to sit and enjoy chatting. It is no wonder why the hot tubs in Iceland are so popular as it truly is a rejuvenating experience to sit in an outdoor tub.

FUTURE RESEARCH

Although the application of heat is associated with therapeutic benefits, harm can also occur when overdone. Future research on heat applications is needed to for the following:

- Identify technologies that can signal when tissue damage may occur and to stop therapy to prevent injury
- Determine the target tissue temperature measurements reflecting ideal therapy according to the purpose for which it was applied

■ Determine potential beneficial effects, through large rigorous randomized controlled trials (RCTs) for pain relief and quality of life of patients with dysmenorrhea

COLD

Cryotherapy (freezing or cold therapy) is often used for acute injury. Ice may be used following intense muscle use/high-intensity exercise to reduce or prevent inflammation and swelling. Cryotherapy is also used for treating actinic keratosis, a precancerous skin condition occurring from sun damage among fair-skinned people.

DEFINITION

The sensation of cold is experienced when the temperature of a substance is lower than the tissues to which the substance is applied. The temperature of the skin surface of the torso can be regarded as the neutral point and is usually about 33.9 °C (93 °F). When water is used as a therapeutic agent, it is called *tepid* if its temperature is between 26.7 °C and 33.9 °C (80°F–93 °F), *cool* when between 18.3 °C and 26.7 °C (65 °F–80 °F), *cold* when between 12.8 °C and 18.3 °C (55 °F–65 °F), and *very cold* when below 12.8 °C (55 °F; Bierman, 1955).

SCIENTIFIC BASIS

Cold is used to prevent swelling, relieve pain, and preserve tissues such as inducing hypothermia after cardiac arrest and cooling the heart in open-heart surgery. Vasoconstriction slows blood flow, tissue metabolism, enzyme activity, and local nerve conduction velocity. Its anti-inflammatory effects reduce erythema and edema, thereby facilitating tissue repair and healing. Cold therapy also has antispasmodic and analgesic effects. A proposed mechanism of action for its salutary effects on pain is encompassed in the gate control theory (Mendell, 2014). According to this theory, a nonpainful stimulus (such as cold) "closes the gates" to painful stimuli. This closure prevents a pain sensation from traveling the central nervous system to the higher cerebral cortex (brain) where it is perceived as pain. Thus, cold application is able to suppress pain.

INTERVENTION

When an ice bag is applied to the calf, it can lower the skin temperature by 5 °C (41 °F), lower subcutaneous tissue by –4.4 °C (24 °F), and the deep muscle mass temperature by –7.2 °C (19 °F; Bierman, 1955). Cold therapy produces vasoconstriction by reflexes mediated by the central nervous system. The blood and body temperature may be reduced by lowering the temperature in venous blood through the cold-treated area. Cold may numb the limb, so sensitivity is diminished, and muscles become less efficient.

After injury, ice is used for the first 2 to 3 days to minimize swelling. Ankle sprain is a common injury. Following injury, a quick response is important. Steps for application of cold for treating an ankle sprain or a new injury are summarized in Exhibit 22.3.

> ### Exhibit 22.3 *Technique for Application of Ice Following Ankle Sprain*
>
> - Assess the injury and pain experienced.
> - Elevate limb to decrease blood flow that is adding to congestion.
> - Obtain an ice pack (often the quickest, most readily available source of ice is a package of frozen vegetables).
> - Place a thin cloth barrier between the source ice pack and tissue to prevent irritation.
> - Quickly apply the pack to the site of the injury. The more rapid the response, the greater chance the ice will reduce inflammation and prevent/reduce internal bleeding, thus reducing healing time.
> - Limit icing sessions to 20 minutes as needed over the next 24 to 48 hours to avoid skin irritation or injury.
> - If swelling persists, seek medical attention.

Using a cold pack, ice bag, or cold compress on a newly injured joint can reduce existing swelling or prevent fluid buildup. Applying a cold pack can reduce joint pain through its effects on nerve endings, inflammatory response, and reduction of circulatory flow and pressure from fluid buildup in the surrounding tissues. Cold should not be used on an already stiff joint that is not moving well.

USES

Cold therapy is useful to reduce pain and swelling associated with new or acute injuries. Athletes use cold as a mainstay to prevent swelling. See Exhibit 22.4 for recent evidence on the therapeutic effects of cold applications with various patient populations including cardiovascular, orthopedic, and surgical.

MEASUREMENT OF OUTCOMES

Intended health-related physiological outcomes of the application of cold include reduced pain or pain sensitivity and swelling; improved joint mobility and healing time; decreases in the extent of bruising; and decreased need/requests for analgesia.

PRECAUTIONS

Equipment malfunction may result in injury (skin tears), thermal injury, or hypothermia. Special precautions are necessary for young children, older adults, and vulnerable persons who lack sensory perception and/or the ability to communicate regarding potential tissue injury. Cold therapy should be avoided or used with caution in individuals with circulatory problems, including older persons or persons with diabetes. One cold application—whole-body cryotherapy—has been touted to relieve pain in conditions such as rheumatoid arthritis, fibromyalgia, migraines, or chronic pain. Athletes also use this therapy to reduce inflammation and muscle spasms, as well we speed up injury recovery. However, this cold therapy lacks evidence and poses more risk than benefit (Food and Drug Administration, 2016). Excessive cold on the body surface results in the

Exhibit 22.4 *Effects of Cold Applications in Various Populations*

POPULATION	INTERVENTION	OUTCOMES	LEVEL OF EVIDENCE
CARDIOVASCULAR			
SQ heparin injection Rupam et al. (2018)	Dry cold (ice bag covered with linen) over injection site for 20 minutes after SQ administration	• ↓ pain • ↓ bruising at 12, 48 & 72 hours	II
Wang et al. (2020)	Ice bag or cold gel pack applied 5–20 minutes before & after abdominal SQ injections	• ↓ pain immediately after injection • ↓ bruising at 48 hours • ↓ size bruises at 12, 24, 48 & 72 hours	I
Cardioversion Yava et al. (2012)	Reusable silicone gel pads applied over apical & sternal paddle areas for 10 minutes followed by 5 minutes rest; procedure repeated for 1 hour	• ↓ pain/sensitivity • ↓ burn incidence	I
ORTHOPEDIC			
Soft tissue ankle injury Mutlu and Yilmaz (2020)	Cold gel pack applied to affected ankle	• ↓ pain with 20 minutes of cold therapy	I
Neck/back sprain Garra et al. (2010)	Cold pack for 30 minutes to strained area	• ↓ pain	I
SURGICAL			
Thyroidectomy Temiz et al. (2020)	On day of surgery, cold gel pack applied over surgical drain area for 20 minutes 3 hours after TID analgesic doses; procedure repeated for 20 minutes after drain removed on POD 1	• ↓ analgesic requirements on day of surgery & POD 1 • ↓ pain after drain removed	I
Cardiac surgery Removal of chest tubes; Hasanzadeh et al. (2016)	Cooling gel pack applied around chest tube dressing while being undressed; pack then placed on top of pericardial tubes until skin temperature of 12.8 °C (55 °F) reached; tubes removed 1–2 minutes later	• ↓ pain at 5, 10 & 15 minutes after chest tube removal (but not statistically lower than other treatment groups) • ↓ anxiety immediately after tube removal when cold therapy was augmented with essential oils	I

SQ = subcutaneous; TID = three times daily; POD = postoperative day.

development of wheals, skin that has been frozen is red and tender with desquamation and pigmentation occurring.

To utilize cold therapy, place a cloth or towel between the cold pack and skin to prevent skin irritation or damage. As a general rule, never leave the cold application on the skin for greater than 20 minutes to prevent the skin from becoming too cold. Prolonged exposure to cold may also cause muscle tension and increase muscle contraction. When using a cold application, always monitor for any adverse effects, including numbness, blistering, or changes in color to bright red. Also, inspect the area after the therapy for signs of damage following treatment.

CULTURAL APPLICATIONS

Cold is used therapeutically around the world and has been with us since ancient times. The Egyptians used cryotherapy for the treatment of inflammation and injuries since 2500 BCE. Hippocrates used cold in 400 BCE for pain and swelling. Other cultures across time have tapped its healing abilities. For instance, some cultures believe health results from a "hot–cold" balance. The Latino and Asian cultures believe hot conditions, such as a sore throat or gastroesophageal reflux, should be treated with cold therapies, and cold conditions, like headaches and menstrual cramps, should be managed with hot therapies. On the other hand, cold is typically not used in traditional Chinese medicine as it, too, is founded on the principle of maintaining a harmonious balance. In Chinese Medicine, this balance is between the body's yin (cold) and yang (hot; Juckett, 2005). As a result, the application of cold to the body stops the flow of chi.

FUTURE RESEARCH

Like heat, the application of cold is associated with therapeutic benefits, but harm can occur if overused or inappropriately used. Future research on cold therapy applications is needed to discover the following:

- What other therapies can be combined with the application of cold to enhance the reduction of pain?
- What other integrative therapies can be combined with cold therapies to protect the skin from potentially detrimental procedural effects?

HEAT AND COLD

Combination therapy utilizes applications of both heat and cold. In this approach, heat and cold applications are used in an alternating manner to create a pumping action, markedly stimulating local circulation. Cold is applied to restrict circulation and, thereby, to reduce swelling as previously discussed with cold therapy. Then circulation is increased to the affected area with the application of heat bringing nutrients to the affected area and relaxing smooth muscles. This alternating pattern may increase flexibility by improving range of motion, expediting recovery, and reducing pain. Exhibit 22.5 outlines current evidence on the therapeutic effects of combination heat/cold therapy in various patient populations, including orthopedic and obstetric/gynecologic.

Heat and cold combination therapy is often used when heat or cold alone has not been effective and when an injury is at least a week old. These therapies are simple, reliable, and economical. Similar precautions as heat and cold therapy (described previously) should be used with these alternating treatments.

Exhibit 22.5 *Effects of Alternating Heat and Cold Applications in Various Populations*

POPULATION	INTERVENTION	OUTCOMES	LEVEL OF EVIDENCE
ORTHOPEDIC			
Osteoarthritis knee Abd elFatah et al. (2019)	Contrast hydrotherapy – Alternating wrapping knee with heating pads for 1–2 minutes, followed by cold packs for 20 minutes BID (a.m. & p.m.)	• ↓ pain • ↑ function	II
Aciksoz et al. (2017)	Hot vs. cold pack applied to affected knee for 20 minutes BID (a.m. & p.m.) for 3 weeks	• ↓ pain • ↑ functional status • ↑ quality of life	I
Heel pain Arankalle et al. (2016)	Hot moist compress applied to heel for 15–20 minutes, followed by cold moist compress for 30 seconds-1 minute	• ↓ foot function disability	III
OB/GYN			
Labor Sugandary et al. (2018)	Intermittent alternating hot water bag at 37.8 °C–40 °C (100 °F–104 °F) and cold pack at 15 °C–17.8 °C (59 °F–64 °F); first applied to abdomen, then lower abdomen & then back (duration 10 minutes each site, with both packs covered with towel)	• ↓ pain • ↓ duration of stage 1 & 2 labor	II

FUTURE RESEARCH

Future research on the combination of heat and cold therapy application is needed to discover the following:

■ For what other pain syndromes or health conditions can combination therapy be tested to determine its effect on pain reduction?
■ What other integrative therapies can be used as an adjunct with the combination heat and cold therapy to increase analgesic effects?

CONCLUSION

The application of hot and cold have been used across time in cultures around the world. Heat is used to alleviate discomfort associated with conditions like joint stiffness, muscle spasms, bursitis, and low back pain, while cold is the gold standard for managing acute injuries to reduce inflammation and pain. Newer applications of the combination of heat and cold therapy have been used to stimulate circulation and, thereby, increase the supply of nutrients to support healing while at the same time relaxing smooth muscles and increasing flexibility of surrounding tissues to alleviate pain and discomfort.

WEBSITES

Reputable websites for information about heat and cold therapies include the following:

- American Society for Surgery of the Hand
  /www.assh.org/handcare/condition/heat-treatment-cold-treatment
- Cleveland Clinic
  https://health.clevelandclinic.org/should-you-use-ice-or-heat-for-pain
  -infographic/
- Merck Manual
  www.merckmanuals.com/home/fundamentals/rehabilitation/treatment
  -of-pain-and-inflammation
- WebMD
  www.webmd.com/pain-management/when-use-heat-ice
  www.webmd.com/arthritis/heat-and-cold-therapy-for-arthritis-pain

REFERENCES

Abd elFatah, M. I., Weheida, S. M., & Mekkawy, M. M. (2019). Effect of cold application versus contrast hydrotherapy on patient's knee osteoarthritis outcomes. *American Journal of Nursing, 8*(4), 145–152. https://doi.org/10.11648/j.ajns.20190804.14

Aciksoz, S., Akyuz, A., & Tunay, S. (2017). The effect of self-administered superficial local hot and cold application methods on pain, functional status and quality of life in primary knee osteoarthritis patients. *Journal of Clinical Nursing, 26*(23–24), 5179–5190. https://doi.org/10.1111/jocn.14070

Arankalle, D., Wardle, J., & Nair, P. M. (2016). Alternate hot and cold application in the management of heel pain: A pilot study. *The Foot, 29*, 25–28. https://doi.org/10.1016/j.foot.2016.09.007

Bierman, W. (1955). Therapeutic use of cold. *Journal of the American Medical Association, 157*(14), 1189–1192. https://doi.org/10.1001/jama.1955.02950310015003

Cohen, M. (2020). Turning up the heat on COVID-19: Heat as a therapeutic intervention. *F1000Research, 9*, 292. https://doi.org/10.12688/f1000research.23299.2

Demirel, & Cakir, F. (2020). Heat, cold application and women's health. In P. Chernopolski, N. Shapekova, B. Ak, & B. Sancar (Eds.), *Advances in health sciences research* (pp. 243–256). St. Kliment Ohridski University Press.

Food and Drug Administration (United States). (2016). *Whole body cryotherapy (WBC): A "cool trend that lacks evidence, poses risks.* https://www.fda.gov/consumers/consumer-updates/whole-body-cryotherapy-wbc-cool-trend-lacks-evidence-poses-risks

French, S. D., Cameron, M., Walker, B. F., Reggars, J. W., & Esterman, A. J. (2006). A Cochrane review of superficial heat or cold for low back pain. *Spine, 31*(9), 998–1006. https://doi.org/10.1097/01.brs.0000214881.10814.64

Garra, G., Singer, A. J., Leno, R., Taira, B. R., Gupta, N., Mathaikutty, B., & Thode, H. J. (2010). Heat or cold packs for neck and back strain: A randomized controlled trial of efficacy. *Academic Emergency Medicine, 17*(5), 484–489. https://doi.org/10.1111/j.1553-2712.2010.00735.x

Garrett, M. T., Torres-Rivera, E., Brubaker, M., Portman, T. A. A., Brotherton, D., West-Olatunji, C., Conwill, W., & Grayshield, L. (2011). Crying for a vision: The Native American sweat lodge ceremony as therapeutic intervention. *Journal of Counseling & Development, 89*(3), 318–325. https://doi.org/10.1002/j.1556-6678.2011.tb00096.x

Hampton, I. (1893). *Nursing, its principles and practice for hospitals and private use.* E.C. Koechert.

Hasanzadeh, F., Kashouk, N. M., Amini, S., Asili, J., Emami, S. A., Vashani, H. B., & Sahebkar, A. (2016). The effect of cold application and lavender oil inhalation in cardiac surgery patients undergoing chest tube removal. *EXCLI Journal, 15,* 64–74. https://doi.org/10.17179/excli2015-748

Jo, J., & Lee, S. H. (2018). Heat therapy for primary dysmenorrhea: A systematic review and meta-analysis of its effects on pain relief and quality of life. *Scientific Reports, 8,* 16252. https://doi.org/10.1038/s41598-018-34303-z

Juckett. (2005). Cross-cultural medicine. *American Family Physician, 72*(11), 2267–2274. https://www.aafp.org/afp/2005/1201/afp20051201p2267.pdf

Lehmann, J., & de Lateur, B. (1982). Therapeutic heat. In J. Lehmann (Ed.), *Therapeutic heat and cold* (pp. 404–562). Williams & Wilkins.

Lehmann, J. F. (Ed.). (1990). *Therapeutic heat and cold.* Williams & Wilkins.

Mendell, L. M. (2014). Constructing and deconstructing the Gate Theory of Pain. *Pain, 155*(2), 210–216. https://doi.org/10.1016/j.pain.2013.12.010

Mobily, P. R., Herr, K. A., & Nicholson, A. C. (1994). Validation of cutaneous stimulation interventions for pain management. *International Journal of Nursing Studies, 31*(6), 533–544. https://doi.org/10.1016/0020-7489(94)90063-9

Mutlu, S., & Yılmaz, E. (2020). The effect of soft tissue injury cold application duration on symptoms, edema, joint mobility, and patient satisfaction: A randomized controlled trial. *Journal of Emergency Nursing, 46*(4), 449–459. https://doi.org/10.1016/j.jen.2020.02.017

Nightingale, F. (1992). *Notes on nursing.* Lippincott. (Original work published in 1859).

Potur, D. C., & Kömürcü, N. (2014). The effects of local low-dose heat application on dysmenorrhea. *Journal of Pediatric and Adolescent Gynecology, 27*(4), 216–221. https://doi.org/10.1016/j.jpag.2013.11.003

Rupam, S., Sheoran, P., & Sharma, T. (2018). Effectiveness of dry cold application on pain intensity and bruise at the subcutaneous injection site among patients admitted in selected hospital of Mullana Ambala. *Research Journal of Pharmacy and Technology, 11*(4), 1559–1562. https://doi.org/10.5958/0974-360X.2018.00290.1

Sugandary, M., Dash, M., & Chitra, A. F. (2018). Effectiveness of intermittent heat and cold application on labour pain and duration of labour among the intranatal mothers. *Journal of Public Health and Diseases, 1*(3), 49–55. https://integrityresjournals.org/journal/JPHD/article-full-text-pdf/7FE5D6562

Temiz, Z., Sayilan, A. A., Kanbay, Y., & Akarsu, C. (2020). The effect of cold application on drain-related pain control after thyroidectomy. *Hacettepe Üniversitesi Hemşirelik Fakültesi Dergisi, 7*(3), 226–231. https://doi.org/10.31125/hunhemsire.834077

Toro, V., Siquier-Coll, J., Bartolomé, I., Pérez-Quintero, M., Raimundo, A., Muñoz, D., & Maynar-Mariño, M. (2021). Effects of twelve sessions of high-temperature sauna baths on body composition in healthy young men. *International Journal of Environmental Research and Public Health, 18*(9), 4458. https://doi.org/10.3390/ijerph18094458

Türkmen, H., & Oran, N. T. (2021). Massage and heat application on labor pain and comfort: A quasi-randomized controlled experimental study. *Explore, 17*(5), 438–445. https://doi.org/10.1016/j.explore.2020.08.002

Vannier, M. L., & Thompson, B. A. (1929). *Nursing procedures: A manual used in the teaching of the principles and practice of nursing in the Associated Hospitals in the University of Minnesota School of Nursing.* University of Minnesota Press.

Wang, H., Guan, J., Zhang, X., Wang, X., Ji, T., Hou, D., Wang, G., & Sun, J. (2020). Effect of cold application on pain and bruising in patients with subcutaneous injection of low-molecular-weight heparin: A meta-analysis. *Clinical and Applied Thrombosis/Hemostasis, 26,* 1–10. https://doi.org/10.1177/1076029620905349

Yava, A., Koyuncu, A., Tosun, N., & Kiliç, S. (2012). Effectiveness of local cold application on skin burns and pain after transthoracic cardioversion. *Emergency Medicine Journal, 29*(7), 544–549. https://doi.org/10.1136/emj.2010.098053

Yıldırım, N., Filiz Ulusoy, M., & Bodur, H. (2010). The effect of heat application on pain, stiffness, physical function and quality of life in patients with knee osteoarthritis. *Journal of Clinical Nursing, 19*(7–8), 1113–1120. https://doi.org/10.1111/j.1365-2702.2009.03070.x

23

Healing Touch

LAUREN JOHNSON, CYNTHIA LEE DOLS FINN, MARILYN BACH, SUSAN HEITZMAN, AND ALEXA W. UMBREIT

All cultures, both ancient and modern, have developed some form of touch therapy as part of people's desire to heal and care for one another. The oldest written evidence of the use of touch to enhance healing comes from Asia more than 5,000 years ago (Jackson & Latini, 2016). This therapeutic use of the hands has been passed on from generation to generation as a tool for healing. However, philosophical and cultural differences have influenced the way touch has been used throughout the world. The Eastern viewpoint has based its touch-healing practices on energy channels (meridians), energy fields (auras), and energy centers (chakras). Expert practitioners of energetic touch therapies use their hands to influence this flow of energy to promote balance and healing. The Western viewpoint focuses on physiological changes that occur at the cellular level from touch therapies that are believed to influence healing. A blending of both Eastern and Western techniques has led to an explosion of a wide variety of touch therapies (Jackson & Latini, 2016). Nursing has used touch throughout its history, and today's nurses are integrating many touch techniques into their practice. One of these therapies is healing touch (HT), "a relaxing, nurturing, heart-centered energy therapy that uses gentle, intentional touch that assists in balancing physical, emotional, mental, and spiritual well-being" (Healing Beyond Borders, 2021a, para. 1). HT is taught internationally at universities, medical and nursing schools, and other settings.

DEFINITION

HT is an integrative health mind and body practice that works in harmony with and is complementary to standard medical care. HT uses gentle touch and energy-based techniques to influence and support the human biofield within the body (energy centers) and surrounding the body (energy fields) to support and promote the body's natural ability to heal (Healing Beyond Borders, 2021a; Healing Touch Program, 2022). Based on a holistic view of health and illness, HT focuses on creating an energetic balance of the whole body at the physical, emotional, mental, and spiritual levels rather than on dysfunctional parts of the body to create an environment that is conducive to self-healing.

Umbreit (2000) describes the work of the HT practitioner as observation, assessment, and repatterning of the client's energy field, which is disrupted when there is disease, illness, psychological stressors, and pain. Practitioners describe these disruptions in the energy field as blockages, leaks, imbalances, or congestion. The goal of the HT practitioner is to open these blockages, release congestion, seal the leaks, and rebalance the energy field to symmetry.

Through the interaction of the energy fields between practitioner and client, the use of the HT practitioner's hands, an intention focusing on the client's highest good, and a centering process, noninvasive HT techniques specific to the client's needs are used to create this energetic balance (Umbreit, 2000). Krieger (1979) describes the centering process as a meditation in which one eliminates all distractions and concentrates on that place of quietude within which one can feel truly integrated, unified, and focused. Finding this "place of quietude within" is achieved by many through deep belly breathing, prayer, meditation, or any other technique that slows one down, calms the mind, and accesses a deeper spirit of compassion and strength. To be centered is to be fully present with another person or situation and engaged with heart and mind, deeper feelings, and thoughts. The centered state of mind is maintained throughout the HT treatment.

EARLY ROOTS IN THERAPEUTIC TOUCH

HT evolved from the pioneering work of the Therapeutic Touch (TT) community that was started in 1972 by a nurse, Dr. Dolores Krieger, and Dora Kunz, a natural intuitive healer, who assisted many physicians with perplexing patient cases (Krieger, 1993). Together they established TT, described as a "contemporary interpretation of several ancient healing practices ... [consisting of learning] skills for consciously directing or sensitively modulating human energies" (Krieger, 1993, p. 11). Foundational to the practice of TT, is the assumption that humans comprise complex energy fields that are imbalanced with disease. Practitioners use their hands to smooth, repattern, or boost areas that need attention to restore balance to the body, mind, and spirit. The five steps of TT follow: Center in the present moment, assess the energy field, clear and mobilize the energy field, direct energy toward wholeness, and evaluate the response (Krieger, 1993).

Dr. Krieger and others conducted early research studies on the effects of TT (Easter, 1997; Heidt, 1981; Krieger, 1993; Quinn, 1988; Wirth, 1992). These studies found significant responses in recipients of TT, with improvements in hemoglobin levels, wound healing and relaxation responses, and decreases in anxiety. In healthcare, TT philosophy, practice, and research have become the basis for many newer energetic modalities, including HT.

HISTORY AND EVOLUTION OF HEALING TOUCH CURRICULA

Healing Touch programs were started in 1989 by Janet Mentgen who provided energy healing in private practice for more than ten years. She joined other nurse members of the American Holistic Nurses Association (AHNA) to develop the curriculum for Healing Touch taught through the AHNA's Healing Touch Program (Hover-Kramer, 1996). Healing Touch International (HTI) was founded in 1996 as a nonprofit professional educational organization to oversee the HT certification process, continuing education, and code of ethics/standards. Subsequently, two AHNA-endorsed organizations emerged that offer HT classes and certification: Healing Touch Program and Healing Beyond Borders (formerly HTI).

Presently, the HT curriculum has six levels of education (Healing Beyond Borders, 2021b). The six-level HT educational curriculum in energy-based practice moves from beginning to advanced practice, certification, and instructor levels. Advanced practice requires at least 100 hours of workshop instruction plus a 1-year rigorous and comprehensive course of study involving an extensive reading program and education on a wide variety of complementary therapies. In addition, there is work on case studies, mentoring, ethics, client–practitioner relationships, the development of higher sense perception, and the establishment of a practice. Emphasis is based on self-care and the development of the student (Healing Beyond Borders, 2021c; Wardell et al., 2014a). Upon completion, students may apply for certification. Instructor status requires more education and mentoring. The HT coursework is open to registered nurses, body-oriented therapists, psychotherapists, licensed healthcare professionals, and individuals who desire an in-depth understanding and practice of healing work using touch and energy-based concepts (Healing Touch Program, 2021b).

IMPORTANCE OF HT TO NURSES' SELF-CARE

It is vital for a nurse to have a strong positive sense of well-being in order to be fully present to the patient and ensure care of the highest quality and safety. The link between a healthcare professional's sense of well-being and patient safety outcomes is well supported in the literature (Adimando, 2018; Hall et al., 2016; Linton & Koonmen, 2020; Melnyk et al., 2018). Self-care is vital to developing a sense of well-being. Moreover, the American Nurses Association (ANA, 2015) views self-care as an ethical responsibility. Strategies to support self-care include meditation, spirituality, intentionality, self-awareness, and energy field therapies as evidence-based approaches for reducing the stress response and enhancing well-being (Church, 2018; Crane & Ward, 2016; McTaggart, 2017). HT is a readily available therapy that can be used to reduce stress and anxiety and enhance the well-being of nurses/nursing students.

SCIENTIFIC BASIS

The nursing profession has long been described as dedicated to the art and science of human caring. Nurse theorists have also emphasized the promotion of health and well-being, taking into account the individual's constant interaction with the environment. It was this concern that led nurse-theorist Rogers to develop her concepts of the nature of individuals and the environment as energy fields in constant interplay, which affects the health of human beings (Eschiti, 2014). Rogers' theoretical framework (Rogers, 1990) postulates that all living things are composed of energy, and there is a continual exchange of energy among them as they strive toward the goal of balance and universal order. Using the hands, intention, and centering, the HT practitioner assesses the client's energy field and helps direct it to a more open, symmetrical pattern that enhances the client's ability to self-heal. The nursing diagnosis used for HT and other biofield therapies is defined as an "Imbalanced Energy Field [state in which a] disruption of the flow of energy surrounding a person's being results in a disharmony of the body, mind, and/or spirit" (Herdman et al., 2021).

The concept of energy systems as part of the human interactive environment and healing has been part of many cultures for centuries. It is believed by traditional societies that a life force is involved in the interchange between humans and their surroundings. This life force is called by many names in different cultures: Chinese, *qi*; Japanese, *ki*; Greek, *pneuma*; Tibetan, *lung*; Native American, *oki, orenda, ton*; Hindu, *prana*; and Western, *biofield* (Wilson, 2020), to name a few. The common principle is that an imbalance in this energy force can result in illness.

Although we are able to measure or evaluate some of the effects of energy-based healing interactions on illness and symptoms, it is still not clear how biofield/energy field modalities, including HT, influence the energy patterns of recipients or how recipients use the energy to enhance their self-healing processes. Physicists continue to further analyze Einstein's premise that everything is energy and organized in energy fields. Experts in the fields of physics, engineering, biology, and physiology continue to conduct research in this area of energy exchange in an attempt to explain what occurs during an energetic interaction (Oschman, 2016b). Studies of photon emission could provide evidence that enhances the assessment of health and could be used to evaluate the impact of different types of interventions, which could help explain how photonic energy exchanges occur between practitioners' hands and diseased body tissues (Ives et al., 2014; Oschman, 2016a).

The growing study of psychoneuroimmunology suggests a more integrative body system and the existence of extensive two-way communication between the brain and body (Anderson, 2016). Increased understanding and study of these communication pathways may help better explain the relaxation response and the physiological effects of mind–body therapies, including HT.

Historically, a number of instruments have been invented to directly measure the human energy field (e.g., Kirlian photography, gaseous discharge visualization, and poly-contrast interference). In 2008, Oschman reported that various energy therapies stimulate tissue healing by the production of pulsating electromagnetic fields that induce currents to flow within the body's tissue (Oschman, 2008). It was proposed that these currents are generated via the heartbeat and move throughout the circulatory system and the "living matrix," which Oschman (2008) describes as an informational nervous system of the body where electron movement occurs, producing these waves. He stated that the heart generates the body's largest electromagnetic field, which can be measured in the space around the body using the superconducting quantum interference device (SQUID). The SQUID is a sensitive magnetometer used to measure extremely subtle magnetic fields, and it has been used to measure the biomagnetic fields emanating from the hands of energy field practitioners who use TT, qigong, yoga, and meditation. It has been found that low electromagnetic frequencies (a coherent pattern) can be emitted from a trained energy healer's hands at a rate needed for tissue healing, which has the possibility to convert a stalled healing process to active repair by restoring coherence to the tissue (Oschman, 2008). However, existing methods are not sufficiently accurate or sensitive to definitively measure the potentially subtle effects of therapies such as HT. Until accurate, direct measurement of the human energy field is possible, the potential effects of HT on the energy field will need to be measured by more indirect methods.

It is unknown precisely how symptoms are affected by HT interventions. And since there is limited experimental data, many explanations for healing touch remain theoretical. There continues to be much to learn and understand about the human biofield, the effects of energy therapies on the biofield, and the ways and reasons that these effects occur.

Systematic reviews of studies and randomized controlled trials (RCTs) and a synthesis of best evidence focusing on biofield therapies, including HT, describe studies of medium quality overall. The reviews suggest moderate to strong evidence that HT reduces pain per self-report for those with pain (Anderson & Taylor, 2011; Hammerschlag et al., 2014). Some studies specific to HT interventions focus on managing the symptoms of pain, anxiety, nausea, and stress; decreasing the side effects of cancer treatments; promoting postprocedural recovery; improving mental health, including posttraumatic stress disorder (PTSD); using HT with older adults to manage pain and improve appetite, sleep, behavior patterns, and functional abilities; increasing relaxation; and promoting a sense of well-being (Darbonne, 2012; FitzHenry et al., 2014; Hardwick et al., 2012; Jain et al., 2012a, 2012b; Lu et al., 2013a, 2013b, 2016; Megel et al., 2012; Ostuni & Pietro, 2012). In pediatrics, several small research studies (Bhardwaj & Koffman, 2017; Cone et al., 2014; James et al., 2019; Wong et al., 2013) examined the effects of HT on cancer fatigue, the sleep of burn patients, and, in a surgical setting, measures of pain, anxiety, sleep, and anesthesia emergence.

A proposed theoretical description of how an HT practitioner may promote positive changes in client symptoms follows. A trained HT practitioner uses the hands to assess, sense or evaluate the client's biofield. The practitioner then sends coherent energy waves from the provider's hands to the client that, in turn, affects the incoherent energy patterns that cause disease or imbalance in the client's energy field and body. Due to a resonant effect, the incoherent energy pattern shifts to a healthier, coherent pattern affecting the client's circulatory, endocrine, and nervous systems and/or other unidentified mechanisms, promoting positive client responses with the potential to restore optimal health. The HT practitioner moves and repatterns a client's energy field, promoting a more open and symmetric pattern to enhance the client's perceived sense of well-being. This movement of energy may stimulate physiological, neurochemical, and psychological changes that promote positive effects on pain, anxiety, wound healing, immune system function, depression, and sense of well-being.

INTERVENTION

TECHNIQUES

Nearly 30 techniques are taught in the HT curriculum, from the simple to the complex, ranging from localized to full-body techniques. The HT practitioner determines which technique to use after an assessment of the client's expressed needs, symptoms, and results of an energy field hand scan. Each technique begins with determining the client's specific need for HT and obtaining client permission.

Table 23.1 *Basic Healing Touch (HT)Sequence*

Techniques	Indications	Brief Description of Procedure Steps
Basic HT sequence	Influences the human energy field. Used for: promoting relaxation; reducing pain; lowering anxiety, tension, and stress; facilitating wound healing; promoting restoration of the body; promoting a sense of well-being	1. Center, ground, and set intention. 2. Assess the client's energy field for disturbances with a hand scan over the body. 3. Based upon the assessment findings, determine the best technique to use with the client and implement the HT technique/s. 4. Assess the client's energy field with a hand scan to determine the effects of the intervention. 5. Ground the client to the present moment and to a connection to the earth. 6. Assess the client's perception of the effectiveness of the intervention.

Source: Adapted from Anderson, J. G., Anselme, L. C., & Hart, L. K. (2017). *Foundations and practice of healing touch.* Healing Beyond Borders.

Mutual goals are set. This is followed by the basic HT sequence (Table 23.1), including the practitioner physically and psychologically centering, grounding, and setting the intention for the client's highest good; assessing client's energy field; selecting and deliverinf of the specific HT intervention technique; evaluating the energy field to evaluate intervention effects; grounding the client; and assessing for the effects of the HT intervention.

Table 23.2 lists several full-body techniques along with indications and brief descriptions of the procedures. Table 23.3 describes several localized HT techniques. These techniques, which treat a wide range of client symptoms, should be practiced in a supervised setting with an instructor before working with a client. Most of the HT techniques involve basic hand actions called field repatterning. The practitioner uses "intent" to facilitate a transfer of energy to the specific body part of the client from a "universal source" of energy, with the practitioner as the conduit of this energy.

Although several HT techniques can be done with the client in a seated position, most are done while the client is lying down and fully dressed in the most relaxed state possible to promote a more profound effect. The practitioner briefly describes HT and the procedure plan, invites the client to ask any questions at any time, and receives permission to do the treatment and to touch the client. HT therapists use the principles of holistic communication, which calls forth the full use of self in interacting with another. Thornton and Mariano (2016) describe this as the acknowledgment of "the infinite and sacred nature of Being; the use of centering, grounding, intention, and intuition; and caring, healing, [and] transcendent presence" (p. 477) as key elements. They also state, "Holistic communication invites us to engage our higher Self as we meet another in that transcendent space where profound healing occurs" (p. 477). Both the practitioner and the client are enriched and nurtured during this process.

Table 23.2 *Selected Full-Body Basic Healing Touch Techniques*

Techniques	Indications	Brief Description of Procedure
Chakra Connection and Chakra Energizing (Anderson et al., 2017)	Connects, opens, and balances the energy centers (chakras), enhancing the flow of energy throughout the body. Used for balancing, before and after medical–surgical procedures; after injuries, promoting relaxation, diminishing pain, easing anxiety, post-chemotherapy or radiation, promoting general well-being	1. Center, ground, and set intention. 2. Assess client's energy field. 3. Place hands on or over the minor energy centers (chakras) on the extremities and the major energy centers (chakras) on the trunk in a defined sequential manner, holding each area for at least 1 minute. 4. Reassess client's energy field. 5. Ground the client.
Chakra spread (Kunz, 1995)	Opens the energy centers (chakras), producing a deep clearing of energy blocks. Used for physical or emotional pain, before and after medical procedures or surgery, severe stress reactions, terminal illness, stress, assisting in coping with various life transitions	1. Ground, center, and set intention. 2. Assess the client's energy field. 3. Hold the client's feet; then hands, one by one, in a gentle embrace for at least 1 minute. 4. Start at the head at the crown chakra. Place hands (palms down) above each energy center (chakra), moving the hands slowly downward toward the chakra, then spreading the hands outward as far as possible; motion is repeated three times for each energy center, moving from the upper to the lower chakras. 5. Repeat the entire sequence two more times. 6. Reassess client's energy field. 7. End treatment with holding the client's hand and heart center (procedure is done in silence and takes 10–15 minutes; is used very carefully by experienced practitioners for special needs and sacred moments in healing).
Field Repatterning	Influences the human energy field and is used to move and balance one's energy.	1. Center, ground, and set intention. 2. Assess the client's energy field. 3. Starting from the head, use the hands to brush down and away from the body in a calm and gentle manner. Repeat until energy is cleared. 4. Reassess the client's energy field. 5. Ground the client.

(continued)

Table 23.2 *Selected Full Body Basic Healing Touch Techniques (continued)*

Techniques	Indications	Brief Description of Procedure
Modified Mesmeric Clearing (Anderson et al., 2017)	Clears the body of congestion and emotional debris in the field. Used for history of drug use, postanesthesia, reducing pain, clearing out toxins, posttrauma; systemic disease, after breathing polluted air, history of smoking, environmental sensitivities, emotional clearing and release of unresolved feelings (e.g., anger, fear, worry, tension), easing nausea, chemotherapy or radiation, and kidney dialysis	1. Center, ground, and set intention. 2. Assess the client's energy field. 3. Place hands 12–18 inches above the top of the client's head with fingers spread, relaxed, and curled, thumbs touching or close together. 4. Move hands very slowly in long continuous raking motions over the body from above the head to off the toes, 1–6 inches above the body, each sweep taking about 30 seconds (work the middle of the body first, followed by each side). 5. Repeat the procedure until energy is cleared. 6. Reassess client's energy field. 7. Ground the client.

Source: Adapted from Anderson, J. G., Anselme, L. C., & Hart, L. K. (2017). *Foundations and practice of healing touch.* Healing Beyond Borders.

DISTANCE HEALING

Distance healing touch, also known as remote healing touch, is a way for healers to connect with those clients or patients who are not or cannot be in the same physical location (Kagel, 2014a; Moreno et al., 2018). The person receiving the distance HT session could be in the next room, city, state, country, or continent, and sessions are sometimes provided to people with whom the practitioner has never spoken or met. Distance HT traverses space and time and can be provided to individuals or groups. Some practitioners posit that distance healing is easier because there are no physical distractions and the practitioner is linked directly to the energetic field (Kagel, 2014a). Distance HT provides opportunities for individuals who don't readily have access to healing touch practitioners, such as those isolated during a pandemic or those in rural areas where healing touch practitioners may not exist. Distance HT may be easier for practitioners, and their clients who have physical limitations since neither need to leave their homes and the HT session can be done in any position.

Distance HT sessions mirror in-person HT sessions in process and ethical considerations. Permission should be obtained from the receiver prior to giving a distance HT session (Kagel, 2014a). Practitioners can engage with their clients through a wide range of visual electronic formats, via personal text messages, or over the phone. All can be effective. When providing a distance HT session, the same basic HT sequence that is used for an in-person session is completed while incorporating steps to accommodate the distance aspects. Setting intention is crucial in distance healing touch and is thought to work through nonlocal intention (Schwartz, 2017) and nonlocal mind (Dossey, 2015). The healing session's length

Table 23.3 *Selected Localized Healing Touch Techniques*

Techniques	Indications	Brief Description of Procedure
Beak Fingers	Breaks up congestion, energy patterns, and blockages. Used for easing pain; assists in stopping internal bleeding and bruising, sealing lacerations, healing fractures, and joint injuries; eye or ear issues; accelerating healing; tumors; swelling; inserting intravenous catheters, helping to bring blood vessels to skin surface; stimulating return of bowel motility after surgery	1. Center, ground, and set intention. 2. Assess local energy field. 3. Hold the thumb and first and second fingers together, directing energy from the palm down the fingers. 4. Imagine a beam of light coming from the fingers of one hand into the client's body. 5. Move the hand in any direction over the affected part, continuously moving for 1–3 minutes. 6. Reassess energy field.
Field Repatterning	Influences the human energy field and is used to move and balance one's energy.	1. Center, ground, and set intention. 2. Assess client's energy field. 3. Place hands 1–6 inches above the skin or clothing. 4. Identify the congested area or blockage. Over the area, use the hands to brush down and away from the area in a calm and gentle manner to remove the blockage. Movements may be short and rapid or slow and sweeping. Repeat until the congestion or blockage is cleared. **OR** 5. Identify the congested area. Hold the hands still on the body or above the congested area to stimulate energy flow. Hold for 1 to several minutes until energy is cleared. 6. Reassess the client's energy field. 7. Ground the client. Note: This technique can also be used on the full body using a sweeping technique from head to toe.

(continued)

Table 23.3 *Selected Localized Healing Touch Techniques (continued)*

Techniques	Indications	Brief Description of Procedure
Noel's Mind clearing (Noel, 2011)	Promotes mental clarity, peace, and calm Used for quieting the mind, promoting clarity in thinking and facilitating insights, for deep relaxation, deepening intuition, promoting sleep, attention-deficit/hyperactivity disorder, stress reduction, promoting stroke and aphasia recovery	1. Center, ground, and set intention. 2. Assess local energy field. 3. Hold fingertips or palms on designated parts of the neck and head, holding each part 1–3 minutes in a designated sequence. 4. End with lightly placing both hands over the heart chakra and brushing up over the shoulder. 5. Reassess the energy field. 6. Ground the client.
Siphon (Bruyere, 1989)	Draining pain or energy congestion Used for acute or chronic pain	1. Center, ground, and set intention. 2. Assess the local energy field 3. Place the left hand on the area of pain or energy congestion and the right-hand palm down and lower that the area needing siphoning and away from the body. 4. Siphon off congested energy from the painful area through the left hand and out the right hand. 5. Place the right hand on the painful or congested area and place the left-hand palm upward in the air to bring in healing energy from the universal energy field (each position is generally held 3–5 minutes). 6. Reassess the local energy field. 7. Ground the client.
Sword Fingers Energetic laser	Cuts, seals, and breaks up congestion in the energy field. Used for relieving pain, stopping bleeding from a laceration, assisting in wound repair, fractured bones, joint injuries and surgeries, tumors, eye and ear problems	1. Center, ground, and set intention. 2. Assess the client's localized energy field. 3. Hold one or more fingers still and pointed toward the problem area. 4. Use for a few seconds to a minute. 5. Reassess local energy field. 6. Ground the client.

(continued)

Table 23.3 *Selected Localized Healing Touch Techniques (continued)*

Techniques	Indications	Brief Description of Procedure
Wound healing	Repairs energy field tears or leaks that occur from physical trauma. Used for ongoing pain at the site of surgery, trauma, wounds, after childbirth; after radiation; or with clients who report extreme fatigue	1. Center, ground, and set intention. 2. Hand scan body above a scar or injury to determine whether any leaks of energy are felt coming from the site (may feel like a column of cool air). 3. Move hands over the area, gathering energy. 4. Bring gathered energy down into the wound/leak, once the leak is filled, hold hands on or close to the area for up to 1 minute to seal the leak. 5. Rescan the area to determine the energy field feels evenly symmetrical over the entire body. 6. Ground the client.

Source: Adapted from Anderson, J. G., Anselme, L. C., & Hart, L. K. (2017). *Foundations and practice of healing touch*. Healing Beyond Borders.

will vary based on the needs and assessment findings of the client. Sessions can range from a few minutes to an hour. The practitioner can use a variety of objects that represent the client. These objects can include a doll or teddy bear, a picture of a human body, or a table set up with clothes used to represent the individual receiving the session.

MEASUREMENT OF OUTCOMES

Outcomes that are measured to evaluate the effectiveness of HT session(s) must reflect the specific client need and presenting symptoms, and the particular HT technique used. Depending on the setting and purpose of the evaluation (e.g., clinical versus research), standardized instruments (e.g., the Geriatric Depression Scale, PHQ-9, or PROMIS® measures) may be selected, nurse observation, or simple verbal subjective self-report may be used. HT outcomes that have been measured have included such things as patient/client satisfaction, anxiety and stress, mood (e.g., depression), fatigue, nausea, sleep length and quality, and pain reduction. Often a sense of well-being and health-related quality of life, and length of hospitalization have also been measured. Symptoms of PTSD, hostility, and cynicism have been measured in post-deployed active military when HT sessions are offered. A number of physiological and biological measures have been used including blood pressure, blood glucose, salivary immunoglobulin A, oxygen saturation, polysomnographic data, and natural killer cell activity or other measures of immune function. Agitation levels and disruptive behavior of persons with cognitive deficits/dementia have been measured, as well as the functional status of people with mobility issues.

It is difficult to determine whether the outcome of the HT intervention is due solely to the treatment or to other factors such as a placebo effect, the effect of the practitioner's presence, or other uncontrolled or unknown/unmeasured variable. Such potential confounding is not unique to HT, but potential confounds may also be present with many other nursing interventions that are assessed for their effectiveness.

PRECAUTIONS

Precautions to be aware of when using HT techniques include the following:

- The energy fields of infants, children, older people, the extremely ill, and the dying are sensitive to energy work, so treatments should be gentle and time-limited.
- Gentle energy treatments are required for pregnant women because the energy field also includes the fetus.
- Energy work with a cancer patient should be focused on balancing the whole field rather than concentrating on a particular area.

The effect of medications and chemicals in the body may be enhanced with energy work, so one must be alert to the possibility of side effects and sensitivity reactions to these substances.

It is recommended that experienced practitioners work with clients in the previously discussed situations. However, to help develop a knowledgeable practice, a student or an apprentice in HT can provide treatments in these situations if supervised by a mentor. HT is not considered a curative treatment and is often complementary to conventional medical care. However, some practitioners report that clients express experiencing a sense of healing at a more holistic level of mind, body, and spirit, even if a cure is not possible. Umbreit (2000) reports anecdotal comments from clients that include feeling "wonderful," "relaxed," "peaceful," "in a meditative state," "warm," "soothed," "safe," "reassured," "more balanced," "mellow," "happier with life," "as if all my tension was melting," and a "sense of inner peace." Reduced stress, increased energy, vitality, and well-being may also be experienced. Because HT is a noninvasive intervention, these responses have the potential for use for stress reduction and improving well-being and quality of life—especially for patients, families, nurses, and nursing students in the COVID era.

USES

HT interventions can be used with all age groups, from the neonate to the older adult. Models of delivering services range from volunteer to staff-provided programs. HT is being used within diverse healthcare facilities: hospitals, long-term care facilities, private practices, hospices, outpatient clinics, home care, communities, church-related health and spiritual ministry departments, and spas (Healing Beyond Borders, 2021a; Kagel & Anselme, 2014). Table 23.4 lists selected research studies supporting the effectiveness of HT interventions for various patient populations/clinical situations. Also, many HT practitioners add HT interventions such as chakra connection for self-care, self-field repatterning, and sword fingers energetic laser to their routine self-care practices.

CULTURAL APPLICATIONS

As with other healthcare and medical practices, ethnic and cultural factors and attitudes can influence people's perceptions and experiences with HT. Ghiasuddin et al. (2015) studied HT interventions with a small group of pediatric oncology patients in Hawaii. Most of the subjects were of Asian or Pacific Island heritage. Responses from children and families indicated that all parents were

Table 23.4 *Selected Recent Studies Using Healing Touch Interventions*

Healing Touch Uses	Selected Sources
Anxiety/stress/mood	Goldberg et al. (2016); Hendricks & Wallace (2017); Running & Hildreth (2016)
Cancer pain and treatment	Gentile et al. (2018, 2021); Lu et al. (2016)
Critical care	Davis et al. (2020)
Mental Health	Mangione et al. (2017)
Pain	Anderson et al. (2015); Gentile et al. (2021)
Pediatrics	Bhardwaj & Koffman (2017); James et al. (2019)
Postsurgical/postprocedural care	Foley et al. (2016)
Posttraumatic stress syndrome	Reeve et al. (2020)

enthusiastically interested in using healing touch for their children. Interestingly, in a couple of cases, the children did not share their parents' interest in using HT.

HT is being taught and practiced in countries around the world, including impoverished communities with few economic resources; people in more countries continue to request HT education each year. It is noted that "the richness of HT is that it lends itself to flowing to and across continents and cultures and maintains its standardization while it melds with the flavor of the area it serves" (Van Aken, 2014, p. 5).

HT appropriately adapts to the culture and available resources (Wardell et al., 2014b). HT students are able to use their skills in their communities: hospitals, clinics, homes, rural areas, villages, and places where healthcare may be limited, medications lacking, and living conditions very difficult. Even in impoverished places of the world, where strife, abject poverty, and hidden hopelessness pervade daily life, learning and practicing HT has helped empower people to address their serious social and public health issues by decreasing their suffering, especially where people are underserved or marginalized.

Frost (2014) reported on her HT experiences in South Africa, teaching caregivers of people suffering and dying of AIDS and some of the millions of orphaned children in Africa. Many live in desperately inadequate settlement camps, and the caregivers were so appreciative to learn the basic HT technique to use as part of the care to support their ill patients. Frost (2014) also writes about helping to set up an HT clinic for women and children of the "first" peoples from the Kalahari Desert region. Techniques taught addressed the women's main complaints of headaches and body pain. After the HT classes, they reported an easing of pain, feeling relaxed, and feeling good.

Kagel (2014b) reported her experiences and the challenges of teaching HT in several poor rural locations around Ecuador. Some of her students spoke Spanish, some Quichua (a local dialect), often in the same class, so one or two translators were needed. Many students did not read, so the translator created pictorial references easily distributed to the students to support their future practice. Kagel reports that teaching in Ecuador was very different than in the United States.

Community leaders controlled the scheduling of classes in Ecuador, and all HT classes had to be approved by government officials after interviews, explanations of the work, and intended benefits to the community were presented. Once approved, officials set the days and times of the classes; classes had to start after work (3 p.m.) and finish before dark "so that the women would not 'disappear' walking home." Women were given a day off during the weekend to cook, wash clothes in the open-air laundry tubs, care for their families, and be ready for the new work week" (p. 54). Kagel shares her story about teaching in Ecuador in Sidebar 23.1. Chris Lepoutre describes the status and limited access to energy healing therapies in the context of healthcare and broader sociopolitical culture in France (Sidebar 23.2).

Sidebar 23.1 *Teaching Healing Touch in Rural Ecuador*

Sue Kagel

We were escorted in and out of dangerous communities, teaching in churches, community buildings, and in one situation, the second floor of a small police department. Our classrooms often had no heat or bedding. We were creative and used whatever was available. One room had only chairs, so we taught techniques for chair use, a few used gym mats or thin mattresses on the floor and we worked kneeling. In another class, I demonstrated techniques sitting on the floor with one of our teen volunteers lying on the cold linoleum floor. A church setting had desks and benches, so we pushed them together to create space for people to recline and used chairs. Roosters crowed; kids ran in and out; babies cried, nursed, and slept; rooftops rattled and flapped in the wind. We held the energy for the class and stayed in a flexible, loving, healing presence.

In one location, the class swelled the second day as excited students brought their family members and friends. Rather than moving to the next technique sequences, we brought the new members up to speed and advanced the students at the same time. They were so grateful to have new tools to use as medical care was scarce.

Several communities were located on the mountainside, so pain-relief techniques for legs and shoulders were taught to address the problems incurred from carrying huge loads up and down steep slopes. Techniques to address the problems of family and domestic violence issues were also taught. At the lower altitudes, headaches and dehydration from the heat were addressed at the people's request. For the day-care workers, we focused on heart-centered presence, energetic balancing, pain management, and calming techniques for the children rather than corporal punishment. All classes needed to be short and focused. Class sizes changed unexpectedly, so constant adjustments had to be made. Those we served noted decreased emotional stress, relief of physical symptoms, and a decrease in aggressive, violent behaviors in families who took the Healing Touch classes. Grounding, centering, body awareness, and breathing became tools used in community gatherings and individually to continue supporting their well-being.

Sidebar 23.2 *Energy Healing in France*

Chris Lepoutre

Energy healing is not a part of the occidental (Western) healthcare system in France. It would be highly unusual for a physician to request that an energy healer work with a patient. Patients or their family may ask an energy healer to visit a patient in the hospital, but this request is not made by the hospital staff.

Being an energy healer is not freely shared with others. Some see energy healers as witches. If it is known that you are an energy healer, you may be shunned. In the Judeo-Christian culture, energy healers are often viewed as the hand of the devil. A Catholic priest, who was using energy healing, was told by his bishop to end this activity or resign.

However, many people go to energy healers for therapy, although it is an underground activity. Some physicians may informally advise a person to go for healing to an energy healer, but this is never a formal referral. More often it is a nurse who will whisper about the therapy to the patient or family. This is particularly true for some specific illnesses such as shingles or burns.

It is not uncommon for a person who has had energy healing to share their experience with friends. The person may recommend this therapy to friends for the treatment of specific health issues through word of mouth. In these cases, sessions are typically paid for with cash as an "underground" economy.

There is no formal well-publicized education program for energy healing in France. Information on 2-day education sessions can be found on the Internet. At the end of the 2-day course, the person receives a certificate. However, there is no government recognition for preparation in healing touch.

As an indication that interest in and use of energy healing is growing in France, some energy healers have recently begun to open offices to provide this therapy. However, these are viewed as stores and not as a medical business.

FUTURE RESEARCH

Research on biofield therapies is growing, and we are seeing an increase in the number and quality of HT research studies (Hess et al., 2020). Many of the studies and anecdotal cases in HT offer promising, yet certainly not conclusive, data on the positive outcomes of this complementary therapy. The research continues to be controversial because the exact mechanism of action cannot be seen or easily explained in our Western view of what constitutes sound scientific research, and few double-blind studies have been done in this area. Until a reliable and readily available tool is developed to measure changes in the energy system, objective measurement of changes in the flow of an energy field is not possible. However, skilled practitioners do report a change in clients' energy fields that they perceive through the use of their senses, most commonly through touch. Qualitative responses from clients have been especially important in helping guide the direction of the research and may provide insight into the phenomenon of energy exchange in the future. Some of the problems encountered in nursing research include insufficient funding to support the work, multiple variables that are hard to control in a clinical setting versus a laboratory setting, and the use of small sample sizes that can be easily affected by highly variable data and sampling error.

There is the additional difficulty of testing the efficacy of an energy-based therapy in which the energy exchange between practitioner and client cannot be seen by most people but is only observed as subjective responses from clients. The whole conceptual framework of energy fields and energy exchange does not fit the cause–effect model that Western science is focused on. Rogers's theory (1990) speaks about energy changing, exchanging, and patterning, one moment in time never replicating itself. The focus is on nature's restoring universal order and balance, and restoring energy balance is the goal of HT. This is an area of research that obviously will require a multidisciplinary effort by Western and Eastern medicine, quantum physics, biology, psychology, philosophy, spirituality, and nursing. Outcome studies, as well as studies of mechanism, will help support the development and understanding of the phenomenon of energy exchange. Mediating factors may contribute to a decrease in pain intensity, anxiety reduction, acceleration of healing, immune system enhancement, diminished depression, and increased sense of well-being. More studies that measure some of these mediating mechanisms are recommended.

The choice of valid instruments for measuring outcomes is critical in HT studies. Results can be skewed in either direction if the instruments are not reliable. However, to obtain subject cooperation when working with those who are ill, measurement instruments must be easy to use and not burdensome to patients who are already facing difficulties.

Other challenges to be controlled in conducting HT research studies include the experience of the HT practitioner, the phenomenon of the caregiver's presence, the type of HT treatment modality chosen, the duration and number of treatments, the time when the treatment is done, the time when measurements are done, and long-term effects of HT. There is a wide range of skill levels of HT practitioners from novices to certified practitioners, and comparable skill level is important in planning a research study since the expertise of the healer may affect the length and depth of the healing.

The phenomenon of the presence of the HT practitioner may also affect the outcome of the research and needs to be controlled in the study design. Because many HT interventions can be used, a research study needs to be consistent in the type of therapy chosen. The challenge with duration and number of treatments is that, under normal circumstances, an HT intervention is not used for a prescribed length of time or number of treatments. The work is done until the practitioner intuitively determines that it is time to stop or that no more treatments are needed. Research could restrict this professional decision-making process. Choosing when to give an HT treatment, when to measure outcomes, and ascertaining how long the outcome may last continue to be challenging. Experienced HT practitioners must have input into determining these timelines by observing patterns they may typically see in their own professional practice.

There continues to be some criticism within the scientific community of current energy/biofield therapy research, pointing to study quality and limitations such as small subject numbers, controls for placebo effect, possible Hawthorne effect, and nonblinding of participants. The effects of HT interventions have been supported by only a limited number of rigorous research studies. Some reports are anecdotes or case studies (Wardell et al., 2014c). Some studies are missing controls or lack vital information, which leads to problems with both internal and external validity.

Researchers can design future studies with more rigor or using designs to overcome some of these limitations, for example, placebo-controlled studies. Goals of future HT research include increasing the number of studies and RCTs that are replicable and that have larger numbers of participants using standardized, reliable, and valid instruments. In addition, investigators can conduct studies that help determine the optimal amount, techniques, or protocol of HT to alleviate various symptoms and conditions.

The next steps for research must build on the studies already completed. Replication of studies would help strengthen the scientific base underlying HT. Questions that researchers might investigate in the future include the following:

- Is HT equally effective in acute versus chronic pain? How long and how frequently do treatments need to be for the client to report a decrease in pain? How long does this improvement last?
- Is HT an effective nonpharmacological option to opioids in the treatment/management of pain?
- How is postoperative recovery affected by administering HT (pain relief, wound healing, restored bowel function, ease of physical activity, length of stay in the hospital)?
- Does HT have a positive effect on symptoms caused by degenerative diseases such as arthritis, multiple sclerosis, fibromyalgia, and other inflammatory-based diseases?
- What effects does HT have in the care and treatment of the health issues of the aging population and those with mental health conditions?
- Can HT reduce symptoms and assist in managing the side effects of treatments in cancer patients?
- What is the impact of HT as a complement to help eliminate PTSD and depression in our military and others who have experienced trauma?
- What tools exist that are effective in measuring a change in energy in the recipient before and after HT or an exchange of energy between practitioner and recipient?
- Does HT reduce medical costs for pharmaceuticals, hospital stays, and clinic time?
- Does the use of HT as a patient-centric intervention improve patient satisfaction scores?

In the quest to examine the impact of HT scientifically, care must be taken to not be too quick to dismiss the positive client feedback from its clinical application. Creativity is necessary when conducting research on this phenomenon that may not be seen by the naked eye but that is felt by the human spirit.

WEBSITES

INFORMATION ON HT

- American Holistic Nurses Association (AHNA): www.ahna.org
- Healing Beyond Borders (HBB): www.healingbeyondborders.org

- Healing Touch Program (HTP): www.healingtouchprogram.com
- Consciousness and Healing Initiative: www.CHI.is
- YouTube: Intro to Healing Touch with Sue Kagel: www.youtube.com/watch?v=HhrMiMlWx4E

HBB INTERNATIONAL AFFILIATE HT ORGANIZATIONS

- Australian Foundation for Healing Touch Inc.: https://healingtouch.org.au
- Healing Touch Canada Inc.: https://healingtouchcanada.net
- Healing Touch Association of Canada: https://healingtouchassociation.ca
- Healing Touch Sweden: https://healingtouch.se
- Healing Touch Netherlands: https://healingtouch.nl
- Healing Touch New Zealand Inc.: https://healingtouchnz.com
- Healing Touch Peru: https://prosh-promoviendosaludholistica.blogspot.com

INFORMATION ON THERAPEUTIC TOUCH

- Therapeutic Touch International Association: www.therapeutictouch.org

REFERENCES

Adimando, A. (2018). Preventing and alleviating compassion fatigue through self-care. *Journal of Holistic Nursing, 36*(4), 304–317. https://doi.org/10.1177/0898010117721581

American Nurses Association. (2015). *Code of ethics for nurses with interpretive statements.* http://www.nursingworld.org/MainMenuCategories/EthicsStandards/CodeofEthicsforNurses/Code-of-Ethics-For-Nurses.html

Anderson, J. G. (2016, October). *A deep dive into psychoneuroimmunology* [Paper presentation]. Healing Beyond Borders Conference, Colorado Springs, CO, USA.

Anderson, J. G., Anselme, L. C., & Hart, L. K. (2017). *Foundations and practice of healing touch.* Healing Beyond Borders.

Anderson, J. G., Suchicital, L., Lang, M., Kukic, A., Mangione, L., Swengros, D., Fabian, J., & Friesen, M. A. (2015). The effects of healing touch on pain, nausea and anxiety following bariatric surgery: A pilot study. *Explore: The Journal of Science and Healing, 11*(3), 208–216. https://doi.org/10.1016/j.explore.2015.02.006

Anderson, J. G., & Taylor, A. G. (2011). Effects of healing touch in clinical practice. *Journal of Holistic Nursing, 29*(3), 221–228. https://doi.org/10.1177/0898010110393353

Bhardwaj, T., & Koffman, J. (2017). Non-pharmacological interventions for management of fatigue among children with cancer: Systematic review of existing practices and their effectiveness. *BMJ Supportive and Palliative Care, 7*(4), 404–414. https://doi.org/10.1136/bmjspcare-2016-001132

Bruyere, R. L. (1989). *Hands of light.* Bantam.

Church, D. (2018). *Mind to matter: The astonishing science of how your brain creates material reality.* Hay House Inc.

Cone, L., Gottschlich, M. M., Khoury, J., Simakajornboon, N., & Kagan, R. J. (2014). The effect of healing touch on sleep patterns of pediatric burn patients: A prospective pilot study. *Journal of Sleep Disorders: Treatments and Care, 3*(2), 1–6. https://doi.org/10.4172/2325-9639.1000136

Crane, P. J., & Ward, S. F. (2016). Self-healing and self-care for nurses. *AORN Journal, 104*(5), 386–400. https://doi.org/10.1016/j.aorn.2016.09.007

Darbonne, M. (2012). The effects of healing touch modalities on patients with chronic pain. In M. Megel, J. G. Anderson, D. Lu, & N. Strybol (Eds.), *Healing touch research survey* (14th ed., pp. 76–77). Healing Touch International.

Davis, T. M., Lindgren, V., Jackson, R., Mangione, L., Swengros, D., & Anderson, J. G. (2020). The effect of healing touch on critical care patients' vital signs: A pilot study. *Holistic Nursing Practice, 34*(4), 244–251. https://doi.org/10.1097/HNP.0000000000000394

Dossey, L. (2015). Nonlocal mind: A (fairly) brief history of the term. *Explore (NY)*, *11*(2), 89–101. https://doi.org/10.1016/j.explore.2014.12.001

Easter, A. (1997). The state of research on the effects of therapeutic touch. *Journal of Holistic Nursing*, *15*(2), 158–175. https://doi.org/10.1177/089801019701500207

Eschiti, V. (2014). Martha Rogers: The science of unitary human beings in foundational aspects of healing work. In D. Wardell, S. Kagel, & L. Anselme (Eds.), *Healing touch: Enhancing life through energy therapy* (pp. 76–68). iUniverse LLC.

FitzHenry, F., Wells, N., Slater, V., Dietrich, M. S., Wisawatapnimit, P., & Chakravarthy, A. B. (2014). A randomized placebo-controlled pilot study of the impact of healing touch on fatigue in breast cancer patients undergoing radiation therapy. *Integrated Cancer Therapies*, *13*(2), 105–113. https://doi.org/10.1177/1534735413503545

Foley, M. K., Anderson, J., Mallea, L., Morrison, K., & Downey, M. (2016). Effects of healing touch on postsurgical adult outpatients. *Journal of Holistic Nursing*, *34*(3), 271–279. https://doi.org/10.1177/0898010115609486

Frost, M. (2014). South Africa. In D. Wardell, S. Kagel, & L. Anselme (Eds.), *Healing touch: Enhancing life through energy therapy* (pp. 57–61). iUniverse LLC.

Ghiasuddin, A., Wong, J., & Siu, A. M. (2015). Ethnicity, traditional healing practices, and attitudes towards complementary medicine of a pediatric oncology population receiving healing touch in Hawaii. *Asia-Pacific Journal of Oncology Nursing*, *2*(4), 227–231. https://doi.org/10.4103/2347-5625.158015

Gentile, D., Boselli, D., O'Neill, G., Yaguda, S., Bailey-Dorton, C., & Eaton, T. A. (2018). Cancer pain relief after healing touch and massage. *Journal of Alternative and Complementary Medicine*, *24*(9–10), 968–973. https://doi.org/10.1089/acm.2018.0192

Gentile, D., Boselli, D., Yaguda, S., Greiner, R., & Bailey-Dorton, C. (2021). Pain improvement after healing touch and massage in a breast center: An observational retrospective study. *International Journal of Therapeutic Massage and Bodywork*, *14*(1), 12–20. https://doi.org/10.3822/ijtmb.v14i1.549

Goldberg, D. R., Wardell, D. W., Kilgarriff, N., Williams, B., Eichler, D., & Thomlinson, P. (2016). An initial study using healing touch for women undergoing a breast biopsy. *Journal of Holistic Nursing*, *34*(2), 123–134. https://doi.org/10.1177/0898010115585414

Hall, L. H., Johnson, J., Watt, I., Tsipa, A., & O'Connor, D. B. (2016). Healthcare staff well-being, burnout, and patient safety: A systematic review. *PLoS One*, *11*(7), e0159015. https://doi.org/10.1371/journal.pone.0159015

Hammerschlag, R., Marx, B. L., & Aickin, M. (2014). Nontouch biofield therapy: A systematic review of human randomized controlled trials reporting use of only nonphysical contact treatment. *Journal of Alternative and Complementary Medicine*, *20*(12), 881–892. https://doi.org/10.1186/1472-6882-12-S1-P98

Hardwick, M. E., Pulido, P. A., & Adelson, W. S. (2012). Nursing intervention using healing touch in bilateral total knee arthroplasty. *Orthopedic Nursing*, *31*(1), 5–11. https://doi.org/10.1097/NOR.0b013e31824195fb

Healing Beyond Borders. (2021a). *About. What is healing touch?* https://www.healingbeyondborders.org/index.php/what-is-healing-touch

Healing Beyond Borders. (2021b). *Statement of scope of practice: HTI healing touch certificate program.* https://www.healingbeyondborders.org/index.php?option=com_content&view=article&id=88:scope-of-practice&catid=89:about&Itemid=536

Healing Beyond Borders. (2021c). *Vision and mission.* https://www.healingbeyondborders.org/index.php/about?id=99:vision-and-mission

Healing Touch Program. (2022). *What is healing touch?* https://www.healingtouchprogram.com/about/what-is-healing-touch

Heidt, P. (1981). Effect of therapeutic touch on the anxiety level of hospitalized patients. *Nursing Research*, *30*(1), 32–37. https://doi.org/10.1097/00006199-198101000-00014

Hendricks, K., & Wallace, K. F. (2017). Pilot study: Improving patient outcomes with healing touch. *Advances in Peritoneal Dialysis*, *33*(2017), 65–67. https://doi.org/10.15761/NRD.1000135

Herdman, T. H., Kamitsuru, S., & Lopes, C. T. (Eds.). (2021). *NANDA International nursing diagnoses: Definitions & classification, 2021–2023*. Thieme.

Hess, S. M., Lu, D-F., Mangione, L., Friesen, M. A., Allen, S. & Anderson, J. G. (2020). *Healing touch research brief: A summary of topics on research and strategies for the future*. Healing Beyond Borders.

Hover-Kramer, D. (1996). *Healing Touch; A resource for Health Care Providers*. Delmar.

Ives, J. A., van Wijk, E. P. A., Bat, N., Crawford, C., Walter, A., Jonas, W. B., van Wijk, R., & van der Greef, J. (2014). Ultraweak photon emission as a non-invasive health assessment: A systematic review. *PLoS ONE, 9*(2), e87401. https://doi.org/10.1371/journal.pone.0087401

Jackson, C., & Latini, C. (2016). Touch & hand mediated therapies. In B. Dossey & L. Keegan (Eds.), *Holistic nursing: A handbook for practice* (7th ed., pp. 299–319). Jones & Bartlett.

Jain, S., McMahon, G. F., Hasen, P., Kozub, M. P., Porter, V., King, R., & Guarneri, E. M. (2012a). Healing touch with guided imagery for PTSD in returning active duty military: A randomized controlled trial. *Military Medicine, 177*(9), 1015–1021. https://doi.org/10.7205/milmed-d-11-00290

Jain, S., Pavlik, D., Distefan, J., Bruyere, R. L., Acer, J., Garcia, R., Coulter, I., Ives, J., Roesch, S. C., Jonas, W., & Mills, P. J. (2012b). Complementary medicine for fatigue and cortisol variability in breast cancer survivors: A randomized controlled trial. *Cancer, 118*(3), 777–787. https://doi.org/10.1002/cncr.26345

James, L. E., Gottschlich, M. M., Nelson, J. K., Cone, L. C., & McCall, J. E. (2019). Pediatric perioperative measures of sleep, pain, anxiety and anesthesia emergence: A healing touch proof of concept randomized clinical trial. *Complementary Therapies in Medicine, 42*, 264–269. https://doi.org/10.1016/j.ctim.2018.11.027

Kagel, S. (2014a). Distance healing. In D. Wardell, S. Kagel, & L. Anselme (Eds.), *Healing touch: Enhancing life through energy therapy* (pp. 303–308). iUniverse LLC.

Kagel, S. (2014b). Ecuador. In D. Wardell, S. Kagel, & L. Anselme (Eds.), *Healing touch: Enhancing life through energy therapy* (pp. 53–57). iUniverse LLC.

Kagel, S., & Anselme, L. (2014). Integrating from self to family, community, & the world. In D. Wardell, S. Kagel, & L. Anselme (Eds.), *Healing touch: Enhancing life through energy therapy* (pp. 332–335). iUniverse LLC.

Krieger, D. (1979). *The therapeutic touch: How to use your hands to help or to heal*. Simon & Schuster.

Krieger, D. (1993). *Accepting your power to heal*. Bear & Co.

Kunz, D. (1995). *Spiritual healing: Doctors examine therapeutic touch and other holistic treatments*. Theosophical Publishing House.

Linton, M., & Koonmen, J. (2020). Self-care as an ethical obligation for nurses. *Nursing Ethics, 27*(8), 1694–1702. https://doi.org/10.1177/0969733020940371

Lu, D-F., Hart, L. K., Lutgendorf, S. K., Oh, H., & Schilling, M. (2013a). Slowing progression of early stages of AD with alternative therapies: A feasibility study. *Geriatric Nursing, 34*(6), 457–464. https://doi.org/10.1016/j.gerinurse.2013.07.003

Lu, D-F., Hart, L. K., Lutgendorf, S. K., Oh, H., & Silverman, M. (2016). Effects of healing touch and relaxation therapy on adult patients undergoing hematopoietic stem cell transplant: A feasibility pilot study. *Cancer Nursing, 39*(3), E1–E11. https://doi.org/10.1097/NCC.0000000000000272

Lu, D-F., Hart, L. K., Lutgendorf, S. K., & Perkhounkova, Y. (2013b). The effect of healing touch on the pain and mobility of persons with osteoarthritis: A feasibility study. *Geriatric Nursing, 34*(4), 314–322. https://doi.org/10.1016/j.gerinurse.2013.05.003

Mangione, L., Swengros, D., & Anderson, J. G. (2017). Mental health wellness and biofield therapies: An integrative review. *Issues in Mental Health Nursing, 38*(11), 930–944. https://doi.org/10.1080/01612840.2017.1364808

McTaggart, L. (2017). *The power of 8: Harnessing the miraculous energies of a small group to heal others, your life, and the world*. Altria Books, Simon and Schuster.

Megel, M. E., Anderson, J. G., Lu, D-F., & Strybol, N. (2012). *Healing touch research survey* (14th ed.). Healing Touch International.

Melnyk, B. M., Orsolini, L., Tan, A., Arslanian-Engoren, C., Melkus, G. D., Dunbar-Jacob, J., Hill Rice, V., Millan, A., Dunbar, S., Braun, L. T., Wilbur, J., Chyun, D., Gawlik, K., & Lewis, L. M. (2018). A national study links nurses' physical and mental health to medical errors and perceived worksite wellness. *Journal of Occupational and Environmental Medicine, 60*(2), 126–131. https://doi.org/10.1097/jom.0000000000001198

Moreno, M., Stephen, S., Mazon, S., Gerhard, I., Huber, C., Koren, N., & Endler, P. C. (2018). Distant resonance of Brennan Healing Science® practitioners to different states: A contribution to fundamental research. *Journal of Alternative Medicine Research, 10*(3), 223–228.

Noel, R. (2011). *The Huggin' Healer*. Publish America.

Oschman, J. (2008, September). *Validating the heart's work*. Paper presented at the Healing Touch International Conference, Milwaukee, WI.

Oschman, J. (2016a, October). *Scientific basis of energy medicine*. Paper presented at the Healing Beyond Borders Conference, Colorado Springs, CO.

Oschman, J. L. (2016b). *Energy medicine: The scientific basis* (2nd ed.). Elsevier.

Ostuni, E., & Pietro, M. J. (2012). Effects of healing touch on nursing home residents in later stages of Alzheimer's. In M. Megel, J. G. Anderson, D-F. Lu, & N. Strybol (Eds.), *Healing touch research survey* (14th ed., pp. 47–48). Healing Touch International.

Quinn, J. F. (1988). Building a body of knowledge: Research on therapeutic touch 1974–1986. *Journal of Holistic Nursing, 6*(1), 37–45. https://doi.org/10.1177/089801018800600110

Reeve, K., Black, P. A., & Huang, J. (2020). Examining the impact of a healing touch intervention to reduce posttraumatic stress disorder symptoms in combat veterans. *Psychological Trauma: Theory, Research, Practice, and Policy, 12*(8), 897–903. https://doi.org/10.1037/tra0000591

Rogers, M. (1990). Nursing: Science of unitary, irreducible, human beings: Update 1990. In E. A. M. Barrett (Ed.), *Vision of Rogers' science-based nursing* (pp. 5–11). National League for Nursing.

Running, A., & Hildreth, L. (2016). Bio-energy during finals: Stress reduction for a university community. *Journal of Community Health Nursing, 33*(4), 209–217. https://doi.org/10.1080/07370016.2016.1227214

Schwartz, S. A. (2017). The manipulation of perceived reality through nonlocal intention. *Explore: The Journal of Science & Healing, 13*(1), 12–15. https://doi.org/10.1016/j.explore.2016.10.012

Thornton, L., & Mariano, C. (2016). Evolving from therapeutic to holistic communication. In B. Dossey & L. Keegan (Eds.), *Holistic nursing: A handbook for practice* (7th ed., p. 477). Jones & Bartlett.

Umbreit, A. (2000). Healing touch: Applications in the acute care setting. *AACN Clinical Issues, 11*(1), 105–119. https://doi.org/10.1097/00044067-200002000-00012

Van Aken, R. (2014). An international perspective. In D. Wardell, S. Kagel, & L. Anselme (Eds.), *Healing touch: Enhancing life through energy therapy* (pp. 3–4). iUniverse LLC.

Wardell, D. W., Kagel, S., & Anselme, L. (2014a). History of healing touch education and certification. In D. W. Wardell, S. Kagel, & L. Anselme (Eds.), *Healing touch: Enhancing life through energy therapy* (pp. 63-67). iUniverse LLC.

Wardell, D. W., Kagel, S., & Anselme, L. (2014b). An international perspective. In D. W. Wardell, S. Kagel, & L. Anselme (Eds.), *Healing touch: Enhancing life through energy therapy* (pp. 1–5). iUniverse LLC.

Wardell, D. W., Kagel, S., & Anselme, L. (2014c). Healing touch through the life continuum: Clinical application. In D. W. Wardell, S. Kagel, & L. Anselme (Eds.), *Healing touch: Enhancing life through energy therapy* (pp. 211–245). iUniverse LLC.

Wilson, D. R. (2020). Energetic interconnectedness. In Shields, D. A., Avino, K. M., & Rosa, W. E. (Eds.), *Dossey & Keegan's holistic nursing: A handbook for practice* (8th ed., pp. 253–261). Jones & Bartlett Learning.

Wirth, D. P. (1992). The effect of non-contact therapeutic touch on the healing rate of full thickness dermal wounds. *Subtle Energies, 1*(1), 1–20.

Wong, J., Ghiasuddin, A., Kimata, C., Patelesio, B., & Siu, A. (2013). The impact of healing touch on pediatric oncology patients: *Integrative Cancer Therapies, 12*(1), 25–30. https://doi.org/10.1177/1534735412446864

Reiki

DEBBIE RINGDAHL

The Reiki principles:

- Just for today, I will live in the attitude of gratitude.
- Just for today, I will not worry.
- Just for today, I will not be angry.
- Just for today, I will do my work honestly.
- Just for today, I will show love and respect for every living being. (Miles, 2006, p. 91)

Reiki is an energy-healing method that can be used as an integrative therapy for a broad range of acute and chronic health problems. Increasingly, it is gaining acceptance as an adjunct to the management of chronic conditions with significant symptom burden in oncology, palliative care, and hospice settings. Additionally, Reiki self-practice enables applying it to symptom exacerbation, stress reduction, and relaxation. This aspect of Reiki practice is particularly useful for those managing chronic health conditions and individuals pursuing a daily self-care practice. Evidence of increasing healthcare delivery complexity also supports the use of Reiki for stress reduction among healthcare workers (Kentischer et al., 2017). Reiki offers whole-person healing through regular self-Reiki practice and through the Reiki Principles, which provide guidelines for present-moment living (Lipinski & Van De Velde, 2020).

The 2010 Complementary and Alternative Medicine Survey of Hospitals (Ananth, 2011) reported that Reiki and therapeutic touch (TT) were offered in 21% of inpatient settings surveyed. Reiki use in hospitals has likely experienced increased acceptance since this survey was conducted, but without mandatory registry for Reiki programs, this is difficult to quantify. Many prominent academic medical centers offer Reiki services: Portsmouth (New Hampshire) Regional Hospital, Brigham and Women's Hospital (Massachusetts), California Pacific Medical Center, Yale New Haven Hospital (Connecticut), Hartford Hospital (Connecticut), M. D. Anderson Cancer Center (Texas), Memorial Sloan Kettering Cancer Center (New York), Mayo Clinic (Minnesota; Baldwin, 2020). Reiki in hospitals is frequently offered through volunteer Reiki programs or the hospital's integrative medicine department, but some hospitals offer Reiki training to nursing staff who can incorporate Reiki into direct care (Baldwin, 2020; Miles, 2021). This author notes that six large healthcare facilities in the metropolitan Minneapolis–St. Paul area incorporate Reiki into their healthcare delivery in a variety of settings, including chemotherapy units, hospice, labor and delivery, a pediatric bone and marrow transplant unit, and long-term care.

According to the National Center for Complementary and Integrative Health (NCCIH, 2021a), Reiki falls into the subgroup of mind and body practices, a diverse group of modalities or techniques that can be practiced or taught by a trained practitioner or teacher. The NCCIH (2021b) defines *Reiki* as "a *complementary health approach* in which practitioners place their hands lightly on or just above a person, with the goal of facilitating the person's own healing response" (para. 1). Reiki, TT, and healing touch (HT) are all therapies that are used to support the healing process. Although each has its own history, techniques, and practice standards, they share many similarities. All three traditions include the fundamental assumption that a universal life force sustains all living organisms, that human beings have an energetic and spiritual dimension that is a part of the healing process, and that positive energetic influences exist in human interactions. The focus is on balancing the total energies of a person and stimulating the body's own natural healing ability rather than on treating specific physical diseases (Engebretson & Wardell, 2012). The common thread that exists among these modalities lies in their capacity to reduce stress, promote relaxation, and mitigate pain. All three of these energy practices have been introduced into clinical care over the past few decades, representing a renewed interest in the therapeutic use of intentional touch in clinical practice. An additional important consideration is the high safety profile that exists with energy-healing practices: To date, there have been no negative side effects identified in energy therapy outcomes. They are noninvasive and can be used safely in conjunction with other therapies (Baldwin, 2020).

A Reiki practitioner does not need to be prepared as a healthcare practitioner; however, nurses, physical therapists, massage therapists, and physicians who practice Reiki may have greater access and acceptability within the healthcare system in performing hands-on treatments. In addition, Reiki practice by nurses supports a high-touch practice model in a high-tech practice environment. The Institute of Medicine (IOM) 2009 Summit on Integrative Medicine and the Health of the Public identified that empathy and compassion enhanced care and improved outcomes with grade A evidence (IOM, 2010). Although this evidence is not specific to physical touch, research suggests that recipients of touch therapies frequently experience an integration of mind, body, and spirit that promotes feelings of well-being (Engebretson & Wardell, 2012). Watson's conceptualization of the reciprocal nature of caring also supports the value of Reiki touch in providing nursing care (Watson, 2011). Reiki offers nurses an avenue for caring for themselves and creating an optimal caring and healing environment for their patients and clients (Lipinski & Van DeVelde, 2020; Shepherd-Gentle, 2001). Reiki is not commonly reimbursed by health insurance plans, but some insurance companies may cover Reiki when delivered by a nurse or a licensed professional (Lipinski & Van DeVelde, 2020).

Reiki began as an oral tradition and relied on practitioners to pass on the method developed by the founder, Mikao Usui. Reiki historians generally agree that its roots may stem from hands-on healing techniques that were used in Tibet or India more than 2,000 years ago. Reiki emerged in modern times around

1900 through the work of a Japanese businessman and practitioner of Tendai Buddhism, Mikao Usui (Miles, 2006). Usui had a transformative experience that resulted in the development of Reiki, and this resulted in the precise format he established for administering Reiki. One of Dr. Usui's students, Chujiro Hayashi, opened up a Reiki clinic in Tokyo, further developing Reiki as a hands-on healing practice. Hawayo Takata, a Japanese American living in Hawaii, attended this clinic and studied with Hayashi after her recovery. Takata is credited with the spread of Reiki in the Americas and Europe (Stiene & Stiene, 2005). Reiki is now practiced throughout North and South America, Europe, New Zealand, Australia, and other parts of the world (Oschman, 2016), including Japan.

In recent years, several additional branches of Reiki have developed: Karuna Reiki, Holy Fire Reiki (International Center for Reiki Training [ICRT], 2021a), Seichem Reiki (Reiki and Seichem Association, 2021), and Temari Reiki (Townsend, 2013). There are currently no uniform standards in Reiki education or board certification for Reiki practitioners, either at the national or international level. Because of the noninvasive nature of the treatments, this does not present problems in Reiki hands-on practice but may contribute to variable levels of professionalism among practitioners. This lack of standardization may also pose problems when working to develop practice standards for integrating Reiki into the conventional healthcare system. Membership in a professional Reiki association supports adherence to professional and ethical standards (Baldwin, 2020).

DEFINITION

The word *Reiki* is composed of two Japanese words—*rei* and *ki*. *Rei* is usually translated as "sacred" or "spiritual." *Ki* refers to the life force energy that flows throughout all living things, known in certain other parts of the world as *chi*, *prana*, or *mana* (Stiene & Stiene, 2005). When *ki* energy is unrestricted, there is thought to be less susceptibility to illness or imbalances of the mind, body, or spirit (Lubeck et al., 2001). In its combined form, the word *Reiki* is taken to mean "spiritually guided life force" energy or "universal life force energy." Hyakuten Inamoto, Japanese Buddhist monk and Reiki Master, describes Reiki as twofold; a healing and spiritual practice (Inamoto, 2019).

The mind–body component of Reiki healing is evidenced in the underlying belief that the deepest level of healing occurs through the spirit. The emphasis is on healing, not curing, which is believed to occur by Reiki energy connecting individuals to their own innate spiritual wisdom and "highest good," creating a harmonization among the mind, body, spirit. Reiki is considered a nondirective healing tradition: Reiki energy flows through, but is not directed by, the practitioner, leaving the healing component to the individual receiving Reiki. Reiki is not only a healing technique but also a philosophy of living that acknowledges mind–body–spirit unity and human connectedness to all things. It is not a religion and is without religious creed or doctrine (Lipinski & Van De Velde, 2020).

The ability to practice Reiki is transmitted in stages directly from teacher to student via initiations called *attunements*. This attunement process differentiates Reiki from other hands-on healing methods. During attunements, teachers open the students' energy channels by using specific visual symbols that were revealed to Dr. Usui. There are three degrees of attunement preparatory to achieving the status of Master Teacher, at which stage the practitioner is considered fully open to the flow of universal life force energy. By tradition, the Usui Reiki symbols and their Japanese names are confidential. This arises from the sacred nature of the techniques rather than from proprietary motives; the symbols are believed not to convey Reiki energy if used by noninitiates.

Level I Reiki is taught as a hands-on technique that includes basic information about Reiki history, application, principles, and hand positions. At level II, students are taught symbols that allow the transfer of energy through space and time, also known as *absentee* or *distance healing*. The higher vibration of energy available at Level II is considered to work at a deeper level of healing and with greater intuitive awareness. Level III, or the mastery level, was traditionally achieved through an apprenticeship with a Reiki master and includes more in-depth study of Reiki practice and teaching. Increasingly, the mastery level is achieved through 3- to 5-day workshops. It is also common to add a mastery teacher level in order to focus on teaching skills (Baldwin, 2020). At all levels, Reiki skill develops through years of committed practice. It is prudent to seek Reiki teachers and practitioners who demonstrate commitment through daily self-practice, 1 to 2 years of dedicated practice, and affiliation with a professional Reiki organization. The International Association for Reiki Practitioners (https://iarp.org/) and the ICRT (www.reiki.org/) both offer referral services for teachers on their websites (Lipinski & Van De Velde, 2020).

Increasingly, Reiki classes are offered in an online format. This was initially introduced for easier access but further accelerated during the COVID-19 pandemic. In order to prevent COVID-19 exposure from travel and hands-on practice, this author reconfigured all three levels of Reiki classes into an online format in order to continue offering required Reiki classes for graduate nursing students. This was achieved by developing videos demonstrating Reiki practice and reconfiguring class activities, assignments, and class intervals. Advances in technology allowed for smooth and easy class interactions. This online format was well received, and learning outcomes were very similar to in-person instruction. The ICRT has reported similar outcomes with online Reiki education (Benelli, 2020).

SCIENTIFIC BASIS

Biofield science is an emerging field of study that views energy as a part of a complex system that has the capacity to influence the whole system. The biofield model is based on the principle that all living things contain a vital life force that creates an invisible field of energy (biofield) around them (Singg, 2015). According to Rubik et al. (2015), "The biofield or biological field, a complex organizing energy field engaged in the generation, maintenance, and regulation of biological homeodynamics, is a useful concept that provides the rudiments of a scientific foundation for energy medicine and thereby advances the research and practice of it" (p. 8). Reiki, as an energy-healing tradition, is consistent with a human biofield modality. Biofield theory suggests that complex interactions involving energy-healing modalities may be mediated by forces and processes yet to be discovered and understood. As other examples in science and medicine have revealed, theories once viewed as implausible over time become accepted through research and science (Kafatos et al., 2015). It is also important to consider that precise mechanisms for some common medications have postdated usage: The anti-inflammatory mechanism of action for salicylic acid wasn't discovered until 1971 (Baldwin, 2020).

Researchers have attempted to study the biological effects of biofields on biomolecules, in vitro cells, bacteria, plants, and animals, as well as the clinical effects on hemoglobin, immune functioning, and wound healing (Movaffaghi & Farsi, 2009). There is increasing evidence that living systems are sensitive to bioinformation and that biofield therapies can influence diverse cellular and biological systems. The notion that cellular and molecular changes occur within the energy spectrum of biofields is congruent with the view that subtle energy shifts may manifest as a physiological cause or effect and play a role in intercellular and intracellular communication (Movaffaghi & Farsi, 2009). Morse and Beem (2011) reported a case with an increase in absolute neutrophil count following Reiki, resulting in toleration of interferon and subsequent clearance of hepatitis C virus. Kent et al. (2020) demonstrated that Reiki significantly increased cell photon emission in stressed mouse intervertebral disc cells post-Reiki, compared with pretreatment and sham Reiki. The Reiki group also showed an increase in extracellular matrix proteins, suggesting improved cellular function (Kent et al., 2020).

There have also been studies focused on identifying the physical properties of biofields to determine potential mechanisms of action (Baldwin, 2020). An emerging body of evidence confirms the existence of energy fields and suggests new ways of measuring energy, although these are not specific to Reiki. Traditional electrical measurements, such as electrocardiograms and electroencephalograms, can now be supplemented by biomagnetic field mapping to obtain more accurate information about the human condition. Electromagnetic information has been used to both diagnose and treat disease (Oschman, 2016). Some evidence supports Reiki mediation through an electromagnetic biofield, but this doesn't explain the mechanism for distant Reiki (Baldwin, 2020). Baldwin (2020) suggests the most rational model for explaining the biological mechanism of Reiki is the Oschman theory; Reiki flow in the practitioner is triggered by an environmental source, which entrains and amplifies the brain waves.

Studies conducted to ascertain the impact of biofields on Reiki practitioners have been inconclusive. Baldwin et al. (2013) used a superconducting quantum interference device (SQUID) to measure the electromagnetic field from the hands and heart of three Reiki masters and four volunteers using Reiki on the self and were unable to demonstrate consistent high-intensity magnetic fields. SQUIDs have been used to show the effect of disease on the magnetic field of the body, and pulsating magnetic fields have been used to improve healing (Oschman, 2016). There is now evidence that the heart and brain both generate measurable electromagnetic fields (biofields) that extend away from the body (Baldwin, 2020), and disturbances in the electromagnetic parts of the biofield can significantly impact health processes (Muehsam et al., 2015).

Rogers's Science of Unitary Human Beings has been used as a theoretical framework for understanding the experience of Reiki. This theory connects scientific principles of energy as matter to the human energy field and energetic interconnections that occur in the environment (Ring, 2009). These concepts are similar to those of experts who suggest that rather than identifying the unique characteristics of each subtle energy field, we should view biofield theory as a unifying concept for understanding the wide range of forces that influence health and well-being on the physical, emotional, social, and spiritual levels (Kreitzer & Saper, 2015).

Recipients' subjective feelings during a Reiki session are not considered indications of effectiveness. Patients may feel sensations similar to those of the practitioner, but they may also feel nothing. Sensations may include heat, cold, numbness, involuntary muscle twitching, heaviness, buoyancy, trembling, throbbing, static electricity, tingling, color, and heightened or decreased awareness of sound (Engebretson & Wardell, 2002). It is not uncommon for clients to fall asleep during a treatment, with reports of increased relaxation and peacefulness. These subjective feelings are supported in research studies that demonstrate physiological and psychological evidence of stress reduction following a Reiki session (Bukowski, 2015; McManus, 2017; Thrane et al., 2017). A Reiki session commonly elicits the relaxation response, presumably by downregulating the body's autonomic nervous system to move from sympathetic to parasympathetic mode, which lowers blood pressure and relieves tension and anxiety (Díaz-Rodríguez et al., 2011; Salles et al., 2014). The relaxation response releases physical and mental tension, reducing the impact of stress, and returning the body to a state of balance (Lipinski &Van De Velde, 2020). To date, the strongest support for the measurable physiological effect of Reiki was demonstrated in an animal model (Baldwin et al., 2008).

Methodological problems, which hinder the interpretation of results, have been identified in a number of studies. Although case studies and anecdotal examples have been relatively consistent in reporting positive responses to Reiki treatments, they do not represent the scientific rigor that is demanded within an evidence-based healthcare system. Efforts to strengthen research design and mitigate the confounding effects of human touch led to the development of sham or placebo Reiki (Mansour et al., 1999), now frequently incorporated into randomized controlled trials (RCTs). McManus (2017) reviewed 13 peer-reviewed studies published between 1998 and 2016 that included hands-on Reiki, a "sham" Reiki, or placebo control, with 20 or more participants in the Reiki arm and found that Reiki was more effective than placebo in 8 studies. Four studies found no difference between Reiki and placebo, and one study in which neither Reiki nor the placebo had any beneficial effect. McManus (2017) concluded that Reiki is better than placebo in activating the parasympathetic nervous system and reducing pain, anxiety, and depression and in improving self-esteem and quality of life.

Although both hands-on healing and distance healing are forms of energy healing, the presence of touch has the capacity to confound the research results, as all touch may have some healing properties. An overview of the scientific evidence on distant healing therapies identified both methodological limitations and positive outcomes meriting further study (Hammerschlag et al., 2014; Radin et al., 2015). Distance studies conducted between 2015 and 2017 showed pain, stress, and fatigue reduction following chemotherapy (Demir et al., 2015); decreased stress among software engineers (Vasudev & Shastri, 2016); and decreased incision pain following coronary artery bypass grafting (Shaybak et al., 2017), but Baldwin (2020) concluded these data were insufficient to draw positive conclusions.

In 2009, the Center for Reiki Research (CRR) was founded in order to develop procedures to evaluate the state of Reiki research that are available to public, academic, and medical communities and provide guidelines for conducting high-quality Reiki research. From 1989 to 2019, there were 77 original Reiki research articles published in peer-reviewed scientific journals. Of the 77 current peer-reviewed published research articles, CRR placed 33 of them in the top tier for quality (Baldwin, 2020). According to Baldwin (2020), "the higher quality research indicates that Reiki shows some promise as a noninvasive tool for healing at the physical and nonphysical levels, particularly regarding the alleviation of pain, depression, and anxiety and the maintenance of well-being" (p. 15).

A significant consolidation of research and scholarship exists in the 2020 publication of *Reiki in Clinical Practice: A Science Based Guide*, authored by Ann Baldwin, a pioneer and dedicated researcher on Reiki. This book provides well-developed and current information on key elements of Reiki practice, including evidence of clinical efficacy and mechanism of action, current theoretical frameworks, and practical considerations for practitioners and healthcare systems. Many of her research findings are cited in this chapter and provide the best updated resource for the status of clinical research on Reiki.

INTERVENTION

The Reiki practitioner acts as a conduit for this healing-intended energy to the self or others. In this section, we discuss the intervention continuum for nursing practice, guidelines for conducting a Reiki session, and outcomes used to measure physiological and psychological effectiveness.

INTERVENTION CONTINUUM FOR NURSING PRACTICE

Increasingly, there is evidence that many integrative approaches facilitate the natural healing process, including Reiki practice. In the recent publication of the text *Integrative Nursing*, Kreitzer and Koithan (2018) provide a set of six principles that further guide nursing practice in promoting the natural healing process. Principle 5 focuses on using evidence to utilize "the full range of therapeutic modalities, moving from least intensive and invasive to more, depending on need" (p. 12). This means that nurses employ a variety of interventions to support the natural healing process, from touch and presence to specific integrative therapies to medication. The principle of "least intensive and invasive to more" guides nurses to start with an intervention that has fewer side effects, less potential to do harm, and a greater likelihood that the natural healing processes will be supported. An "intervention continuum" represents the range of interventions that can be used when managing a symptom, starting from the least invasive/intensive and moving to the most invasive/intensive. Another way of viewing the intervention continuum is through a risk/benefit lens. The lower risk interventions fall at the beginning of the continuum, and those higher risk interventions move to the right. Evidence that Reiki has no adverse effects and reduces pain and anxiety suggests that Reiki could be utilized as a least intensive nursing intervention with the capacity to potentiate presence, breathwork, and touch for symptom management. The opioid crisis and the recent Joint Commission charge to offer nonpharmacologic methods for pain relief in hospitals, ambulatory care, and surgical centers further support Reiki practice as an essential pain management strategy (Joint Commission on Accreditation of Healthcare Organizations, 2017a, 2017b, 2018a, 2018b, 2018c).

GUIDELINES FOR HANDS-ON REIKI SESSION

One of the hallmarks of Reiki practice is its relative simplicity. In Mikao Usui's words, "Everyone can learn and practice Reiki" (Lubeck et al., 2001). Reiki energy flows through the hands without using cognitive, emotional, or spiritual skills.

The attunement process provides access to the energy without requiring ongoing practice or conscious intention. This makes Reiki particularly easy to learn and simple to use. For the nursing profession, the simplicity of Reiki has great potential for daily use, easy incorporation into direct care, and potentiating the natural healing process. The recipient may sit or lie down, and either method is suitable for Reiki practice. Because Reiki tends to be very relaxing, it is often preferable to lie down, but a seated session may be more practical if a table or bed is not available. Patients typically remain clothed. A massage table or hospital bed for a full session is ideal, providing comfort for both patient and practitioner. After practitioners establish the intent to heal with Reiki, the energy flows automatically from their hands without cognitive effort. The hands rest gently on the person's body, with the fingers touching so that each hand functions as a unit. Reiki can also be provided with the hands 2 to 3 inches off the body. The sequence of hand positions may vary but generally includes all seven major chakras and the endocrine glands. The success of a Reiki treatment does not depend on the use of certain hand positions, for the *ki* energy goes where it is needed.

A Level I Reiki practitioner typically uses a series of 12 to 15 hand positions for a full session and six to seven hand positions for a seated session, but all hand positions can be modified or adapted for each session (see Exhibit 24.1). A level II Reiki practitioner also uses hand positions but may use various Reiki symbols to focus the *ki* energy or perform distance healings. If touch is contraindicated for any reason, the hands can be held 1 to 4 inches above the body. A full Reiki session usually lasts 45 to 60 minutes, and a seated session usually lasts 15 to 20 minutes. Reiki practitioners, especially if they are nurses working in a clinical setting, often do not have the luxury of providing a full session. At such times, shorter and more targeted treatments may be offered for specific purposes. In *The Original Reiki Handbook of Dr. Mikao Usui* (Petter, 1999), the use of particular hand positions is recommended for addressing specific health problems. Although Reiki practitioners often provide Reiki sessions to individuals with specific health problems, Reiki practice is not intended to diagnose or treat a health condition but rather support balance restoration.

In clinical practice, four basic principles of physical touch should be considered: (a) Ask permission to touch, (b) provide basic information about what you

---

Exhibit 24.1 *Reiki Seated Session*

(Each hand position is held for approximately 2–3 minutes.)

1. General approach: Use Reiki practice competencies: apply hands for approximately 2–3 minutes of light touch in each hand position; vary positions and duration based on individual needs
2. Hands on shoulders (introduction to light touch)
3. One hand on forehead, one hand on upper nape of neck
4. One hand on chest, other hand on upper back
5. One hand on abdomen, other hand on lower back
6. One hand around each ankle
7. Hands on shoulders (conclusion to light touch)

will be doing, (c) describe anticipated benefits and range of outcomes, and (d) ensure the right to decline or discontinue receiving physical touch. Standards of practice have been developed by several professional Reiki organizations and include ethics related to intention, healing environment, healing principles, and the nondiagnostic nature of the work (International Association of Reiki Professionals [IARP], 2021; ICRT, 2021b, 2021c). The American Holistic Nurses Association and American Nurses Association (2015) developed the scope and standards of practice for holistic nursing, but these are not specific to any one integrative therapy. In the book *Creating Healing Relationships: Professional Standards for Energy Therapy Practitioners*, Hover-Kramer (2011) describes parameters for level of competence, record keeping, professional responsibility, boundaries, confidentiality, marketing, and informed consent. Although Reiki is not considered a religious practice, some believe that a spiritual consent form should be used to protect individual cultural, spiritual, and religious beliefs/practices (Arvonio, 2014). General competencies for Reiki practice are provided in Exhibit 24.2.

As more healthcare institutions offer complementary therapies, policies and guidelines must be developed that provide standards for implementation. Reiki practice at a Magnet®-designated facility in Pennsylvania requires evidence of competency in practice and adherence to written hospital policy when administering Reiki (Kryak & Vitale, 2011). A protocol for Reiki use in the operating room was developed at a hospital in New Hampshire following a request to have a Reiki practitioner be present during surgery (Sawyer, 1998). This author developed a Reiki protocol for use by nurses providing care to chemotherapy patients (Ringdahl, 2008). Vitale (2014) provides an outline for starting a Reiki program in a healthcare facility using a business model approach; she discusses institutional congruence, business plan development, and Reiki program start-up. Jurkovich and Watson (2020) describe the implementation of a volunteer Reiki program at an academic medical center, using a person-centered holistic care model and applying an evidence-based practice model. This included Reiki training by a Reiki master with holistic nursing board certification, a careful selection of volunteers, comprehensive orientation including using a Reiki criterion checklist, monthly follow-up meetings, and pre/post-Reiki data collection assessing pain, general

---

Exhibit 24.2 *Reiki Practice Competencies*

- Ask permission to touch before any encounter.
- Provide basic information about what you will be doing, including the use of light touch, basic hand positions, and the length of the session.
- Describe the areas of the body you will be touching and what sensations the patient may experience. Ask whether there are areas they would prefer not to be touched.
- Describe anticipated benefits and range of outcomes.
- Let them know you will stop at any time. Ask whether they prefer to be wakened if they fall asleep.
- Create an environment that promotes feelings of safety. If possible, ensure privacy. In a hospital setting, consider putting a sign on the door asking to not be disturbed.
- Clearly communicate that Reiki practice is not diagnostic or used to treat specific disease conditions.

discomfort, anxiety, insomnia, and nausea. This Reiki program demonstrated positive outcomes and continues to recruit more volunteers in order to meet the growing demand for access to Reiki in all hospital units.

MEASUREMENT OF OUTCOMES

Physiological outcome measures examined in other studies involving touch, such as hematological tests, blood pressure and heart rate, cortisol levels, bioelectric measures, wound-healing rate, inhibition of harmful microorganisms, and body temperature changes, are also appropriate for Reiki. Psychological measures, including perceived pain, stress, cognitive function, memory, and levels of anxiety, depression, or quality of life, are equally important. To date, Reiki research outcomes are focused primarily on reducing stress and pain, increasing relaxation, and an overall sense of well-being, particularly in the area of chronic disease and pain management.

According to Baldwin (2020), a leading expert in Reiki research and scholarship, rigorous data suggests positive effects of Reiki practice in four areas: (a) acute and chronic pain; (b) pain and well-being during cancer treatment; (c) stress, anxiety, and depression; and (d) practitioner well-being. Selected recent studies are summarized in Table 24.1.

Table 24.1 *Application and Evidence of Effective Uses of Reiki*

Author	Condition & Setting	Intervention	Conclusions
Santos et al. (2020)	Anxiety, depression, fear prior to cardiac surgery in cardiology hospital	Intervention group received 2 Reiki sessions prior to surgery (31); control group usual care (59)	Reiki group: (1) lower anxiety & depression (w/o statistical significance); (2) increased spiritual well-being
Bondi et al. (2021)	Pain & anxiety in women hospitalized for obstetric and/or gynecologic conditions	199 Reiki sessions performed by nine Reiki practitioners for women with pain >0	Statistical and clinical improvement in pain (92%) and anxiety (96%) scores following Reiki therapy
Buyukbayram and Saritas (2020)	Pain & fatigue in oncology patients	180 oncology patients in 3 groups: Reiki (×3 days), guided imagery (×3 days), control	Statistical improvement in pain and fatigue for Reiki and guided imagery groups, not in control
Jurkovich and Watson (2020)	Pain, anxiety, fatigue, general discomfort in medical/surgical/obstetrical patients	1,278 patients received 1 session	90% reported improvements in pain, anxiety, general discomfort, insomnia, or nausea

(continued)

Table 24.1 *Application and Evidence of Effective Uses of Reiki (continued)*

Author	Condition & Setting	Intervention	Conclusions
Gantt and Orina (2020)	Feasibility & acceptance of Reiki by military healthcare beneficiaries with chronic pain	30 beneficiaries with chronic pain received 6 sessions over 2–3 weeks	Significant reduction in pain, pain-related stress, and pain's interference with general activity, relationships, sleep, and enjoyment of life
Topdemir and Saritas (2020)	Anxiety levels of patients receiving pre-op Reiki for elective surgery	Intervention group (105) received 1 session prior to surgery and control group (105) received usual care.	Anxiety level in Reiki group unchanged and control group had increased anxiety
Dyer et al. (2019)	Physical/psychological health measures among clients receiving Reiki in private-practice setting	1411 participants received session & were assessed for physical & psychological state before/after session	All outcome measures (mood, pain, drowsiness, fatigue, anxiety, depression, shortness of breath, well-being) showed statistical improvement
Zucchetti et al. (2019)	Feasibility & efficacy using Reiki to reduce pain in children receiving hematopoietic stem cell transplantation	9 patients received 3 sessions/week over a month and assessed for pain control	Improvement in pain control in short/medium term but not long term
Zins et al. (2019)	Feasibility & efficacy of Reiki intervention to reduce pain, fatigue, depression in hemodialysis patients	15 patients received 2 sessions/week for 4 weeks of dialysis	Significant reduction in pain, depression, fatigue with no reduction in standard of care
Baldwin et al. (2017)	Reducing pain, anxiety, & blood pressure in patients undergoing knee replacement surgery	45 post-op patients in 3 groups: Reiki, sham, "quiet time"	Significant trend in pain reduction only seen in Reiki group

(continued)

Table 24.1 *Application and Evidence of Effective Uses of Reiki (continued)*

Author	Condition & Setting	Intervention	Conclusions
Chirico et al. (2017)	Reducing anxiety & improving mood: impact of coping skills & self-efficacy on outcomes in women with new breast cancer diagnosis	Intervention group (55) received 1 session day before surgery and control group (55) received standard care	Reiki prior to surgery effective in improving general well-being, greater coping skills were associated with less anxiety & correlated with better outcomes.
Thrane et al. (2017)	Feasibility & acceptability using Reiki for children 7–16 receiving palliative care and effect on pain, anxiety, relaxation	16 children/mothers received 2 sessions 1–3 days a part	Pain, anxiety, heart rate, respiratory rate decreased but not statistically significant
Alarcão and Fonseca (2016)	Impact on quality of life (QoL) with Reiki vs. sham Reiki in blood cancer patients	Reiki (58) & sham Reiki (42) 2 sessions/week × 4 weeks	Reiki group showed significantly more improvements in physical, environmental, & social dimensions of QoL
Erdogan and Cinar (2014)	Evaluate effect of reiki on depression in elderly people living in nursing homes	30 received Reiki 1× week, 30 received sham Reiki 1× week, 30 received no hands-on therapy.	Statistically significant decrease in Geriatric Depression Scale scores for Reiki group week 4, 8, 12, compared with week 1
Kirshbaum et al. (2016)	Perception & experience of Reiki in women following cancer treatment: quality of life	10 women completed cancer treatment & received Reiki sessions at local spa or hospice were interviewed	Increased wellbeing, reduced fatigue, mood disturbances, pain, anxiety following Reiki
Midilli and Gunduzoglu (2016)	nursing application: effect of Reiki on post-c/s incision pain, anxiety, & hemodynamic parameters (blood pressure, respirations, pulse) pre/post measures	90 women hospitalized for planned or unplanned c/s: Control (rest only) & Reiki	Patients in Reiki group had significantly less pain (66.75%) & anxiety (29.61%) & Reiki group needed significantly fewer analgesics than control group

(continued)

Table 24.1 *Application and Evidence of Effective Uses of Reiki (continued)*

Author	Condition & Setting	Intervention	Conclusions
Notte et al. (2016)	Effect of Reiki on pain perception of patients undergoing total knee arthroplasty looking at pain reduction and reducing pain meds	Reiki ($n = 23$), one session before surgery, 1 session after surgery, and daily session for 3 post-op or non-Reiki ($n = 20$) received usual care	Reiki sessions significantly reduced pain except sessions in a post anesthesia care unit immediately following surgery. No statistical difference in pain meds used
Siegel et al. (2016)	Explore whether individualized Reiki given to cancer patients improved symptoms and well-being	36 patients received Reiki sessions, and 14 patients were in the comparison group	Reiki practice delivered as integrative care produced clinically significant effects, although not statistically significant, for more than half of the patients
Iacorossi et al. (2017)	Evaluate how Reiki can help manage radiotherapy-related symptoms in head and neck cancer patients	Reiki was integrated into a cancer setting to evaluate its use to manage radiotherapy related symptoms with head and neck cancer	Reiki treatment provided psychological support together with integrated support toward pain therapy
Yüce and Taşcı (2021)	Effect of Reiki on the stress level of caregivers of patients with cancer	42 women primary caregivers of patients with cancer randomized to Reiki and sham Reiki groups	Reiki reduced stress levels of caregivers, effective in regulating blood pressure and pulse rate, no significant change in saliva cortisol level, provides relief to caregivers

The application of Reiki for anxiety and/or pain management among patients with cancer, chronic pain, and those undergoing surgery has been the focus of several recent studies (Alarcão & Fonseca, 2016; Baldwin et al., 2017; Billot et al., 2019; Bondi et al., 2021; Buyukbayram & Sanitas, 2020; Chirico et al., 2017; DiScipio, 2016; Gantt & Orina, 2020; Iacorossi et al., 2017; Jurkovich & Watson, 2020; Kirshbaum et al., 2016; Midilli & Gunduzoglu, 2016; Notte et al., 2016; Rosenbaum & Van de Velde, 2016; Santos et al., 2020; Siegel et al., 2016; Thrane et al., 2017; Topdemir & Saritas,

2020; Yüce & Taşcı, 2021; Zins et al., 2019; Zucchetti et al., 2019), all demonstrating clinically significant reduction of symptoms studied, and only two without statistical significance.

The most recent meta-analysis of the effect of Reiki on pain was conducted by Demir Dogan (2018), reviewing four studies that used the visual analogue scale (VAS) for assessing pain levels. Reiki was observed to cause a statistically significant decrease in VAS score when comparing 104 receiving Reiki compared with 108 in the control group. The largest study (1,411 participants), to date, that examined Reiki outcomes in a private-practice setting demonstrated statistical improvement in mood, pain, drowsiness, fatigue, anxiety, depression, shortness of breath, and well-being following a 45- to 90-minute Reiki session (Dyer et al., 2019).

A Cochrane review conducted to evaluate the efficacy of Reiki for depression and anxiety described the results of three RCTs (Joyce & Herbison, 2015); none had sufficient evidence to demonstrate a positive or negative effect on anxiety and depression. An integrative review conducted by Mangione et al. (2017) summarized the effects of HT and Reiki in research published between 2014 and 2016 in terms of anxiety, mood, and wellness with a special focus on mental health wellness. A total of 19 relevant articles on Reiki and 11 on HT were reviewed; biofield therapies showed safety and promise in reducing anxiety, improving mood, and cultivating mental health and wellness (Mangione et al., 2017). Erdogan and Cinar (2016) studied the effects of Reiki on depression in elderly persons living in nursing homes by conducting an RCT of 90 older adults diagnosed with depression through the Geriatric Depression Scale (GDS). Thirty received Reiki once a week for 12 weeks, 30 received sham Reiki once a week, and 30 received no hands-on therapy. There was a statistically significant decrease in depression scores in the Reiki group on Weeks 4, 8, and 12 and not in the other two groups. Charkhandeh et al. (2016) compared the effectiveness of cognitive behavior therapy (90 min 2 × week for 12 weeks) to Reiki (20 min 1 × week for 12 weeks) in reducing symptoms of depression in adolescents and found both groups had a reduction in depression compared to the waitlist group, with greater significance for the cognitive behavior therapy group.

Achieving institutional approval for Reiki use requires evidence of safety and effectiveness. Additionally, using Reiki within healthcare delivery requires evidence of feasibility: Is it possible to offer Reiki to patients in a variety of clinical settings with specific health conditions without interfering with healthcare delivery or incurring significant costs? This author served as coinvestigator in a study testing the feasibility, acceptability, and safety of Reiki touch for premature infants (Duckett, 2008), demonstrating that application of Reiki in a neonatal intensive care unit (NICU) was feasible, accepted by parents and healthcare providers, and safe to use for a premature infant population. Radziewicz et al. (2018) conducted a pilot study using Reiki therapy for 30 newborns at risk for neonatal abstinence syndrome and concluded that Reiki is feasible and safe when administered to this high-risk population.

In their exploration of the use of Reiki in a dialysis unit, Ferraresi et al. (2013) suggest that healthcare providers should consider not only efficacy but also side effects, availability, cost, and patient request when evaluating Reiki (and other integrative modalities) for pain management. In addition to the impact of Reiki on pain reduction following knee replacement surgery, Notte et al. (2016) verified that participants receiving Reiki were satisfied with Reiki and their hospital experience. Notably, four feasibility studies have been conducted in the past 3 years, addressing the feasibility of Reiki practice in a variety of settings and populations: feasibility and acceptability of Reiki use in-home palliative care for children (Thrane et al., 2021), feasibility and acceptance of Reiki by military healt care beneficiaries with chronic pain (Gantt & Orina, 2020), feasibility and efficacy using Reiki to reduce pain in children receiving hematopoietic stem cell transplantations (HSCTs; Zucchetti et al., 2019), and feasibility and efficacy of Reiki intervention to reduce pain, fatigue, depression in hemodialysis patients (Zins et al., 2019). All these studies demonstrated that Reiki was feasible, acceptable, and well tolerated and resulted in significant improvements in symptom burden for each population studied.

Another recent trend in Reiki research is to compare or combine Reiki with other integrative modalities in order to further evaluate efficacy. Jahantiqh et al. (2018) compared physiotherapy versus Reiki in relieving lower back pain and improving activities of daily living (ADLs) in intervertebral disc hernia patients, finding no significant difference in pain or ADLs between Reiki and physiotherapy groups but a significant difference between the standard of care (pain medication only) and Reiki groups. Vergo et al. (2018) compared massage therapy to Reiki in reducing pain, nausea, fatigue, anxiety, and depression and improving well-being for hospitalized patients and found significant symptom relief reported with both modalities but greater improvement with Reiki for fatigue and anxiety. Kurebayashi et al. (2016) compared the effects of massage with or without Reiki to reduce stress and anxiety and found that massage and Reiki produced better results than massage and rest, suggesting synergy between the effects of Reiki and massage therapy. Rosenbaum and Van de Velde (2016) compared the effects of yoga, massage, and Reiki on patient well-being at a cancer resource center and found that all three services decreased stress and anxiety and improved mood, but Reiki had a greater effect on pain reduction. DiScipio (2016) studied the perception of relaxation using restorative yoga and Reiki versus yoga alone in cancer survivors, finding that Yoga with Reiki subjects had a greater perceived depth of relaxation than Yoga alone, also suggesting synergy between the effects of Reiki and Yoga. Buyukbayram and Saritas (2020) found that Reiki and guided imagery both decreased pain and fatigue in oncology patients when compared to a control group. Bremner et al. (2016) studied the effect of Reiki with music (RMG) versus music only (MOG) on pain, stress, anxiety, depression among people living with HIV and found MOG pain levels unchanged, but RMG pain decreased significantly, another potential synergistic effect.

Many research models, including the RCTs, are not complex enough to capture the subjective experience of a Reiki session. Using a qualitative research design, Engebretson and Wardell (2002) found that participants had a diverse and descriptive language that accompanied their experience, creating a more complete picture of the subjective experience of a Reiki session and secondary qualitative analysis of this data validated the taxonomy of spiritual experiences that emerged during a Reiki session (Engebretson & Wardell, 2012). Using a qualitative approach to describe Reiki experiences in women who have cancer, Kirshbaum et al. (2016) demonstrated that Reiki had multiple positive effects that could significantly impact the quality of life for this population.

PRECAUTIONS

No serious adverse effects of Reiki treatments have been published. Some patients, however, may experience an emotional release that may be uncomfortable or disturbing. Therefore, practitioners must be prepared to provide necessary assistance and appropriate referrals if emotional distress persists. Moreover, some individuals may dislike being touched. Practitioners can avoid this discomfort by assessing the person's level of comfort with touch, selective hands-off practice as indicated, and by carefully accounting for gender and cultural considerations. Few patients who are fully informed object to the therapy; this is true even among vulnerable populations such as victims of torture (Kennedy, 2001) or those with long-term mental health problems (Charkhandeh et al., 2016; Erdogan & Cinar, 2014; Mangione et al., 2017), in whom responses to Reiki have been favorable.

USES

An increasing body of literature supports the use of Reiki as a stress-reduction and relaxation technique. Therapies that contribute to a relaxation response have the potential for enhancing overall well-being and reducing the physiological effects of stress. The range of potential practical applications with patients is broad and depends on the setting. Reiki has been used for preoperative and postoperative patients; in oncology, hospice, and palliative care; for pain management, rehabilitation, and long-term care; for stress and anxiety reduction; for self-care and stress reduction for healthcare providers and caregivers; and for pediatric symptom management. In addition, this author has anecdotal evidence and experience working with nursing students who practice Reiki in a variety of specialty settings, including pediatric and adult bone marrow transplant units, labor and delivery suites, emergency departments, chemotherapy infusion units, chemical dependency inpatient units, Huntington's chorea units, and veteran's health facilities (see Table 24.2 on Reiki experiences of positive benefit to healthcare providers and patients).

Energy touch therapies are considered to be within the scope of nursing practice and touch is recognized in the Nursing Interventions Classification Code (Butcher et al., 2018). In the past 25 years, many professional organizations and state boards of nursing have developed statements that provide parameters for integrative therapy use by nurses, reinforcing the notion that integrative nursing care is often accompanied by the use of specific integrative modalities. Several authors have documented the effective use of Reiki in the direct provision of nursing care (Frisch et al., 2018; Lipinski & Van De Velde, 2020; Ringdahl, 2008; Ringdahl & Voss, 2016). The authors of a qualitative research study conducted to provide a theoretical construct for Reiki concluded that Reiki was congruent with nursing modalities (Ring, 2009). Bremner et al. (2014) described a project designed to introduce nursing students to a more holistic care model through engagement in a nurse-managed community clinic by assessing needs and evaluating Reiki outcomes.

Increased evidence of efficacy and support for integrative nursing practice supports a shift to greater nursing engagement in Reiki practice, including informal application in all clinical encounters. The common theme described in many

Table 24.2 *Excerpts of Healthcare Providers' Descriptions of Positive Benefits of Reiki Practice*

"Energy often seems palpable in the hospice setting, for patients and caregivers, making the energetic practice of Reiki ideal in this space. After a reiki session with a patient experiencing terminal agitation, the patient's son stated, 'Reiki just pours love into people when they need it.' Looking at the now sleeping patient, I agreed."

—Julie, hospice nurse

"During a time when there was nothing left to be done, when all measures of life support were maximized, when the end of suffering and death were imminent, I turned to the practice of Reiki. As I laid one hand on his heart and another on his abdomen, I watched his respiratory rate slow down, his tense body relax, and his ventilator stop alarming. For a brief moment, the chaos was gone, and I felt a sense of balance and purpose for the work I was doing."

—Angelica, COVID-19 ICU nurse

"Cancer disrupts the balance of the body's energetic pathways. Having the knowledge and training to do Reiki therapy allows me to connect with my oncology patients on a deeper level. I have the opportunity to help restore patients physical, emotional, and spiritual balance and promote comfort and healing throughout all stages of cancer treatment."

—Maggie, oncology nurse

"Using Reiki in a transitional care unit enriched my passion for nursing. In moments when there were limited medication or treatment options for the physical, mental, and emotional challenges of illness or injuries, Reiki was a method that allowed me to still provide the comfort, care, and peace that is innate to nursing practice."

—Anne, TCU nurse

"As a respiratory therapist working in a pediatric pulmonary function lab, there are many opportunities to use Reiki for the patient and their caregivers. When the Reiki takes hold there is a deep sense of calm and relaxation. The patient is better able to focus on the task at hand and I believe we get better effort and more accurate test results."

—Jo, respiratory therapist

"For a woman admitted in the antepartum unit for a high-risk pregnancy, she described Reiki as giving her a sense of calm, warmth, and feeling supported. For a woman in labor, intentional touch with Reiki is healing and supportive. Reiki allows me to renew my own spirit so that I can provide the compassionate care that I want to give my patients."

—Loryanne, labor and delivery nurse

"I use Reiki in my nurse practitioner practice for geriatric patients in residential facilities for comfort and emotional support. A wheelchair-bound elderly patient with high anxiety was having a particularly "bad" day. After I spoke with her a few minutes I offered to hold her hand, and as the patient's anxiety began to subside, she asked me to put my hand on her forehead. Her anxiety continued to decrease, and she was able to finally relax after hours of debilitating anxiety."

—Dianne, geriatric nurse practitioner

Reiki programs is the benefit of Reiki for pain relief, stress and anxiety reduction, and promoting relaxation (Hahn et al., 2014). In a survey conducted by Frisch et al. (2017), 424 nurses responded to the item "Please provide a description of the kinds of patient conditions where you use energy-based modalities (EBM) in your practice." Content analysis revealed four themes: EMBs are (a) caring modalities used to treat a wide range of identified nursing concerns, (b) implemented across the life span and to facilitate life transitions, (c) support care for the treatment of specific medical conditions, and (d) the use of EBMs transcend labels of "conditions" and are used within a holistic framework. Integrative approaches to direct care increase nurse agency and options for symptom management. Using an "intervention continuum" provides an avenue for clinical decision-making that further supports 'a least to most' pathway for the management of these common symptoms.

Within hospitals, the introduction of Reiki into patient care has been initiated primarily through volunteers; however, increasingly, there is support for embedding these modalities into direct care through educational programs for healthcare providers (Clark, 2013; Frisch et al., 2018; Kryak & Vitale, 2011; Lipinski & Van De Velde, 2020; Ringdahl, 2008). Access to Reiki within a hospital setting may also exist through an integrative health team that provides a variety of services through a nurse and physician referral system that includes Reiki. Ambulatory care models for integrative therapies exist primarily through contracting with integrative practitioners to provide specific services. These services may exist within an integrative care clinic that has a specialty focus, such as oncology or women's health. In a biomedical treatment setting, Reiki is best seen as a complementary healing modality, whereas in other circumstances, it can either be used alone or with other approaches.

Several recent studies have been conducted on the use of Reiki with children, focusing on symptom management, particularly in children with serious health problems. Thrane et al. (2017) conducted a pilot study using Reiki for symptom management for children receiving palliative care and demonstrated a decrease in pain, anxiety, heart, and respiratory rates following two Reiki sessions received at home and validated the acceptability and feasibility of Reiki use among this population (Thrane et al., 2021). Zucchetti et al. (2019) demonstrated the feasibility and efficacy of using Reiki to reduce pain in children receiving HSCT. A case report of a 9-year old girl with a history of several chronic conditions demonstrated that twice-weekly Reiki sessions over a period of 6 weeks reduced stress in both mother and child and improved the child's sleep (Bukowski & Berardi, 2014). The use of Reiki among parent caregivers also has the potential for mitigating parental stress by reducing their child's stress. A recent pilot program demonstrated that teaching Reiki to caregivers of hospitalized pediatric patients improved patient comfort, provided relaxation, reduced pain and assisted the caregivers in becoming active participants in their child's care. A participation rate of 94.4% was achieved by offering shorter and more frequent classes, as well as adapting classes to take place in their child's room (Kundu et al., 2013). A similar format was used by the author when offering a Reiki class to parents of children at a pediatric bone marrow transplant unit, demonstrating that Reiki has the capacity to reduce stress for both child and caregivers in the hospital and during recovery at home (see Exhibit 24.3).

> **Exhibit 24.3** *Teaching Reiki to Parents in a Pediatric Bone Marrow Transplant Unit*
>
> Following a comprehensive needs assessment, a pilot program was designed to teach the parent/family caregivers of pediatric bone marrow transplant patients how to practice Reiki. Reiki was selected because the integrative nurse clinician identified significant symptom relief when using Reiki on these patients and the parents identified that learning relaxation techniques would be the most helpful additional support provided during their child's hospitalization. The Reiki curriculum was redesigned to meet the unique needs of this group. Many significant outcomes were achieved: (a) It was readily apparent that each attendee experienced an internal shift in personal well-being throughout the 3 weeks. (b) Many parents reported using Reiki on themselves for their own stress management and to aid in falling asleep. (c) Furthermore, the intervention not only seemed to give parents the permission to take time for themselves but also provided a meaningful way to connect with their child (Ringdahl & Voss, 2016).

SELF-TREATMENT AND PRACTITIONER BENEFITS

One of the more unique features of Reiki therapy is its capacity for self-use. Reiki practitioners can place their hands on the head, abdomen, chest, or other areas of the body, reducing pain and/or increasing a sense of relaxation. A study conducted among college students demonstrated that after 20 weeks of performing self-Reiki twice a week, there was a significant reduction in stress levels (Bukowski, 2015). The concepts of empowerment and self-treatment have particular value when considering chronic health problems. For some Reiki practitioners, teaching Level I Reiki provides the clients with a greater sense of control over some of their health problems, including pain management and stress reduction. This author teaches levels I and II to students with a variety of health problems, including fibromyalgia, mood disorders, cancer, and neurological problems such as advanced amyotrophic lateral sclerosis. Clients with physical limitations may gain particular benefits from learning Level II, or distance healing.

In addition, those using Reiki receive the benefits of the therapies while performing them on patients. Reiki practitioners report feeling energized, relaxed, and/or more centered after performing a Reiki treatment. Research on Reiki use by nurses has demonstrated positive effects on the practitioner, including greater job satisfaction and an increase in caring behaviors (Brathovde, 2006, 2017). The increased sense of well-being that occurs when giving and receiving Reiki may influence the patient–nurse relationship and create a less stressful work environment. The use of integrative therapies by nurses working in the acute care setting may create an environment in which the patient feels more caring and the nurse feels more fulfilled in their role as a caregiver (Bondi et al., 2021).

Reiki may also be used for healthcare providers' and students' self-care, with the potential for reducing stress. Several research studies have shown beneficial effects of Reiki for nurses and other healthcare providers in positively influencing well-being, stress reduction, and burnout. Cuneo et al., 2011 administered the Perceived Stress Scale tool prior to attending a Reiki I class and 3 weeks after practicing self-Reiki and found a statistically significant decrease in perceived stress. Rosada et al. (2015) demonstrated reduced burnout among community mental health clinicians in the Reiki versus sham group using the Maslach Burnout Inventory. Yüce and Taşcı (2021) studied the effects of Reiki and sham Reiki on primary caregivers of patients with cancer and demonstrated a reduction in stress levels of caregivers receiving Reiki using blood pressure, pulse rate, and a Caregiver Strain Index (CSI) measurements.

CULTURAL APPLICATIONS

Energy and touch therapies are found in the health traditions of most cultures. A hands-off healing tradition, johrei, also originated in Japan and is currently practiced by millions of people worldwide. Johrei means purification of the spirit and aims to cure illness and create balance and happiness. Both Reiki and Johrei are recognized in Brazil as practices that can complement conventional treatment and are included in the National Policy on Integrative and Complementary Practices (de Melo et al., 2021). Although healthcare workers may find that some of the energy and healing practices used in non-Western cultures differ greatly from Western health practices and even from the more frequently used integrative therapies, respecting the person's belief in these practices is important in the healing process. Sidebar 24.1 details the current use of Reiki in Japan, the country in which the therapy originated.

Sidebar 24.1 *Reiki Practice in Japan*

Contributions by Ikuko Ebihara and Hyakuten Inamoto

Reiki was started in Japan by Dr. Mikao Usui in the early 1920s. After World War II, many of the healing arts in Japan, including Reiki, were discouraged, and secret societies were developed for those committed to retaining the tradition. Reiki was imported back from abroad in the 1990s, and traditional Usui Reiki has been regaining popularity in Japan since then, but acceptance has been slow. According to H. Inamoto (personal communication, July 22, 2017), "Reiki practice in Japan is like a developing country."

People in Japan find Reiki practitioners and masters by word of mouth and internet searches. The common reason for seeking Reiki practice is to restore mind and body balance; it is not for seeking remedies for physical discomfort. Reiki does not have any national standards; it is not recognized as a medical or physiotherapeutic practice.

There are numerous traditional medicines in Japan, but only a limited number of therapies are nationally recognized. Judo therapies, acupuncture, and moxibustion are examples of nationally recognized practices; they have national certification systems. Insurance and reimbursement are available for such therapies; however, even though they are reimbursable, they are not usually provided at hospitals. Western medicine and Japanese traditional medicines are governed by different regulations. Patients may visit both care providers. In Japan, as in most Western countries, Western and alternative practices are rarely provided by the same healthcare organizations.

FUTURE RESEARCH

Reiki research has enjoyed a significant acceleration and increased rigor within the past 20 years and researchers are developing more improved methodology and research designs. The CRR website and the Touchstone Process provide a clearinghouse for disseminating current Reiki research information for practitioners and researchers. The Touchstone Project has a process for systematically analyzing published, peer-reviewed studies of Reiki and has results from 77 studies accessible online, with the majority of studies conducted since 2010 (Baldwin et al., 2010; CRR, 2021a, 2021b). Analysis of these studies has generated data supporting Reiki as a noninvasive tool for healing at the physical and nonphysical levels, particularly in alleviating pain, depression, and anxiety.

However, many published studies on Reiki have been conducted with small, nonrandom convenience samples, raising questions about the validity and generalizability of findings. There are currently 26 peer-reviewed research articles published between 2015 and 2019, but all except three are pilot studies (Baldwin, 2020). There are three large scale Reiki clinical research studies that have been published in the past 6 years (Charkhandeh et al., 2016; Chirico et al., 2017; Kurebayashi et al., 2016) that all support the use of Reiki for reducing pain, depression, and anxiety, but more large studies are needed. Further experiments are required with greater numbers of subjects to provide the statistical power necessary for meaningful interpretation (Baldwin, 2020). Outcomes for touch therapies such as Reiki are typically not disease-specific and establishing an appropriate time frame for detecting effect is variable (Engebretson & Wardell, 2007). New models of research that enlarge the definition of outcomes need to be explored. Clinical evaluation of Reiki represents a challenge using current standards of assessment. Combining subjective and physiological measures in such research studies will allow for a broader assessment of the effects of Reiki. Because the goals of Reiki may be broader than symptom relief and include concepts of physiological and psychological balance, qualitative studies that can address values and meaning are also important, as evidenced in the research by Engebretson and Wardell (2002) and Kirshbaum et al. (2016).

Vitale (2007) identified limitations in research design and the use of linear research methods as problematic in conducting Reiki research. Current outcome measures may not accurately reflect or measure all aspects of a Reiki treatment. A lack of standardization in Reiki practice also impacts reliability and validity. Some research studies do not identify all components of the Reiki intervention used, including the length of treatment, the type of treatment, or the level/training of the Reiki practitioner. Another consideration in improving research accuracy is to evaluate energy practitioner competency. Connor et al. (2021) tested 213 subjects through use of 13 empirical outcome measures and found some consistency in using Acoustimeter, Tri Axial ELF magnetic field meter, and pH levels.

There is a need to develop research designs that consider more subtle and longer lasting outcomes than those that have typically been used. If energy treatment works on a different level from the conventional medical model, the results may not be as dramatic and may require larger groups and a longer treatment period to show a positive outcome. Little research has explored the spiritual dimension of Reiki practice, yet recipients of a Reiki session often describe feelings associated with spiritual well-being (Engebretson & Wardell, 2012).

Hospitals are exploring the use of integrative modalities as an adjunct to pain management in response to healthcare provider and consumer demands for integrative models of care, and The Joint Commission has developed new guidelines for pain management standards, including nonpharmacologic approaches for pain. The Hospital Consumer Assessment and Healthcare Providers System survey are publicly reported by the Centers for Medicare and Medicaid Services, and patients' perception of pain management during the hospital stay is a critical survey item (www.hcahpsonline.org). These growing trends in practice and regulatory environments further increase the need for more research into the effectiveness of Reiki as a supportive therapy in surgical and nonsurgical pain management among nurses and other healthcare professionals (Baldwin et al., 2017).

Within a clinical setting, Reiki practice has the potential for (a) reducing stress and anxiety, (b) promoting health and well-being, (c) promoting trust, (d) potentiating drug therapy, (e) reducing medication use and medication side effects, and (f) reducing recovery time. Reiki may have a particular application for people suffering from chronic physical and mental health conditions. There is also the potential for reducing stress and burnout and promoting positive well-being and competency among both formal and informal caregivers. Only a few of these areas of Reiki practice have been explored in the research literature.

Suggested questions for future research include the following:
- What outcome measures and study designs best capture the complexity and efficacy associated with Reiki practice?
- What kind of longitudinal studies and outcome measures would best demonstrate the effectiveness of self-Reiki for stress reduction?
- What is the best way to use Reiki in providing stress and burnout reduction for healthcare providers?
- What populations would most benefit from learning Reiki as a stress-reduction strategy?
- How can Reiki be incorporated into nursing clinical practice?

WEBSITES

Additional information about Reiki can be obtained from the following websites:
- Center for Reiki Research (www.centerforreikiresearch.org)
- International Association of Reiki Professionals (IARP) (www.iarp.org)
- International Center for Reiki Training (ICRT) (www.reiki.org)
- Reiki online module, Taking Charge of Your Health, University of Minnesota Center for Spirituality and Healing (www.takingcharge.csh.umn.edu/explore-healing-practices/reiki)
- The Touchstone Process (https://centerforreikiresearch.com/touchstone-process/)

REFERENCES

Alarcão, Z., & Fonseca, J. R. (2016). The effect of Reiki therapy on quality of life of patients with blood cancer: Results from a randomized controlled trial. *European Journal of Integrative Medicine, 8*(3), 239–249. https://doi.org/10.1016/j.eujim.2015.12.003

American Holistic Nurses Association & American Nurses Association. (2015). *Holistic nursing: Scope and standards of practice* (3rd ed.). http://Nursebooks.org

Ananth, S. (2011). *2010 Complementary and alternative medicine survey of hospitals*. Samueli Institute.

Arvonio, M. (2014). Cultural competency, autonomy, and spiritual conflicts related to Reiki/ CAM therapies: Should patients be informed? *Linacre Quarterly, 81*(1), 47–56. https://doi.org/ 10.1179/2050854913Y.0000000007

Baldwin, A. L. (2020). *Reiki in clinical practice: A science-based guide.* Handspring Publishing.

Baldwin, A. L., Rand, W. L., & Schwartz, G. E. (2013). Practicing Reiki does not appear to routinely produce high-intensity electromagnetic fields from the heart or hands of Reiki practitioners. *Journal of Alternative and Complementary Medicine, 19*(6), 518–526. https://doi.org/10.1089/acm.2012.0136

Baldwin, A. L., Vitale, A., Brownell, D., Scicisnski, J., Kearns, M., & Rand, W. (2010). The touchstone process: An ongoing critical evaluation of Reiki in the scientific literature. *Holistic Nursing Practice, 24*(5), 260–276. https://doi.org/10.1097/HNP.0b013e3181f1adef

Baldwin, A. L., Vitale, A., Brownell, E., Kryak, E., & Rand, W. (2017). Effects of Reiki on pain, anxiety, and blood pressure in patients undergoing knee replacement: A pilot study. *Holistic Nursing Practice, 31*(2), 80–89. https://doi.org/10.1097/HNP.0000000000000195

Baldwin, A. L., Wagers, C., & Schwartz, G. E. (2008). Reiki improves heart rate homeostasis in laboratory rats. *Journal of Alternative and Complementary Medicine, 14*(4), 417–422. https://doi .org/10.1089/acm.2007.0753

Benelli, C. (2020, Winter). The evolution of teaching Reiki online. *Reiki News Magazine,* pp. 21–23.

Billot, M., Daycard, M., Wood, C., & Tchalla, A. (2019). Reiki therapy for pain, anxiety and quality of life. *BMJ Supportive & Palliative Care, 9*(4), 434–438. https://doi.org/10.1136/bmjspcare-2019 -001775

Bondi, A., Morgan, T., & Fowler, S. B. (2021). Effects of reiki on pain and anxiety in women hospitalized for obstetrical-and gynecological-related conditions. *Journal of Holistic Nursing, 39*(1), 58–65. https://doi.org/10.1177/0898010120936437

Brathovde, A. (2006). A pilot study: Reiki for self-care and healthcare providers. *Holistic Nursing Practice, 20*(2), 95–101. https://doi.org/10.1097/00004650-200603000-00010

Brathovde, A. (2017). Teaching nurses Reiki energy for self-care. *International Journal for Human Caring, 21*(1), 20–25.

Bremner, M., Bennett, D., & Chambers, D. (2014). Integrating Reiki and community-engaged scholarship: An interdisciplinary educational innovation. *Journal of Nursing Education, 53*(9), 541–543. https://doi.org/10.3928/01484834-20140820-02

Bremner, M. N., Blake, B. J., Wagner, V. D., & Pearcey, S. M. (2016). Effects of Reiki with music compared to music only among people living with HIV. *Journal of the Association of Nurses in AIDS Care, 27*(5), 635–647. https://doi.org/10.1016/j.jana.2016.04.004

Bukowski, E. (2015). The use of self-Reiki for stress reduction and relaxation. *Journal of Integrative Medicine, 13*(5), 336–340. https://doi.org/10.1016/S2095-4964(15)60190-X

Bukowski, E., & Berardi, B. (2014). Reiki brief report: Using Reiki to reduce stress levels in a nine-year-old child. *Explore: The Journal of Science & Healing, 10*(4), 253–255. https://doi .org/10.1016/j.explore.2014.02.007

Butcher, H., Bulechek, G., Dochterman, J. M., & Wagner, C. (2018). *Nursing Interventions Classification (NIC)* (7th ed.). Mosby.

Buyukbayram, Z., & Saritas, S. C. (2020). The effect of Reiki and guided imagery intervention on pain and fatigue in oncology patients: A non-randomized controlled study. *EXPLORE, 17*(1), 22–26. https://doi.org/10.1016/j.explore.2020.07.009

Center for Reiki Research. (2021a). *Reiki research study summaries.* https://centerforreikiresearch .com/reiki-research-summaries/

Center for Reiki Research. (2021b). *The touchstone process.* https://centerforreikiresearch.com/ touchstone-process/

Charkhandeh, M., Talib, M. A., & Hunt, C. J. (2016). The clinical effectiveness of cognitive behavior therapy and an alternative medicine approach in reducing symptoms of depression in adolescents. *Psychiatry Research, 239,* 325–330. https://doi.org/10.1016/j.psychres.2016.03.044

Chirico, A., D'Aiuto, G., Penon, A., Mallia, L., DE Laurentiis, M., Lucidi, F., Botti, G., & Giordano, A. (2017). Self-efficacy for coping with cancer enhances the effect of Reiki treatments during the pre-surgery phase of breast cancer patients. *Anticancer Research, 37*(7), 3657–3665. https:// doi.org/10.21873/anticanres.11736

Clark, C. (2013). An integral nursing education experience: Outcomes from a BSN Reiki course. *Holistic Nursing Practice, 27*(1), 13–22. https://doi.org/10.1097/HNP.0b013e318276fdc4

Connor, M. H., Connor, C. A., Eickhoff, J., & Schwartz, G. E. (2021). Prospective empirical test suite for energy practitioners. *Explore (NY), 17*(1), 60–69. https://doi.org/10.1016/j.explore.2020.07.010

Cuneo, C., Cooper, M., Drew, C., Naoum-Heffernan, C., Sherman, T., & Walz, K. (2011). The effect of Reiki on work-related stress of the registered nurse. *Journal of Holistic Nursing, 29*(1), 33–43. https://doi.org/10.1177/0898010110377294

De Melo, M., Rodrigues, C., Santos, D., Melo, J., & Tokeshi, H. (2021). Alternative treatment with Johrei: A controlled randomized study evaluating seed physiological potential. *Explore (NY), 17*(1), 32–39. https://doi.org/10.1016/j.explore.2020.07.012

Demir Dogan, M. D. (2018). The effect of Reiki on pain: A meta-analysis. *Complementary Therapies in Clinical Practice, 31*, 384–387. https://doi.org/10.1016/j.ctcp.2018.02.020

Demir, M., Can, G., Kelam, A., & Aydiner, A. (2015). Effects of distant Reiki on pain, anxiety and Fatigue in oncology patients in Turkey: A pilot study. *Asian Pacific Journal of Cancer Prevention, 16*(2), 4859–4862. https://doi.org/10.7314/apjcp.2015.16.12.48

Díaz-Rodríguez, L., Arroyo-Morales, M., Cantarero-Villanueva, I., Férnandez-Lao, C., Polley, M., & Fernandez-de-las-Peñas, C. (2011). The application of Reiki in nurses diagnosed with burnout syndrome has beneficial effects on concentration of salivary IgA and blood pressure. *Latin American Journal of Nursing, 19*(5), 1132–1138. https://doi.org/10.1590/s0104-11692011000500010

DiScipio, W. (2016). Perceived relaxation as a function of restorative yoga combined with Reiki for cancer survivors. *Complementary Therapies in Clinical Practice, 24*, 116–122. https://doi.org/10.1016/j.ctcp.2016.05.003

Duckett, L. (2008). *Testing feasibility, acceptability, and safety of Reiki touch for premature infants.* University of Minnesota IRB application.

Dyer, N. L., Baldwin, A. L., & Rand, W. L. (2019). A large-scale effectiveness trial of Reiki for physical and psychological health. *The Journal of Alternative and Complementary Medicine, 25*(12), 1156–1162. https://doi.org/10.1089/acm.2019.0022

Engebretson, J., & Wardell, D. W. (2002). Experience of a Reiki session. *Alternative Therapies, 8*(2), 48–53. https://www.researchgate.net/publication/11473710_Experience_of_a_Reiki_session

Engebretson, J., & Wardell, D. W. (2007). Energy-based modalities. *Nursing Clinics of North America, 42*, 243–259. https://doi.org/10.1016/j.cnur.2007.02.004

Engebretson, J., & Wardell, D. W. (2012). Energy therapies: Focus on spirituality. *Explore: The Journal of Science & Healing, 8*(6), 353–359. https://doi.org/10.1016/j.explore.2012.08.004

Erdogan, Z., & Cinar, S. (2016). The effect of Reiki on depression in elderly people living in nursing home. *Indian Journal of Traditional Knowledge, 15*(1), 35–40. http://nopr.niscair.res.in/bitstream/123456789/33556/1/IJTK%2015%281%29%2035-40.pdf

Ferraresi, M., Clari, R., Moro, I., Banino, E., Boero, E., Crosio, A., Dayne, R., Rosset, L., Scarpa, A., Serra, E., Surace, A., Testore, A., Colombi, N., & Piccoli, G. B. (2013). Reiki and related therapies in the dialysis ward: An evidence-based and ethical discussion to debate if these complementary and alternative medicines are welcomed or banned. *BMC Nephrology, 14*, 129. https://doi.org/10.1186/1471-2369-14-129

Frisch, N., Butcher, H. K., Campbell, D., & Weir-Hughes, D. (2018). Holistic nurses' use of energy-based caring modalities. *Journal of Holistic Nursing, 36*(3), 210–217. https://doi.org/10.1177/0898010116665447

Gantt, M., & Orina, J. A. T. (2020). Educate, try, and share: A feasibility study to assess the acceptance and use of Reiki as an adjunct therapy for chronic pain in military health care facilities. *Military Medicine, 185*(3–4), 394–400. https://doi.org/10.1093/milmed/usz271

Hahn, J., Reilly, P., & Buchanan, T. (2014). Development of a hospital Reiki training program: Training volunteers to provide Reiki to patients, families, and staff in the acute care setting. *Dimensions of Critical Care Nursing, 33*(1), 15–21. https://doi.org/10.1097/DCC.0000000000000009

Hammerschlag, R., Marx, B., & Aickin, M. (2014). Nontouch biofield therapy: A systematic review of human randomized controlled trials reporting use of only nonphysical contact treatment.

Journal of Alternative and Complementary Medicine, 20(12), 881–892. https://doi.org/10.1089/acm.2014.0017

Hover-Kramer, D. (2011). *Creating healing relationships: Professional standards for energy therapy practitioners.* Energy Psychology Press.

Iacorossi, L., Di Ridolfi, P., Bigiarini, L., Giannarelli, D., & Sanguineti, G. (2017). The impact of Reiki on side effects in patients with head-neck neoplasia undergoing radiotherapy: A pilot study. *Professioni Infermieristiche, 70*, 214–222. https://pubmed.ncbi.nlm.nih.gov/29460558/

Inamoto, H. (2019). *About Komyo ReikiDo.* Komyo ReikiDo International. https://www.komyoreikido-international.net/hyakuten-inamoto.html

Institute of Medicine. (2010). *Integrative medicine and the health of the public: A summary of the February 2009 summit.* National Academies Press.

International Association of Reiki Professionals. (2021). *Code of ethics for Reiki practitioners and Reiki master teachers.* https://iarp.org/iarp-code-ethics/

International Center for Reiki Training. (2021a). *The birth of holy fire.* https://www.reiki.org/birth-holy-fire

International Center for Reiki Training. (2021b). *Ethical standards.* https://www.reiki.org/ethical-standards

International Center for Reiki Training. (2021c). *ICRT Reiki code of ethics.* https://www.reiki.org/code-ethics

Jahantiqh, F., Abdollahimohammad, A., Firouzkouhi, M., & Ebrahiminejad, V. (2018). Effects of Reiki versus physiotherapy on relieving lower back pain and improving activities daily living of patients with intervertebral disc hernia. *Journal of Evidence-based Integrative Medicine, 23*, 2515690X18762745. https://doi.org/10.1177/2515690X18762745

Joint Commission on Accreditation of Healthcare Organizations. (2017a). Joint Commission enhances pain assessment and management requirements for accredited hospitals. *The Joint Commission Perspectives: Official Newsletter of The Joint Commission, 37*(7), 1–4. https://www.acep.org/globalassets/sites/acep/media/equal-documents/opioids-documents/pain-assessmen-tperspectives.pdf

Joint Commission on Accreditation of Healthcare Organizations. (2017b). *R3 Report: Requirement, rationale, reference: Pain assessment and management standards for hospitals* (Issue 11). https://www.jointcommission.org/-/media/tjc/documents/standards/r3-reports/r3_report_issue_11_2_11_19_rev.pdf

Joint Commission on Accreditation of Healthcare Organizations. (2018a). *R3 Report Issue 14: Pain assessment and management standards for ambulatory care.* https://www.jointcommission.org/-/media/tjc/documents/standards/r3-reports/r3_14_pain_assess_mgmt_ahc_6_20_18_final.pdf

Joint Commission on Accreditation of Healthcare Organizations. (2018b). *R3 Report Issue 15: Pain assessment and management standards for critical access hospitals* (Issue 15). https://www.jointcommission.org/-/media/tjc/documents/standards/r3-reports/r3_15_pain_assess_mgmt_cah_6_22_18_final.pdf

Joint Commission on Accreditation of Healthcare Organizations. (2018c). *Report Issue 16: Pain assessment and management standards for office-based surgeries* (Issue 16). https://www.jointcommission.org/-/media/tjc/documents/standards/r3-reports/r3_16_pain_assess_mgmt_obs_6_20_18_final.pdf

Joyce, J., & Herbison, G. P. (2015). Reiki for depression and anxiety. *Cochrane Database of Systematic Reviews,* (4), CD006833. https://doi.org/10.1002/14651858.CD006833.pub2

Jurkovich, P., & Watson, S. (2020). Implementation of a volunteer Reiki program at an academic medical center in the Midwest. *Journal of Holistic Nursing, 38*(4), 400–409. https://doi.org/10.1177/0898010120907734

Kafatos, M. C., Chevalier, G., Chopra, D., Hubacher, J., Kak, S., & Theise, N. (2015). Biofield science: Current physics perspectives. *Global Advances in Health and Medicine, Biofield Special Issue, 4*(Suppl.), 25–34. https://doi.org/10.7453/gahmj.2015.011.suppl

Kennedy, P. (2001). Working with survivors of torture in Sarajevo with Reiki. *Complementary Therapies in Nursing and Midwifery, 7*(1), 4–7. https://doi.org/10.1054/ctnm.2000.0516

Kent, J. B., Jin, L., & Li, X. J. (2020). Quantifying biofield therapy through biophoton emission in a cellular model. *Journal of Scientific Exploration, 34*(3), 434–454. https://doi.org/10.31275/20201691

Kentischer, F., Kleinknect-Dolf, M., & Spirig, R., Frei, I., & Huber, E. (2017). Patient-related complexity of care: A challenge or overwhelming burden for nurses—A qualitative study. *Scandinavian Journal of Caring Sciences, 32*(1), 204–222. https://doi.org/10.1111/scs.12449

Kirshbaum, M., Stead, M., & Bartys, S. (2016). An exploratory study of Reiki experiences in women who have cancer. *International Journal of Palliative Care Nursing, 22*(4), 166–172. https://doi.org/10.12968/ijpn.2016.22.4.166

Kreitzer, M. J., & Koithan, M. (2018). *Integrative nursing* (2nd ed.). Oxford University Press.

Kreitzer, M. J., & Saper, R. (2015). Exploring the biofield. *Global Advances in Health and Medicine, Biofield Special Issue, 4*(Suppl.), 3–4. https://doi.org/10.7453/gahmj.2015.105.suppl

Kryak, E., & Vitale, A. (2011). Reiki and its journey into a hospital setting. *Holistic Nursing Practice, 25*(5), 238–245. https://doi.org/10.1097/HNP.0b013e31822a02ad

Kundu, A., Dolan-Oves, R., Dimmers, M. A., Towle, C. B., & Doorenbos, A. Z. (2013). Reiki training for caregivers of hospitalized pediatric patients: A pilot program. *Complementary Therapies in Clinical Practice, 19*(1), 50–54. https://doi.org/10.1016/j.ctcp.2012.08.001

Kurebayashi, L. F. S., Turrini, R. N., T., de Souza, T., P., B., Takiguchi, R. S., Kuba, G., & Nagumo, M. T. (2016). Massage and Reiki used to reduce stress and anxiety: Randomized clinical trial. *Revista latino-americana de enfermagem, 24*, e2834. https://doi.org/10.1590/1518-8345.1614.2834

Lipinski, K., & Van De Velde, J. (2020). Reiki: Defining a healing practice for nursing. *Clinics of North America, 55*(4), 521–536. https://doi.org/10.1016/j.cnur.2020.06.017

Lubeck, W., Petter, F., & Rand, W. (2001). *The spirit of Reiki: The complete handbook of the Reiki system.* Lotus Press.

Mangione, L., Swengros, D., & Anderson, J. G. (2017). Mental health wellness and biofield therapies: An integrative review. *Issues Mental Health Nursing, 38*(11), 930–944. https://doi.org/10.1080/01612840.2017.1364808

Mansour, A. A., Beuche, M., Laing, G., Leis, A., & Nurse, J. (1999). A study to test the effectiveness of placebo Reiki standardization procedures developed for a planned Reiki efficacy study. *Journal of Alternative and Complementary Medicine, 5*(2), 153–164. https://doi.org/10.1089/acm.1999.5.153

McManus, D. E. (2017). Reiki is better than placebo and has broad potential as complementary health therapy. *Journal of Evidence Based Complementary Alternative Medicine, 22*(4), 1051–1057. https://doi.org/10.1177/2156587217728644

Midilli, T., & Gunduzoglu, C. (2016). Effects of Reiki on pain and vital signs when applied to the incision area of the body after cesarean section surgery: A single-blinded, randomized, double-controlled study. *Holistic Nursing Practice, 30*(6), 368–378. https://doi.org/10.1097/HNP.0000000000000172

Miles, P. (2006). *Reiki: A comprehensive guide.* Jeremy P. Tarcher/Penguin.

Miles, P. (2021). *Reiki in hospitals: An update.* https://reikiinmedicine.org/clinical-practice/reiki-in-hospitals-an-update/

Morse, M. L., & Beem, L. A. W. (2011). Benefits of Reiki therapy for a severely neutropenic patient with associated influences on a true random number generator. *Journal of Alternative and Complementary Medicine, 17*(12), 1180–1190. https://doi.org/10.1089/acm.2010.0238

Movaffaghi, Z., & Farsi, M. (2009). Biofield therapies: Biophysical basis and biological regulations? *Complementary Therapies in Clinical Practice, 15*, 35–37. https://doi.org/10.1016/j.ctcp.2008.07.001

Muehsam, D., Chevalier, G., Barsotti, T., & Gurfein, B. (2015). An overview of biofield devices. *Global Advances in Health and Medicine, 4*(Suppl.), 52–57. https://doi.org/10.7453/gahmj.2015.022.suppl

National Center for Complementary and Integrative Health. (2021a). *Complementary, alternative, or integrative health: What's in a name?* https://www.nccih.nih.gov/health/complementary-alternative-or-integrative-health-whats-in-a-name

National Center for Complementary and Integrative Health. (2021b). *Reiki.* https://www.nccih.nih.gov/health/reiki

Notte, B., Fazzini, C., & Mooney, R. (2016). Reiki's effect on patients with total knee arthroscopy: A pilot study. *Nursing, 46*(2), 17–23. https://doi.org/10.1097/01.NURSE.0000476246.16717.65

Oschman, J. (2016). *Energy medicine: The scientific basis* (2nd ed.). Elsevier.

Petter, F. (1999). *The original Reiki handbook of Dr. Mikao Usui.* Lotus Press.

Radin, D., Schlitz, M., & Baur, C. (2015). Distant healing intention therapies: An overview of the scientific evidence. *Global Advances in Health and Medicine, 4*(Suppl.), 67–71. https://doi.org/10.7453/gahmj.2015.012.suppl

Radziewicz, R. M., Wright-Esber, S., Zupancic, J., Gargiulo, D., & Woodall, P. (2018). Safety of Reiki therapy for newborns at risk for neonatal abstinence syndrome. *Holistic Nursing Practice, 32*(2), 63. https://doi.org/10.1097/HNP.0000000000000251

Reiki and Seichem Association. (2021). *What is Seichem?* http://reikiseichem.org/WhatIsSeichem.php

Ring, M. E. (2009). Reiki and changes in pattern manifestation. *Nursing Science Quarterly, 22*(3), 250–258. https://doi.org/10.1177/0894318409337014

Ringdahl, D. (2008). *Implementation of a hospital-based Reiki program* (Unpublished University of Minnesota DNP project). University of Minnesota.

Ringdahl, D., & Voss, M. (2016). *Teaching Reiki to caregivers of children receiving bone marrow transplants* (Unpublished University of Minnesota DNP project). University of Minnesota.

Rosada, R. M., Rubik, B., Mainguy, B., Plummer, J., & Mehl-Madrona, L. (2015). Reiki reduces burnout among community mental health clinicians. *Journal of Alternative and Complementary Medicine, 8*, 489–495. https://doi.org/10.1089/acm.2014.0403

Rosenbaum, M. S., & Van de Velde, J. (2016). The effects of yoga, massage, and Reiki on patient well-being at a cancer resource center. *Clinical Journal of Oncology Nursing, 20*(3), E77–E81. https://doi.org/10.1188/16.CJON.E77-E81

Rubik, B., Muehsam, D., Hammerschlag, R., & Jain, S. (2015). Biofield science and healing: History, terminology, and concepts. *Global Advances in Health and Medicine, Biofield Special Issue, 4*, 8–15. https://doi.org/10.7453/gahmj.2015.038.suppl

Salles, L., Vannucci, L., Salles, A., & Sliva, M. A. (2014). The effect of Reiki on blood hypertension. *Acta Paulista de Enfermagem, 27*(5), 479–84. https://doi.org/10.1590/1982-0194201400078

Santos, C. B. R. D., Gomes, E. T., Bezerra, S. M. M. D. S., & Püschel, V. A. D. A. (2020). Reiki protocol for preoperative anxiety, depression, and well-being: A non-randomized controlled trial. *Revista da Escola de Enfermagem da USP, 54*. https://doi.org/10.1590/S1980-220X2019012403630

Sawyer, J. (1998). The first Reiki practitioner in our OR. *AORN Journal, 67*(3), 674–676. https://doi.org/10.1016/S0001-2092(06)62838-

Shaybak, E., Abdollahimohammad, A., Rahnama, M., Masinaeinezhad, N., Azadi-Ahmadabadi, C., & Firouzkohi, M. (2017). Effects of Reiki energy therapy on saphenous vein incision pain: A randomized clinical trial study. *Der Pharmacia Lettre, 9*(1), 100–109. https://www.scholarsresearchlibrary.com/articles/effects-of-reiki-energy-therapy-on-saphenous-vein-incision-pain-a-randomized-clinical-trial-study.pdf

Shepherd-Gentle, L. (2001). Insurance payments for reiki treatments. *International Center for Reiki Training.* https://www.reiki.org/articles/insurance-payments-reiki-treatments

Siegel, P., da Motta, P. M. R., da Silva, L. G., Stephan, C., Lima, C. S. P., & de Barros, N. F. (2016). Reiki for cancer patients undergoing chemotherapy in a Brazilian Hospital. *Holistic Nursing Practice, 30*(3), 174–182. https://doi.org/10.1097/HNP.0000000000000146

Singg, S. (2015). Use of Reiki as a biofield therapy: An adjunct to conventional medical care. *Clinical Case Report Review, 1*(3), 54–60. https://doi.org/10.15761/CCRR.1000121

Stiene, B., & Stiene, F. (2005). *The Japanese art of Reiki.* O Books.

Thrane, S. E., Maurer, S. H., & Danford, C. A. (2021). Feasibility and acceptability of Reiki therapy for children receiving palliative care in the home. *Journal of Hospice & Palliative Nursing, 23*(1), 52–58. https://doi.org/10.1097/NJH.0000000000000714

Thrane, S. E., Maurer, S. H., Ren, D., Danford, C. A., & Cohen, S. M. (2017). Reiki therapy for symptom management in children receiving palliative care: A pilot study. *American Journal of Hospice and Palliative Care, 34*(4), 373–379. https://doi.org/10.1177/1049909116630973

Topdemir, E. A., & Saritas, S. (2020). The effect of preoperative Reiki application on patient anxiety levels. *Explore (NY), 17*(1), 50–54. https://doi.org/10.1016/j.explore.2020.01.003

Townsend, J. S. (2013). Temari Reiki: A new hands-off approach to traditional Reiki. *International Journal of Nursing Practice, 19*(Suppl. 2), 34–38. https://doi.org/10.1111/ijn.12206

Vasudev, S. S., & Shastri, S. (2016). Effect of distance Reiki on perceived stress among software professionals in Bangalore. *The International Journal of Indian Psychology, 3*, 136–142. https://doi.org/10.25215/0304.055

Vergo, M. T., Pinkson, B. M., Broglio, K., Li, Z., & Tosteson, T. D. (2018). Immediate symptom relief after a first session of massage therapy or Reiki in hospitalized patients: A 5-year clinical experience from a rural academic medical center. *The Journal of Alternative and Complementary Medicine, 24*(8), 801–808. https://doi.org/10.1089/acm.2017.0409

Vitale, A. (2007). An integrative review of Reiki touch therapy research. *Holistic Nursing Practice, 21*(4), 167–179. https://doi.org/10.1097/01.HNP.0000280927.83506.f6

Vitale, A. (2014). Initiating a Reiki or CAM program in a healthcare organization—Developing a business plan. *Holistic Nursing Practice, 28*(6), 376–380. https://doi.org/10.1097/HNP.0000000000000052

Watson, J. (2011). *Nursing: Human science and human care* (2nd ed.). Jones & Bartlett.

Yüce, U. O., & Taşcı, S. (2021). Effect of Reiki on the stress level of caregivers of patients with cancer: Qualitative and single-blind randomized controlled trial. *Complementary Therapies in Medicine, 58*, 102708. https://doi.org/10.1016/j.ctim.2021.102708

Zins, S., Hooke, M. C., & Gross, C. R. (2019). Reiki for pain during hemodialysis: A feasibility and instrument evaluation study. *Journal of Holistic Nursing, 37*(2), 148–162. https://doi.org/10.1177/0898010118797195

Zucchetti, G., Candela, F., Bottigelli, C., Campione, G., Parrinello, A., Piu, P., Vassallo, E., & Fagioli, F. (2019). The power of Reiki: feasibility and efficacy of reducing pain in children with cancer undergoing hematopoietic stem cell transplantation. *Journal of Pediatric Oncology Nursing, 36*(5), 361–368. https://doi.org/10.1177/1043454219845879

Acupressure

PAMELA WEISS-FARNAN

Touch has been central to the practice of nursing since its inception. This chapter describes a form of touch—and its application in nursing care—known in traditional Chinese medicine (TCM) as acupressure. This method of treatment is common in many cultures. As Dossey et al. (2000) note, "all cultures have demonstrated that some form of rubbing, pressing, massaging or holding are [*sic*] natural manifestations of the desire to heal and care for one another" (p. 615). Acupressure is also integral to the practice of shiatsu, tui na, tsubo, and jin shin jiyutsu.

DEFINITIONS

To assist the reader, the following definitions are provided:

- **acupressure:** An "ancient healing art that uses the fingers to press certain points on the body to stimulate the body's self-curative abilities" (Gach, 1990, p. 3).
- **acupuncture:** The term *acupuncture* describes a family of procedures involving the stimulation of points on the body using a variety of techniques, usually sterile needles. The acupuncture technique that has been most often studied scientifically involves penetrating the skin with thin, solid, metallic needles that are manipulated by the hands or by electrical stimulation. Acupuncture has been practiced in China and other Asian countries for thousands of years, acupuncture is one of the key components of TCM (National Center for Complementary and Integrative Health [NCCIH], 2021).
- **auricular acupuncture:** A microacupuncture technique similar to reflexology in which points in the ear are stimulated with pressure that stimulates the central nervous system through the cranial nerves/spinal nerves on the auricle of the ear (Fan et al., 2016).
- **jin shin jyutsu:** A physiophilosophy that involves the application of the hands for gently balancing the flow of life energy in the body; more generally, it is the awakening to awareness of complete harmony within the self and the universe (Lamke et al., 2014).
- **meridians:** Meridional theory identifies meridians as a system of channels through which vital energy, or *Qi*, flows. (Longhurst, 2010).
- **qi:** The force that animates and controls the observable functions of living beings (acufinder.com, 2017).

■ **shiatsu:** This term means "finger pressure" in Japanese; in practice, a practitioner uses touch, comfortable pressure, and manipulative techniques to adjust the body's physical structure and balance its energy flow (www.shiatsu.com).

TRADITIONAL CHINESE MEDICINE

TCM is an ancient system of health developed more than 3,000 years ago in Asia. This system is based on the concept that qi flows throughout the body and that balance of yin and yang forces represents health and well-being. As Kaptchuck (1984) describes it,

> this system of care is based on ancient texts and is the result of a continuous process of critical thinking, as well as extensive clinical observation and testing. It represents a thorough formulation and reformulation of material by respected clinicians and theoreticians. It is also, however, rooted in the philosophy, logic and sensibility, and habits of a civilization entirely foreign to our own. It has therefore developed its own perception of the body and health and disease. (p. 2)

The focus of care within this system is to restore balance in the body. To do so, yin and yang must be balanced. Yin aspects are associated with cold, passivity, interiority, and decreases. Yang aspects are associated with warmth, activity, external forces, and increases. Yin and yang are always in relation to each other (Kaptchuk, 1983). According to this conceptualization, they are in continuous flux, and there is always yin within yang and yang within yin.

Unschuld (1999) reflects that TCM theory is a mixture of beliefs that pathogenic influences from the outside combine with the lack of balance or harmony within the person and result in illness. TCM is also concerned with the concept of qi. Qi flows in the body through specific pathways identified as meridians or channels. If the qi is blocked or diminished, a person experiences pain or illness.

According to TCM theory, there are 12 bilateral meridians and eight extra meridians. All meridians have an exterior and an interior pathway and are named according to the organ system. Located on the meridians are specific points. In the 12 major meridians, the points are bilateral and in the West are called acupuncture points. This nomenclature implies that the points are designated for needle insertion and does not fully reflect the TCM concept of the point.

Acupuncture points are also used for acupressure. The points do not have a corresponding anatomical structure but are described by their location relative to other anatomical landmarks. This contributes to the skepticism of many Western-trained scientists about their existence. In Chinese, the name of the point usually is descriptive of its function or location. Mistranslation over the years has often limited the importance of the anatomical basis for the nomenclature of points and the apparent knowledge of anatomy of Chinese scholars (Schnorrenberger, 1996).

There are 365 (Kaptchuk, 1983) to 700 (Yang, 2006) major points on the meridians. Yang (2006) stated that 108 points could be stimulated using the fingers. In a traditionally formulated TCM treatment plan, whether the modality is needles or pressure, the points are combined to achieve maximal benefit for the patient. Rarely is only one point used. There are also points that should not be stimulated, especially during pregnancy, which are referred to as forbidden points. These points according to Betts and Budd (2011) are LI4, SP6, GB21, BL32, BL60, and BL67.

SCIENTIFIC BASIS

Western medicine is the dominant system of healthcare in the United States. It is characterized by hospitals, clinics, pharmaceutical resources, and a workforce of physicians, nurses, specialized therapists, and various support service personnel. There are many differences between Western medicine and TCM that become more evident as nurses seek to add TCM modalities to their practice. Western medicine emphasizes disease, causal agents, and treatments that are designed to control or destroy the cause of disease (Kaptchuk, 1983). Once a causal agent or mechanism is identified, treatment plans are developed that focus on the agent or mechanism as a consistent factor in all human manifestations of the disease. In Western journals, almost all studies using the modality of acupuncture and acupressure emphasize the specific effects of needling one point known to address a specific symptom. Medical researchers are eager to find the mechanism by which acupuncture alleviates the symptoms.

Some mechanisms of action of acupuncture and/or acupressure have been suggested through Western medical research. As research has expanded into the mechanism, other researchers have hypothesized that the therapeutic effects produced by stimulation of the points with needles or with pressure may be due to the following:

- local effects, including activation of the diffuse, noxious, inhibitory response that is induced with an immediate suppression of pain transmission
- conduction of electromagnetic signals that may start the flow of pain-killing biochemicals, such as endorphins, and of immune system cells to specific sites in the body that are injured or vulnerable to disease
- activation of opioid systems, which also reduces pain
- changes in brain chemistry, sensation, and involuntary responses by changing the release of neurotransmitters and neurohormones in a health-promoting way (Huang et al., 2012; Liang et al., 2012)
- changes in the response of the fascia, producing a relaxation effect (Cheng, 2009, 2014; Dale, 1997; Han, 2003; Kawakita & Okada, 2014; Lund & Lundeberg, 2016; MacPherson et al., 2016; Takeshige, 1989; Wu et al., 1994)
- patient expectations, reassurance from the practitioner, or noninsertive physiological stimulation (Cherkin et al., 2009)

The scientific research into an underlying mechanism demonstrates one of the differences between Western medicine and the TCM system. The focus in TCM is the imbalance in the patient, and the causality is always multifactorial. The function of the points is described in terms of TCM diagnosis. For example, Western medicine research has focused on pericardium 6, or nei guan, for the treatment of nausea. In English, its name means "inner border gate." Lade (1986) describes the point:

> The name refers to the point's role as the gateway or connecting point of the triple burner channel and the yin-linking vessel. Inner refers to the palmar aspect of the forearm and to the point's location on the yin channel. The actions of this point are: to regulate and tonify the heart, transform heart phlegm, facilitate qi flow, regulate the yin-linking vessel and clear heart fire, redirect rebellious qi downward, expand and relax the chest and benefit the diaphragm. The indications for use

of the point are: asthma, bronchitis, pertussis, hiccups, vomiting, diaphragmatic spasms, intercostal neuralgia, chest fullness, and pain and
dyspnea. (pp. 196, 197)

Whereas Western medicine focuses on the treatment of nausea for this point,
the TCM paradigm suggests multiple uses. In TCM theory, nausea is considered
rebellious qi (qi that flows in the wrong direction). Nausea and vomiting are
examples of this. Nei guan (pericardium 6) is used as one of the points in the
treatment of a patient with nausea. In TCM theory, nausea is considered one of
the external manifestations of the imbalance; however, in an authentic TCM treatment, a practitioner would evaluate the imbalances that set up the manifestation
and treat the underlying condition. Therefore, a combination of points to treat
nausea would be used, possibly including other primary points for antiemesis
(Hoo, 1997): Stomach 36 on the stomach meridian located on the knee, Ren 12 on
the ren/conception meridian located on the upper abdomen, or Spleen 4 on the
spleen meridian located on the foot. The application of multiple acupoints may
be more effective for the treatment of nausea; however, in Western medicine, the
focus on finding the single active point or the mechanism creates an almost insur-
mountable challenge to the fullest application of the therapy.

In 1997, the National Institutes of Health (NIH) held the first consensus conference on acupuncture. The conference members concluded that

> acupuncture is effective in the treatment of adult nausea and vomit-
> ing in chemotherapy and probably pregnancy and in postoperative
> dental pain. The conference members stated there is an indication
> that acupuncture may be helpful in the treatment of addiction, stroke
> rehabilitation, headache, menstrual cramps, tennis elbow, fibromy-
> algia, myofascial pain, osteoarthritis, low back pain, carpal tunnel
> syndrome, and asthma, in which acupuncture may be useful as an
> adjunct treatment or an acceptable alternative or be included in a com-
> prehensive management program. (NIH, 1997, para. 5)

Since that original statement, the conditions that can be treated successfully
have expanded in number. NCCIH/NIH remain cautious about broadly endors-
ing acupuncture for a wide range of conditions. Instead, however, NCCIH has
continued to fund research in numerous areas in efforts to scientifically document its efficacy in the treatment of specifically targeted conditions.

Following the NIH statement, studies completed for the treatment of nausea and vomiting included the use of devices to apply pressure or stimulation to
pericardium 6 (P6) increased. These devices included an elastic bracelet with a
pressure button called a Sea-Band (trade brand) or an electrical stimulation device
called a ReliefBand (trade brand). Bands to stimulate P6 are manufactured and
distributed by numerous companies. Most devices are expandable wristbands
with a button or a magnetic closure that places pressure on P6. A few of the models also provide electrical stimulation that provides a more intense treatment. All
the products are available as over-the-counter products and do not require a physician's order.

Gach and Henning (2004) have expanded their self-care guide to the use
of acupressure to include trauma, stress, and common emotional imbalances.
Also, in recent years, research related to the use of acupressure has expanded,

incorporating the study of a wide range of points and techniques. Multiple studies now include auricular acupuncture as the primary intervention. Research has examined a variety of Western-diagnosed conditions that have been treated with by acupressure utilizing different modalities and pressure points.

SELECTED STUDIES

Table 25.1 presents a brief summary of selected recent studies examining the use of acupressure to treat a range of patient conditions. The conditions in the table include such things as postoperative and cancer-related nausea and

Table 25.1 *Sample of Studies Using Acupressure and Combined Interventions*

Author	Condition	Modality	Findings/ Conclusions
Perkins et al. (2020)	Palliative care patients	Sea-Bands on Ps6	No statistically significant decrease in nausea episodes.
Solt Kirca and Kanza Gul (2020)	Nausea and vomiting of pregnancy	Acupressure taught to pregnant women in a double-blind randomized trial	Techniques of acupressure reduced nausea and vomiting
Li et al. (2018)	Symptomatic knee osteoarthritis	Randomized trial of outpatients who performed acupressure five times per week for 8 weeks	Statistically significant improvement in knee pain
Susana et al. (2020)	Cervical (neck) pain of benign origin	Randomized controlled trial of self-applied acupressure to specified points	Visual analog pain scores were lower, and quality of life utility index scores were higher in intervention group
Soylu and Tekinsoy (2021)	Postop pain after laparoscopic cholecystectomy	Acupressure stimulation of Neiguan (P6) and Hegu (LI4) applied by nurses	Acupressure reduced pain and shortened time to defecation
Asgari et al. (2020)	Pain and limitations of movement of carpal tunnel	Acupressure taught to patients for 1 month prior to planned surgery date	Severity of clinical symptoms was reduced, and hand function improved
Hsieh et. al. (2019)	Adverse reactions of antituberculosis drug therapy	Participants were taught self-care acupressure to administer before taking the medication	Acupressure can prevent and relieve adverse gastrointestinal drug reactions

vomiting, pain of dysmenorrhea, labor and delivery, and pain experienced in other settings, as well as anxiety, insomnia, and health promotion in older adults. A variety of pressure-related modalities were used in these studies to assess their efficacy in providing relief. Numerous studies were done outside of the United States, where the cultural barriers about the use of this ancient type of medicine are lower likely because the use of acupressure is an accepted part of the cultural health practices.

META-ANALYSES

Meta-analyses published by the Cochrane Collaborative and others conclude that the use of acupressure for the treatment of a number of symptoms may be useful, however more rigorous trials are required (Hu, 2015; Smith et al., 2020). The

Table 25.2 *Meta-Analyses of the Use of Acupressure or Acupuncture for Various Conditions*

Authors	Condition	Intervention or Modality	Findings/Conclusion
Garcia et al. (2021)	Chemotherapy-induced nausea and vomiting	Electrical stimulation to PC6	Meta-analysis of 14 articles indicated a reduction in the number of episodes of acute nausea and vomiting
He et al. (2020)	Improvement of cancer pain	Acupressure/acupuncture combined to provide pain relief	Analysis of 25 articles indicated that the combination of therapies can increase the reduction of pain
Chen et al. (2020)	Health promotion in older adults	Acupressure was taught to older community-living adults	Sleep quality and cognitive functioning improved; slight increase in alleviating constipation and moderate pain relief
Smith et al. (2020)	Pain management during labor	Acupuncture or acupressure	Acupressure showed promise for alleviating symptoms. More rigorous study designs are needed
Godley and Smith (2020)	Chronic low back pain	Acupressure applied on specific points	Meta-analysis of 150 studies found acupressure to be a feasible, effective, and low-cost method to treat low back pain
Fu et al. (2021)	Postoperative nausea and vomiting	Protocols of acupuncture or acupressure	Acupuncture was superior to placebo and usual care to manage postoperative nausea and vomiting
Raana and Fan (2020)	Pain during the first stage of labor	Acupressure at prescribed points by practitioner	Acupressure can provide significant pain relief during labor. Future trials need standardized protocols

quality of the articles in the reviews limits conclusions and scientific, theoretical, and clinical advancement related to the use of acupressure. In the studies, the small numbers of participants and the lack of clear explanations of interventions to test the efficacy of the interventions remain problematic (see Table 25.2).

Pediatric patients have not been studied extensively using acupressure as an intervention; however, in the framework of TCM, children are considered sensitive to any type of energy and may enjoy the same benefits that are found in adult populations. Acupressure is less invasive than other treatments and may be more acceptable to pediatric patients. The number of studies that use acupressure as a modality but in the form of auricular acupuncture or combined interventions of acupressure and acupuncture has increased.

Methodological problems persist in the study of acupressure. This may result from funding issues or remaining skepticism about a simple intervention improving health and well-being. In order to overcome the small sample sizes and research design flaws, several meta-analyses have been completed. The growing concern over pharmacological interventions and the motivation for nurses to provide innovative and easily implemented treatments will only increase the interest in other modalities. A nurse can apply acupressure as part of the intervention plan using Western diagnoses. The employer may provide incentives for nurses to consider incorporating acupressure techniques into their practices. Acupressure techniques are easily learned, are minimally invasive, and have a salutary positive impact on patient outcomes. How to intervene using acupressure is further explained below using two of the most important points of the body, Hegu (large intestine 4) and Neiguan (P6).

INTERVENTION

A TCM practitioner would follow a multistep diagnostic process to choose the correct points to stimulate. Nurses can use a Western, symptom-based system of determining the points that will provide relief for the patient's suffering. The nurse will also be able to teach the patient and the family to implement acupressure techniques to assist the patient in reducing symptoms and stimulating the body's own healing strengths.

GUIDELINES FOR USE

Nurses can incorporate acupressure into the care of patients by using some common points that have specific actions to relieve common symptoms. The nurse can treat the patient with acupressure or teach the patient or family members to use acupressure as part of a care plan.

Prior to touching patients, the nurse must assess the patients' readiness to be touched. Shames and Keegan (2000) recommend the following assessment of patients:

- perception of mind–body situation
- pathophysiological problems that may require referral
- history of psychological disorders
- cultural beliefs about touch
- previous experience with body therapies (p. 264)

Each point is located using an anatomical marker. Many books describe point locations. The standard measure is the cun, which is different for each individual. One cun for a particular patient is defined as the "width of the interphalangeal joint of the patient's thumb" or as "the distance between the two radial ends of the flexor creases of a flexed middle finger of the patient. Two cun is the width of the index finger, the middle finger, and the ring finger" (Hoo, 1997).

STIMULATING THE POINT

Several different types of techniques are used to stimulate the points, according to Gach (1990):

- firm stationary pressure—using the thumbs, fingers, palms, sides of hands, or knuckles
- slow-motion kneading—using the thumbs and fingers with the heels of the hands to squeeze large muscle groups
- brisk rubbing—using friction to stimulate the blood and lymph
- quick tapping—using the fingertips to stimulate muscles of unprotected areas of the body such as the face (p. 9)

EVALUATING ACUPRESSURE'S EFFECT

Gach (1990) has developed guidelines for assessing results. The elements of the assessment include the following:

- identifying the problems being addressed with acupressure
- identifying the points being used for the treatment
- determining the length of time for the acupressure
- identifying what makes the condition worse (e.g., standing, cold weather, menstruation, constipation, lack of exercise, stress, traveling, other variables)
- describing the changes experienced by the patient after 3 days and after 1 week of treatment
- describing the changes in the condition and overall feeling of well-being (Gach, 1990, p. 13)

ACUPRESSURE FOR SELECT CONDITIONS

Nausea

Point: Pericardium 6 (P6; Nei Guan, "Inner Gate")

Location: Pericardium 6 is located on the inner aspect of the wrist 2 cun (units) proximal to the transverse crease of the wrist between the tendons of the palmaris longus and flexor carpi radialis muscles (Lade, 1986). The patient should place the middle three fingers (index, middle, and ring fingers) on the opposite hand that is palm upward. The point under the ring finger between the two tendons is pericardium 6 (see Figure 25.1).

Functions: Its functions were outlined previously in the discussion on the research on this point.

Method of Stimulation: The point can be stimulated using firm pressure either with a rotating pattern with the thumb or the static pressure of a Sea-Band.

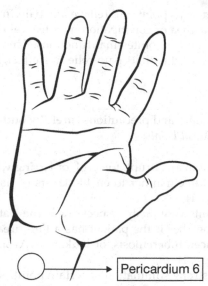

Figure 25.1 Pressure point Pericardium 6. This point has multiple functions and is one of the most important points.

Indications in Nursing: This point can be used for the treatment of nausea in many situations, but research, as cited previously, has focused on postoperative nausea, nausea of pregnancy, and nausea accompanying chemotherapy.

PAIN AND GASTROINTESTINAL DISORDERS

Point: Large Intestine 4 (LI4; Hoku, "Joining the Valley")

Location: This point is on the back of the hand halfway between the junction of the first and second metacarpal bones, which form a depression or valley when the thumb is abducted (Lade, 1986). There are two ways to locate this point easily. The patient holds the hand with the thumb touching the index finger; when the hand is held at eye level, the highest mound at the base of the thumb and index finger is the location of LI4. Alternately, the nurse instructs the patient to place the thumb of one hand in the web between the thumb and index finger of the opposite hand. The patient should match the first crease on the thumb of one hand to the web of the other and then rotate the thumb to touch the fleshy area between the index finger and the thumb. The point is where the tip of the thumb touches the area between the thumb and the index finger.

Functions: This point has multiple functions and is one of the most important points of the body. It alleviates pain, tones qi, and generates protective qi (in Western medicine this would be considered an immune system–building function); moistens the large intestine and in so doing relieves diarrhea or constipation; clears the nose; regulates the lungs in asthma, bronchitis, or the common cold; and expedites labor. This point is contraindicated in pregnancy because of the latter function (Lade, 1986, pp. 40–41).

Method of Stimulation: Firm pressure can be applied on this point with a rotating thumb massage technique. This point is often sensitive, and the patient reports a feeling of discomfort. This is normal and not indicative of a problem.

Indications in Nursing: This point will relieve any pain in the body. In addition, individuals with diarrhea or constipation may feel relief because stimulating the point balances the gastrointestinal functions. This point can be used to induce labor and, coupled with its pain-relieving effect, may be helpful.

PRECAUTIONS

There are overall guidelines and precautions carefully outlined by Gach (1990) in his book, *Acupressure Potent Points*:

- Never press any area in an abrupt, forceful, or jarring way. Apply finger pressure in a slow, rhythmic manner to enable layers of tissues and the internal organs to respond (p. 11).
- Use abdominal points cautiously, especially if the patient is ill. Avoid the abdominal area altogether if the patient has a life-threatening disease, especially intestinal cancer, tuberculosis, or leukemia. Avoid the abdominal area during pregnancy (pp. 11–12).
- During pregnancy, strong stimulation of certain points should be avoided: LI4 (fourth point on the large intestine meridian), K3 (third point on the kidney meridian), and SP6 (sixth point on the spleen meridian). Each of these points may have an effect on the pregnancy (p. 192).
- Lymph areas such as the groin, the area of the throat just below the ears, and the outer breast near the armpits are very sensitive. Touch these areas lightly (p. 12).
- Do not work directly on a serious burn, ulcer, or area of infection.
- Do not work directly on a newly formed scar. New surgical or other wounds should not be touched directly. Continuous holding on the periphery of the injury will stimulate the injury to heal (p. 12).
- After an acupressure treatment, tolerance to cold is lowered and the energy of the body is focused on healing, so advise the patient to wear warm clothes and keep out of drafts (p. 12).
- Use acupressure cautiously in individuals with a new acute or serious illness (p. 12).
- Acupressure is not a sole treatment for cancer, contagious skin disease, or sexually transmitted disease (pp. 11–12).
- Brisk rubbing, deep pressure, or kneading should not be used for patients with heart disease, cancer, or high blood pressure (p. 9).

CULTURAL APPLICATIONS

Nurses work with patients from differing cultural backgrounds. Multiple cultures throughout the world use manual therapies to either promote or maintain health or to treat illness. Although the therapies are part of the Indigenous healing methods used by different groups of people, they are classified as complementary and alternative medicine (CAM) in the United States. However, within many cultures, individuals and families treat manual therapies as mainstream and integral to their health practices. Such remains the case in mainland China. The contemporary widespread use of acupressure in China and internationally is described in Sidebar 25.1.

Folk and Indigenous healing practices are common not only for the people of Asian origin but also for almost every other culture. The practices include

Sidebar 25.1 *Acupressure and Its International Appeal*

Fang Yu, Arizona State University, Phoenix, AZ, USA (PR China)

On a weekend in the spring of 2017, I was showing off the renowned Mall of America in Bloomington, Minnesota, to my nephew, who was a high school student at the time. While strolling around, both of our eyes were caught by a prominent Chinese reflexology picture of a massage parlor. The reflexology picture depicted the common acupressure points and their linkage to different organs. Acupressure is a practice of traditional Chinese medicine (TCM) to heal diseases for more than 3,000 years. Ancient healers found that applying certain techniques of rubbing and pressing the acupressure points could relieve symptoms such as hemorrhage, pain, and swelling. The acupressure points used may or may not be in the same area of the body where the targeted symptoms occur, which is known as reflexology. The selection of the acupressure points for acupressure depends on how they are theorized to rebalance *yin* and *yang* as well as *Qi* (life energy in TCM) and blood to stimulate the channels and collaterals to induce symptom relief. Fingers and knuckles used for rubbing and pressing can be a single finger (often a thumb or a middle finger), double fingers (e.g., two thumbs), or multiple fingers.

Acupressure was widely used for the treatments of common ailments and diseases, especially in rural regions where there was a shortage of doctors and limited access to healthcare. Many practitioners learned from their parents and local elders to use acupressure to treat back pain, headache, stomach pain, and *Bi Zheng* (a painful obstruction syndrome). The recent three decades have witnessed an unimaginable popularity and momentum in acupressure use in China as a heightened awareness of health and wellness promotion, as well as disease prevention and treatment, has fueled business growth in self-care practices based on acupressure and other TCM practices such as cupping. Spas and massage parlors have become increasingly popular and affordable for the Chinese as places to relax and socialize, and they are readily accessible in every Chinese city. For example, it was estimated that foot acupressure parlors dot the streets of Shanghai every 1,500 feet.

As I stood in front of the massage parlor inside the Mall of America waiting for my nephew to decide if he wanted to purchase an acupressure session, I recalled how I would fit a visit to a foot massage parlor into my schedule at the first chance I got when I visited China. I had been so delighted to come across similar parlors in my trips to the large U.S. cities, such as Washington, D.C., and New Orleans, where I would indulge myself with an acupressure session. In 2017, I realized that accessible acupressure had come to my town! During the COVID-19 pandemic, I relocated to Arizona State University in Phoenix, Arizona. When the summer of 2021 rolled around, I needed to buy some clothes, so I went shopping at San Tan Village in Gilbert, Arizona. As I window-shopped, the sight appearance of a foot massage parlor unexpectedly greeted me. At that moment, it dawned on me that acupressure had truly transcended borders and come to life internationally. At that moment, I felt a deep appreciation of my Chinese roots and culture.

massage: pressure, rubbing, stretching, and pulling the skin, with and without herbal preparations, oils, or poultices. For example, many indigenous practices are focused on preparing for childbirth. To illustrate, in Oaxaca (a Mexican state), a practice called sobada massage is used as a diagnostic tool for gestational age, for relieving the aches and pain of pregnancy and delivery, and then stimulating the baby immediately after birth. In India, infant massage with various oils is a regular practice, and recent research has confirmed that massage with coconut oil enhances the baby's weight gain (Sankaranarayanan et al., 2005).

Although Western-trained nurses may not understand how different cultural groups incorporate skin massage and rubbing and may misinterpret what they may observe, it is important for them to allow the family to express the types of practices they use as part of their routine caring for each other and their children (Davis, 2000). Struthers (2008) emphasized that there is a "need for nurses and other healthcare providers to become knowledgeable regarding traditional indigenous healthcare that their clients may be receiving—to foster open communication" (p. 74). What the practices are called varies from one cultural group to another, but each uses skin stimulation as part of health routines and family bonding.

NURSING SELF CARE IN THE COVID-19 ERA

Nurses are also humans, and any intervention of acupressure used for patients to improve their conditions will also improve the conditions by the application of acupressure with nurses and student nurses. Acupressure also improves the quality of life among nurses who have chronic back pain (Najafabad et al., 2019). Both as self-treatments and for treatment of COVID-19 patients, acupuncture and acupressure can help stimulate and improve the environment of healing. Nursing has recently had a great challenge in the COVID-19 pandemic. The extent of psychological stress on nurses has been difficult to measure. Acupressure may contribute to the ability of the nurse to manage stressful situations and or may be helpful for patients and nurses alike. A Korean study demonstrated that meridian acupuncture was effective in reducing nurses' stress, fatigue, and anxiety (Youngmi et al., 2021). Acupressure can be used to promote relaxation and can improve mental health in an older population (Chen et al., 2020); it is possible that acupressure could be used to support nurses' mental health and relaxation as well. One study protocol has been published that aims to determine whether acupressure can ease the side effects of COVID-19 vaccine injections (Fu et al., 2021).

PHONE APPS

Smartphone apps are available that can be used to guide a person through specific acupressure protocols; they are easy for nurses to use and for nurses to teach the techniques to their patients (Hofmeyer et al., 2020). These acupressure techniques can assist the nurse in self-care processes as well as assist patients in their routine self-care or during acute COVID-19 experiences and often lengthy recoveries. For example, one free app, *Point Acupressure Selfcare app* (https://apps.apple.com/us/app/point-acupressure-selfcare-app/id1528501360), has been designed for the iPhone by Press Health, LLC. This app was created with the expertise of board-certified and licensed acupuncturists to provide basic, portable guidance to stimulate acupressure points for relief of stress, pain and anxiety anytime, anywhere. It can be purchased through the Mac app store. Other phone apps exist for free or for purchase. Consumers should read the available product ratings and reviews and make app selections or purchases according to product quality and suitability for the purpose for which the consumer is seeking to address.

Acupressure is used by millions of people around the world. Incorporating this technique into nursing care plans will unite us in the commonality we share—the desire to relieve human suffering.

FUTURE RESEARCH

There are many areas of research in which the methods of TCM and the underlying theory are being tested using the research techniques of Western medicine. Research questions about the usefulness of acupressure strategies can be proposed in many areas of nursing, including use for palliative care, rehabilitation nursing, support of women in labor, and health-promotion and disease-prevention programs. In the Western-based models, acupressure and acupuncture using various methods of stimulation (with injections, electrical stimulation, and manual pressure) are common. While many interesting questions pertaining to the use of acupressure in healthcare remain to be answered through the process of rigorous research, a few are offered here that are particularly relevant to nursing:

- Can the use of a smartphone app of selected pressure points for anxiety and stress relief, as part of nurses/nursing student self-care, be effective in promoting their well-being and reducing stress-related illness?
- Would the use of acupressure as a routine part of patient care be associated with higher levels of patient satisfaction?
- Could the use of acupressure reduce the amount of postoperative pain medication required to promote comfort and relieve postoperative pain?
- Can acupuncture be effective when taught to patients to reduce pain and aid in emotional and physical recovery after hospital discharge?

WEBSITES

- Accupressure.com (www.acupressure.com)

This is the website of Dr. Michael Reed Gach, an expert who has written extensively on acupressure. (A list of his publications appears on the website.) It includes a list of online courses that will yield certification in acupressure interventions. Point locations for treatment based on symptoms or Western medical diagnosis are also available at this site.

- Acupuncture and Acupressure for Pregnancy and Childbirth (https://acupuncture.rhizome.net.nz)

This website, maintained by `Debra Betts (2018), provides details on the use of acupressure in pregnancy and childbirth. She offers multiple brochures for patients and practitioners in numerous languages.

REFERENCES

Acufinder.com. (2017). *The definition of "Qi."* https://www.acufinder.com/Acupuncture+ Information/Detail/The+Definition+of+Qi+Acupuncture.com

Asgari, M. R., Vafaei-Moghadam, A., Babamohamadi, H., Ghorbani, R., & Esmaeili, R. (2020). Comparing acupressure with aromatherapy using Citrus aurantium in terms of their effectiveness in sleep quality in patients undergoing percutaneous coronary interventions: A randomized clinical trial. *Complementary Therapies in Clinical Practice, 38,* 101066. https://doi.org/10.1016/j.ctcp.2019.101066

Betts, D. (2018). *Acupuncture and acupressure for pregnancy and childbirth.* https://acupuncture.rhizome.net.nz/download-booklet

Betts, D., & Budd, D. (2011). Forbidden points in pregnancy: Historical wisdom? *Acupuncture in Medicine, 29,* 137–139. https://doi.org/10.1136/aim.2010.003814

Chen, M. C., Yang, L. Y., Chen, K. M., & Hsu, H. F. (2020). Systematic review and meta-analysis on using acupressure to promote the health of older adults. *Journal of Applied Gerontology, 39*(10), 1144–1152. https://doi.org/10.1177/0733464819870027

Cheng, K. J. (2009). Neuroanatomical basis of acupuncture treatment for some common illnesses. *Acupuncture in Medicine, 27*(2), 61–64. https://doi.org/10.1136/aim.2009.000455

Cheng, K. J. (2014). Neurobiological mechanisms of acupuncture for some common illnesses: A clinician's perspective. *Journal of Acupuncture and Meridian Studies, 7*(3), 105–114. http://www.jams-kpi.com/article/S2005-2901(13)00174-X/fulltext#sec2.4

Cherkin, D. C., Sherman, K. J., Avins, A. L., Erro, J. H., Ichikawa, L., Barolow, W. E., Delaney, K., Hawkes, R., Hamilton, L., Pressman, A., Khalsa, P. S., & Deyo, R. A. (2009). A randomized trial comparing acupuncture, simulated acupuncture, and usual care for chronic low back pain. *Archives of Internal Medicine, 169*(9), 858–866. https://doi.org/10.1001/archinternmed.2009.65

Davis, R. (2000). Cultural health care or child abuse? The Southeast Asian practice of cao gio. *Journal of the Academy of Nurse Practitioners, 3*(2), 125–131. https://onlinelibrary.wiley.com/doi/epdf/10.1111/j.1745-7599.2000.tb00173.x

Dossey, B. M., Keegan, L., & Guzzetta, C. E. (2000). *Holistic nursing: A handbook for practice.* Aspen.

Fan, S. (2016). *Auricular acupuncture.* http://acupuncturewellnessfan.com/therapy/acupuncture-in-dc-va-md/auricular-acupuncture-in-dc-va-md

Fu, Q., Xie, H., Zhou, L., Li, X., Liu, Y., Liu, M., Wang, C., Wang, X., Wang, Z., Tang, J., Xiao, H., Xiao, Z., Zhou, J., Feng, C., Wang, L., Ao, Z., Chen, X., Su, C., Wu, X., Zhao, M., … Jiang, L. (2021). Traditional Chinese medicine auricular point acupressure for the relief of pain, fatigue, and gastrointestinal adverse reactions after the injection of novel coronavirus-19 vaccines: a structured summary of a study protocol for a multicentre, three-arm, single-blind, prospective randomized controlled trial. *Trials, 22*(1), 162. https://doi.org/10.1186/s13063-021-05138-3

Gach, M. R. (1990). *Acupressure's potent points: A guide to self-care for common ailments.* Random House. https://www.penguinrandomhouse.com/books/57326/acupressures-potent-points-by-michael-reed-gach/9780553349702/

Gach, M. R., & Henning, B. A. (2004). *Acupressure: A self-care guide for trauma, stress, and common emotional imbalances.* Bantam Books.

Garcia, G. T., Ribeiro, R. F., Faria Santos, I. B., Gomes, F. C., & de Melo-Neto, J. S. (2021). Electrical stimulation of PC 6 to control chemotherapy-induced nausea and vomiting in patients with cancer: A systematic review and meta-analysis. *Medical Acupuncture, 33*(1), 22–44. https://doi.org/10.1089/acu.2020.1431

Godley, E., & Smith, M. A. (2020). Efficacy of acupressure for chronic low back pain: A systematic review. *Complementary Therapies in Clinical Practice, 39,* 101146. https://doi.org/10.1016/j.ctcp.2020.101146

Han, J-S. (2003). Acupuncture: Neuropeptide release produced by electrical stimulation of different frequencies. *Trends in Neuroscience, 26*(1), 17–22. https://pubmed.ncbi.nlm.nih.gov/12495858/

He, Y., Guo, X., May, B. H., Zhang, A. L., Liu, Y., Lu, C., Mao, J. J., Xue, C. C., & Zhang, H. (2020). Clinical Evidence for Association of Acupuncture and Acupressure with Improved Cancer

Pain: A Systematic Review and Meta-Analysis. *JAMA Oncology, 6*(2), 271–278. https://doi
.org/10.1001/jamaoncol.2019.5233

Hofmeyer, A., Taylor, R., & Kennedy, K. (2020). Knowledge for nurses to better care for themselves so they can better care for others during the Covid-19 pandemic and beyond. *Nurse
Education Today, 94,* 104503. https://doi.org/10.1016/j.nedt.2020.104503

Hoo, J. J. (1997). Acupressure for hyperemesis gravidaum. *American Journal of Obstetrics and
Gynecology, 176*(6), 1395–1396. https://doi.org/10.1016/s0002-9378(97)70369

Hsieh, C. J., Su, W. J., Wu, S. C., Chiu, J. H., & Lin, L. C. (2019). Efficacy of acupressure to prevent adverse reactions to anti-tuberculosis drugs: Randomized controlled trials. *Journal of
Advanced Nursing, 75*(3), 640–651. https://doi.org/10.1111/jan.13881

Hu, R-F., Jiang, X-Y., Chen, J., Zeng, Z., Chen, X. Y., Li, Y., Huining, X., & Evans, D. J. W. (2015).
Non-pharmacological interventions for sleep promotion in the intensive care unit. *Cochrane
Database of Systematic Reviews, 2015*(10). https://doi.org/10.1002/14651858.CD008808.pub2

Huang, W., Pach, D., Napadow, V., Park, K., Long, X., Neumann, J., & Fleckenstein, J. (2012).
Characterizing acupuncture stimuli using brain imaging with fMRI—a systematic review
and meta-analysis of the literature. *Deutsche Zeitschrift für Akupunktur, 55*(3), 26–28. https://
doi.org/10.1016/j.dza.2012.08.008

Kaptchuck, T. (1983). *The web that has no weaver.* McGraw Hill.

Kawakita, K., & Okada, K. (2014). Acupuncture therapy: Mechanism of action, efficacy, and
safety: A potential intervention for psychogenic disorders? *Biopsychosocial Medicine, 8,* 4.
https://doi.org/10.1186/1751-0759-8-4

Lade, A. (1986). *Images and functions.* Eastland.

Lamke, D., Catlin, A., & Mason-Chadd, M. (2014). "Not just a theory": The relationship between Jin
Shin Jyutsu® self-care training for nurses and stress, physical health, emotional health, and caring efficacy. *Journal of Holistic Nursing, 32*(4), 278–289. https://doi.org/10.1177/0898010114531906

Li, L. W., Harris, R. E., Tsodikov, A., Struble, L., & Murphy, S. L. (2018). Self-acupressure for older
adults with symptomatic knee osteoarthritis: A randomized controlled trial. *Arthritis Care &
Research, 70*(2), 221–229. https://doi.org/10.1002/acr.23262

Liang, F., Chen, R., & Cooper, E. L. (2012). Neuroendocrine mechanisms of acupuncture. *Evidence-
Based Complementary & Alternative Medicine, 2012,* 1–2. https://doi.org/10.1155/2012/792793

Longhurst, J. C. (2010). Defining meridians: A modern basis of understanding. *Journal of
Acupuncture and Meridian Studies, 3*(2), 67–74. https://www.sciencedirect.com/science/article/
pii/S2005290110600143

Lund, I., & Lundeberg, T. (2016, December 15). *Mechanisms of acupuncture.* Science Direct
Elsevier, Research Gate. https://www.researchgate.net/publication/311505128_Mechanisms
_of_Acupuncture

MacPherson, H., Hammerschlag, R., Coeytaux, R. R., Davis, R. T., Harris, R. E., & Kong, J.-T.,
Wayne, P. M. (2016). Unanticipated insights into biomedicine from the study of acupuncture. *Journal of Alternative and Complementary Medicine, 22*(2), 101–107. https://doi.org/10.1089/
acm.2015.0184

Najafabad, M. V., Ghafari, S., Nazari, F., & Valliani, M. (2019). The effect of acupressure on the
quality of life among females with chronic back pain. *Applied Nursing Research, 51,* 151175.
https://doi.org/10.1016/j.apnr.2019.05.020.

National Center for Complementary and Integrative Health. (2021). *Acupuncture: In depth.* https://
nccih.nih.gov/health/acupuncture-in-depth

National Institutes of Health. (1997). Acupuncture. *NIH Consensus Statement Online, 15*(5), 1–34.
https://consensus.nih.gov/1997/1997Acupuncture107html.htm

Perkins, P., Parkinson, A., Parker, R., Blaken, A., & Akyea, R. K. (2020). Does acupressure help
reduce nausea and vomiting in palliative care patients? A double blind randomised controlled trial. *BMJ Supportive & Palliative Care.* Advance online publication. https://doi
.org/10.1136/bmjspcare-2020-002434

Raana, H. N., & Fan, X. N. (2020). The effect of acupressure on pain reduction during first
stage of labour: A systematic review and meta-analysis. *Complementary Therapies in Clinical
Practice, 39,* 101126. https://doi.org/10.1016/j.ctcp.2020.101126

Sankaranarayanan, K., Mondkar, J. A., Chauhan, M. M., Mascarenhas, B. M., Mainkar, A. R., & Salvi, R. Y. (2005). Oil massage in neonates: An open randomized controlled study of coconut versus mineral oil. *Indian Pediatrics, 42*(9), 877–884. https://www.indianpediatrics.net/sep2005/877.pdf

Schnorrenberger, C. C. (1996). Morphological foundations for acupuncture: An anatomical nomenclature of acupuncture structures. *Acupuncture in Medicine, 14*(2), 89–103.

Shames, K., & Keegan, L. (2000). Touch: Connecting with the healing power in 2000. In B. Dossey, L. Keegan, & C. E. Guzzetta (Eds.), *Holistic nursing: A handbook for practice* (3rd ed., pp. 613–635). Aspen.

Smith, C. A., Collins, C. T., Levett, K. M., Armour, M., Dahlen, H. G., Tan, A. L., & Mesgarpour B. (2020). Acupuncture or acupressure for pain management during labor. *Cochrane Database of Systematic Reviews, 2*(2). https://doi.org/10.1002/14651858.CD009232.pub2

Solt Kirca, A., & Kanza Gul, D. (2020). Effects of acupressure applied to P6 point on nausea and vomiting in pregnancy: A double blind randomized controlled. *Alternative Therapies in Health and Medicine,26*(6), 12–17.

Soylu, D., & Tekinsoy, K. P. (2021). The effect on gastrointestinal system functions, pain and anxiety of acupressure applied following laparoscopic cholecystectomy operation: A randomised, placebo- controlled study. *Complementary Therapies in Clinical Practice. May, 43,* 101304. https://doi.org/10.1016/j.ctcp.2021.101304

Struthers, R. (2008). The experience of being an Anishinabe man healer: Ancient healing in the modern world. *Journal of Cultural Diversity, 15*(2), 70–75. https://pubmed.ncbi.nlm.nih.gov/18649444/

Susana, C. T., Maria, T., Pilar, D. S., María, M., Pilar, M. S., Valentín, M. G., & Group EDIDO-CUH (2020). Effectiveness of self-applied acupressure for cervical pain of benign origin (EDIDO-CUH): A randomized controlled clinical trial. *Acupuncture in Medicine, 964528420961398.* https://doi.org/10.1177/0964528420961398

Takeshige, C. (1989). *Mechanism of acupuncture analgesia based on animal experiments: Scientific bases of acupuncture.* Springer-Verlag.

Unschuld, P. U. (1999). The past 1000 years of Chinese medicine. *Lancet, 354,* SIV9. https://doi.org/10.1016/s0140-6736(99)90352-5

Wu, B., Zhou, R. X., & Zhou, M. S. (1994). Effect of acupuncture on interleukin-2 level and NK cell immunoactivity of peripheral blood of malignant tumor patients [in Chinese]. *Zhongguo Zhong Xi Yi Jie He Za Zhi, 14*(9), 537–539. https://pubmed.ncbi.nlm.nih.gov/7866002/

Yang, J-M. (2006). *Chinese quigong massage* (2nd ed.). Jang's Martial Arts Academy (YMAA) Publication Center, Inc.

Youngmi, C., Joo, J-M, Kim, S., & Sok, S. (2021). Effects of meridian acupressure on stress, fatigue, anxiety, and self-efficacy of shiftwork nurses in South Korea. *International Journal of Environmental Research and Public Health, 18,* 4199. https://doi.org/10.3390/ijerph18084199

Reflexology

THÓRA JENNÝ GUNNARSDÓTTIR

Reflexology is a complementary therapy implemented for symptom management and to enhance patient well-being. In this practice, massage techniques are applied to specific areas of hands and feet that reflexology has identified to correspond to other parts of the entire body. Typically, the feet are easier to work with due to their larger surface area, which makes it simpler to find the required corresponding areas than when using the hands. Therefore, this chapter concerns feet reflexology. Holism, on which reflexology is based, has philosophical elements in common with nursing. This makes it a useful technique for nurses in assisting patients, plus there is evidence of its alleviation of some symptoms. Reflexology can be adopted as a key technique to give attentive care as it not only involves making the patient feel whole and better but also expresses the caregiver's compassion. More research into the effects of reflexology is required to bolster the scientific underpinning of this type of therapy.

DEFINITION

Reflexology is a specific pressure technique that works on precise reflex points of the feet that correspond to other body parts as depicted in Figure 26.1. Different definitions have been put forth, but they all convey the basic principle behind reflexology. In the practice of reflexology, it is believed that the extremities are connected to all other parts and internal organs of the human body, and there is a relationship between organs, systems, and processes. Therefore, by using specific pressure techniques on the foot or hand, it may be possible to affect the whole body. The left foot/hand represents the left side of the body and the right foot/hand represents the right side of the body. Different definitions have been set forth and Exhibit 26.1 shows some examples.

SCIENTIFIC BASIS

Reflexology dates back to ancient times, during which pressure therapies were known to both prevent and treat various ailments. Therapeutic foot massage is evident historically within a range of cultures globally. The oldest documented example of reflexology, dating from 2500 to 2330 BCE was uncovered in Egypt.

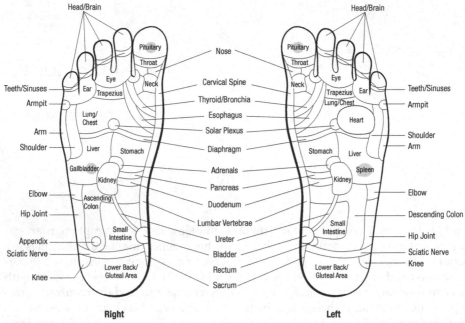

Figure 26.1 Relationship of body parts with reflexology points on the feet.

Exhibit 26.1 *Different Definitions of Reflexology*

- Reflexology is defined as a science concerning the principle that reflex areas in the feet and hands correspond to all the glands, organs, and parts of the body. Stimulating these reflexes properly can help many health problems in a natural way, a type of preventive maintenance (International Institute of Reflexology, 2021).
- Reflexology is a practice in which different amounts of pressure are applied to specific points on the feet or hands. These points are believed to match up with certain other parts of the body (National Center for Complementary and Integrative Health, 2020).
- Foot reflexology is the study and practice of working reflexes in the feet which correspond to other parts of the body. With specific hand and finger techniques, reflexology causes responses (relaxation) in corresponding parts of the body (Kunz & Kunz, 2003).
- Reflexology is a touch therapy based on the theory that different points on the feet, lower leg, hands, face, or ears correspond with different areas of the body (Association of Reflexologists, 2019).

Notably, generations of North American Native peoples have used reflex pressure on the feet to heal.

The reflexology literature comprises two main orthodoxies: traditional Chinese medicine (TCM) and the Western technique of *zone therapy*.

TRADITIONAL CHINESE MEDICINE

The notion that the body in its entirety can be denoted by its parts is ancient. In China, tongue diagnosis has been in use for at least 2,000 years. The iris of the eye, the face, and the ear are other parts of the body said to signify the whole (Maciocia, 2005). Reflexology also aligns with the concept of organ representation from TCM, whereby *the whole represents itself in the parts* (Kaptchuk, 2000). In other words, the feet can be seen as a miniature representation of the body, like a map onto which all body parts, such as glands and organs, are reflected.

TCM suggests that there are unseen energy meridians, or conduits, inside the body, that transport energy known as *qi*, which is the fundamental drive responsible for all processes. All organs are interconnected with one another by this meridian network system that connects all organs, so for a person to keep healthy, energy must flow in a balanced way. Elements that prevent qi from circulating properly are categorized as "excess" and "deficiency." *Excess* is when there is something that is "too much" for the individual to cope with—too much food to consume or too much waste to dispose of, for example. *Deficiency* is the lack of or comparative inadequacy of one or more of the life energies needed to foster well-being and health. If there is a deficiency or excess of life energy, this can cause outside factors to overpower the individual, thus causing pain and illness (Maciocia, 2005).

A healthy person with balance will have soft feet with a consistent texture across all areas. When an area is massaged that feels "empty" or without the same texture as other areas, this suggests a deficiency in the energy in the corresponding organ or body part. A stiff and hard area points to an energy excess. If one area is lacking in energy, another area must have excessive energy; energy must be in balance. Empty areas are treated with a gradual application of aggressive pressure to enhance the energy flow. Meanwhile, areas with too much energy are treated more vigorously, with light but steady pressure. This allows the energy to flow out and away from it, toward another area where there is a deficiency, fixing that inadequacy while also suppressing excess.

ZONE THERAPY

Zone therapy originated in the West at the start of the 20th century, when Dr. William Fitzgerald discovered that applying pressure to some parts of the feet created anesthesia in other body parts. He then found that the feet could be mapped, with the whole body and all its organs corresponding to particular areas on the soles of the feet. He separated the body, head to toe, into 10 longitudinal zones. According to Fitzgerald, parts of the body within a particular zone corresponded with one another; as such, it is called "zone" therapy.

The current form of reflexology was founded by the American therapist Eunice Ingham (1984). Using the zones as guidance, she charted the feet to identify areas to which pressure could be applied to create certain effects in the body. She devised a map of the whole body on the feet and labeled the areas *reflexes*. According to Ingham, when the bloodstream is made impassable by waste or excess acid, calcium deposits begin to take shape in the nerve endings. This then prevents the typical circulation of the blood and causes various body parts to have imbalances, related to the location of the blockage. She contended that reflexology can assist to detect the calcium deposits on the feet, what she called "gritty areas," which may hurt when touched. Ingham calls these "particles of frost" or "crystal blocks" that can be seen when examined using a microscope. Reflexology's massage and pressure techniques are intended to disperse these blockages and dissolve their crystalline structures. The area that corresponds with this nerve ending then gains more of the blood supply. Hence, stimulation of both the circulatory and lymphatic systems occurs, which promotes the discharge and elimination of toxins, and this leads to healing. There are other theories studied in this field; however, these are not included in this chapter.

DIFFERENT PERSPECTIVES

One of the key ideas in reflexology and acupuncture is the TCM energy channels. In both therapies, energy is directed throughout the body, via the meridians or the zones, with both practices claiming that illnesses are the result of energy channels being impeded. In acupuncture/acupressure, energy is aroused or repressed using needles or finger pressure. There are six meridians, which either start or finish in the feet, with the other ends beginning or ending in the fingers; hence, the meridians in the upper and lower areas of the body are linked.

Reflexology applied to the entire foot is also performed on the acupuncture points located there. This can assist to eradicate obstructions in the meridians. Another helpful approach is to proactively push, press, or massage these points to encourage energy in the meridians. This enhances energy movement along the meridians and in the organs to which they are linked. Overall, reflexology as a concept is founded mostly on energy and assessing how it moves within the body. Eunice Ingham's zone therapy is mainly applied in Europe and the United States.

The terms *reflexology, reflex zone therapy,* and *reflexotherapy* all refer to the modern use of the treatment, with distinctions between them being related to different scientific and philosophical views of experts in the field.

INTERVENTION

The patient should lie in a relaxed position, slightly higher than the reflexologist's seat. The patient may have a blanket covering them, and pillows under their knees and head to create comfort. Furthermore, the patient should be barefoot and in a relaxed state, with circulation not impeded by tight clothing. When in position, the patient is evaluated constantly to check their comfort with the degree of pressure being applied. The pressure should be enough to trigger the body's healing abilities, but the patient must also be able to cope with it. Each individual is different, so it is important to pay close attention. Over time, after more treatments, the feet will likely become more sensitive. During the treatment, each area on each foot receives attention; for example, the toe area on the first foot and then the toe area on the second. The treatment continues from one foot to the other until it is complete.

Reflexology emphasizes the treatment of the feet as a whole. However, a specific focus must be given to the body's key systems, for example, the digestive system to escalate appropriate elimination, the lymphatic system to encourage the disposal of waste, the bladder and kidneys to foster urine and energy flow (the kidneys are one origin of qi), the solar plexus (the storage point for feelings and emotions) to allow relaxation, all internal glands to trigger their particular functions, and the lungs to promote oxygen consumption. The reflexologist, by implementing reflexology, is simultaneously heightening circulation and elimination and impacting the flow of qi, as meridians link all organs with each other.

Further research is needed to determine the exact effect of the actions prescribed by reflexology, but it has definitely demonstrated significant physiological results. These may, in part, be due to the patient relaxing as a reaction to the therapeutic engagement and as a response to touch. Other aspects and practices including aromatherapy, calming music, and a tranquil setting can also enhance the use of reflexology. The International Institute of Reflexology asserts that its purpose is not to treat or diagnose any specific medical disorder but to promote better health and well-being (International Institute of Reflexology, 2021).

TECHNIQUES

Learning reflexology requires specific training, although its application is quite easy, and it can be applied in many circumstances. There are several techniques used, depending on what area of the feet is worked on. One hand is used to support the foot while the fingers and the thumb of the other are used to massage the skin. A period of 45 minutes to 1 hour is estimated to be enough time to perform reflexology on both feet and allows for extra time for work on specific areas that need further care. It is important not to forget any area and to finish one area before starting the next one. At the end of each session, the client is encouraged to relax for several minutes.

USING REFLEXOLOGY FOR SELF-CARE

Self-administered foot reflexology is easy to learn and apply and may well help improve perceived stress, fatigue, and depression (Song et al., 2015). Increasing personal wellness using reflexology for self-care can be done. Using specific grips with your fingers and hands on the feet you can give yourself reflexology. You can also use a foot roller, available at most health food stores, for a few minutes every day. It is good to have a map of reflexology points nearby and explore how the sole of the feet represents the whole body. When starting the massage, some points may be sore but applying pressure to them can release the tenderness. Hardly any harm can be done as long as you use a soft touch and pressure that is tolerable. By lying in a bed or sitting in a chair, it is possible to give reflexology to yourself, alternating the position of the feet.

Reflexology is given with the fingers and different techniques and grips can be used. Exhibit 26.2 presents some descriptions of the use of a grip technique, thumb-walking technique, and how to use a roller. It is good to prepare the feet before by doing some exercises or rotation by circling the feet in both directions.

PRECAUTIONS

Patients report that reflexology is largely a pleasant experience, that leaves them both calm and relaxed. However, many do not like to have their feet touched, so approval from the patient is needed before starting. Before starting reflexology, the condition of the feet must be examined for swelling, color, ulcerations, toe deformities, and odor. The physical condition of the person is also very important; hence, their health history should be reviewed. If there is a problem regarding the blood flow to the limbs because of diabetes, neurological diseases, or

---

Exhibit 26.2 *Self-Care Using Reflexology Techniques*

The Grip

The grip techniques are an extension of the natural ability to grasp; with them, you can vary the power grip to exert pressure to pinpoint an area or areas. The finger or thumb tip is the point of contact for the pressure. The single finger grip technique is used to pinpoint areas of the hand or foot. The tip of the finger is placed on the area to be worked, but the palm of the working hand rests on top of the hand being worked.

Thumb Walking

The goal of the thumb-walking technique is to apply constant, steady pressure to the surface of the foot or the hand:

1. With the other hand (holding hand) stretch the sole of the foot. Rest your working thumb on the sole and your fingers on the top of the foot. Drop your wrist to create leverage, which exerts pressure with the thumb.
2. Bend and unbend the thumb's first joint, moving it forward a little bit at a time. When your working hand feels stretched, reposition it and continue walking it forward. Take a little step forward with each unbend. The goal is to work with a small area in each step to create a feeling of constant, steady pressure. Always walk in a forward direction, not backward. Keep your thumb slightly cocked as you work to prevent overextending it.

Using a roller

1. Place the foot on the roller. Reposition the foot from inside to center to outside to roll the entire foot.
2. Place the heel of the opposite foot on the toe to be worked and roll. The heel provides leverage. Reposition the heel to work each toe.
3. Roll using a heel on top of the foot for increased pressure. Angle the foot from outside to center to inside to work the whole area.
4. Roll, angling the foot from outside to center to inside. Pressure may be increased by crossing the legs.
5. The heel is a tough area, and the roller will easily slip away. For these reasons, you may want to cross your legs while rolling this area to exert pressure and to control the roller.

Source: Adapted from Kunz B., & Kunz, K. (2003). *Reflexology: Health at your fingertips.* DK Publishing.

---

arteriosclerosis, the therapist must be careful about the pressure of the massage. Older adults may need special precautions because of concerns such as restricted movement, incontinence, arthritis, and aching joints. When dealing with such conditions, it may be better to consider the person's comfort and feel of the touch as the primary goals.

Some symptoms of adverse effects after undergoing a complementary therapy such as reflexology are often referred to as *healing crises*. Healing crises are said to happen frequently during and immediately following a treatment such as reflexology and are experienced as localized or distal pain, perspiration or shivering, and changes in the heart rate, respiration, or temperature. This phenomenon is also described as a cleansing process because the treatment is believed to activate the body's healing power, whereby accumulated waste products and toxins, which have often lain dormant in the body, are then released into the bloodstream. In one study on the effects of reflexology on fibromyalgia syndrome, the participants were specifically observed and asked about healing crises as part of the reflexology treatment (Gunnarsdottir & Jonsdottir, 2010). The participants, six women who were given 10 reflexology treatments, described several symptoms as a healing crisis: headaches, increased thirst, increased pain, increased urination, more frequent bowel movements, aggravated skin conditions, increased perspiration, fatigue, feverishness, dizziness, exhaustion, and increased energy. These symptoms appeared during the early stages and lasted for a day or two each time. Because of reports of such reactions, reflexologists may need to be very careful when performing reflexology on people who are seriously ill (e.g., cancer patients), as they may not tolerate healing crises. It is also important to explain to people what can be expected after a treatment.

There may also be problems with localizations of reflexology points. One researcher, a nurse, Jenny Jones, has looked specifically at the localization of the heart point and surveyed members of the Association of Reflexologists in the United Kingdom (Jones et al., 2012). The findings showed a lack of clarity and consistency regarding the indication of reflexology for cardiac patients, inconsistencies in reflexology teaching literature, and marked inconsistencies in the heart point placement.

USES OF REFLEXOLOGY

The publication of research on the effect of reflexology has been increasing over the last 10 years. Some conditions for which it has been recently used have been selected and are listed in Exhibit 26.3.

The methods used in the studies differ and are often not adequately explained. The length and frequency of sessions vary, and the principle behind reflexology states that it can affect the body as a whole. Also, it may be more difficult to have an effect on chronic symptoms. Topcu et al. (2020) did not find any clinical effects when adding reflexology to conventional treatment in asthma, and it did not have an affect on reducing blood pressure in patients with Stage 2 hypertension (Kotruchin et al., 2021). Subjective reports about receiving reflexology frequently describe relaxation, calm, and comfort as benefits, indicating that the experience is mostly positive (Dyer et al., 2013). Reflexology can be used in combination with other complementary therapies, such as massage and aromatherapy (Candy et al., 2020). In this chapter, self-care techniques using reflexology have been described. In a study of self-administered foot reflexology, Song et al. (2015) found that objective outcomes showed limited significance in statistical results, but subjective outcomes, such as perceived stress, fatigue, and depression, showed significant improvements. Numerous schools of reflexology have been established throughout the world. Interestingly, there seems to be growing interest in reflexology research in countries such as Malaysia, Thailand, Taiwan, India, Iran, and Turkey, as evident by a growing number of studies on reflexology from these countries, which will be interesting to follow up in the future.

Exhibit 26.3 *Uses of Reflexology*

- Reduce anxiety and pain during dressing change in burn patients (Davodabady et al., 2021)
- Effective in reducing crying duration and symptoms in infants with colic (Karatas & Dalgic, 2021)
- Improve sleep quality of adults with sleep disturbances (Huang et al., 2021)
- Decrease anxiety and depression in patients with cancer (Mantoudi et al., 2020).
- Improve constipation in patients with multiple sclerosis (Sajadi et al., 2020)
- Reduces pain and fatigue in patients after kidney transplant (Samarehfekri et al., 2020)
- Helpful in decreasing reported pain among women with advanced breast cancer (Sikorskii et al., 2020)
- Reduce pain and anxiety in children suffering from persistent or chronic pain (Bertrand et al., 2019)
- Reduce fatigue and pain and improve the quality of sleep in patients with lymphoma (Rambod et al., 2019)
- Some positive effects on anxiety among patients undergoing cardiovascular procedures (Chandrababu et al., 2019)
- Decrease fatigue and pain in patients with rheumatoid arthritis in a rheumatoid clinic (Metin & Ozdemir, 2016)
- Decrease menopausal period problems (Gozuyesil & Baser, 2016)
- Decrease pain in patients with fibromyalgia (Korhan et al., 2016)
- Improve sleep and fatigue in hemodialysis patients (Unal & Akpinar, 2016)
- Decrease fatigue in women with multiple sclerosis (Nazari et al., 2015)

CULTURAL APPLICATIONS

The roots of reflexology are embedded in ancient history, when pressure therapies were recognized as preventive and therapeutic. Evidence indicates that therapeutic foot massage has been practiced throughout history by a variety of cultures. The oldest documentation depicting the practice of reflexology was unearthed in Egypt and dated from around 2500 to 2330 BCE. The use of reflex pressure applied to the feet as a healing therapy has been practiced by the North American Native peoples for generations.

As discussed earlier in the chapter, there are different perspectives on the effects of reflexology in Eastern and Western cultures. Zone therapy, as developed by Eunice Ingham, is mostly practiced in Europe and the United States.

Numerous schools of reflexology have been established throughout the world. Interestingly, there seems to be much interest in the use and research of reflexology in countries such as Malaysia, Thailand, India, Iran, and Turkey, as evident by a growing number of studies on reflexology from these countries.

REFLEXOLOGY IN SCANDINAVIA

Reflexology is quite popular in Scandinavia, especially Norway, Sweden, and Denmark (Hansen et al., 2005). The greatest use is in Denmark, where it is one of the most frequently used complementary therapies and it is practiced in both private clinics and health communities. Reflexology in Denmark is further described in Sidebar 26.1.

Sidebar 26.1 *Reflexology in Denmark*

Leila Eriksen, **Denmark**

Reflexology has been a very popular complementary therapy in Denmark. It is practiced in both private clinics and in health communities. A number of private insurance companies support reflexology treatments. Danish reflexologists have 300 hours of education in, for example, anatomy and physiology besides theoretical and practical education. More than one in five people in Denmark have used reflexology. However, it is unknown why particular age groups seek reflexology and what specific issues they seek to address. A national survey was completed by 490 Danish reflexologists that included data from 2,368 clients. The data showed that a majority of reflexology clients request treatment for muscle pain (44%). Other problems include stomach pain/digestive problems, headache/migraine, fatigue, and hormonal problems. One in five clients (22%) chooses to have reflexology on their own initiative. In another survey (unpublished study, Leila Eriksen), it was shown that 26 of 58 (approximately 45%) Danish children with cancer have used reflexology.

FUTURE RESEARCH

What are the specific effects of reflexology, and how do these effects compare with other complementary therapies? How can these specific effects be captured in research? It is important to keep these questions in mind when researching reflexology. It is difficult to evaluate if one or two sessions can make much difference in symptoms, and therefore, it is important to measure the effect of reflexology over a number of sessions to gain insight into its overall benefits (Gunnarsdottir & Peden-Mc-Alpine, 2010). Also, if the design uses a sham method, it is important that said method does not enhance the same effect as reflexology. Practitioners need to be critical and acknowledge the value of research and inquiry in this process. It has been argued that more randomized controlled trials are needed using rigorous methodology, appropriate sample size, and adequate randomization (Wang et al., 2020).

In a summary article of the current practice of reflexology, it is argued that qualitative research may assist in understanding the impact of the context and process of reflexology intervention (Embong et al., 2015). The principle behind reflexology states that it can affect the body as a whole. However, it is not clear how these holistic changes come about. There is an urgent need to explore the experience of having reflexology to try to gain more information about what occurs during sessions and how the framework from which it is derived and delivered supports the intervention.

The scientific basis for reflexology is growing, and promising results of its use to alleviate some symptoms are beginning to emerge, but more rigorous research is needed if reflexology is to be used effectively by nurses in healthcare settings. Nurses are in a primary position to research reflexology because their holistic background is in tune with its philosophies.

WEBSITES

■ International Institute of Reflexology: www.reflexology-usa.net

This is the only school licensed to teach the Original Ingham Method. Reflexology has grown to international proportions under the able direction of Ingham's nephew, Dwight Byers, today's leading authority. The school also has branches around the world.

■ International Council of Reflexologists: www.icr-reflexology.org

Established in Toronto, it holds an international conference on reflexology every other year.

■ Association of Reflexologists in the United Kingdom: www.aor.org.uk

This is a good resource that includes a list of worldwide reflexology organizations, as well as interactive information on reflexology products and practice.

REFERENCES

Association of Reflexologists. (2019). *What is reflexology?* http://www.aor.org.uk/what-is
-reflexology/

Bertrand, A., Mauger-Vauglin, C., Martin, S., Goy, F., Delafosse, C., & Marec-Berard, P. (2019). Evaluation of efficacy and feasibility of foot reflexology in children experiencing chronic or persistent pain. *Bulletin du Cancer, 106*(12), 1073–1079. https://doi.org/10.1016/j.bulan.2019.05.008

Candy, B., Armstrong, M., Flemming, K., Kupeli, N., Stone, P., Vickerstaff, V., & Wilkinson, S. (2020). The effectiveness of aromatherapy, massage and reflexology in people with palliative care needs: A systematic review. *Palliative Medicine, 34*(2), 179–194. https://doi.org/10.1177/0269216319884198

Chandrababu, R., Rathinasamy, E. L., Suresh, C., & Ramesh, J. (2019). Effectiveness of reflexology on anxiety of patient undergoing cardiovascular interventional procedures: A systematic review and meta-analysis of randomized controlled trials. *Journal of Advanced Nursing, 75*, 43–53. https://doi.org/10.1111/jan.13822

Davodabady, F., Naseri-Salahshour, V., Sajadi, M., Mohtarami, A., & Rafiei, F. (2021). Randomized controlled trial of the foot reflexology on pain and anxiety severity during dressing change in burn patients. *BURNS, 47*, 215–221. https://doi.org/10.1016/j.burns.2020.06.035

Dyer, J., Thomas, K., Sandsund, C., & Shaw, C. (2013). Is reflexology as effective as aromatherapy massage for symptom relief in an adult outpatient oncology population? *Complementary Therapies in Clinical Practice, 19*, 139–146. https://doi.org/10.1016/j.ctcp.2013.03.002

Embong, N. H., Soh, Y. C., Ming, L. C., & Wong, T. W. (2015). Revisiting reflexology: Concept, evidence, current practice, and practitioner training. *Journal of Traditional and Complementary Medicine, 5*, 197–206. https://doi.org/10.1016/j.jtcme.2015.08.008

Gozuyesil, E., & Baser, M. (2016). The effect of foot reflexology applied to women aged between 40 and 60 on vasomotor complaints and quality of life. *Complementary Therapies in Clinical Practice, 24*, 78–85. https://doi.org/10.1016/j.ctcp.2016.05.011

Gunnarsdottir, T. J., & Jonsdottir H. (2010). Healing crisis in reflexology: Becoming worse before becoming better. *Complementary Therapies in Clinical Practice, 16*, 239–243. https://doi.org/10.1016/j.ctcp.2010.01.005

Gunnarsdottir, T. J., & Peden-McAlpine, C. (2010). Effects of reflexology on fibromyalgia symptoms: A multiple case study. *Complementary Therapies in Clinical Practice, 16*, 167–172. https://doi.org/10.1016/j.ctcp.2010.01.006

Hansen, B., Grimsgaard, S., Launsø, L., Fønnebø, V., Falkenberg, T., & Rasmussen, N. K. (2005). Use of complementary and alternative medicine in the Scandinavian countries. *Scandinavian Journal of Primary Health Care, 23*, 57–62. https://doi.org/10.1080/02813430510018419

Huang, H., Chen, K., Kuo, S., & Chen, I. (2021). Can foot reflexology be a complementary therapy for sleep disturbances? Evidence appraisal through a meta-analysis of randomized controlled trials. *Journal of Advanced Nursing, 77*, 1683–1697. https://doi.org/10.1111/jan.14699

Ingham, E. D. (1984). *Stories the feet can tell thru reflexology/Stories the feet have told thru reflexology*. Ingham Publishing.

International Institute of Reflexology. (2021). *Facts about reflexology*. http://www.reflexology-usa.net/facts.htm

Jones, J., Thomson, P., Lauder, W., & Leslie, S. J. (2012). Reported treatment strategies for reflexology in cardiac patients and inconsistencies in the location of the heart reflex point: An online survey. *Complementary Therapies in Clinical Practice, 18*, 145–150. https://doi.org/10.1016/j.ctcp.2012.04.001

Kaptchuk, T. J. (2000). *The web that has no weaver: Understanding Chinese medicine*. Contemporary Books.

Karatas, N., & Dalgic, A. I. (2021). Is foot reflexology effective in reducing colic symptoms in infants: A randomized placebo-controlled trial. *Complementary Therapies in Medicine, 59*, 102732. https://doi.org/10.1016/j.ctim.2021.102732

Korhan, E. A., Uyan, M., Eyigör, C., Yönt, G. H., & Khorshid, L. (2016). Effects of reflexology on pain in patients with fibromyalgia. *Holistic Nursing Practice, 30*(6), 351–359. https://doi.org/10.1097/HNP.0000000000000178

Kotruchin, P., Inoun, S., Mitsungnern, T., Aountrai, P., Domthaisong, M., & Kario. K. (2021). The effects of foot reflexology on blood pressure and heart rate: A randomized clinical trial in stage-2 hypertensive patients. *The Journal of Clinical Hypertension, 23*, 680–686. https://doi.org/10.1111/jch.14103

Kunz, K., & Kunz, B. (2003). *Reflexology: Health at your fingertips*. DK Publishing.

Maciocia, G. (2005). *The foundations of Chinese medicine* (2nd ed.). Elsevier.

Mantoudi, A., Parpa, E., Tsilika, E., Batistaki, C., Nikoloudi, M., Kouloulias, V., Kostopoulou, S., Galanos, A., & Mystakidou, K. (2020). Complementary therapies for patients with cancer: Reflexology and relaxation in integrative Palliative care. A randomized controlled comparative study. *Journal of Alternative and Complementary Medicine, 26*(9), 792–798. https://doi.org/10.1089/amc.2019.0402

Metin, Z. G., & Ozdemir, L. (2016). The effects of aromatherapy massage and reflexology on pain and fatigue in patients with rheumatoid arthritis: A randomized controlled trial. *Pain Management Nursing, 17*(2), 140–149. https://doi.org/10.1016/j.pmn.2016.01.004

National Center for Complementary and Integrative Health. (2020). *Reflexology*. http://nccam.nih.gov/health/reflexology

Nazari, F., Shahreza, M. S., Shaygannejad, V., & Valiani, M. (2015). Comparing the effects of reflexology and relaxation on fatigue in women with multiple sclerosis. *Iran Journal of Nursing and Midwifery Research, 20*(2), 200–204.

Rambod, M., Pasyar, N., & Shamsadini, M. (2019). The effect of foot reflexology on fatigue, pain, and sleep quality in lymphoma patients: A clinical trial. European *Journal of Oncology Nursing, 43*, 101678. https://doi.org/10.1016/j.ejon.2019.101678

Sajadi, M., Davodabady, F., Naseri-Salahshour, V., Harorani, M., & Ebranimi-monfared, M. (2020). The effect of foot reflexology on constipation and quality of life in patients with multiple sclerosis. A randomized controlled trial. *Complementary Therapies in Medicine, 48*, 102270. https://doi.org/10.1016/j.ctim.2019.102270

Samarehfekri, A., Dehghan, M., Arab, M., & Ebadzadeh, M. R. (2020). Effect of foot reflexology on pain, fatigue, and quality of sleep after kidney transplantation surgery: A parallel randomized controlled trial. *Evidence-based Complementary and Alternative Medicine, 2020*, 5095071. https://doi.org/10.1155/2020/5095071

Sikorskii, A., Niyogy, P. G., Victorson, D., Tamkus, D., & Wyatt, G. (2020). Symptom response analysis of a randomized controlled trial of reflexology for symptom management among women with advanced breast cancer. *Support Care Cancer, 28*(3), 1395–1404. https://doi .org/10.1007/s00520-019-04959-y

Song, H. J., Son, H., Seo, H., Lee, H., Choi, S. M., & Lee, S. (2015). Effect of self-administered foot reflexology for symptom management in healthy persons: A systematic review and meta-analysis. *Complementary Therapies in Medicine, 23*, 79–89. https://doi.org/10.1016/j .ctim.2014.11.005

Topcu, A., Løkke, A., Eriksen, L., Nielsen, L. P., & Dahl, R. (2020). Evaluation the effect on asthma quality of life of added reflexology or homeopathy to conventional asthma management – An investigator-blinded, randomised, controlled parallel group study. *European Clinical Respiratory Journal, 7*(1). https://doi.org/10.1080/20018525.2020.1793526

Unal, K. S., & Akpinar, R. B. (2016). The effect of foot reflexology and back massage on hemo-dialysis patients' fatigue and sleep quality. *Complementary Therapies in Clinical Practice, 24*, 139–144. https://doi.org/10.1016/j.ctcp.2016.06.004

Wang, W., Hung, H., Chen, Y., Chen, K., Yang, S., Chu, C., & Chan, Y. (2020). Effect of foot reflex-ology intervention on depression, anxiety and sleep quality in adults: A meta-analysis and meta-regression of randomized controlled trials. *Evidence-Based Complementary and Alternative Medicine, 2020*, 2654353. https://doi.org/10.1155/2020/2654353

VI

Practice, Education, and Research

AVIS JOHNSON-SMITH

In 2014, the National Institutes of Health (NIH) changed the name of its division that focuses on complementary therapies to the National Center for Complementary and Integrative Health (NCCIH). The name change aligns with the realization that complementary therapies are now becoming an integral part of Western health (NIH, 2014). Complementary therapies, which were once only viewed as conventional healthcare outliers, are now being seamlessly woven into the fabric of education (Chapter 27), practice (Chapter 28), and research (Chapter 29). Nurses have been instrumental in this seamless integration. Although great strides have been made, proponents of complementary and alternative therapies must remain vigilant in order to ensure that holistic healthcare is available to all people.

Public demand and emerging preferences for complementary therapies to treat illness and improve health and well-being continue to grow. Given the unique worldwide health challenges of the 21st century (including the COVID-19 pandemic), the interest in exploring the use of traditional and complementary medicine is burgeoning (World Health Organization, 2019). Whether these are well-known therapies, such as music and yoga, or ones that seem quite foreign to many, such as the Alexander technique and smudging ceremonies, health systems are looking very different from the way they were 25 or even 10 years ago. As research continues to substantiate the benefits of complementary therapies, the health professions integrate more content on these therapies into program curricula and healthcare systems continue to reflect more holistic care.

Concerns about the safety and efficacy of many of the complementary therapies continue. Funding for research on complementary therapies by the NCCIH has increased, thus providing a greater foundation for evidence-based practice.

Other NIH institutes are also funding research on complementary therapies. Not only is the increase in research important, but reviews and meta-analyses of studies on specific procedures also provide invaluable assistance to practitioners, educators, and researchers. New methods of inquiry and measurements for outcomes are needed for numerous therapies, particularly those practiced in non-Western and Indigenous cultures. With the emergence of new methods of inquiry and measurements for outcomes, healthcare workers will have increased opportunities to gain knowledge and expertise about the health practices of indigenous people.

Guidelines for using complementary treatments have been developed by professional organizations such as the American Holistic Nurses Association (n.d.) and the Oncology Nursing Society (2021) and address safety in the use of complementary therapies. In addition, many state boards of nursing have delineated guidance for the use of complementary therapies within nursing practice.

As noted in Chapter 27, professional nursing education organizations have specifications for content on complementary therapies that should be incorporated into the various curricula. If these are to be truly implemented, many more faculty members versed in complementary therapies are needed to teach nursing students, both at the basic and the graduate levels. Faculty are also at the forefront of conducting research on complementary therapies.

In not only the United States but also across the globe, greater attention is being given to the integration of complementary therapies into healthcare. As has been noted numerous times in this text, the mobility of individuals globally for travel or education, coupled with the mobility of immigrants and refugees globally is requiring that nurses and other health professionals become more conversant regarding the broad diversity in healthcare practices used around the world. Nurses, as caring, competent professionals, have an opportunity as well as a charge to be leaders in these efforts.

Parting words are found in Chapter 30. In this chapter, final remarks are made as trends across the therapies are observed and implications for the future of complementary therapies as an integral part of healthcare and self-care are reflected on. Words of caution are stated as therapies are often used without strong evidence or with only limited evidence. Examining available but credible information combined with honest and open communication among patients and providers is essential for the safe use of complementary therapies in healthcare or self-care. With the increasing availability of new and emerging information-gathering technologies and valid research related to complementary therapies and their delivery, nurses and nursing students are well equipped to obtain up-to-date information or deliver therapies at local, state, national, or global levels. We envision a bright future for the use of complementary therapies in integrative care models and the impact this will have on nursing education and practice, as well as patient outcomes and satisfaction. Future challenges to be mastered by the profession and exciting opportunities for leadership and change are outlined, as we share our dreams and visions for a preferred future that embraces and normalizes the utilization of sound evidence-based complementary therapies within the education, practice, and research arenas.

REFERENCES

American Holistic Nurses Association. (n.d.) *Resources to enhance practice*. https://www.ahna
.org/Resources

National Institutes of Health. (2014). *NIH complementary and integrative health agency gets new name*. U. S. Department of Health and Human Services. https://www.nih.gov/news-events/
news-releases/nih-complementary-integrative-health-agency-gets-new-name

Oncology Nursing Society. (2021). *Explore resources*. https://www.ons.org/explore-resources

World Health Organization. (2019). *WHO global report on traditional and complementary medicine 2019*. https://www.who.int/publications/i/item/978924151536

27

Integrating Complementary Therapies Into Nursing Education

CARIE A. BRAUN

Nursing curricula must constantly evolve to improve patient care quality and keep pace with the ever-changing healthcare environment. The impact of globalization and technological advancements and the increasing complexity of patient care have heightened the need to seamlessly integrate complementary and alternative therapies into holistic patient care (Boz et al., 2017; Solomon et al., 2016). This is primarily due to the proliferative use of complementary and alternative therapies by the public, safety issues with combining conventional and alternative modalities, cultural humility and the emphasis on patient-centered care, and increasing evidence of the positive impact of interprofessional collaboration and integrative healthcare systems on healthcare outcomes (Chandler, 2016; Rosenthal et al., 2019; Vega et al., 2020). Hritz et al. (2018) assert, however, that there is a notable gap between the prevalence of using complementary and alternative therapies by the public and integrating these therapies into education.

The National Academy of Medicine (NAM), formerly the Institute of Medicine, prepared a consensus report on *The Future of Nursing 2020–2030: Charting a Path to Achieve Health Equity* (National Academies of Sciences, Engineering and Medicine [NASEM], 2021). In this report, the NAM (2021) calls for nursing education to prepare students to address the determinants of health, promote health equity, and become advocates for the well-being of the population. The report (NASEM, 2021) calls for quality nursing education that prepares a diverse nursing workforce focused on the health and wellness of all people. In addition, *Healthy People 2030* (U.S. Department of Health and Human Services, 2020) guides nurse educators to assure future professional nurses promote health and wellness across the life span, including utilization of alternative and complementary therapies when appropriate. These influential initiatives have created a directive for nurse educators to respond to the needs of the population and to work to integrate alternative and complementary therapies into nursing education.

The licensure examination for nurses and other regulatory influences have also played an important role. The NCLEX-RN®, a reflection of entry-level nursing practice and one indicator of nursing program quality, has required basic knowledge of complementary therapies for entry-level registered nurses (RNs) since 2004 (Stratton et al., 2007). Today, the detailed test plans for the NCLEX-RN® continue to require the application of health promotion and maintenance, including the safe integration of complementary therapies into the patient's plan of care (National Council of State Boards of Nursing, 2019). For example, knowledge of herbal remedies and their interactions with other pharmacologic treatments continues to be a significant expectation for the NCLEX-RN®.

Complementary therapy education expectations are also evident in various boards of nursing (BONs) documents within the states and territories of the United States that regulate nursing practice to ensure patient safety. Of the 53 BONs surveyed in 2001, 47% had statements or positions that included specific complementary therapies or examples of these practices, 13% had them under discussion, and 40% had not formally addressed the topic but did not necessarily discourage these practices (Sparber, 2001). Although this survey has not been updated, the percentage of BON with formal position statements is likely on the rise. BONs are increasingly aware of and supportive of the integration of complementary therapies into nursing practice, and they are continuously clarifying what is within the scope of nursing practice and identifying basic education and competencies required for nursing practice. The American Holistic Nurses Association (AHNA) provides a resource for finding a state's position on holistic nursing practice at www .ahna.org/Resources. For example, the Minnesota Board of Nursing reaffirmed in 2017 a *Statement of Accountability for Utilization of Integrative Therapies in Nursing Practice*. An excerpt from this statement is as follows:

> Complementary and alternative practices and integrative therapies may address health needs by promoting comfort, healing and well-being, and may be adjunctive or primary interventions in nursing care. The Board believes the utilization of integrative therapies and alternative healthcare practices within the practice of nursing should be consistent with the consumer expectation for public safety, without undue regulation or restriction on the integrative therapies desired by consumers. (p. 1)

Internationally, similar nursing regulatory agencies have articulated the role of the RN and/or advanced practice nurse in understanding and practicing complementary therapies. For example, the Government of Western Australia's Community Midwifery Program (2015) has published a standard protocol for use of complementary therapies in midwifery practice. The guidelines indicate that "only midwives who have undertaken post-registration educational qualifications in specialized techniques and modalities of the recognized complementary and alternative medicine (CAM) should administer or advise pregnant women" (p. 1). Selecting and verifying the educational program in the specific complementary therapy are the responsibility of the midwife.

The inclusion of complementary and alternative therapies is also driven by the scope of practice and professional nursing standards. The American Nurses Association (ANA, 2021), in its *Nursing: Scope and Standards of Practice*, fourth edition, spells out the practice parameters and responsibilities for all professional RNs in the United States. This document indicates that nurses must be knowledgeable about and sensitive to a range of health practices in order to promote holistic nursing care (ANA, 2021). The practice standards of assessment, diagnosis, outcome identification, planning, implementation, and evaluation drive nursing education and allow for an individualized plan of care that is sensitive to diverse healthcare practices for all patients. The professional performance standards of quality of practice, practice evaluation, education, collegiality, collaboration, ethics, research, resource utilization, and leadership commit nurses constantly to improve knowledge, skills, and competencies appropriate to the nursing role (ANA, 2021).

The American Association of Colleges of Nursing (AACN) specifically identifies entry-level and advanced-level nursing education to focus on person-centered, holistic, and individualized care (AACN, 2021). Nurses must have a global perspective, demonstrate appropriate clinical judgment based on a broad knowledge base, focus their practice on healing and wellness, demonstrate cultural sensitivity, and integrate culturally relevant best practice interventions (AACN, 2021). Advanced-level nurses are called to lead systems change to promote optimal health and well-being to individuals, families, populations, and communities and to lead the translation of evidence, such as the evidence articulated throughout this text, into practice (AACN, 2021). All these entry-level and advanced-level expectations include integrating alternative and complementary therapies into nursing education. Likewise, the National League for Nursing (2017) published its *Vision for Expanding US Nursing Education for Global Health Engagement* to highlight the need for nurses to be knowledgeable about diverse cultural beliefs and practices.

The *ANA Scope and Standards* (ANA, 2021) and professional organizations recognize the need for holistic nursing practice but do not identify specific therapies that nurses may or may not incorporate into nursing practice. Specific therapies, which are within the realm of nursing, are included in the Nursing Interventions Classification (Butcher et al., 2018). This document identifies acupressure, animal-assisted therapy, aromatherapy, art therapy, biofeedback, massage, music therapy, self-hypnosis facilitation, and therapeutic touch as appropriate nursing interventions (Butcher et al., 2018). Although the knowledge base for many complementary therapies may be part of the educational program, performance proficiency is often not achieved during undergraduate or even graduate nursing education.

Nurses are increasingly aware of the need to holistically integrate complementary and alternative therapies to improve patient outcomes (Hall et al., 2017). Accordingly, the questions around nursing education and the integration of alternative and complementary therapies have shifted over time. In the 1990s, educators wondered whether complementary therapies *should* be taught in nursing. In the 2000s and early 2010s, the question focused on *what* should be included. Now, nurse educators, committed to the integration, are establishing *ways to deepen the integration* of complementary therapies within a holistic patient-care paradigm (Ben-Arye et al., 2017; Van Sant-Smith, 2015). The challenge for nurse educators today is to promote socially responsive and flexible nursing education while expanding the integration of complementary and alternative therapies, which has always had a fundamental role in quality nursing care (Salmon, 2010).

STUDENT AND FACULTY PERSPECTIVES

There is ample evidence to suggest that nursing education programs are inconsistently attending to the knowledge base needed and to the understanding of the role of complementary therapies in healthcare. For example, multiple studies have confirmed that nursing faculty and students believe that complementary therapies must be integrated into the nursing curriculum and that nurses must be prepared to advise patients regarding best practices in integrative health-care (Ae-Kyung, 2017; Geisler et al., 2015; Kessack, 2015; Kinchen & Loerzel, 2019; Poreddi et al., 2016). However, nursing students, upon graduation, do not feel pre-pared to integrate complementary therapies, rate their knowledge as "average," and are overwhelmed by the expectation that they provide these therapies (Avino, 2011; Nevins & Sherman, 2016). Although students report comfort in caring for patients who are using various complementary and alternative therapies, they are astutely aware that more education is needed (Balouchi et al., 2018; Kinchen & Loerzel, 2019; Nevins & Sherman, 2016; Poreddi et al., 2016; Topuz et al., 2015). This is similar to other studies of students and practicing nurses in Turkey, India, Croatia, Iran, and South Africa, which indicated they had varied personal knowl-edge, limited use, and lacked formal education but believed these therapies were effective and wanted to learn more (Camurdan & Gül, 2013; Kavurmaci et al., 2018; Pirincci et al., 2018; Poreddi et al., 2016; Racz et al., 2019; Van Rensburg et al., 2020; Zeighami & Soltani-Nejad, 2020).

Nursing faculty are also aware that integration is important, but this must be balanced with the risk of content overload in curricula. In the most recent sur-veys of nursing faculty in the United States, Burman (2003), Dutta et al. (2003), Fenton and Morris (2003), and Richardson (2003) determined the extent to which the schools integrated complementary and alternative modalities into their cur-ricula. For all four studies, a large percentage already included complementary therapies in the curriculum (49%–85%), and almost all the programs were plan-ning to incorporate additional complementary therapies in the future. Very few of the responding faculty had a separate required course on complementary therapies (11%–15%), whereas most faculty offered a separate elective course (37%–84%) and approximately one third offered a continuing education option. Therapies most often included in curricula were spirituality/prayer/meditation, relaxation, guided imagery, herbals, acupuncture, massage, and therapeutic touch. International studies also demonstrate high levels of faculty interest and intent with infusing complementary therapies into the curriculum. A decade ago, only 13% of nursing colleges in Saudi Arabia introduced complementary thera-pies briefly within a course. None of the respondents reported having a dedicated complementary therapies course, continuing education related to complementary therapies, or faculty interest/expertise in complementary therapies (Al-Rukban et al., 2012). Eight years later, access to formal courses in complementary and alter-native therapies grew to about 37% (Khan et al., 2020). In 2014 in Brazil, only about a third of public institutions offer courses related to complementary and alternative therapies, of which only a quarter were compulsory (Salles et al., 2014). However, in 2019, Azevedo and colleagues affirmed nurses and nurse educators are leading the implementation of complementary and alternative therapy education in Brazil.

COMPLEMENTARY THERAPY CORE COMPETENCIES

In response to the demand for greater integration of holistic nursing practices at the entry and advanced levels of nursing, the ANA and the AHNA have jointly developed the *Scope and Standards of Practice for Holistic Nursing* (ANA & AHNA,

2019), designed to "articulate the scope and standards of the specialty practice of holistic nursing and to inform holistic nurses, the nursing profession, and other healthcare providers and disciplines, employers, third-party payors, legislators, and the public about the unique scope of knowledge and the standards of practice and professional performance of the holistic nurse" (p. xi). The intent of the ANA/AHNA standards is to build upon the ANA Scope and Standards described previously to illustrate the specialty role of the holistic nurse. The document designates core values that include (a) holistic philosophy, theories, and ethics; (b) holistic nurse self-reflection, self-development, and self-care; (c) holistic caring process; (d) holistic communication, therapeutic relationship, healing environment, and cultural care; and (e) holistic *education* and research (ANA & AHNA, 2019). These core values are translated into competencies suitable for holistic nursing, which build on professional nurse education for the entry-level and advanced-level nurse. These competencies, which are elevated to achieve a higher level of holistic and integrated patient care outcomes, include health counseling, health literacy, therapeutic communication, cultural sensitivity, patient teaching/learning principles, motivational interviewing, and coaching. The ANA and AHNA (2019) noted that "because of the lack of intentional focus on integration, unity, and healing, the educational exposure of most nursing students is not adequate preparation for assuming the specialty role of a holistic nurse" (p. 43).

To fill this gap, the American Holistic Nurses Credentialing Corporation (AHNCC) published the *Foundations, Competencies, and Curricular Guidelines for Basic to Doctoral Holistic Nursing Education* (AHNCC, 2017). The guidelines provide the essential requirements for basic and advanced holistic nursing. At the basic level, holistic RNs must hold an associate or baccalaureate degree. Advanced-practice holistic nurses must hold a minimum of a master's degree. The educational foundations for the holistic nurse encompass several curricular threads. These threads include (a) scientific underpinnings of holistic nursing, (b) clinical scholarship and application of analytical methods, (c) ethics of holistic nursing practice, and (d) holistic nursing within and across delivery systems (AHNCC, 2017). In addition, essential requirements, including required skills, knowledge, attitudes, and behaviors of the basic and advanced holistic nurse, are articulated in the *Guidelines*, including competencies for the advanced holistic nurse related to holistic nursing prescriptive authority (AHNCC, 2017).

Education programs in nursing that desire to meet the essential requirements and commit to promoting the advancement of a holistic paradigm in nursing education can apply to the AHNCC for endorsement as a holistic nursing program (AHNCC, 2021). The AHNCC functions to approve academic entry-level and graduate nursing programs that meet their defined criteria and uphold curricula that meet the ANA and AHNA's (2019) *Scope and Standards of Practice for Holistic Nursing*. Endorsement of a program seeks to identify and recognize colleges and universities that produce transformational leaders with the skills, knowledge, attitudes, and behaviors to advance the holistic nursing agenda (AHNCC, 2021, para 1). In 2021, 16 programs were endorsed by AHNCC (see Websites at the end of this chapter for a link to endorsed programs).

Graduates of endorsed programs and others interested in becoming certified, who pass the NCLEX and obtain their RN license are eligible for certification in holistic nursing. Certification involves successfully passing the AHNCC

Holistic Nursing Certification examination (AHNCC, 2021). At present, AHNCC recognizes four levels of certification for holistic nurses: (a) the nonbaccalaureate, (b) baccalaureate, (c) advanced, and (d) advanced practice levels. Basic and advanced certification leads to a credential, such as Holistic Nurse Baccalaureate, Board Certified (HNB-BC), which indicates successful completion of the preparation and examination.

IMPLEMENTATION MODELS

INTEGRATIVE CURRICULA

In a systematic review, Balouchi and colleagues (2018) determined that nurses had about "average" knowledge of complementary and alternative therapies (62%), with close to two thirds reporting use of these therapies with patients, primarily for stress and anxiety. This gap between knowledge needed and knowledge achieved calls for greater integration of complementary and alternative therapies in nursing curricula. The 16 nursing programs endorsed by the AHNCC represent a series of robust ways in which nursing programs have fully integrated complementary and alternative therapies into the nursing curriculum. Each of these programs has implemented a model of holistic nursing practice that meets the standards and expectations of the AHA and AHNA. Examples of nursing programs that have achieved endorsement follow:

- Drexel University (https://drexel.edu/cnhp/academics/graduate/MS-Com plementary-Integrative-Health/) offers multiple programs leading to a credential in integrative health, including a Master of Science, and several certificate programs in advanced study related to integrative health.
- The University of Connecticut offers a three-course online graduate certificate in holistic nursing (https://holistic.nursing.uconn.edu/#). The program includes a basic course in holistic nursing, advanced course, and holistic nursing practicum.
- Pacific College of Health and Sciences offers a holistic nursing RN to BSN, MSN, and holistic nursing certificate program (www.pacificcollege.edu/nursing/). The MSN program has three tracks: Nurse Coach, Nurse Educator, and Professional Development Specialist.
- Metropolitan State University (St. Paul, MN), as per Dr. Karen Gutierrez, demonstrates a deep commitment to holistic nursing. Three of the four nursing programs are endorsed, including the RN-BSN, Minnesota Alliance for Nursing Education baccalaureate (MANE), and an entry-level MSN. Faculty are also currently seeking holistic nursing endorsement for the BSN and an entry-level MSN to DNP/Family Nurse Practitioner programs. Metropolitan State University's nursing programs incorporate holistic theories, concepts, and interventions to guide students in learning how to practice as a professional holistic nurse. Courses, such as Advanced Integrative Nursing Care, guide students around knowledge and use of complementary and alternative therapies in clinical practice and for self-care. Through evidence-based practice assignments, students evaluate complementary and alternative therapies and apply this knowledge to design lifestyle interventions that promote health and wellness. Students select one therapy, conduct a literature review focused on the therapy, and experience

the therapy culminating in a class presentation. Knowledge is also threaded into both medical–surgical courses, Holistic Nursing Care of the Adult I and Holistic Nursing Care of the Adult II. In these courses, students develop plans of care that integrate their knowledge of integrative therapies.

■ St. Catherine University, in Case Study 27.1, provides a deeper explanation of the integration of complementary and alternative therapies by this AHNCC-endorsed program.

The CAM Education Program, started in 2000, is now completed, but the impact continues. This project was designed to incorporate CAM information into the curricula of selected health profession schools (Pearson & Chesney, 2007) and has been influential in providing models for integrating complementary and alternative therapies into healthcare education (Nedrow et al., 2007b). The 75-plus-member Consortium for Academic Health Centers for Integrative Medicine (www .imconsortium.org) coordinates integrative health systems, including integrative education, research, policy, and patient care. The mission of the consortium is to advance integrative healthcare within academic institutions.

At least four programs in the CAM Education Project created integrative curricula in nursing. For example, the School of Nursing at the University of Minnesota and the Center for Spirituality and Healing (Minneapolis, MN)

Case Study 27.1 *Integration of Complementary and Alternative Therapies at St. Catherine University*

Joyce Perkins

At St. Catherine University College for Adults Bachelor of Science in Nursing program, faculty begin by ordering levels and kinds of information available to human beings conscious of a broad horizon of meaning embedded within a benevolent cosmic design. In other words, we embrace and bring order to the complexity of human endeavors, pandimensional consciousness, many ways of knowing, and numerous worldviews. Our conceptual framework of Unitary Human Caring Science (Perkins, 2021) melds the art, science, and spirit of nursing as one universal perspective that calls forth the highest good in relationships of all kinds. Based on an understanding of the energetic foundation of all creation (Merrick, 2010; Rogers, 1992), the paradigms of nursing (Newman et al. 1991, 2008), expanding human consciousness (Newman, 1994), caring science (Smith, 2020; Watson, 2018; Watson & Smith, 2002), complexity science (Zimmerman et al., 2008), plasma cosmology, and quantum physics, we are able to reveal a coherent, harmonious and synchronous unfolding of cosmic design. This choice of compassionate alignment with the order of the natural world brings forth a rich tapestry of healing potentials. The healing practices of indigenous peoples inform diverse multicultural perspectives on healing alongside Western medicine.

(continued)

Case Study 27.1 *Integration of Complementary and Alternative Therapies at St. Catherine University (continued)*

The healing potentials within this broad landscape of meaning are operationalized by the degree of certainty and agreement (Stacey matrix) around any course of action mutually decided on by patient and provider. The healing modality chosen for any circumstance depends on the consciousness of the patient and provider, as well as on the level of disturbance to be addressed. A physical, mental, emotional, and/or spiritual approach may be in order. Students learn through coming to know their own bodies, minds, and hearts by practicing some form of meditation or contemplative practice, reflection, and self-care consistently for 2 years throughout the program of study. They are introduced to various practices and perspectives through guest speakers and the direct experience of each modality. Students then integrate their learning directly with patients in clinical and lab situations.

References

Merrick, R. (2010). *Harmonically guided evolution*. http://interferencetheory.com/files/Harmonic_Evolution.pdf

Newman, M. A. (1994). *Health as expanding consciousness* (2nd ed.). National League for Nursing.

Newman, M. A., Sime, A., & Corcoran-Perry, S. (1991). The focus of the discipline of nursing. *Advances in Nursing Science, 14*(1), 1–6.

Newman, M., Smith, M., Pharris, M., & Jones, D. (2008). The focus of the discipline revisited. *Advances in Nursing Science, 31*(1), E16–E27. https://doi.org/10.1097/01.ANS.0000311533.65941.f1

Perkins J. B. (2021). Watson's caritas processes© with the lens of unitary human caring science. *Nursing Science Quarterly, 34*(2), 157–167. https://doi.org/10.1177/0894318420987176

Rogers, M. E. (1992). Nursing science and the space age. *Nursing Science Quarterly, 5*(1), 27–34. https://doi.org/10.1177/089431849200500108

Smith, M. (2020). Marlaine Smith's theory of unitary caring. In M. C. Smith & D. L. Gullett (Eds.), *Nursing theories and nursing practice* (5th ed.). F. A. Davis.

Watson, J. (2018). *Unitary caring science: Philosophy and praxis of nursing* (pp. 493–502). University Press of Colorado.

Watson, J., & Smith, M. C. (2002). Caring science and the science of unitary human beings: A trans-theoretical discourse for nursing knowledge development. *Journal of Advanced Nursing, 37*(5), 452–461. https://doi.org/10.1046/j.1365-2648.2002.02112.x

Zimmerman, B., Lindberg, C., & Plsek, P. (2008). *Chapter 1. In Primer in Edgeware: Lessons from complexity science for health care leaders* (2nd ed.). Plexus Institute.

revised curricula to incorporate complementary and alternative therapies into baccalaureate, master's, doctoral, and continuing education programs (Halcón et al., 2001). The curricular revisions strengthened didactic and experiential learning to encompass complementary therapies theory and research, supported interdisciplinary courses as part of the graduate minor in complementary therapies and healing practices, and incorporated self-care concepts. These programs have continued and expanded (www.csh.umn.edu/education/focus-areas/integrative-nursing). The University of Minnesota offers an Integrative Health and Healing specialty within the Doctor of Nursing Practice (DNP) program to prepare students to develop integrated approaches to health and wellness (www.nursing.umn.edu/doctor-nursing-practice-program/specialty-areas/integrative-health-and-healing).

Faculty and practitioners have also created interdisciplinary integrative curricula around specialty patient populations. Zick and colleagues (2018) reported on an integrative scholars program to facilitate collaborative education for 100 integrative oncology leaders while forming partnerships with complementary and alternative therapy practitioners. The program is well underway. Karim and colleagues (2021) further describe three in-person sessions at the University of Michigan and the completion of several eLearning modules on "cancer-related symptoms where integrative oncology therapies may have a role (i.e., fatigue, sleep, sexual health, pain, mood disorders), description and evidence for a variety of integrative medicine modalities (diet, exercise, mind–body therapies, and natural health products), and communication skills for discussing integrative therapies with patients and complementary providers" (p. 854).

Nursing programs throughout the world are implementing integrative educational models to build the complementary therapy knowledge base of generalist nurses. Helms (2006) proposed a sustainable model in which every course included complementary therapy content, with course objectives reflective of complementary and alternative therapy integration in patient care. For example, healthcare system or policy courses included the history of and philosophical basis for complementary and alternative therapies and health systems. Health assessment courses included history taking inclusive of complementary and alternative therapies. Pharmacology courses were a logical placement for herbal medicines, essential oils, and homeopathic preparations. Nutrition courses added dietary/biologically based therapies. Psychiatric nursing courses emphasized cognitive behavioral therapy or meditation. And nursing research courses included all aspects of complementary therapy efficacy through the lens of evidence-based practice. In addition, the use of simulation, which emphasizes integrative healthcare is an expected addition to nursing curricula.

MAJOR AND MINOR FIELDS OF STUDY

Following the lead of the CAM Education Project, colleges and universities throughout the United States are offering major or minor studies in integrative health, nursing, medicine, and other disciplines from the bachelor's degree to the doctorate. In 2016, Tollefson and colleagues reported on the characteristics of students who enroll in the Metropolitan State University of Denver in Colorado, the first university to offer a Bachelor of Science in integrative healthcare in the United States (Tollefson et al., 2016). "With a foundation in the basic sciences, including general biology, chemistry, anatomy and physiology, and pathophysiology, the student progresses into the core curriculum, composed of complementary and alternative medicine, holistic health, healthcare ethics, stress and sleep, and healthcare research methods. The students learn about various complementary medicine modalities and gain a holistic approach to the lifespan through their coursework" (Tollefson et al., 2016, p. 167). The University of Arizona also provides a Bachelor of Science program in integrative health, which provides a foundation for integrative health and focuses on the mind, body, and spirit (https://nursingandhealth.asu.edu/

integrative-health). Multiple examples of integrative health majors or minors are available to students interested in complementary and alternative therapies.

COURSES IN COMPLEMENTARY THERAPIES

Another potential approach for learning about complementary and alternative therapies is through specific courses. Calado and colleagues (2019) described a 36-hour university graduate course in complementary and alternative therapies in Brazil. The course included theory, active and reflective learning methodologies, seminars, and completion of practical experiences in auriculoacupuncture/auriculotherapy and Reiki. Groft and Kalischuk (2005) described a 13-week, 3-hour-per-session undergraduate elective course on health and healing. Students explored a range of complementary and alternative therapies commonly used by patients. The course was determined to be highly effective in aiding students' understanding of healing and wholeness. Van der Reit et al. (2011) implemented and evaluated an elective course for undergraduate students that included a study tour to Thailand, where students learned the techniques of Thai massage and other complementary therapies. The course was positively evaluated and improved global health awareness. Countless courses are offered throughout the United States and beyond to facilitate learning about complementary therapies from general principles to specialized knowledge about specific therapies.

CONTINUING EDUCATION OFFERINGS

Practicing nurses also have multiple opportunities to expand their knowledge of complementary therapies through continuing education opportunities. The AHNA, through its Education Provider Committee, is responsible for developing continuing nurse education (CNE) activities and has reportedly increased these offerings over time (Roberts, 2019). Examples of activities include education within its publications, monthly educational webinars, national and regional conferences, a Foundation of Holistic Nursing self-study course, and the Integrative Healing Arts Program in Holistic Nursing (IHAP), offered as a certification preparatory course (Roberts, 2019). In addition, AHNA has endorsed several continuing-education modules and certification programs that promote holistic nursing practice.

The National Center for Complementary and Integrative Health (NCCIH, 2021), with its mission to "determine, through rigorous scientific investigation, the fundamental science, usefulness, and safety of complementary and integrative health approaches and their roles in improving health and health care" (para. 20), has been instrumental in facilitating education about complementary and alternative therapies among practicing professionals. Among the nine major divisions of the Center, the Office of Communications and Public Liaison manages activities pertaining to implementing integrative healthcare education and outreach initiatives. The NCCIH hosts a wealth of educational resources, including its free online continuing education series (see Websites at the end of this chapter).

EXPERIENTIAL LEARNING

Active learning, whether in the clinical setting, simulation laboratory, or a study abroad immersion, is recommended for any students interested in complementary therapies. Bell (2017) described a pediatric clinical experience for senior nursing students where students used therapeutic touch with patients with significant disabilities. Bell (2017) is certified as a holistic nurse and guided students using therapeutic touch with positive results. Chan and Schaffrath (2017) conducted a study of nursing students, who provided foot reflexology, lavender aromatherapy, and mindful breathing, in various settings (home, lab, and clinical) and found that learning modalities are best supported through self-reflection, building presence, and role-modeling by a nurse faculty member with expertise in delivering these modalities. Johnson (2014) studied the use of aromatherapy that, when used by nursing students, was shown to decrease test anxiety.

In 2005, Chlan et al. (2005) studied the influence of skills laboratory practice on nursing student confidence levels in performing select complementary therapy skills. Student confidence in the performance of the five therapies (hand massage, imagery, music interventions, reflexology, breathing/mindfulness) increased after the session. The greatest increases in confidence were seen with hand massage, reflexology, and imagery. This study demonstrated the immense value of bringing the practical application of CAM into undergraduate nursing education. Similarly, Adler (2009) and Cook and Robinson (2006) implemented an intensive massage therapy experience to promote nursing student competence. Most student participants indicated that the experience was valuable in their development as nurses by contributing to the nurse–patient relationship and holistic patient care.

Clinical experiences have also been described that allow students to participate through assessment and observation of the application of Reiki (Bremner et al., 2014). Conroy and Taggart (2016) noted in a study-abroad cultural immersion program in China that students demonstrated a greater appreciation for culture, including the complementary and alternative therapies used. Participants reflected on their experiences and noted a greater likelihood of supporting holistic nursing care for all (Conroy & Taggart, 2016).

INTERNATIONAL EXEMPLARS

Sok et al. (2004) reported that more than 10 universities in the United Kingdom offered students full-time degree programs in complementary and alternative therapies, such as osteopathy, chiropractic medicine, herbal medicines, acupuncture, and homeopathy. Hon et al. (2006) reported that the regulatory body for nursing in Hong Kong now requires the nursing curriculum to contain 20 hours devoted to traditional Chinese medicine (TCM). Similarly, Yeh and Chung (2007) investigated the current and expected levels of competence in TCM that baccalaureate nurses should possess in Taiwan. In Korea, one college of nursing science now has a 1-year program that leads to a certificate in complementary and alternative therapies for clinical nurses and researchers (Sok et al., 2004). The Improving the Nursing Care with Best Complementary Therapy Strategies Based on European Union Standards (BestCARE) project was conducted in collaboration with nurses in Turkey and Europe to provide education via online learning and in a simulation laboratory to promote knowledge and skills around complementary therapies used in women's health and oncology (Ozer et al., 2019). The project results in greater integration of complementary therapies, including the development of a university course, a simulation module, training videos, and dissemination materials (Ozer et al., 2019). Toygar and colleagues (2020) also determined a 14-week course in complementary and alternative therapies promoted positive attitudes among nursing students in Turkey.

Karin Gerber, a nurse educator from South Africa, details the inclusion of complementary therapies within the curriculum at Nelson Mandela Metropolitan University (NMMU). Content from an interview is found in Sidebar 27.1.

Sidebar 27.1 *Integration of Traditional Healers With Nursing Education in South Africa*

Karin Gerber

Throughout the world, nurse educators are responding to the need to integrate complementary and traditional healing into nursing curricula, including South Africa, the "Rainbow Nation," where health practices are as diverse as the people. In an interview with two nurse educators from Nelson Mandela Metropolitan University (NMMU), located in Port Elizabeth, South Africa, it was affirmed that traditional African healing practices are presented to the nursing students alongside Western modalities. The nurse educators teach students to be open to various methods of healing but to always seek best practices in their nursing care. The nursing program is science-oriented but inclusive of a broad view of therapies based on patient and family preferences. Of particular note is the collaboration of nursing education with traditional healers within the Nguni and Xhosa societies of South Africa: the diviner (*sangoma* or *amagqirha*) and the herbalist (*inyanga* or *ixwele*).

The diviners and herbalists are highly respected and serve approximately 60% of the people of South Africa. Traditional healers in South Africa greatly outnumber Western-medicine doctors at a rate of 8:1 (Truter, 2007). The distinction between the two types of healers is often blurred; however, in general, the herbalist is concerned with medicines made from plants and animals, and the diviner is a spiritualist, using divination for healing purposes. Herbalists make use of more than 3,000 botanical, zoological, and mineral products to bring healing (van Wyk et al., 1999). These products are used as a bathwater or steaming preparation, ingested (often with a goal to induce vomiting), or inserted as an enema; are placed into incisions in the skin; or inhaled nasally (van Wyk et al., 1999). The diviner, through ancestral channeling, prayer, purification, throwing of the bones, use of incense, dream interpretation, or animal sacrifice with a goal of appeasing the spirits, seeks to establish a positive relationship and restitution between the ill person and the spirits causing the illness (Campbell, 1998). The Traditional Health Practitioners Act of 2007 (Republic of South Africa, Government Gazette, 2008) legally recognizes diviners, herbalists, traditional surgeons, and traditional birth attendants as traditional health practitioners. Western-medicine providers continue to study the efficacy of the herbal remedies used, including those for HIV/AIDS, pneumonia, and diarrhea, all major causes of death in South Africa.

(continued)

Sidebar 27.1 *Integration of Traditional Healers With Nursing Education in South Africa (continued)*

Clearly, public acceptance and use of traditional healers have a major influence on the integration of course content at NMMU. The nurse educators noted that each of the nursing courses has relevant content related to traditional healing, and students often talk about their own personal experiences with the healing modalities. Students are made aware of the risks of the various healing practices because some are known to be toxic, particularly to the kidneys, causing patients to require dialysis. Students are taught how to work together with traditional healers in situations in which traditional healing and Western medicine are complementary, such as in the induction of labor. Nurse educators also work with students in the communities to promote optimal health in areas where ritualistic cutting in initiations or as part of traditional healing has led to high rates of infection and mortality. Overall, there is a conscientious effort to help students understand what is helpful and what can be harmful and how to intervene to promote optimal patient care.

References

Campbell, S. (1998). *Called to heal.* Lotus Press.

Republic of South Africa, Government Gazette. (2008, January 10). *Traditional Healers Act of 2007 (511 No. 42).* http://www.info.gov.za/view/DownloadFileAction?id=77788

Truter, I. (2007). African traditional healers: Cultural and religious beliefs intertwined in a holistic way. *South Africa Pharmaceutical Journal, 74,* 56–60.

van Wyk, B., van Oudtshoorn, B., & Gericke, N. (1999). *Medicinal plants of South Africa.* Briza.

FACILITATING AND EVALUATING STUDENT LEARNING

Increasingly, nursing programs are integrating complementary therapies into nursing education, beginning with the development of appropriate learner outcomes, activities, and evaluation strategies. Multiple authors have suggested specific content applicable to the undergraduate and graduate nursing curriculum that align with nursing's scope and standards (Booth & Kaylor, 2018; Gaster et al., 2007; Kreitzer et al., 2008; Lee et al., 2007). The following is a compilation of suggested student learner outcomes that address the necessary dimensions for generalist nursing practice:

- Describe the prevalence and patterns of complementary therapy use by the public.
- Compare and contrast the underlying principles and beliefs in Western belief systems and alternative health belief systems.
- Communicate effectively with patients and families about complementary and alternative therapies.
- Critique the scientific evidence available for the most used complementary and alternative therapies.
- Identify reputable sources of information to support continued learning about complementary and alternative therapies.

- Explore the roles, training, and credentialing of complementary and alternative therapy practitioners.
- Reflect on and improve self-care measures and wellness to incorporate complementary therapies for self, where applicable.

In addition, fully integrated curricula should include learner outcomes written at the depth necessary for holistic nursing practice. For example, Pacific College of Health and Science, one of the AHNCC-endorsed programs, indicates these outcomes for its RN to BSN program:

- Empower patients/clients/families by teaching whole person healing and self-care practices for a healthier lifestyle.
- Assist individuals and families to manage stress, make healthy changes, and prevent disease by improving health and well-being.
- Guide individuals and families between the conventional allopathic medical system and complementary/alternative/integrative therapies and systems.
- Incorporate holistic integrative CAM modalities with other nursing interventions.
- Work on integrated health teams.
- Practice in numerous settings.
- Integrate reflection and self-care into personal and professional life.

Active and creative pedagogies are needed to facilitate student learning and support effective teaching of complementary therapies. Swanson et al. (2012) reported that online case-based modules were an effective method of teaching graduate nursing students about the clinical issues surrounding complementary and alternative therapies. According to Lee et al. (2007), CAM Education Project schools used a variety of instructional delivery strategies to help students learn about complementary therapies, including classroom-based programs, online modules, and experiential learning. These authors also recognized that personal reflection and self-care are critical components of student learning. At the course level, traditional student learning evaluation methods, such as written papers, examinations, and other projects, were used along with explorative methods, such as through interviews, focus groups, and 1-minute feedback papers, to gain course evaluation information for course improvement (Stratton et al., 2007). Sutch (2017) encourages educators to integrate complementary and alternative therapies regularly into the class to facilitate learning about these therapies. For example, hosting alternative therapy practitioners to speak to students, using a diffuser, practicing mindfulness in class, or facilitating animal-assisted therapy during finals week (Sutch, 2017). Matthias-Anderson and Reid (2019) from Metropolitan State University (Minneapolis, MN), one of the AHNCC-endorsedschools, describe an interactive role-play simulation to teach assessment to nursing students.

FACULTY QUALIFICATIONS AND DEVELOPMENT

Kessack (2015) determined experts in complementary and alternative therapies should teach content in the didactic prelicensure nursing classroom. Although the majority of nursing programs in the United States and throughout the world integrate complementary therapies in some way, the greatest challenges have included finding qualified faculty, making space in an already crowded curriculum, a lack of definition for "best practices" in integrative care, and sustainability of complementary therapy content within the curriculum (Homberg & Stock-Schröer, 2021). In one study, the top three therapies for which additional training was desired by faculty included nutritional supplements, herbal medicine, and massage (Avino, 2011). However, Khan and colleagues (2020) noted students "acquired more information about CAM from media (55%), books (56%), friends/relatives (59.7%), and other health professionals (58.4%), however, very little information from formal CAM courses or training (36.7%)" (p. 1).

Stratton et al. (2007) identified essential faculty development needed to facilitate learning in integrative healthcare. First and foremost, a critical mass of knowledgeable faculty is essential to the successful integration and sustainability of complementary therapies into a nursing curriculum. Viewing complementary therapy information through the lens of evidence-based practice can facilitate acceptance and provide an opportunity for faculty to become more familiar with complementary therapy principles and research (Stratton et al., 2007). Faculty development requires time and resources, access to scholarly writings, reference and research resources, reassigned time, consultations, collaboration, continuing education, and support. Ideally, continuing-education workshops or conferences should be structured using a collaborative approach representing the varying perspectives of complementary and alternative therapy practitioners. Encouraging and supporting faculty research in complementary therapies is another mechanism of generating a team of qualified faculty.

The University of Washington School of Nursing (Seattle), in partnership with Bastyr University (Kenmore, WA; San Diego, CA), provided faculty development on complementary therapies through a summer educational program (Booth-LaForce et al., 2010; Fenton & Morris, 2003; Nedrow et al., 2007a). Faculty used what they learned to support the integration of complementary therapies throughout the nursing curriculum. As a result of this implementation project, about half of the faculty incorporated complementary therapy content in class, and more than half indicated that their complementary therapy knowledge increased by a moderate or great extent. A higher number of students (70%) indicated that their knowledge of complementary therapies improved, with intended self-reported competencies increased throughout the grant period.

CONCLUSION

Linderman (2000) predicted that the future of nursing education would include "greater diversity in clinical experiences to provide contact with people from different cultures, ethnic groups, economic levels, and with alternatives to [W]estern medicine" (p. 11). This certainly has been the case. In their 2016 national convention resolutions, the National Student Nurses Association called for nursing schools to implement holistic nursing components into the curricula, noting that "it is important that the nursing schools are integrating the philosophy of holism into their curricula because it prepares nurses to provide holistic patient care, enhances the nurse–patient relationship which improves patient outcomes, and enables nurses to better understand the relationships between mind and body and the effects they have on a person's entire life" (National Student Nurses Association, 2016, p. 87). Nursing education bears a significant responsibility in the movement toward integrative health. Koithan (2015) describes what this looks like:

> In adopting this principle, our care becomes individualized, tailored, and meaningful. We do not recommend therapies, whether biomedical, mind–body, or manipulative, that a person cannot afford or access. We do not ask the impossible of our clients or their families. We consider the full ramifications of our interventions on the ecological (environmental) and social (communities and organizations) systems within which we exist. As such, our practice becomes sustainable and moral, one that is mindful and respectful of the complexities of life. We listen more and talk less, recognizing that personal wisdom may be just as important as professional knowledge as together we identify and strengthen resources (biopsychosocial–spiritual) that restore and replenish and ultimately support the emergence of health and well-being. (p. 194)

In 2019, there were almost 150,000 graduates of baccalaureate nursing programs in the United States, with approximately 50,000 additional graduates of master's and doctoral programs in nursing (AACN, 2020). That is a formidable influence on the potential integration of complementary and alternative therapies in the nursing workforce. Homberg and Stock-Schröer (2021) argued that knowledge of complementary and alternative therapies, developed through interprofessional education, was essential for holistic patient-centered care and was the best approach for preparing future students. The same researchers noted the challenges of such an endeavor, including uncritical teaching, content overload, and a lack of receptiveness by students (Homberg & Stock-Schröer, 2021). Despite these challenges, Hart (2019) acknowledged "holistic nurses will play a vital role in increasing understanding of holistic principles, practices, healing environments, and integrative therapies" (p. 54).

With care paradigms shifting away from diseases to health and healing that integrates holistic health practices, nurse educators must thoughtfully reflect curricula, adherence to the scope and standards of practice for nurses, and educational and healthcare influences as we continue to move forward. In addition, teaching clinicians how to conduct disciplinary and interdisciplinary research on complementary and alternative therapies and increasing the capacity to research in this way is another avenue of education worthy of development (Bradley et al., 2019; Dicianno et al., 2016).

Despite constant change, however, integrative health is fundamentally connected to the past, present, and future of nursing education, research, and practice (Salmon, 2010). Koithan (2015) recognized that the integration of complementary therapies in nursing education requires little or no shift in philosophical paradigm because issues such as wellness, prevention, and holistic health have long been at the core of nursing practice. It is through this foundation that nursing education continues to evolve in the depth and intensity with which it demonstrates this fundamental connection.

WEBSITES

There is an abundance of reputable resources to facilitate effective teaching and student learning in complementary and alternative therapies. A beginning list follows:

- American Holistic Nurses Association-Educational Resources (www.ahna.org/Resources)
- American Holistic Nurses Credentialing Corporation (AHNCC) endorsed nursing programs (www.ahncc.org/school-endorsement-program/current-endorsed-nursing-programs/)
- Center Institute for Research and Education in Integrative Medicine (www.healthandhealingny.org/professionals/nurse.asp)
- CINAHL: Cumulative Index to Nursing & Allied Health Literature (www.ebsco.com/products/research-databases/cinahl-plus-full-text)
- Consortium for Academic Health Centers for Integrative Medicine (www.imconsortium.org)
- National Center for Complementary and Integrative Health-Online Continuing Education Series (https://nccih.nih.gov/training/videolectures)

REFERENCES

Adler, P. (2009). Teaching massage to nursing students of geriatrics through active learning. *Journal of Holistic Nursing, 27*, 51–56. https://doi.org/10.1177/0898010108329132

Ae-Kyung, K. (2017). Acceptance of complementary and alternative therapy among nurses: A Q-methodological study. *Korean Journal of Adult Nursing, 29*, 441–449. https://doi.org/10.7475/kjan.2017.29.4.441

Al-Rukban, M., AlBedah, A., Khalil, M., El-Olemy, A., Khalil, A., & Alrasheid, M. (2012). Status of complementary and alternative medicine in the curricula of health colleges in Saudi Arabia. *Complementary Therapies in Medicine, 20*, 334–339. https://doi.org/10.1016/j.ctim.2012.05.006

American Association of Colleges of Nursing. (2020). *2019–2020 enrollment and graduations in baccalaureate and graduate programs in nursing.* https://www.aacnnursing.org/Store/product-info/productcd/IDSR_20ENROLLBACC.

American Association of Colleges of Nursing. (2021). *The essentials: Professional core competencies for professional nursing education.* https://www.aacnnursing.org/Portals/42/AcademicNursing/pdf/Essentials-2021.pdf

American Holistic Nurses Credentialing Corporation. (2017). *Foundations, competencies, and curricular guidelines for basic to doctoral holistic nursing education* (1st ed.). https://www.ahncc.org/wp-content/uploads/2018/10/Foundations-Competencies-Curricular-Guidelines.pdf

American Holistic Nurses Credentialing Corporation. (2021). *Certification…the path to personal growth and professional recognition.* https://www.ahncc.org/

American Nurses Association. (2021). *Nursing: Scope and standards of practice* (4th ed.). American Nurses Association.

American Nurses Association and American Holistic Nurses Association. (2019). *Holistic nursing: Scope and standards of practice* (3rd ed.).

Avino, K. (2011). Knowledge, attitudes, and practices of nursing faculty and students related to complementary and alternative medicine. *Holistic Nursing Practice, 25*, 280–288. https://doi.org/10.1097/HNP.0b013e318232c5aa

Azevedo, C., deCastro Moura, C., Pinheiro Correa, H., Ferreira de Mata, L., Lopes Chaves, E., & Machado Chianca, T. (2019). Complementary and integrative therapies in the scope of nursing: Legal aspects and academic-assistance panorama. *Esc Anna Nery, 23*, 9. https://doi.org/10.1590/2177-9465-EAN-2018-0389

Balouchi, A., Mahmoudirad, G., Hastings-Tolsma, M., Afshin Shorofi, S., Shahdadi, H., & Abdollahimohammad, A. (2018). Knowledge, attitude and use of complementary and alternative medicine among nurses: A systematic review. *Complementary Therapies in Clinical Practice, 31,* 146–157. https://doi.org/10.1016/j.ctcp.2018.02.008

Bell, K. (2017). Teaching therapeutic touch to pediatric nursing students in chronic care. *Beginnings, 37*(5), 18–19.

Ben-Arye, E., Shulman, B., Eilon, Y., Woitiz, R., Cherniak, V., Shalom Sharabi, I., Sher, O., Reches, H., Katz, Y., Arad, M., Schiff, E., Samuels, N., Caspi, O., Lev-Ari, S., Frenkel, M., Agbarya, A., & Admi, H. (2017). Attitudes among nurses toward the integration of complementary medicine into supportive cancer care. *Oncology Nursing Forum, 44,* 428–434. https://doi.org/10.1188/17.ONF.428-434

Booth, L., & Kaylor, S. (2018). Teaching spiritual care within nursing education. *Holistic Nursing Practice, 32,* 177–181. https://doi.org/10.1097/HNP.0000000000000271

Booth-LaForce, C., Scott, C., Heitkemper, M., Cornman, J., Lan, M., Bond, E., & Swanson, K. (2010). Complementary and alternative (CAM) attitudes and competencies of nursing students and faculty: Results of integrating CAM into the nursing curriculum. *Journal of Professional Nursing, 26,* 293–300. https://doi.org/10.1016/j.profnurs.2010.03.003

Boz, I., Ozer, Z., Teskereci, G., & Turan Kavradim, S. (2017). Learning experiences of nurses as part of a European Union project on complementary therapies: A multinational qualitative study. *Holistic Nursing Practice, 31,* 42–49. https://doi.org/10.1097/HNP.0000000000000171

Bradley, R., Booth-LaForce, C., Hanes, D., Scott, C., Sherman, K., Lin, Y., & Zwickey, H. (2019). Design of a multidisciplinary training program in complementary and integrative health clinical research: Building research across interdisciplinary gaps. *The Journal of Alternative and Complementary Medicine, 25,* 509–516. https://doi.org/10.1089/acm.2018.0454

Bremner, M., Bennett, D., & Chambers, D. (2014). Integrating Reiki and community-engaged scholarship: An interdisciplinary educational intervention. *Journal of Nursing Education, 53,* 541–543. https://doi.org/10.3928/01484834-20140820-02

Burman, M. (2003). Complementary and alternative medicine: Core competencies for family nurse practitioners. *Journal of Nursing Education, 42,* 28–34. https://doi.org/10.3928/0148-4834-20030101-07

Butcher, H., Bulechek, G., Dochterman, J., & Wagner, C. (Eds.). (2018). *Nursing interventions classification (NIC)* (7th ed.). Elsevier.

Calado, R., Silva, A., Oliveira, D., Silva, G., Silva, J., Silva, L., Lemos, M., & Santos, R. (2019). Teaching of integrative and complementary practices in nursing graduation. *Journal of Nursing UFPE Online, 12,* 261–267. https://doi.org/10.5205/1981-8963-v13i01a237094p261-267-2019

Camurdan, C., & Gül, A. (2013). Complementary and alternative medicine use among nursing and midwifery students in Turkey. *Nurse Education in Practice, 13,* 350–354. https://doi.org/10.1016/j.nepr.2012.09.015

Chan, R., & Schaffrath, M. (2017). Participatory action inquiry using baccalaureate nursing students: The inclusion of integrative health care modalities in nursing core curriculum. *Nurse Education in Practice, 22,* 66–72. https://doi.org/10.1016/j.nepr.2016.12.003

Chandler, D. (2016). Integrated care and leprosy in India: A role for Indian systems of medicine and traditional health practice in the eradication of leprosy. *Current Science, 111,* 351–355. https://doi.org/10.18520/cs/v111/i2/351-355

Chlan, L., Halcón, L., Kreitzer, M., & Leonard, B. (2005). Influence of an experiential education session on nursing students' confidence levels in performing selected complementary therapy skills. *Complementary Health Practice Review, 10,* 189–201. https://doi.org/10.1177/1533210105284044

Conroy, S. F., & Taggart, H. M. (2016). The impact of a cultural immersion study abroad experience in traditional Chinese medicine. *Journal of Holistic Nursing, 34*(3), 229–235. https://doi.org/10.1177/0898010115602995

Cook, N., & Robinson, J. (2006). Effectiveness and value of massage skills training during preregistration nurse education. *Nurse Education Today, 26,* 555–563. https://doi.org/10.1016/j.nedt.2006.01.010

Dicianno, B., Glick, R., Sowa, G., & Boninger, M. (2016). Processes and outcomes from a medical student research training program in integrative, complementary and alternative medicine. *American Journal of Physical Medicine & Rehabilitation, 95*, 779–786. https://doi.org/10.1097/PHM.0000000000000508

Dutta, A., Bwayo, S., Xue, Z., Akiyode, O., Ayuk-Egbe, P., Bernard, D., Daftary, M. N., & Clarke-Tasker, V. (2003). Complementary and alternative medicine instruction in nursing curricula. *Journal of National Black Nurses Association, 14*, 30–33.

Fenton, M., & Morris, D. (2003). The integration of holistic nursing practices and complementary and alternative modalities into curricula of schools of nursing. *Alternative Therapies, 9*, 62–67. https://web-s-ebscohost-com.ezp2.lib.umn.edu/ehost/pdfviewer/pdfviewer?vid=3&sid=02690f86-692a-4819-b7f1-79fc05bfa1a8%40redis

Gaster, B., Unterborn, J., Scott, R., & Schneeweiss, R. (2007). What should students learn about complementary and alternative medicine? *Academic Medicine, 82*, 934–938. https://doi.org/10.1097/ACM.0b013e318149eb56

Geisler, C., Cheung, C., Johnson Steinhagen, S., Neubeck, P., & Brueggeman, A. (2015). Nurse practitioner knowledge, use, and referral of complementary/alternative therapies. *Journal of the American Association of Nurse Practitioners, 27*, 380–388. https://doi.org/10.1002/2327-6924.12190

Government of Western Australia Department of Health. (2015). *Standard protocols: Use of complementary therapies.* http://www.health.wa.gov.au

Groft, J., & Kalischuk, R. (2005). Nursing students learn about complementary and alternative health care practices. *Complementary Health Practice Review, 10*, 133–146. https://doi.org/10.1177/1533210105280367

Halcón, L., Leonard, B., Snyder, M., Garwick, A., & Kreitzer, M. (2001). Incorporating alternative and complementary health practices within university-based nursing education. *Complementary Health Practice Review, 6*, 127–135. https://doi.org/10.1177/153321010100600203

Hall, H., Leach, M., Brosnan, C., & Collins, M. (2017). Nurses' attitudes towards complementary therapies: A systematic review and meta-synthesis. *International Journal of Nursing Studies, 69*, 47–56. https://doi.org/10.1016/j.ijnurstu.2017.01.008

Hart, J. (2019). The expanding field of holistic nursing—A growing trend. *Alternative and Complementary Therapies, 25*(1), 53–55. https://doi.org/10.1089/act.2018.29199.jha

Helms, J. (2006). Complementary and alternative therapies: A new frontier for nursing education? *Journal of Nursing Education, 45*, 117–123. https://doi.org/10.3928/01484834-20060301-05

Homberg, A., & Stock-Schröer, B. (2021). Interprofessional education on complementary and integrative medicine. *The Clinical Teacher, 18*, 152–157. https://doi.org/10.1111/tct.13280

Hon, K., Twinn, S., Leung, T., Thompson, D., Wong, Y., & Fok, T. (2006). Chinese nursing students' attitudes toward traditional Chinese medicine. *Journal of Nursing Education, 45*, 182–185. https://doi.org/10.3928/01484834-20060501-08

Hritz, S., Wang, Y., & Akkarawongvisit, C. (2018). Exploring cultural health practices at a Midwestern university. *Holistic Nursing Practice, 32*, 268–274. https://doi.org/10.1097/HNP.0000000000000287

Johnson, C. (2014). Effect of aromatherapy on cognitive test anxiety among nursing students. *Alternative and Complementary Therapies, 20*, 84–87. https://doi.org/10.1089/act.2014.20207

Karim, S., Benn, R., Carlson, L. E., Fouladbakhsh, J., Greenlee, H., Harris, R., Henry, N. L., Jolly, S., Mayhew, S., Spratke, L., Walker, E. M., Zebrack, B., & Zick, S. M. (2021). Integrative oncology education: An emerging competency for oncology providers. *Current Oncology, 28*, 853–862. https://doi.org/10.3390/curroncol28010084

Kavurmaci, M., Tan, M., & Kavurmaci, Z. (2018). Nursing, midwifery, and dietetics students' attitudes to complementary and integrative medicine and their applications, *Medical Journal of Bakırköy, 14*, 300–305. https://doi.org/10.5350/BTDMJB.20170606124143

Khan, A., Ahmed, M., Aldarmahi, A., Zaidi, S., Subahi, A., Al Shaikh, A., Alghamdy, Z., & Alhakami, L. (2020). Awareness, self-use, perceptions, beliefs, and attitudes toward complementary and alternative medicines (CAM) among health professional students in King

Saud bin Abdulaziz University for Health Sciences Jeddah, Saudi Arabia. *Evidence-Based Complementary and Alternative Medicine, 2020,* 11. https://doi.org/10.1155/2020/7872819

Kessack, M. (2015). *Teaching complementary and alternative therapies to prelicensure nursing students: A faculty assessment using a basic qualitative research approach* [Doctoral Dissertation]. Capella University. ProQuest Dissertations Publishing. 3681159. https://www.proquest.com/openview/c71bef578e0115c45b69143bb8d196f9/1?pq-origsite=gscholar&cbl=18750

Kinchen, E., & Loerzel, V. (2019). Nursing students' attitudes and use of holistic therapies for stress relief. *Journal of Holistic Nursing, 37,* 6–17. https://doi.org/10.1177/0898010118761910

Koithan, M. (2015). The promise of integrative nursing. *Creative Nursing, 21,* 193–199. https://doi.org/10.1891/1078-4535.21.4.193

Kreitzer, M., Mann, D., & Lumpkin, M. (2008). CAM competencies for the health professions. *Complementary Health Practice Review, 13,* 63–72. https://doi.org/10.1177/1533210107310165

Lee, M., Benn, R., Wimstatt, L., Cornman, J., Hedgecock, J., Gerick, S., Zeller, J., Kreitzer, M. J., Allweiss, P., Finkelstein, C., & Haramati, A. (2007). Integrating complementary and alternative medicine instruction into health professions education: Organizational and instructional strategies. *Academic Medicine, 82,* 939–945. https://doi.org/10.1097/ACM.0b013e318149ebf8

Linderman, C. A. (2000). The future of nursing education. *Journal of Nursing Education, 39,* 5–12. https://doi.org/10.3928/0148-4834-19991201-11

Matthias-Anderson, D., & Reid, C. (2019). Holistic nursing Standard 1 demonstrated in an interactive role play simulation: Teaching holistic assessment to nursing students. *Beginnings, 39,* 12–13.

Minnesota Board of Nursing. (2017). *Statement of accountability for utilization of integrative therapies in nursing practice.* https://mn.gov/boards/assets/Intgrtv_Therapies_Stmt_2017_7-19_tcm21-37140.pdf

National Academies of Sciences, Engineering and Medicine. (2021). *The future of nursing 2020–2030: Charting a path to achieve health equity.* National Academies Press. http://nap.edu/25982

National Center for Complementary and Integrative Health. (2021). *Complementary, Alternative, or Integrative Health: What's in a Name?* Health Information. https://www.nccih.nih.gov/health/complementary-alternative-or-integrative-health-whats-in-a-name

National Council of State Boards of Nursing. (2019). *NCLEX-RN® Examination: Test plan for the national council licensure examination for registered nurses.* NCSBN, Inc. https://www.ncsbn.org/2019_RN_TestPlan-English.htm

National League for Nursing. (2017). *A vision for expanding US nursing education for global health engagement.* NLN Vision Series. https://www.nln.org/docs/default-source/about/nln\-vision-series-(position-statements)/vision-statement-a-vision-for-expanding-us-nursing-education.pdf

National Student Nurses Association. (2016). *Resolutions 2016.* NSNA. https://www.dropbox.com/s/h1un2ns0wcybh2p/NSNA%20Resolutions%202016.pdf?dl=0

Nedrow, A., Heitkemper, M., Frenkel, M., Mann, D., Wayne, P., & Hughes, E. (2007a). Collaborations between allopathic and complementary and alternative medicine health professionals: Four initiatives. *Academic Medicine, 82,* 962–966. https://doi.org/10.1097/ACM.0b013e31814a4e2c

Nedrow, A., Istvan, J., Haas, M., Barrett, R., Salveson, C., Moore, G. Hammerschlag, R., & Keenan, E. (2007b). Implications for education in complementary and alternative medicine: A survey of entry attitudes in students at five health professional schools. *Journal of Alternative and Complementary Medicine, 13,* 381–386. https://doi.org/10.1089/acm.2007.6273

Nevins, C., & Sherman, J. (2016). Self-care practices of baccalaureate nursing students. *Journal of Holistic Nursing, 34,* 185–192. https://doi.org/10.1177/0898010115596432

Ozer, Z., Boz, I., Kavradim, S., & Teskereci, G. (2019). European Union Project 'BestCARE': Improving nursing care with best complementary therapy strategies. *International Nursing Review, 66,* 112–121. https://doi.org/10.1111/inr.12469

Pearson, N., & Chesney, M. (2007). The CAM education program of the National Center for Complementary and Alternative Medicine: An overview. *Academic Medicine, 82,* 921–926. https://doi.org/10.1097/ACM.0b013e31814a5014

Pirincci, E., Kaya, F., Cengizhan, S., & Onal, F. (2018). Nursing department students' knowledge and use of complementary and alternative medicine methods. *Journal of Turgut Ozal Medical Center*, 25(1), 22–29. https://doi.org/10.5455/jtomc.2017.07.099

Poreddi, V., Thiyagarajan, S., Swamy, P., Gandhi, S., Thimmaiah, R., & BadaMath, S. (2016). Nursing student attitudes and understanding of complementary and alternative therapies: An Indian perspective. *Nursing Education Perspectives*, 37, 32–37. https://doi.org/10.5480/14-1319

Racz, A., Crnković, I., & Brumini, I. (2019). Attitudes and beliefs about integration of CAM education in health care professionals training programs in Croatia. *International Multidisciplinary Scientific Conference on Social Sciences & Arts SGEM*, 6, 399–406. https://doi.org/10.5593/sgemsocial2019V/2.1

Richardson, S. (2003). Complementary health and healing in nursing education. *Journal of Holistic Nursing*, 21, 20–35. https://doi.org/10.1177/0898010102250273

Roberts, T. (2019). Our commitment to continuing education & competency in holistic nursing. *Beginnings*, 37, 4–5.

Rosenthal, B., Gravrand, H., & Lisi, A. (2019). Interprofessional collaboration among complementary and integrative health providers in private practice and community health centers. *Journal of Interprofessional Education and Practice*, 15, 70–74.

Salles, L., Homo, R., & Silva, M. (2014). The situation of the teaching of holistic and complementary practices in undergraduate courses in nursing, physiotherapy, and medicine. *Cogitare Enferm*, 19, 682–687.

Salmon, M. (2010). The commons: Nursing education, societal relevance, and going it together. *Alternative Therapies in Health and Medicine*, 16(5), 18.

Sok, S., Erlen, J., & Kim, K. (2004). Complementary and alternative therapies in nursing curricula: A new direction for nurse educators. *Journal of Nursing Education*, 43, 401–405. https://doi.org/10.3928/01484834-20040901-12

Solomon, D., Singleton, K., Zhiyuan, S., Zell, K., Vriezen, K., & Albert, N. (2016). Multicenter study of nursing role complexity on environmental stressors and emotional exhaustion. *Applied Nursing Research*, 30, 52–57. https://doi.org/10.1016/j.apnr.2015.08.010

Sparber, A. (2001). State boards of nursing and scope of practice of registered nurses performing complementary therapies. *Online Journal of Issues in Nursing*, 6. http://www.nursingworld.org/MainMenuCategories/ANAMarketplace/ANAPeriodicals/OJIN/TableofContents/Volume62001/No3Sept01/ArticlePreviousTopic/CmplementaryTherapiesReport.html

Stratton, T., Benn, R., Lie, D., Zeller, J., & Nedrow, A. (2007). Evaluating CAM education in health professions programs. *Academic Medicine*, 82, 956–961. https://doi.org/10.1097/ACM.0b013e31814a5152

Sutch, K. (2017). My path as educator: Holism in the nursing classroom. *Beginnings*, 37, 14–15.

Swanson, B., Zeller, J., Keithley, J., Fung, S., Johnson, A., Suhayda, R., Phillips, M., & Downie, P. (2012). Case-based online modules to teach graduate-level nursing students about complementary and alternative medical therapies. *Journal of Professional Nursing*, 28, 125–129. https://doi.org/10.1016/j.profnurs.2011.11.005

Tollefson, M., Wisneski, L., Sayre, N., Helton, J., Matuszewicz, E., & Jensen, C. (2016). Integrative healthcare: An exploration of students who choose this undergraduate major. *The Journal of Alternative and Complementary Medicine*, 22(2), 166–170. https://doi.org/10.1089/acm.2015.0219

Topuz, S., Uysal, G., & Yilmaz, A. (2015). Knowledge and opinions of nursing students regarding complementary and alternative medicine for cancer patients. *International Journal of Caring Sciences*, 8, 656–664. http://www.internationaljournalofcaringsciences.org/docs/17_Topuz_original_8_3.pdf

Toygar, I., Hancerlıoglu, S., Gul, I., Yondem, S., & Yilmaz, I. (2020). Effect of educational intervention on nursing students' attitudes toward complementary and alternative therapies. *International Journal of Caring Sciences*, 13, 1305–1312. http://www.internationaljournalofcaringsciences.org/docs/55_1_toygar_original_13_2.pdf

U.S. Department of Health and Human Services. (2020). *Health People 2030: Building a healthier future for all*. Office of Disease Prevention and Health Promotion. https://health.gov/healthypeople

van der Reit, P., Francis, L., & Levett-Jones, T. (2011). Complementary therapies in healthcare: Design, implementation, and evaluation of an elective course for undergraduate students. *Nurse Education in Practice, 11*, 146–152. https://doi.org/10.1016/j.nepr.2010.10.002

Van Rensburg, R., Razlog, R., & Pellow, J. (2020). Knowledge and attitudes towards complementary medicine by nursing students at a University in South Africa. *Health SA Gesondheid, 25*, a1436. https://doi.org/10.4102/hsag.v25i0.1436

Van Sant-Smith, D. (2015). Supporting the integrative health care curriculum in schools of nursing. *Holistic Nursing Practice, 28*, 312. https://doi.org/10.1097/HNP.0000000000000042

Vega, A., North, S., Ruggeri, B., Beck, B., Liveris, M. Castro, A., Boyington, N., Leveille, W., St. George, T., & Hopp, J. (2020). A cross-cultural integrative health interprofessional practice model using innovative case study and academic Hispanic community partnership approaches. *Cogent Medicine, 7*, 1767347. https://doi.org/10.1080/2331205X.2020.1767347

Yeh, Y., & Chung, U. (2007). An investigation into competence in TCM of BSN graduates from technological universities in Taiwan. *Journal of Nursing Research, 15*, 310–317. https://doi.org/10.1097/01.JNR.0000387627.25801.12

Zick, S. M., Czuhajewski, C., Fouladbakhsh, J. M., Greenlee, H., Harris, R. E., Henry, N. L., Jolly, S., Khabir, T., Perlmutter, J., Remington, T., & Snyder, D. (2018). Integrative oncology scholars program: A model for integrative oncology education. *The Journal of Alternative and Complementary Medicine, 24*(9–10), 1018–1022. https://doi.org/10.1007/s13187-020-01829-8

Zeighami, M., & Soltani-Nejad, S. (2020). Knowledge, attitude, and practice of complementary and alternative medicine: A survey of Iranian nurses. *Journal of Research in Nursing, 25*, 380–388. https://doi.org/10.1177/1744987120925852

Integrating Complementary Therapies Into Practice Settings

CYNTHIA LEE DOLS FINN

Complementary therapies are increasingly being offered across the continuum of healthcare. Nurses are essential leaders for maximizing the use of complementary and integrative therapies that support holistic healthcare. Holistic healthcare in nursing recognizes the humanistic, caring, healing nature of interventions and often uses many complementary and integrative modalities to support the mind–body–spirit on its healing journey (Clark, 2012; Courdeau, 2020).

This chapter provides examples of strategies that nurses use to incorporate complementary therapies into their practices. Healthcare settings across the country are used to demonstrate the integration of complementary therapies into both inpatient and outpatient hospital nursing practice. The hospitals include Abbott Northwestern Hospital, Broward Health Imperial Point, and the University Medical Center of Southern Nevada. Broward Health Imperial Point and the University Medical Center of Southern Nevada have received the American Holistic Nurses Association Holistic Practice Institutional Award for Excellence in Practice. In addition to traditional nursing roles in hospital settings, examples included in this chapter of nurses incorporating complementary and integrative therapies into community-based care, holistic health and wellness centers, care provided to military veterans, and professional practice self-care show the breadth of opportunities for integration into nursing practice.

Healthcare facilities in the United States are not alone in integrating complementary therapies; this is being done across the world as well (World Health Organization, 2019). The World Health Organization (2019) reports that of its 179 members, 88% report using complementary therapies. Sidebar 28.1 illustrates the use of complementary therapies in Brazil.

MEDICAL CENTER SETTINGS

As complementary therapies become more widely used in the United States, many nurses seek strategies to incorporate them into their nursing practice. Several different healthcare settings across the country including Abbott Northwestern Hospital, Broward Health Imperial Point, and the University Medical Center of

Sidebar 28.1 *Use of Complementary Therapies in Brazil*

Milena Flória-Santos

According to the *Pan American Health Organization* (*PAHO*), which works with the countries of the Americas to improve the health and quality of life of their populations, traditional, complementary and integrative medicines (TCIMs) are an important model of healthcare (Almeida, 2021). In some countries of Latin America, TCIMs are the main provision of services to the population, and in others, they are complementary to the conventional system. Taking this into consideration, an international webinar "Articulation of the Integrative and Complementary Practices in Health in the Health Systems of the Americas: Regulation and Policies" brought together researchers and authorities from 12 countries (Almeida, 2021). During the event, they presented initiatives for the insertion of integrative practices in their health systems and for intercultural dialogue to strengthen the relationship between conventional medicine and the traditional knowledge of Native peoples. At the event, organizers of the webinar, in conjunction with the Brazilian Academic Health Consortium Integrative, launched the book Experiences and Reflections on Traditional, Complementary and Integrative Medicines in Health Systems in the Americas (Sousa et al., 2021). The Brazilian Unified Health System (in Portuguese, Sistema Único de Saúde [SUS]) is considered an example of health system innovation for Latin America and a model for the world, and one of the reasons is because it is entirely free for any person, including foreigners; in other words, it is a publicly funded healthcare system (Castro et al., 2019).

TCIMs have been contemplated by the SUS since the 1980s; however, it is worth highlighting that they received enormous support through the Ordinance 971 of 2006, which established the National Policy on Integrative and Complementary Practices (NPICP) recently reformulated and extended by resolutions 145 and 849 of 2017 and 702 of 2018, in accordance with other national policies, such as primary care, health promotion, and humanization (Azevedo et al., 2019). The NPICP established the insertion of integrative and complementary practices into Brazilian primary healthcare, and currently, more than half of Brazilian municipalities (78%) offer TCIMs to the population in individual and collective care. There are 17,300 health establishments in the country, including primary care and medium- and high-complexity services offering some type of TCIM, and most of them are in primary care, distributed in 4,297 municipalities (Ministry of Health, 2020). The NPICP also enabled nonmedical professionals, including nurses, to practice complementary medicine through accreditation and remuneration by the SUS (Souza & Tesser, 2017).

It is very important to emphasize that the Brazilian Council of Nursing approved, in 2018, the list of nursing specialties (COFEN, 2018). In this context, Nursing in Integrative and Complementary Practices was recognized as a nursing specialty, which allows nurses to work with 12 kinds of therapies: phytotherapy, homeopathy, orthomolecular therapy, floral therapy, foot reflexology, reiki, yoga, therapeutic touch, music therapy, chromotherapy, hypnosis, and acupuncture.

Sidebar 28.1 *Use of Complementary Therapies in Brazil (continued)*

Since then, Brazilian nurses who practice at primary, secondary, or tertiary levels of care in a variety of practice settings, such as community centers, hospitals, or academia, have legal support to apply TCIMs.

The scientific literature of Brazilian nurses focused on TCIMs has grown in recent years. More than 300 scientific articles on this topic were published in the last 20 years by Brazilian nurses and were retrieved through a brief nonsystematic literature review, searching the main databases. Malta et al. (2021) conducted an integrative review to highlight the integrative and complementary practices in the fields of education and performance of nurses described in the Brazilian scientific literature. They found that regarding the types of research, the most cited were qualitative (62.5%), quantitative (15%), and a review of the literature (15%), as well as descriptive and exploratory (7.5%). Furthermore, there are few studies that focus on the discussion of the effectiveness and safety of integrative and complementary practices. The majority of studies focused on the benefits of certain practices, such as herbal medicine and acupuncture, highlighting the almost nonexistence of studies that address other practices, such as aromatherapy, thermalism, and group practices.

Andres et al. (2020) performed descriptive, quantitative field research, with 508 nurses from 19 Brazilian states, most of them female, working in hospitals, with 1 to 5 years of training and experience. Most were familiar with TCIM and the policy of these therapies; the best known were acupuncture, homeopathy, and music therapy. The most available in health services were acupuncture, reiki, and yoga. The authors concluded that it is essential that nurses have training related to TCIMs to expand their knowledge about therapies that promote health and improve the quality of life of individuals.

Azevedo et al. (2019) conducted a documentary study on the legal aspects that support nurses' practice of TCIMs and discussed the scope of teaching, research, extension, and nursing activities regarding those therapies. They found that nurses are prominent professionals in the implementation and use of TCIMs, since the principles of their training are congruent to the paradigms of these therapies. However, in Brazil, there is still only a small contingent of professionals who apply these therapies or have the knowledge to prescribe and refer users to this type of service. The practice and its remuneration in the SUS include acupuncture, corporal practices, and anthroposophical medicine. Nursing has theoretical foundations congruent with TCIMs, and therefore, when nurses are exposed to these practices, they feel an affinity for them.

Finally, it is essential to mention the existence of the Brazilian Association of Acupuncturists Nurses and Integrative Practices Nurses. Their mission is grounded in a social commitment to improving the quality of life of Brazilians, providing the opportunity for holistic care to those who seek acupuncturist nurses, and ensuring that these professionals have a strong voice and essential tools for care and teaching with the organizational support of this association (ABENAH, 2021).

(continued)

Sidebar 28.1 *Use of Complementary Therapies in Brazil (continued)*

References

ABENAH. (2021). *Brazilian Association of Acupuncturists Nurses and Integrative Practices Nurses.* http://abenanacional.org/

Almeida, V. (2021). *ObservaPics.* http://observapics.fiocruz.br/propostas-e-estrategias-para-ampliar -a-articulacao-entre-medicinas-tradicionais-pics-e-politicas-de-saude-nas-americas/Andres

Andres, F. C., Andres, S. C., Moreschi, C., Rodrigues, S. O., & Badke, M. R. (2020). Nurses' knowledge about integrative and complementary health practices. *Research, Society and Development, 9*(7), e969975171. https://doi.org/10.33448/rsd-v9i7.5171

Azevedo, C., Moura, C. C., Corrêa, H. P., Mata, L. R. F., Chaves, É. C. L., & Chianca, T. C. M. (2019). Complementary and integrative therapies in the scope of nursing: legal aspects and academic-assistance panorama. *Escola Anna Nery, 23*(2), e20180389. https://doi.org/10.1590/2177 -9465-EAN-2018-0389

Castro, M. C., Massuda, A., Almeida, G., Menezes-Filho, N. A., Andrade, M. V., de Souza Noronha, K., Rocha, R., Macinko, J., Hone, T., Tasca, R., Giovanella, L., Malik, A. M., Werneck, H., Fachini, L. A., & Atun, R. (2019). Brazil's unified health system: The first 30 years and prospects for the future. *Lancet (London, England), 394*(10195), 345–356. https://doi.org/10.1016/ S0140-6736(19)31243-7

COFEN. (2018). *COFEN Resolution no. 581/2018 -Amended by COFEN Resolution no. 625/2020 and COFEN Decision no. 065/2021.* http://www.cofen.gov.br/resolucao-cofen-no-581-2018_64383 .html

Malta, B. C. S., Malachias, L. B., Magalhães, T. A., Maia, J. S., & Figueiredo, L. P. (2021). Integrative and complementary practices and their applicability in the fields of nurse training and performance. *Pubsaúde, 5*(108), 1–10. https://doi.org/10.31533/pubsaude5.a108

Ministry of Healthy. (2020). *National Monitoring Report on Integrative and Complementary Practices in Health at the Health Information Systems.* http://189.28.128.100/dab/docs/portaldab/ documentos/pics/Relatorio_Monitoramento_das_PICS_no_Brasil_julho_2020_v1_0.pdf

Sousa, I. C., Guimarães, M. B., Gallego-Perez, D. F. (2021). Experiences and reflections on traditional, complementary and integrative medicines in the health systems of the Americas. http:// observapics.fiocruz.br/wp-content/uploads/2021/03/MTCI-America-ObservaPICS-Rede-MTCI.pdf

Souza, I. M. A., & Tesser, C. D. (2017). Traditional and complementary medicine in Brazil: Inclusion in the Brazilian Unified National Health System and integration with primary care. *Cadernos de Saúde Pública, 33*(1), e00150215. https://doi.org/10.1590/0102-311X00150215

Southern Nevada integrate complementary therapies into their nursing practice in conjunction with traditional Western medicine to enhance patient care.

ABBOTT NORTHWESTERN HOSPITAL

Abbott Northwestern Hospital, a part of the Allina Health System, is a 686-bed, tertiary-care, not-for-profit hospital in Minneapolis, Minnesota (Abbott Northwestern Hospital: Internal Medicine Residency, 2021). The nursing department's philosophy at Abbott Northwestern is based on advocacy through caring. In 1999, a complementary and alternative medicine program for cardiovascular inpatients was initiated and has grown into a nationally recognized model for providing integrative care (Sendelbach et al., 2003).

Abbott Northwestern Hospital, in collaboration with the Minneapolis Heart Institute, identified a mission to provide an exceptional healthcare experience for patients with cardiovascular disorders, and to support this initiative, they established a holistic nursing framework for practice. The prevalence of the public's use of complementary and alternative therapies identified in the literature, along with an increasing number of patient and family requests for these interventions, motivated Abbott Northwestern Hospital to initiate its original innovative program, Healing the Hearts, which includes therapeutic interventions such as music and massage (Sendelbach et al., 2003).

Nursing involvement has been critical to the ongoing success of integrative therapies. An Integrative Practice Advisory Board was established in 2001, and one of the three key areas identified for growth was to further develop holistic nursing to complement the interventions received by patients. The interventions were assessed to be congruent with the nursing department's philosophy and the cornerstones of the patient care model. Work was also focused on enhancing a total healing environment that includes developing positive and collaborative relationships between nurses and physicians because this has been shown to positively influence patient outcomes (Sendelbach et al., 2003).

With initial success and institutional support, along with continuing education for providers, the inpatient cardiovascular integrative therapy program developed into a national model for not only inpatient care but also outpatient care, research, and education. The Penny George Institute for Health and Healing (a part of Abbott Northwestern) is a model for enhancing health through an integrative approach. The mission of this innovative program is to transform healthcare locally by providing outstanding integrative care and to transform healthcare nationally through the dissemination of integrative practices that enhance quality and safety and reduce costs. The Penny George Institute has been recognized for its best practices for enhancing care through integrative services (Allina Health, 2021; Bravewell Collaborative, 2015) and is the largest hospital-based integrative healthcare program of its kind in the United States (George Family Foundation, 2021).

The Penny George Institute for Health and Healing offers inpatient services that include acupressure/acupuncture; aromatherapy; energy-based healing; healing arts; and mind/body therapies (Allina Health, 2021). Outpatient services include Oriental medicine/acupuncture, Chinese medicine, energy healing, healing coaching, herbal consultations, integrative medicine physician consultations, integrative nutrition counseling, mind/body therapies, spiritual coaching, massage therapy, therapeutic yoga, classes and workshops on aromatherapy, drum circle, and healing through the arts (Allina Health, 2021).

The holistic nurse clinicians and other members of the integrative therapy team provide ongoing education to the staff. Abbott Northwestern Hospital sponsors physician and nurse practitioner training in integrative medicine and advocates for integrative health in healthcare reform. Education programs are focused on integrative therapies, promotion of self-managed health and wellness, community education classes, transformative nurse training programs (TNT), and local healthcare conferences. Since the inception of the TNT program over 1000 nurses have been trained. The TNT program expanded within the Allina Health System to Children's Hospitals and Clinics of Minnesota, the Mayo Clinic system, and a number of other Minnesota healthcare facilities (George Family Foundation, 2021). Ongoing classes and programs for the community on topics such as yoga, stress reduction, nutrition, and fitness provide up-to-date information to thousands of participants a year (Allina Health, 2021).

Research to measure patient outcomes and identify best practices is also a key to expanding this innovative model. Nurses are involved with ongoing clinical trials using integrative therapies and data analysis to provide sound evidence for integrating complementary and alternative therapies into clinical practice. The impact of integrative therapies has been documented to provide immediate and beneficial effects on pain among hospitalized patients. Following integrative therapy interventions, the average pain reduction was over 55% (Dusek et al., 2010).

BROWARD HEALTH IMPERIAL POINT

Broward Health Imperial Point (BHIP), an award-winning American Nurses Credentialing Center Certified Pathways of Excellence–designated hospital, is located in Fort Lauderdale, Florida. BHIP is a 204-bed acute-care hospital known for its excellent treatment and quality care (Gallison & Kester, 2018). The BHIP theoretical framework for nursing practice is based on the nursing theory of human caring proposed by Dr. Jean Watson. Dr. Watson's theory builds on the concepts of interconnectedness and unitary consciousness that honors every patient as a unique person with the potential to heal holistically. Intentions and presence are cornerstones of creating a healing environment. BHIP has also integrated Watson's 10 Caritas Processes™ as guidelines for clinical practice (Gallison & Curtin, 2016). BHIP is committed to creating a caring environment. Nurses across the continuum of care include complementary therapies as part of the holistic healing process.

Holistic Care Council

In 2014, the BHIP Clinical Services' governance structure established the BHIP Holistic Care Council (HCC) to promote the values of holistic nursing for the individual, patients, and peers. The HCC prioritizes creating an organization-wide healing environment, rooted in the interpersonal relationship to foster quality, holistic care of patients and staff (Gallison & Curtin, 2016; Gallison & Kester, 2018). The HCC promotes the values of kindness, compassion, and care for oneself as well as patients and colleagues; fosters and provides opportunities for self-care practices including meditation and quiet time; and attends to the spiritual, emotional, and physical concerns of nurses as well as their patients and peers (Higgs, 2016). Spiritual support is offered through pastoral care, providing opportunities for staff to connect more deeply with themselves to allow for deeper connections with their patients.

The HCC has developed several successful partnerships to promote connectedness. A partnership with the Human Resources Department has led to programming that supports employees work–life balance. Programming has included salsa lessons, nutritional classes, workplace yoga, and "Zen in 10," which includes meditation, guided imagery, and aromatherapy for staff meetings (Gallison & Curtin, 2016). Other partnerships have led to a variety of resources for staff self-care including donated massage chairs; foot massage devices; the development of a renewal space for staff to center, reflect, and renew; and a space for staff and community members to spend time with puppies and kittens brought in by the local Humane Society. Additionally, a partnership with the local Broward Healing Light Chapter of the American Holistic Nurses Association affords opportunities for a variety of educational sessions led by its membership for BHIP staff on mindfulness-stress reduction, clinical aromatherapy, healing touch, and self-care (Gallison & Curtin, 2016).

The HCC has spearheaded and supports several successful projects for patients. An aromatherapy program was implemented to address postoperative pain, nausea, and anxiety (Gallison & Curtin, 2016). Postoperative patients are offered a selection of aromatherapy options and collaborate with their direct care nurse to choose the oil that would be most appropriate to meet their needs and improve their comfort, well-being, and hospital stay (Gallison & Curtin, 2016). The implementation of aromatherapy has had a positive effect not only on the patients but on family members and staff as well. Nurses have noted a calmness in the workflow with the use of aromatherapy. Several patients shared their experiences at BHIP and have identified receiving traditional medical interventions as well as using yoga and breathwork.

UNIVERSITY MEDICAL CENTER OF SOUTHERN NEVADA

Located in Las Vegas, Nevada, the University Medical Center of Southern Nevada is a 540-bed Level 1 Trauma community hospital. As a result of the administrative support and guidance of Mason Van Houweling, CEO; Debra Fox, CNO; and Margaret Covelli, Assistant CNO, the University Medical Center of Southern Nevada has transformed into an organization that provides traditional and integrative cutting-edge care, empowers employees, and engages the organizational community at all levels. The University Medical Center of Southern Nevada prides itself on providing excellent and specialized care and on being the only Level 1 Trauma Center, the only Designated Pediatric Trauma Center, the only Center for Transplantation, and the first Burn Center in Nevada (UMC: University Medical Center, 2014a). The University Medical Center of Southern Nevada also boasts the first and only hospital-wide, full-time integrative therapies program in Nevada (McKinney & McGrorey, 2019, 2021). Started in 2017, with the support of nursing administration, the Tranquility at UMC integrative program was born. This program uses only evidence-based and researched complementary therapies (McKinney & McGrorey, 2021). Complementary therapies are used in conjunction with standard medical care and patient outcomes are measured and monitored. Stipulations for including any complementary therapy include that the therapy must have research evidence supporting its effectiveness, and evidence supporting its effectiveness within the population for which the modality is used (McKinney & McGrorey, 2021). The integrative modalities include Healing Touch, aromatherapy, the implementation of the Continuous Ambient Relaxation Environment (C.A.R.E.) Channel, breathwork, including the Heart-Focused Breathing (HFB) technique and the 4–7–8 breathing technique, and the implementation of tranquility rooms for staff (McKinney & McGrorey, 2021). (See Case Study 28.1 for a discussion of the tranquility rooms).

The use of these complementary therapies has been extremely successful. Healing touch is provided to all patients across both the age and diagnosis continuum. Data on the outcomes of healing touch have been tracked. Results from 157 patients include an average reduction of pain by 60%, a reduction of stress and tension by 83%, anxiety reduction of 80%, and nausea reduction of 90%. While this was a low level of research, evidence supports that these findings are outside of the placebo effect and warrant further research (McKinney & McGrorey, 2021). McKinney and McGrorey (2021) reported that the use of essential oils was so effective that physicians are routinely consulting the integrative nurses on using it for

Case Study 28.1 *Tranquility Rooms at University Medical Center of Southern Nevada*

Michelle McGrorey & Deborah McKinney

On October 1, 2017, Las Vegas endured the worst mass shooting in U.S. history when a gunman opened fire at the Route 91 Harvest Music Festival held on the famed Las Vegas Strip. A total of 60 people died and more than 800 more were injured. Some of the most critically injured were taken to the University Medical Center of Southern Nevada (UMC), the only Level 1 Trauma Center in Las Vegas and its surrounding areas. The ensuing aftermath and horrific nature of the injuries took a terrible emotional and psychological toll on the hospital's staff. Nurses and physicians, public safety, environmental services, clerks, office personnel, pathology, diagnostics, marketing, administrative staff, and everyone who worked in the hospital were affected by this unbelievable tragedy. Never before had this kind of devastation and immediate demand for critical and acute care been seen on such a massive scale.

As a result of this horrendous ordeal, UMC's Chief Nursing Officer, Debra Fox, launched an impressive hospital-wide effort aimed solely at promoting self-care for the staff so that optimal patient care could be provided. She realized that work hours, burnout, compassion fatigue, overtime, and conflict often make self-care difficult. Because she has been at the forefront in providing stress reduction techniques for staff while on the job, she charged UMC's integrative therapies nurses with creating and furnishing, "tranquility rooms," throughout the hospital. These rooms would be used to provide a brief respite from the stresses of the job for any staff member needing one. Often, having a place of retreat to calm, relax, refresh, regroup, and renew is all it takes to build up enough emotional, physical, and mental resilience to continue working efficiently through the rest of the shift (McKinney & McGrorey, 2021).

A total of four tranquility rooms were created, available to staff 24 hours a day, seven days a week, located in various places throughout the hospital (the cost of one of the rooms was generously paid for by the "Show Me Your Stethoscope" nation of nurses, a nurse-founded and -run organization). The rooms are designed to give staff the opportunity for much-needed self-care. Each Tranquility Room is decorated in a homelike environment, equipped with a computer to access the Continuous Ambient Relaxation Environment (C.A.R.E.) Channel, an essential oil diffuser, ambient lighting, a comfortable reclining chair, coloring books, self-care handouts, and various other modalities known for their abilities to mitigate stress.

In order to determine if the rooms were having an effect on relieving the stress staff were experiencing, data was collected comparing pre- and post–tranquility room use. One hundred thirty- two staff responded using a 0- to 10-point Likert scale, where 0 indicates no stress experienced and 10 indicates worst possible stress experienced. The average stress score

Case Study 28.1 *Tranquility Rooms at University Medical Center of Southern Nevada (continued)*

pre–tranquility room use was 6.83. The average stress score post–tranquility room use was 2.43. Clearly, the rooms were having a decidedly positive effect in reducing the stress experienced by the staff. Staff have provided a tremendous amount of feedback, stating that on numerous occasions, the rooms have, indeed, made a difference!

Because of their effectiveness, UMC's administration is currently looking to create additional tranquility rooms so that even more staff will be able to take advantage of their stress-relieving effects, providing much-needed self-care.

Reference

McKinney, D., & McGrorey, M. (2021). Using holistic modalities in the hospital? You bet! *Energy Magazine, 116,* 14–19. https://www.energy.energymagazineonline.com/content _assets/current-issue/julaug2021-lite.pdf

their patients, and many are incorporating essential oils into their personal use. Nurses at the University Medical Center of Southern Nevada reported using the C.A.R.E. Channel has been effective in assisting some patients in the intensive care unit being weaned off the ventilator, as well as decreasing their sedation requirements (McKinney & McGrorey, 2021). The breathwork techniques have helped with pain, anxiety, stress, and tension. Additionally, the use of complementary therapies was attributed to alleviating some adverse symptoms for some patients leading to improved patient outcomes. One patient with intractable nausea, for whom medications did not work, was taught a complementary modality and was successfully discharged home with the use of the integrative modality (McKinney & McGrorey, 2019). A second patient with hypertension who was not responding to antihypertensive intravenous medications was engaged in a complementary therapy modality and was subsequently able to have surgery (McKinney & McGrorey, 2019). McKinney and McGrorey (2019) also report that hundreds of patients have described remarkable improvement upon receiving an integrative modality session. Further evidence that the integration of complementary therapies is positively impacting patients is the fact that patient satisfaction scores have improved since the inception of the UMC Tranquility Program (McKinney & McGrorey, 2021).

Healthy Living Institute

University Medical Center of Southern Nevada is committed to improving the health and well-being of those living in southern Nevada and to that end created the Healthy Living Institute, which opened in the spring of 2016 (UMC: University Medical Center, 2014b). The Healthy Living Institute brings learning opportunities that promote quality of life and wellbeing. They have a quarterly magazine that fosters healthy living and identifies wellness activities that residents in the area can participate in at no cost. University Medical Center of Southern Nevada believes that well-being is not only one's physical health; it is the ability for one to find a balance in body, mind, and spirit while considering the whole person (UMC: University Medical Center, 2014b). Their goal is to support the community in creating a healthy lifestyle that incorporates complementary evidence-based healing practices. The Healthy Living Institute creates a welcoming environment for all ages and has speakers, activities, and community events that promote healthy lifestyles. Some of the complementary courses and practices offered include yoga, healthy eating, and art therapy (UMC: University Medical Center, 2014b). The healthy prenatal course provides education on both traditional and complementary pain management options for attendees.

COMMUNITY-BASED HEALTHCARE SETTINGS

Complementary therapies are also included as part of patient care in other healthcare settings. Many community-based organizations incorporate integrative healing modalities to enhance patient care. The following examples show how some community-based hospices, clinics, and healing and wellness centers use integrative therapies in their programs.

HOLY REDEEMER HOSPICE

Holy Redeemer Hospice, in southeastern Pennsylvania and New Jersey, provides an innovative model with a team of nurses certified in complementary therapy modalities (Hansen, 2012). This approach enables experienced hospice nurses who are experts in hospice care to have another set of tools in their toolbox. Holy Redeemer Hospice offers a variety of complementary therapies that includes guided imagery and meditation, healing touch, music therapy, pet therapy, massage, and reflexology (Redeemer Health, 2021). Hospice care does not end when the patient who is being cared for dies because nurses continue to provide support to family members following the loss. Complementary therapies can help family members relax and address their stress levels and cope more effectively.

PILLSBURY HOUSE INTEGRATED HEALTH CLINIC

The Pillsbury House Integrated Health Clinic uses student practitioners and serves patients living in South Minneapolis, Minnesota, and the surrounding communities. All services, which are open to the public by appointment, are free of charge. Patients are offered integrative care services and therapies from student interns who are supervised by licensed faculty. The care is planned and delivered by a team of students and providers from several disciplines. These providers and disciplines include chiropractic care, acupuncture, massage therapy, health coaching, mental health counseling, and acupuncture (Northwestern Health Sciences University, 2021). Nursing students from the University of Minnesota and the Center for Spirituality and Healing are involved in providing information at the Pillsbury House. Nurses may be involved in collaborative planning for patients, and nurses who are health-coaching students may also be offering services (Northwestern Health Sciences University, 2021).

HERMITAGE FARM CENTER FOR HEALING

Nurses may work as instructors and practitioners in community-based holistic health and wellness centers. An example of such a community-based program initiated by nurses is the Hermitage Farm Center for Healing in Rochester,

Minnesota. This center was founded by an advanced practice nurse, and several of the practitioners affiliated with the center are nurses with advanced skills in complementary and integrative therapies. These nurses interact and collaborate with other complementary and integrative health practitioners to provide a variety of services. The classes offered are related to energy healing, stress management, and mindfulness-based stress reduction. Practitioners also provide therapies such as Reiki, energy healing, acupuncture, homeopathy, health coaching, and massage (Hermitage Farm Center for Healing, n.d.-a, n.d.-b). The Southeast Minnesota chapter of the American Holistic Nurses Association meets at this location.

PATHWAYS: A HEALING CENTER

Pathways: A Healing Center (Pathways), in Minneapolis, Minnesota, is another example of a community-based holistic wellness center that provides classes focused on the mind, body, heart, and spirit. The focus at Pathways is to enhance healing and Pathways' belief is that healing is always available, even when cure is not (Pathways, 2021a). Volunteers have offered more than 5,000 healing and educational sessions free of charge. Providers include nurses who offer therapies and also teach classes. The Pathways website (2021b) states: "Participants in Pathways holistic care, programs and services provided by volunteer providers have shown improved perceptions of quality of life and well-being and led to more active involvement in the experience of the healing process" (para. 5).

HEALTH COMMONS

Health Commons was started in 2011 and is a free drop-in health and wellness center. Health Commons provides access to health and wellness services, as well as opportunities for enriched community social connections, which help reduce health disparities and improve access to healthcare through creating positive relationships (Augsburg University, n.d.; M Health Now, M Health Fairview, 2019; Redeemer Center for Life, 2021). Services are provided in Minneapolis, Minnesota, in both the Cedar-Riverside community and the North Minneapolis community. The sites primarily serve East African and African American community members, including the Somali community. Services include drop-in hours during which a nurse or doctor is available for one-on-one consultation, massage, aromatherapy, and healthy living classes on topics, such as nutrition, exercise, chronic disease, and emotional health. In 2019, there were 6,512 visits to both sites with a total of 32,057 visits between 2014 and 2019. More than 80% of participants reported making positive lifestyle changes because of Health Commons services (M Health Now, M Health Fairview 2019). Lifestyle changes include healthier eating, increased exercise, and improved stress management. Programming at the Health Commons is supported by several partnerships.

VETERANS HEALTH ADMINISTRATION

Complementary therapies are part of care provided to military veterans. The 2016 Addiction and Recovery Act requires the Veterans Health Administration (VA) to expand research, education, and delivery of complementary therapies to improve the effectiveness of complementary and integrative health services for veterans (Community Anti-Drug Coalitions of America, 2021). Farmer et al. (2021) reported findings related to a national survey of complementary and integrative health (CIH) approaches offered at the VA. According to the survey, respondents described offering 1,568 CIH programs across the United States. Sites offered between 1 and 23 therapies, with an average of five therapies or approaches per program. The five most common CIH approaches provided in the 196 sites were meditation (72% of respondents), mindfulness (other than mindfulness-based stress reduction techniques; 69%), guided imagery (63%), yoga (62%), and meditation (57%) (Farmer et al., 2021).

Elwy et al. (2020) conducted a longitudinal, mixed-hierarchical study on veterans' use of complementary therapies and their related outcomes. Four hundred one surveys were received from 119 veterans. Several complementary therapies were reported to impact patient outcomes. Yoga was related to relieving stress. Tai chi was related to overall improved Patient-Reported Outcome Measurement Information System 28 (PROMIS 28) mental and physical health function, as well as the subscales of anxiety and ability to engage in social role activities. Meditation was associated with the PROMIS 28 subscale of improved physical function. The study findings, in conjunction with other study findings, suggest the importance of offering veterans complementary therapy options to support health and well-being (Elwy et al., 2020).

There is significant interest in using complementary therapies to treat chronic pain and posttraumatic stress disorder (PTSD) because these are growing concerns in the VA. The U.S. Department of Veterans Affairs (2018) estimated that in any given year, 10% to 20% of U.S. service members deployed to Iraq or Afghanistan and 12% of Gulf War U.S. service members experience PTSD. Additionally, it is estimated that 30 out of every 100 Vietnam service members have PTSD in their lifetimes related to their service experience. Another cause of PTSD in the military may be related to sexual assault. The U.S. Department of Veteran Affairs estimates 55% of women and 38% of U.S. service members have experienced sexual assault or harassment while in the military (U.S. Department of Veteran Affairs, 2018). Several complementary therapies have been identified as potentially beneficial for treating PTSD. A review of research evidence for randomized control trials by Niles et al. (2018) identified mindfulness, yoga, and relaxation as three mind-body techniques that are effective interventions for PTSD. The U.S. Department of Veterans Affairs lists complementary treatments on its National Center for PTSD website and provides brochures that highlight the evidence (U.S. Department of Veterans Affairs, 2014). The VA is committed to maximizing the roles that nurses play in comprehensive holistic care for veterans. The Office of Nursing developed the Clinical Practice Program to support nursing clinical practice. Ten specialty advisory committees consisting of a clinical nurse advisor and nurses actively involved in clinical practice focus on identifying and developing recommendations for best practice guidelines and patient care standards and policies (U.S. Department of Veterans Affairs, 2021a). Each of these specialty committees is examining evidence for integrating complementary therapies into comprehensive recommendations.

The VA is working for patient-driven care across its entire system through a Health for Life program. The VA's Whole Health model focuses on empowering the individual's self-healing mechanisms. This model is evidence-based and makes use of all appropriate therapeutic approaches, including complementary and integrative health therapies along with traditional approaches to disease and injury management (U.S. Department of Veterans Affairs, 2021b; Whitehead &

Kligler, 2020). To date, eight complementary therapies have been approved for use in the VA including acupuncture, biofeedback, clinical hypnosis, guided imagery, massage therapy, meditation, tai chi, and yoga (Whitehead & Kligler, 2020). All VA medical facilities, whether at a VA medical center or at a community medical center, are mandated to provide access to these therapies when appropriate. Data support the legitimacy of services offered through the VA's Whole Health model as demonstrated by a decrease in opioid use, greater engagement in self-care practices and in health care, and overall improved well-being of veterans who utilized the Whole Health model services as compared to those who did not utilize these services (Whitehead & Kligler, 2020).

Nurses have led the development and evaluation of Integrative Health Clinics for outcomes on chronic pain and stress, depression, anxiety, and PTSD. One such clinic in Salt Lake City, Utah, concluded that an Integrative Health Clinic and Program was effective at improving chronic pain, stress-related depression, anxiety, and health-related quality of life for veterans. This low-risk, low-cost program used complementary and alternative mind–body skills and was an innovative treatment option that was acceptable to patients and providers (Smeeding et al., 2010).

NURSES USING COMPLEMENTARY THERAPIES

Nurses are key to helping integrate complementary and alternative therapies into clinical practice. They are in a critical position to guide and impact the growth and use of complementary therapies in the continuum of healthcare environments. Nurses have a background and educational curriculum that focuses on holistic mind, body, and spiritual care, although room for improvement regarding knowledge and the use of complementary therapies exists. The nursing profession has long been a strong advocate of holistic nursing care.

A national survey of critical care nurses was conducted by Tracy et al. (2005) to determine attitudes, knowledge, perspectives, and use of complementary and alternative therapies. This study used a random sample of members of the American Association of Critical-Care Nurses, with 726 respondents. The results indicated that most of the respondents were using one or more complementary and alternative therapies in their clinical practice. The most common therapies mentioned were diet, exercise, relaxation techniques, and prayer. A majority of the nurses had some knowledge of more than half of the 28 therapies listed on the survey and desired additional training for 25 therapies (Tracy et al., 2005). The participants generally required more evidence before using or recommending conventional therapy than before using or recommending complementary and alternative therapies. Overall, the respondents viewed complementary and alternative therapies positively, perceived them as legitimate and beneficial to patients for a variety of symptoms, and were open to their use (Tracy et al., 2005).

A majority of respondents desired increased availability of therapies for patients, families, and nursing staff. Respondents' professional use of the therapies was related to additional knowledge about them, the perception of benefits from them, the total number of therapies recommended to patients, personal use, and affiliation with a mainstream religion. This study concluded the benefits of having educational programs that provide information about and evidence for the use of complementary and alternative therapies would increase the appropriate use of these therapies (Tracy et al., 2005).

Lartey et al. (2019) surveyed members of four state School Nurses Associations using a cross-sectional convenience method. There were 209 respondents to the survey. Most of the participants were able to correctly define complementary medicine, but less than 50% indicated an understanding of integrative medicine. A majority of the respondents indicated they believed that music therapy, art therapy, meditation, and yoga were evidence-based. Massage, acupuncture, prayer/spiritual interventions, and chiropractic care were identified as valid therapies by 40% to 50% of the school nurse participants. Alternatively, less than 28% of the participants believed that aromatherapy, hypnotherapy/hypnosis, herbal medicine, and homeopathic therapies were legitimate (Lartey et al., 2019).

The respondents reported little experience with and knowledge of complementary therapies. Less than 20% of school nurses reported that they had seen a variety of complementary therapies used by students in their practice. Complementary therapies that were identified included art therapy, music therapy, yoga, meditation, herbal medicine, homeopathy, massage, and prayer or spiritual interventions (Lartey et al., 2019). Some participants identified that they had safety concerns regarding the use of homeopathy, herbal medicine, hypnotherapy/hypnosis, chiropractic, and acupuncture therapies. Conversely, some school nurses identified they felt comfortable implementing or assisting with some complementary therapies, including music therapy, meditation, prayer/spiritual interventions, yoga, and aromatherapy (Lartey et al., 2019). Additionally, between 17% and 50.3% reported their school district or state board did not allow them to use integrative therapies.

Even though respondents had little experience with complementary therapies, most participants, 100% of certified school nurses and 63% of noncertified nurses, shared that they believed complementary therapies have a role in nursing practice. A significant majority of respondents (82.4%) identified that complementary and integrative therapy education is important and should be incorporated into school nurse training. Most of the respondents thought children should have complementary therapies integrated into their care if the child wanted it. Even though most respondents supported the use of complementary therapies in their practice by school-aged children, only 19% of respondents reported feeling comfortable with assessing the use of alternative therapies. Additionally, only 12% felt comfortable with their knowledge of complementary therapies used by students. This lack of comfort is illustrated by 55% of participants not assessing students for their use of complementary therapies. A lack of knowledge was also identified regarding the school district or state board of nursing policy regarding complementary therapies and student use.

Hall et al. (2017) conducted a systematic review of nurses' attitudes toward complementary therapies. Fifteen articles were included in the analysis representing seven countries. Five themes emerged from the review. One theme addressed the *strengths and weaknesses of conventional medicine*. Although nurses often deferred to Western medicine, complementary therapies were seen by some nurses as a way to address some of the limitations of conventional care. Nurses perceived complementary therapies as viable options especially when Western medicine treatments related to chronic conditions, pain, stress, and sleep problems failed

(Hall et al., 2017). A second theme *included the use of complementary therapies as a way to enhance nursing practice*. Nurses believed that complementary therapies support the values of nursing. Complementary therapies expand the tools nurses have to care for patients and provide opportunities to care for both the soul and the body of the patient at the same time. In addition, providing complementary therapies increased job satisfaction among nurses. The third theme, *patient empowerment and patient-centeredness*, promotes the patient as the center of care and the decision-maker of care. The use of complementary therapies was seen as a patient choice and gave patients greater control (Hall et al., 2017). The fourth theme identified was *cultural barriers and enablers to integration*. Personal experience, collegial skepticism, and institutional culture were related descriptive themes. Nurses who had previous positive experiences with using complementary therapies positively correlated to the use of complementary therapies, while negative perceptions of colleagues and lack of institutional support negatively correlated to the use of complementary therapies in practice. The final theme was *structural barriers and enablers to integration*. One of the descriptive themes was knowledge and skills. More than 50% of the studies reported that a lack of knowledge and skills was a barrier to the implementation of complementary therapies into practice. Only one study identified knowledge and skills as an enabler to implementing complementary therapies into practice. Another barrier included a view that nurses did not have adequate knowledge to promote patients' use of complementary therapies or offer clear recommendations (Hall et al., 2017).

Evidence continues to support findings that there is a need for nurses to have increased education regarding complementary therapies to appropriately support patient use. This need for nursing education regarding the use of complementary therapies is of global concern. In addition to the studies previously presented, several international studies also report nurse's perceived lack of knowledge of complementary therapies and need for education regarding these therapies (Gok Metin et al., 2018; Gyasi, 2018; Hall et al., 2018; Jong et al., 2015; Kim, 2017).

Nursing as a profession is well rooted in understanding the supportive needs of patients to reduce stress and allow for healing from illness or disease. Nurses are exposed to stress in their own lives and in the work environment. They can benefit from incorporating stress-reducing complementary and integrative therapies as a way to prevent professional burnout and improve their own self-care. There is an especially great potential for stress and burnout among new nurses (Boychuk Duchscher & Cowin, 2006; Laschinger et al., 2016). In a study of new nurses with less than 2 years' tenure, 66% were found to have symptoms of burnout, mental exhaustion, and depression (Cho et al., 2006). Laschinger et al. (2016) found that more than half of the respondents experienced high levels of emotional exhaustion. Complementary therapies aimed at stress reduction and relaxation may be helpful in supporting both new and experienced nurses to manage ongoing stressful activities and events.

A study by Tucker and colleagues (2012) on stress ratings and health-promotion practices among more than 2,200 RNs highlighted the importance of continued focus on the health of nurses and recognized a large opportunity for incorporating complementary therapies into nursing self-care. Study results indicated that although overall stress levels of nurses who participated were similar to the national average, the stress levels were inversely correlated with overall health-promotion behavior scores. Nurses with caregiver responsibilities out-side of their nursing roles had higher stress and lower health-promoting behav-ior scores. In a multivariate analysis, health responsibility, spiritual growth, and stress management accounted for most of the variance in perceived stress scores. The findings support work-site interventions that promote nurses' health and wellness and a focus on reducing work and home stress using complementary relaxation and exercise strategies.

Resiliency can counter burnout and can be improved through the integra-tion of complementary practices into self-care. Andersen et al. (2021) found that resiliency increased at four weeks with a sustained effect for 3 months when staff nurses employed a brief activity using a portable resiliency toolkit. The par-ticipants indicated they would continue to use the tool kit even after the study concluded. The toolkit incorporated several complementary therapies, including aromatherapy sticks, gaming, deep breathing exercises, guided meditations, and an activity book (Andersen et al., 2021).

A related study evaluated the results of HeartMath, an approach incorpo-rating complementary therapies into an educational intervention, on the stress of health team members. The compelling imperative for the project was to find a positive and effective way to address the documented stress levels of health-care workers. A pilot study of primarily nurses, including oncology staff (n = 29) and healthcare leaders (n = 15), explored the impact of a positive coping approach on Personal and Organizational Quality Assessment–Revised scores (HeartMath Institute & Caring Management Consulting, 1999–2002) at baseline and at 7 months using paired t tests. Baseline measures of distress demonstrated that stress and its symptoms are problematic issues for hospital and ambulatory clinic staff nurses. This workplace intervention which included complementary therapies was feasible and effective in promoting positive strategies for coping and enhancing well-being, personally and organizationally (Pipe et al., 2011).

By gaining a greater appreciation of the value of complementary therapies for their own well-being, nurses can be very instrumental in further integration of these modalities into comprehensive holistic care for themselves and their patients. Organizations have opportunities to support professional nurses in self-care activities to mitigate stress and build resiliency. Case study 28.1 illuminates how one organization supports its staff in these self-care endeavors.

Nurses can continue serving as strong advocates for patients and families and communicate with interdisciplinary team members, promoting the use of complementary therapies. Motivated nurses influence standards, guidelines, and policies for using complementary therapies in clinical nursing. Nurses can also develop frameworks and practice models for hospital-based complementary alter-native therapy services.

NURSES LEADING INTEGRATION IN HEALTHCARE SETTINGS

Nurses are integral healthcare leaders who provide support for integrating complementary therapies into healthcare practices. It is not easy to bring these practices into the current healthcare environment. There is still a level of skepti-cism about the evidence for such practices. Nurses need to be savvy about how to gather evidence by reviewing the literature and conducting research studies or evidence-based practice projects that can influence healthcare leaders.

The financial challenges in healthcare are great, and these services, although increasingly in demand by patients, are often not covered by insurance and are not seen as generating revenue. This is where nurse administrators and leaders can help meet the challenges of optimizing healing environments in an efficient manner to meet the challenges of an evolving healthcare landscape. This may involve developing clear business models for how these practices align with strategic goals within healthcare systems and benchmarking with other programs that have been able to sustain these models of care over time.

Nurses need to be able to create partnerships with other key leaders in the healthcare environment to be able to influence holistic models of care and highlight the evidence for complementary and integrative therapies. This may include partnering with physicians, administrators, specialty practice leaders, integrative medicine programs, quality improvement specialists, patient experience leaders, volunteer services, and philanthropic or development leaders. Integrating these programs requires significant collaboration, and nurses must be able to establish buy-in across all disciplines.

Nurses need to be aware of their own state board of nursing statements and requirements for being able to integrate complementary therapies into their practice. They should advocate for the inclusion of using such therapies in state board of nursing guidelines. Nurses should also be afforded the opportunity to work within their own nursing departments to create guidelines and resources that enable them to feel comfortable using complementary therapies. Embedding the use of these therapies into the electronic health record so they can be assessed and included in the plan of care for patients is valuable. Nurses should also be aware of reliable and credible electronic applications and resources that can support patient use of complementary and integrative therapies and self-care practices.

CONCLUSION

Nurses and nurse leaders can garner support for incorporating these therapies into a model of the whole person/whole system perspective. The incorporation of complementary therapies must be aligned with their healthcare facilities' values, missions, strategic initiatives, and priority areas, such as pain management and improvement of the patient experience, and nurses need to be at the table for these discussions. Nurses are on the front line of caring for patients daily and are the advocates for providing additional ways to address patients' needs beyond the typical medical management. Future consideration should be on expanding the data and research on the integration of complementary therapies into nursing practice and the creation of greater support for the inclusion of these practices as a standard for nursing education and practice for all nursing roles—entry-level practice, advanced practice, and administration.

REFERENCES

Abbott Northwestern Hospital: Internal Medicine Residency. (2021). *Applicant tour stop 1: About Abbott Northwestern Hospital.* https://anwresidency.com/applicants/hospital.html

Allina Health. (2021). *Penny George Institute for Health and Healing.* http://wellness.allinahealth.org/servicelines/802

Andersen, S., Mintz-Binder, R., Sweatt, L., & Song, H. (2021). Building nurse resilience in the workplace. *Applied Nursing Research, 59,* 151433. https://doi.org/10.1016/j.apnr.2021.151433

Augsburg University. (n.d.). *Health Commons*. https://www.augsburg.edu/healthcommons/

Boychuk Duchscher, J. E., & Cowin, L. S. (2006). The new graduates' professional inheritance. *Nursing Outlook, 54*(3), 152–158. https://doi.org/10.1016/j.outlook.2005.04.004

Bravewell Collaborative. (2015). *Penny George Institute for Health and Healing*. https://bravewell .org/current_projects/clinical_network/institute_health_healing/

Cho, J., Laschinger, H. K. S., & Wong, C. (2006). Workplace empowerment, work engagement and organizational commitment of new graduate nurses. *Canadian Journal of Nursing Leadership, 19*(3), 43–60. https://doi.org/10.12927/cjnl.2006.18368

Clark, C. S. (2012). Beyond holism: Incorporating an integral approach to support caring-healing-sustainable nursing practices. *Holistic Nursing Practice, 26*(2), 92–102. https://doi.org/10.1097/HNP.0b013e3182462197

Community Anti-Drug Coalitions of America. (2021). *Comprehensive addiction and recovery act (CARA): The comprehensive addition and recovery act (Cara)*. https://www.cadca.org/comprehensive-addiction-and-recovery-act-cara

Courdeau, M. A. (2020). Nursing history and the evolution of holistic nursing. In M. A. Blaszko Helming, D. A., Shields, K. M. Avino, & W. E. Rosa (Eds.), *Dossey & Keegan's holistic nursing: A handbook for practice* (8th ed., pp. 3–23). Jones & Bartlett Learning.

Dusek, J. A., Finch, M., Plotnifkoff, G., & Knutson, L. (2010). The impact of integrative medicine on pain management in a tertiary hospital. *Journal of Patient Safety, 6*(1), 48–51. https://doi .org/10.1097/PTS.0b013e3181d10ad5

Elwy, A. R. Taylor, S. L., Zhoa, S., McGowean, M., Plumb, D. N., Westleigh, W., Gaj, L., Yan, G. W., & Bokhour, B. G. (2020). Participating in complementary and integrative health approaches is associated with veterans' patient-reported outcomes over time. *Medical Care, 58*, S125–S132. https://doi.org/10.1097/MLR.0000000000001357

Farmer, M. M., McGowen, M., Yuan, A. H., Whitehead, A. M., Osawe, U., & Taylor, S. L. (2021). Complementary and integrative health approaches offered in the Veterans Health Administration: Results of a national organizational survey. *Journal of Alternative and Complementary Medicine, 27*, S-124–S-130. https://doi.org/10.1089/acm.2020.0395

Gallison, B. S., & Curtin, C. S. (2016). Creating a caring environment illuminates practice potential. *Beginnings (American Holistic Nurses' Association), 36*(1), 20–24. https://doi.org/10.1097/00004650-200505000-00006

Gallison, B. S., & Kester, W. T. (2018). Connecting holistic nursing practice with relationship-based care: A community hospital's journey. *Nurse Leader, 16*(3), 181–185. https://doi.org/10.1016/j.mnl.2018.03.007

George Family Foundation. (2021). *Allina Health*. https://www.georgefamilyfoundation.org/news/nurses-taking-patient-care-to-the-next-level-at-allina-health

Gok Metin, Z., Izgu, N., Karadas, C., & Arikan Donmez, A. (2018). Perspectives of oncology nurses on complementary and alternative medicine in Turkey: A cross-sectional survey. *Holistic Nursing Practice, 32*(2), 107–113. https://doi.org/10.1097/HNP.0000000000000256

Gyasi, R. M. (2018). Unmasking the practices of nurses and intercultural health in Sub-Sahara Africa: A useful way to improve health care? *Journal of Evidence-based Medicine, 23*(1), 1. https://doi.org/10.1177/2515690X18791124

Hall, H., Brosnan, C., Frawley, J., Wardle, J. Collins, M., & Leach, M. (2018). Nurses' communication regarding patients' us of complementary and alternative medicine. *Collegian, 25* (3), 285–291. https://doi.org/10.1016/j.colegn.2017.09.001

Hall, H., Leach, M., Brosnan, C., & Collins, M. (2017). Nurses' attitudes towards complementary therapies: A systematic review and meta-synthesis. *International Journal of Nursing Studies, 69*, 47–56. https://doi.org/10.1016/j.ijnurstu.2017.01.008

Hansen, S. (2012). *Complementary therapy program at hospice puts nurses in unique role*. https://www .nurse.com/blog/2012/09/10/complementary-therapy-program-at-hospice-puts-nurses-in -unique-role-2 This is a broken link

HeartMath Institute & Caring Management Consulting. (1999–2002). *POQA-R personal and organizational quality assessment-revised*.

Hermitage Farm Center for Healing. (n.d.-a). *About Hermitage Farm*. Retrieved February 22, 2022, from https://hermitagefarm.org/about-hermitage-farm/

Hermitage Farm Center for Healing. (n.d.-b). *Home: Welcome to Hermitage Farm*. Retrieved February 22, 2022, from https://hermitagefarm.org/

Higgs, M. (2016). *Spiritual care at Broward Health Imperial Point: Nursing the spirit as the spirit of nursing* (South Florida Hospital News and Healthcare Report). www.southfloridahospitalnews.com

Jong, M., Lundquist, V., & Jong, M. (2015). A cross-sectional study on Swedish licensed nurses' use, practice, perception, and knowledge of complementary and alternative medicine. *Scandinavian Journal of Caring Science, 29*(4), 642–650. https://doi.org/10.1111/scs.12192

Kim, A. K. (2017). Acceptance of complementary and alternative therapy among nurses: A Q-methodological study. *Korean Journal of Adult Nursing, 29*(4), 441–449. https://doi.org/10.7475/kjan.2017.29.4.441

Lartey, G., Sturgeon, L. P., Garrett-Wright, D., Kabir, U. Y., & Eagle, S. (2019). A survey of school nurses' perceptions of complementary, alternative, and integrative therapies. *The Journal of School Nursing: The Official Publication of the National Association of School Nurses, 35*(4), 256–261. https://doi.org/10.1177/1059840518770521

Laschinger, H. K., Cummings, G., Leiter, M., Wong, C., MacPhee, M., Ritchie, J., Wolff, A., Regan, S., Rhéaume-Brüning, A., Jeffs, L., Young-Ritchie, C., Grinspun, D., Gurnham, M. E., Foster, B., Huckstep, S., Ruffolo, M., Shamian, J., Burkoski, V., Wood, K., & Read, E. (2016). Starting out: A time-lagged study of new graduate nurses' transition to practice. *International Journal of Nursing Studies, 57*, 82–95. https://doi.org/10.1016/j.ijnurstu.2016.01.005

M Health Now, M Health Fairview. (2019). *News and stories: Expanded Health Commons will improve healthcare for Cedar-Riverside neighborhood*. M Health.

McKinney, D., & McGrorey, M. (2019). Hoax, hooey, or healing? *Nevada RNformation, 28*(4), 16.

McKinney, D., & McGrorey, M. (2021). Using holistic modalities in the hospital? You bet! *Energy Magazine, 116*, 14–19. https://www.energy.energymagazineonline.com/content_assets/current-issue/julaug2021-lite.pdf

Niles, B. L., Mori, D. L., Polizzi, C., Pless Kaiser, A., Weinstein, E. S., Gershkovich, M., & Wang, C. (2018). A systematic review of randomized trials of mind-body interventions for PTSD. *Journal of Clinical Psychology, 74*(9), 1485–1508. https://doi.org/10.1002/jclp.22634

Northwestern Health Sciences University. (2021). *Pillsbury House Integrated Health Clinic*. https://www.nwhealth.edu/pillsbury-house

Pathways: A Healing Center. (2021a). *About Pathways*. http://www.pathwaysminneapolis.org/about_us

Pathways: A Healing Center. (2021b). *Pathways programming*. https://pathwaysminneapolis.org/programming/

Pipe, T., Buchada, V., Launder, S., Hudak, B., Hulvey, L., Karns, K., & Pendergast, D. (2011). Building personal and professional resources of resilience and agility in the healthcare workplace. *Stress and Health, 28*(1), 11–22. https://doi.org/10.1002/smi.1396

Redeemer Center for Life. (2021). *Health equity: Health commons*. https://www.redeemercenter.org/health-equity

Redeemer Health. (2021). *Compassionate hospice care in NJ & PA*. https://www.redeemerhealth.org/services/home-care/hospice-care

Sendelbach, S., Carole, L., Lapensky, J., & Kshettry, V. (2003). Developing an integrative therapies program in a tertiary care cardiovascular hospital. *Critical Care Nursing Clinics of North America, 15*, 363–372. https://doi.org/10.1016/S0899-5885(03)00002-9

Smeeding, S. J., Bradshaw, D. H., Kumpfer, K., Travithick, S. & Stoddard, G. J. (2010, August). Outcome evaluation of the Veterans Affairs Salt Lake City Integrative Health Clinic for chronic pain and stress-related depression, anxiety, and post-traumatic stress disorder. *Journal of Alternative Complementary Medicine, 16*(8), 823–835. https://doi.org/10.1089/acm.2009.0510

Tracy, M. F., Lindquist, R., Savik, K., Watanuki, S., Sendelbach, S., Kreitzer, M. M., & Berman, B. (2005). Use of complementary and alternative therapies: A national survey of critical care nurses. *American Journal of Critical Care, 14*(5), 404–414. https://doi.org/10.4037/ajcc2005.14.5.404

Tucker, S. J., Weymiller, A. J., Cutshall, S. M., Rhudy, L. M., & Lohse, C. M. (2012). Stress ratings and health promotion practice among RNs at Mayo Rochester: A case for action. *Journal of Nursing Administration, 42*(5), 282–292. https://doi.org/10.1097/NNA.0b013e318253585f

UMC: University Medical Center. (2014a). *About us.* https://www.umcsn.com/Footer/About-UMC-of-Southern-Nevada-Index.aspx?intMenuID=6600&intPageID=305

UMC: University Medical Center. (2014b). *Healthy Living Institute.* https://www.umcsn.com/Medical-Services-at-UMCSN/HealthyLivingInstitute.aspx

U.S. Department of Veterans Affairs. (2014). *Complementary and integrative medicine: A resource for veterans, service members, and their families.* https://www.warrelatedillness.va.gov/education/factsheets/complementary-and-integrative-medicine.pdf

U.S. Department of Veterans Affairs. (2018). *PTSD: National Centers for PTSD: How common is PTSD in veterans?* https://www.ptsd.va.gov/understand/common/common_veterans.asp

U.S. Department of Veterans Affairs. (2021a). *Office of Nursing Services. The clinical practice program.* https://www.va.gov/NURSING/Practice/cpp.asp

U.S. Department of Veterans Affairs. (2021b). *Whole health.* https://www.va.gov/wholehealth

Whitehead, A. M., & Kligler, B. (2020). Innovations in care: Complementary and integrative health in the Veterans Health Administration Whole Health System. *Medical Care, 58*(Suppl 2 9S), S78–S79. https://doi.org/10.1097/MLR.0000000000001383

World Health Organization. (2019). *WHO global report on traditional and complementary medicine 2019.* https://www.who.int/traditional-complementary-integrative-medicine/WhoGlobalReportOnTraditionalAndComplementaryMedicine2019.pdf

Perspectives on Future Research

MARY FRAN TRACY

Nursing's commitment to the generation of high-quality, cost-effective patient outcomes requires that a sound scientific basis for practice be established. Previous chapters have identified existing research related to the therapies reviewed; however, most chapters end with statements that more research is needed. The need for more evidence related to the safety, efficacy, timing, "dose," and specific indications for most therapies is clearly evident. As noted in those chapters and documented in reports from the United States and globally, considerable interest in and use of complementary therapies by the public continues. In a large and comprehensive examination of the use of complementary and alternative therapies, the number of annual visits to providers was found to outnumber visits to primary care physicians (Institute of Medicine [IOM], 2005). Subsequently, the 2012 National Health Interview Survey, a comprehensive in-person survey of Americans regarding their health, found that 33.2% of adults and 11.6% of children surveyed in the United States reported use of a form of complementary and alternative medicine in the preceding 12 months (Black et al., 2015; Clarke et al., 2015). Authors of the 2017 National Health Interview Survey reported significant increases since 2012 in the use of yoga and meditation among both children and adults (Black et al., 2018; Clarke et al., 2018). A 2010 U.S. phone survey of more than 1,000 people aged 50 years and older reported that more than half of the respondents used some form of complementary and alternative medicine; however, only a little more than half of those who reported use said that they had ever discussed their use with their healthcare providers (AARP & National Center for Complementary and Alternative Medicine [NCCAM], 2011). A systematic review of literature comprising 16 studies identified the prevalence rates of the use of complementary and alternative medicine among the general population and health professionals to range from 5% to 74.8% in the countries investigated (Frass et al., 2012). The Pew Center for Research data correspond to this with approximately 50% of Americans having used complementary therapies at least once, 20% having used them in place of conventional therapy, and 33% using them in conjunction with conventional therapy (Pew Research Center, 2017).

The most prevalent use of complementary therapies arguably appears to be by patients dealing with cancer. It has been reported that as many as 45% to 84% of patients use complementary therapies with the intent to cure cancer or for symptom management (Jazieh et al., 2021; Jermini et al., 2019). Consistent with the AARP/NCCAM survey, patient reporting of complementary therapy use to their providers remains concerningly low, ranging from 36% to 58% (Jazieh et al., 2021; Jermini et al., 2019).

One of the most exhaustive data collection on the use of complementary, alternative, and traditional health practices across the globe was published by the World Health Organization (WHO) in 2005 (Ong et al., 2005); it showed a wide range of practices and variability in the degree of use of different therapies. This survey has been repeated twice, with the latest survey in 2018. The WHO reported that 170 member countries acknowledged using traditional (i.e., Indigenous) and complementary medicine (T & CM; WHO, 2019). Of those member countries, 98 reported having national policies on T & CM, 109 had implemented national laws and regulations on T & CM, and 124 had established regulations on herbal products (WHO, 2019).

Interest in complementary therapies is encountered in a broad range of health-care practice settings. Along with public and patient interest, there is a concomitant interest on the part of nurses who not only want to deliver these therapies to patients but also have an interest in the same therapies for their own personal use (Lindquist et al., 2003). The need for this was never more evident than during the COVID-19 pandemic, which only accentuated the reality of stress and burnout for healthcare providers. However, despite provider interest, the therapies most often used by patients are not those that providers are familiar with or that providers most understand (Zhang et al., 2012). In addition to the significant demand and use and a lack of understanding of even commonly used therapies, there is an urgency to increase knowledge among providers and to expand the evidence base that supports the safe and efficacious use of complementary and alternative therapies.

The world is shrinking. "New" therapies or new uses for old therapies are shared across continents. Health providers and researchers are challenged to create and use a solid evidence base to undergird the broad range of complementary therapies used by substantial segments of the United States and populations around the globe. There is an acute need to know and understand the benefits of therapies and whether they work according to the purpose for which they are used; there is also a need to ensure the safety and efficacy of complementary therapies and to understand their effects and interactions when used with other complementary and allopathic therapies. The WHO recognizes these urgent needs in their *Traditional Medicine Strategy 2014–2023* (WHO, 2013). The WHO's strategies fall into three main categories: build the knowledge base; strengthen the quality assurance, safety and proper use, and effectiveness of complementary therapy products; and promote universal health coverage by integrating these therapies in both health systems and self-care through informed consumer choice (WHO, 2013). In this chapter, the need for more evidence to support the expanding use of complementary therapies in practice is presented, research designs appropriate for the study of complementary therapies are explored, the overall state of research on complementary therapies is described, and implications for the state of evidence and expanded use of complementary therapies on future nursing research are identified.

NEED TO EXPAND THE EVIDENCE BASE

The significant documented worldwide interest in and use of alternative and complementary therapies and alternative systems of care have caused healthcare providers to acknowledge the appeal of these therapies to consumers and to carefully consider their safety and efficacy. Concomitantly, questions regarding costs and cost-effectiveness need to be answered for third-party payers and for individuals paying out of pocket. Questions need to be answered through research related to which therapies to select for given conditions, how many treatment sessions are necessary, and what results from the treatment can be expected. The optimal mix and relative cost of the complementary or alternative therapies versus traditional Western treatments must be determined.

With the widespread use of complementary and alternative therapies, there is a reason for concern regarding the safety of their use and their potential interactions with Western medicine. An example is the interaction of herbal remedies such as St. John's wort with prescribed pharmacotherapy, including cyclosporine, oral contraceptives, coumadin, digoxin, and benzodiazepines, as well as others (National Center for Complementary and Integrative Health [NCCIH], 2021b). Contributing to the difficulty is the lack of regulation of complementary and alternative therapies, such as dietary supplements (Ventola, 2010), although increasing attention is being paid to this in an effort to provide guidance for their use to better ensure patient safety (Research Council for Complementary Medicine, 2016). The creation of the WHO's guidelines for the standardization of herbal drugs not only recognizes the value of herbal medicine and its increased use but also acknowledges the concerns about its safety and efficacy (Pradham et al., 2015). Indeed, scientific data in this area are needed by providers to inform their practice. Accurate and reliable knowledge is also needed by consumers who wish to make informed decisions regarding their own health practices.

There are increasing expectations, and indeed a mandate for, evidence-based practice (EBP). *EBP* has been defined as "the use of the best available evidence together with a clinician's expertise and a patient's values and preferences in making healthcare decisions" (Agency for Healthcare Research and Quality [AHRQ], 2018). Nurses and other providers practicing in the context of conventional allopathic care rely on an evidence base. It would be anticipated that they are relying on or requiring similar evidence in their use of complementary therapies, although this may vary among providers. In a national survey, critical care nurses generally reported that they required more evidence for conventional allopathic remedies than they did for complementary and alternative therapies (Tracy et al., 2005).

Resources for accessing knowledge about complementary and alternative therapies must be identified, made available, and used by providers; this information needs to be shared with and accessible by patients and their families (Latte-Naor, 2019). Patients get information and are influenced about complementary therapy use more frequently from family and passed down traditions (Bauml et al., 2015; Latte-Naor, 2019). Decisions about complementary therapy use are made without the input of providers, particularly when providers are perceived as not supportive or knowledgeable about complementary and alternative therapies (Latte-Naor, 2019). An AARP/NCCAM survey (2011) reported that 42% of patient nondisclosures were due to providers not asking. These participants also described not knowing they should disclose, not having enough time during the visit, perceptions of providers' lack of knowledge, or fears of being dismissed by the providers. This lack of bilateral communication can affect patient–provider relationships and treatment choices (Latte-Naor, 2019).

To support informed consumer decision-making, the National Cancer Institute (NCI, 2021) provides informative, though cautionary, data regarding the safety of complementary therapy approaches; this site, as well as the NCCIH website, reminds visitors that "natural does not mean safe" (NCCIH, 2021f). The NCCIH emphasizes to health professionals (NCCIH, 2021e) the need to communicate with their patients and provides resources to consumers (NCCIH, 2021d) about how to identify disinformation and understand complex scientific topics. Research findings regarding the safety and efficacy of therapies must be disseminated broadly to practitioners, who need to be informed so that the safety of patients can be protected, and the potential benefits of therapies realized. A number of smartphone–based resources provide access to authoritative information as a resource for professional practice. Databases of research findings, such as the Cochrane Database of Systematic Reviews (www.cochranelibrary.com/advanced-search), are other good resources for synthesized research findings. As of October 2021, a simple search of "complementary and alternative therapies" on this online resource produced 59 Cochrane reviews related to healing therapies such as healing touch, dietary products, acupuncture, reflexology, meditation, relaxation techniques, herbal medicine, manual therapies, mind–body therapies, hypnosis, aromatherapy, homeopathy, yoga, imagery, and massage. These reviews are an excellent source of well-integrated research-based knowledge about what is known regarding the use of therapies for specific conditions. There were also 1,249 trials registered with the Cochran Central Register of Controlled Trials on complementary therapies. This registry did not include any trials that were initiated related to the COVID-19 pandemic. In addition, websites of government agencies, such as the NCCIH in the National Institutes of Health (NIH; NCCIH, 2021c) and the Office of Cancer Complementary and Alternative Medicine (OCCAM; https://cam.cancer.gov) within the NCI, provide other sources of information on a wide range of complementary and alternative therapies. The Natural Medicines Professional Database provides high-quality information regarding herbs, dietary supplements, natural products, and other complementary therapies used for specific health conditions (Therapeutic Research Center, 2017). The information is graded on a scale ranging from A to F to reflect the level of scientific evidence available.

The NCCIH supports investigator-initiated research and interdisciplinary research training initiatives (NCCIH, 2021g). With a special encouragement of research that focuses on complementary and alternative therapies commonly used by the American public, the NCCIH has begun building a solid foundation from which therapies can be selected and delivered with growing confidence as to their safety and efficacy. To this end, one of their initiatives is a center for excellence for natural product–drug interaction research. This collaboration between Washington State University, the University of Pittsburgh, and the University of North Carolina, Greensboro recommends approaches for assessing the clinical implications of interactions between natural products and drugs, testing those approaches on high-priority combinations, and maintaining a repository for research results on interactions (Hopp, 2021). Unfortunately, while the types of interactions focused on are broad, it is not inclusive due to the sheer number of potential combinations that would need to be tested (Hopp, 2021).

Despite these increasing efforts, much work is yet to be done. The ideal evidence base for complementary therapies would support decision-making in a broad range of complex patient situations. It would differentiate effects on and appropriateness for people with diverse characteristics (e.g., age, gender, body mass) from various cultures (accounting for dietary practices, social acceptability, cultural traditions, and so forth) and genetic makeup, and it would outline the potential differing effects and indications for individuals suffering the full range of pathologies and comorbidities.

There are legitimate safety concerns related to therapy selection, the quality of products (the purity or technique of delivery), dose, timing, duration, and other considerations related to specific therapies such as herbal therapies, nutraceuticals, and supplements. For example, more research is needed to identify potentially adverse drug–herb interactions to answer questions related to whether particular drugs and herbs can be ingested simultaneously; if not, the half-life of herbs in the body, or their "washout" times, need to be determined. Research is also needed to provide data to document the relative risks and benefits of therapies such as the use of diet therapy for hypertension (as opposed to standard allopathic pharmacological therapies) or to consider the potential reduction of the side effects of an allopathic agent if used at a reduced dose but with a complementary therapy.

The growing evidence base provides much-needed information for the consumer and provider. However, additional research is needed to determine the potential beneficial outcomes of complementary therapies. Likewise, studies are necessary to generate findings that protect the public from harm or from needless, costly therapies that have no evidence to support them or no clear evidence of benefit. For example, alternative therapies used to combat cancer cause concern among allopathic providers who fear that the false hope of cure can dissuade patients from seeking legitimate forms of cancer therapy (Latte-Naor, 2019); an additional concern is that the therapy can bleed fortunes from desperate families, despite the fact that there may be no basis for its claims of beneficial effects (NCI, 2021). Extramural funding opportunities and the peer-review system of the NIH ensure the continued accumulation of high-quality evidence and encourage investigators who have the ideas, curiosity, and scientific expertise to explore potential therapies for human use.

RESEARCH DESIGNS FOR THE STUDY OF COMPLEMENTARY THERAPIES

Most scientists would agree that the most rigorous design for testing complementary and alternative therapies is the randomized, placebo-controlled, double-blind design that has long been the standard for testing therapies and advancing fields of inquiry, but randomized controlled trials (RCTs) are not without their limitations (Bothwell et al., 2016). However, this design is not the only one that provides useful information, and data generated from quantitative studies are not the only available evidence base for practice. Other designs and sources of evidence are also important and contribute to knowledge and understanding of patients' responses to therapies, both allopathic and nonallopathic. In addition, even if rigorous studies do not confirm the benefits of a specific complementary therapy approach, they can give insight into how future studies should be designed.

Consumers may be increasingly reluctant to enroll in clinical trials; hence, alternative study designs and strategies for the conduct of clinical research to advance the field are needed (Gul & Ali, 2010). The Committee on the Use of Complementary and Alternative Medicine by the American Public was commissioned by the IOM, the AHRQ, the NCCAM, and 15 other agencies and institutes of the NIH to study and provide specific recommendations regarding complementary and alternative therapies. As part of their report (IOM, 2005), innovative alternative designs for providing information about the effectiveness of therapies were identified, including the following:

- **preference RCTs**—trials that include randomized and nonrandomized arms, which then permit comparisons between patients who chose a particular treatment and those who were randomly assigned to it
- **observational and cohort studies**—studies that involve the identification of patients who are eligible for study and who may receive a specified treatment as part of the study
- **case-control studies**—studies that involve identifying patients who have good or bad outcomes and then "working back" to find aspects of treatment associated with those differing outcomes
- **studies of bundles of therapies**—analyses of the effectiveness, as a whole, of particular packages of treatments
- **studies that specifically incorporate, measure, or account for placebo or expectation effects**—patients' hopes, emotional states, energies, and other self-healing processes are not considered extraneous but are included as part of the therapy's main "mechanism of action"
- **attribute-treatment interaction analyses**—a way of accounting for differences in effectiveness outcomes among patients within a study and among different studies of varying design (p. 3)

EMPLOYING INNOVATIVE RESEARCH DESIGNS

Complementary and integrative approaches are often criticized due to a lack of scientific evidence. Building the scientific evidence base about the usefulness and safety of complementary and integrative approaches is critical for the decision-making of healthcare professionals, including nurses (NCCIH, 2021a). However, it is difficult to investigate the safety, efficacy, and effectiveness of complementary therapies and integrative approaches to care. The NCCIH recently introduced flexible and innovative clinical trial designs to assess complementary and integrative approaches and to help researchers to conduct studies in "real-world" settings (NCCIH, 2021a). These flexible and innovative designs will facilitate investigating the roles of complementary and integrative healthcare strategies in preventing disease, improving health, and managing symptoms (NCCIH, 2021a). In the early stages of clinical research, including pilot and feasibility studies, investigators can use these innovative designs to develop, optimize, and establish intervention protocols and to develop possible resources and strategies for recruiting participants, obtaining measurements, and implementing the study intervention. With the increasing use of electronic health records, hypotheses can be postulated to leverage these large databases regarding complementary therapy use and effectiveness. Larger efficacy or effectiveness studies can use these flexible and innovative designs to assess generalizability in the "real-world" setting. These innovative designs can optimize existing infrastructure for data collection in a cost-effective manner, allowing the NCCIH to fund more large-scale trials (NCCIH, 2021a).

Bayesian approaches are flexible and innovative statistical approaches often used for studying pharmacokinetics/pharmacodynamics, decision-making, toxicity monitoring, efficacy monitoring, and dose-finding (Lee & Chu, 2012). Bayesian approaches are used, for example, when providers decide their preferred option of the therapy to maximize the probability of success from published data. Using a Bayesian approach in a meta-analysis of 65 RCTs, Leng and colleagues (2020) determined that massage and animal-assisted therapy were associated with less agitation in patients with dementia among 11 nonpharmacological interventions. In addition, multiphase optimal strategy designs (MOST) can be used for situations in which mind/body interventions need more refining, for determining which components are necessary to achieve benefit, or for determining which therapies need to stay in multi-therapy interventions (NCCIH, 2021a).

Pragmatic clinical trials can be used to determine the effectiveness of interventions in a normal routine practice, whereas explanatory designs can be used to identify efficacy in the ideal setting (MacPherson, 2004). An example of this is a study that used a pragmatic randomized trial to compare the effectiveness between integral-based Hatha yoga and wait-list groups among sedentary adults with arthritis for the purpose of enhancing the RCT's external validity and allowing flexibility of intervention delivery in "real-world" settings (Moonaz et al., 2015). The NCCIH is encouraging pragmatic trials that have preliminary data from large controlled trials that demonstrate clinical efficacy and effectiveness (NCCIH, 2021a). Another innovative design is sequential multiple assignment randomized trials. These designs can be used to determine the sequencing of interventions or to develop algorithms (NCCIH, 2021a).

In an effort to identify major issues in research design in funding proposals submitted to a specific funding program for clinical trials of complementary and alternative medicine for cancer symptom management, a number of problems with scientific methodology were found (Buchanan et al., 2005). Common issues included "unwarranted assumptions about the consistency and standardization of CAM interventions, the need for data-based justifications for the study hypothesis, and the need to implement appropriate quality control and monitoring procedures during the course of the trial" (Buchanan et al., 2005, p. 6682). Such problems need to be addressed and resolved to ensure the rigor and merit of studies of therapies for managing cancer symptoms and symptoms of other conditions.

ADDRESSING POTENTIAL PLACEBO EFFECTS

Another important and challenging area for investigators involves the placebo effect and placebo/attention control groups (Gross, 2005). The power of the placebo effect, and cautions that it should not be underestimated, have long been appreciated (NCCIH, 2020). Placebo effects may lead to improvements in well over 50% of subjects in trials of medical therapies. There is evidence that the placebo effect in clinical trials of complementary and alternative medicine (CAM) is similar to that in clinical trials of conventional medicine (Dorn et al., 2007). Methods for managing placebo effects must be carefully considered in research on complementary therapies. In addition, when assessing the overall effects of a therapy, the potential added impact of the healer, and the therapeutic relationship on the outcome must be considered. Alternative designs for exploring some therapies are needed, as it is may be difficult to use sham therapy or to identify a suitable control group. In a Delphi study on the development of credible shams for physical intervention research designs, key components were reported as managing expectations, standardization between groups, and ensuring the credibility of the sham (Braithwaite et al., 2020). In addition, the blinding of both participants and researchers is essential to ensure the results are due to the intervention. Shams for other complementary therapies can also be difficult to determine. For example, in the case of the study of aromatherapy to enhance sleep, will subjects remain blinded, or will they detect the aroma? If a "sham" aroma is administered to the control group, may it also have undocumented effects beyond a placebo effect?

Simply knowing that a therapy may be beneficial is not enough. Questions such as the following need to be answered: What are the conditions under which the therapy is effective? What is the dose needed? What dose is too much? How often must a therapy be delivered to achieve a benefit? How long does the effect last? How much therapy should insurers cover? There is a need for studies on the cost-effectiveness of complementary therapies and for research that compares and contrasts complementary therapies with other conventional therapies. There is also a need to examine the safety and effectiveness of complementary therapies when used with or as adjuncts to other allopathic pharmacological or nonpharmacological interventions.

CULTURAL CONSIDERATIONS

Studies of therapies relevant to aging populations, populations at varied ages/ developmental stages, and those having varied cultural backgrounds are also needed. These populations present challenges for the design, recruitment, and implementation of studies. Older subjects often have multiple comorbidities and may be taking multiple medications. Language and a lack of cultural understanding may pose barriers to the inclusion of new immigrants. Access to young children, adolescents, and vulnerable adults and the unique ethical issues surrounding their recruitment and participation may also be perceived as barriers to the inclusion of these groups.

Results from Bauml and colleagues (2015) are consistent with other research findings from the general population—patients with cancer who had higher expectations of results of complementary and alternative therapies tend to be female, younger (<65 years of age), and have some college education. Non-White patients with cancer had the same expectations of benefits from complementary therapies, but also perceived more barriers in being able to access and use them (Bauml et al., 2015). Longer transport times to complementary therapy appointments create disparities in access. These non-White participants were also more concerned about side effects of these therapies than other participants in the study. Beliefs and attitudes about the impact of CAM use accounted for more than demographics (Bauml et al., 2015). This supports the importance of providers querying patients about their interest in or use of complementary therapies and assistance in accessing appropriate approaches.

Research methods and findings from one country can inform the design and implementation of studies in other countries. Findings may be relevant across the globe, or interesting nuances or differences can be identified. It is appropriate that native scholars build a culturally relevant evidence base of complementary and

Sidebar 29.1 *Future Research for Complementary and Alternative Therapy in South Korea*

Sohye Lee

In South Korea, complementary and alternative therapies (CATs) based on Chinese medicine and folk remedies have been used since ancient times. Traditionally, certain types of therapy have been underestimated because of their uncertainty, their side effects, and a lack of scientific evidence. Recently, some types of therapy have been studied and experimentally demonstrated to be effective in the treatment of selected health conditions. Many patients who have chronic conditions, such as cancer, stroke, arthritis, cardiovascular disease, diabetes, and obesity, tend to seek CATs to reduce their pain and alleviate anxiety.

Complementary therapies are practiced by South Korean nurses in the provision of care in many clinical specialty areas. Back, hand, and foot massages, as well as patient position changes, are techniques used by nurses to help patients' body circulation and to prevent patient pressure injuries in many intensive care units. Nurse midwives and obstetrics and gynecological nurses use imagery therapy, aromatherapy, reflexology, or hand massage therapy to reduce patients' pain and anxiety. Anesthesia nurses offer music therapy, aromatherapy, or foot massage to relieve patients' pain and anxiety during and after surgery. Oncology nurses recommend mind therapy (meditation) to their cancer patients for alleviating symptoms and maintaining mental stability.

According to the Korean Nurses Association for Complementary and Alternative Therapy, there are many areas being developed: hand therapy, aromatherapy, foot therapy, alternative dietary therapy, hortitherapy, and hypogastric breathing. Even though the difficulties of applying CATs to patients without strong scientific foundations remain, nurse researchers are trying to develop and test these CATs within nursing's holistic view. They also want to develop these CATs as nursing interventions to help their patients in many areas.

A study reported on Korean research trends in CATs. They found primary articles on foot massage, hand therapy, aromatherapy, acupressure, moxibustion (heat therapy), or combined therapy. They found that foot massage and aromatherapy were effective in improving sleep quality (Kim et al., 2006). As the authors asserted, more research is needed to find scientific evidence for these approaches.

CAT can be used for disease prevention and health promotion. Koreans are getting more interested in healthy eating and physical activity nowadays after the economy has stabilized. Yoga and Pilates are very popular among young women for weight management, stress relief, or posture correction. Stretch exercises, such as tai chi, have been implemented for older adults in public community health centers. Dietary therapies are broadly used for weight loss and management, enhancing the immune system, and maintaining better health.

For prevention, treatment, and rehabilitation, CATs have huge potential to be developed in Korea. The efficacy and safety of these CATs should be examined in order to be used widely.

Reference

Kim, H. J., Lee, K. S., Lee, M. H., Jung, D. S., Yoo, J. S., Han, H. S., & Park, M. S. (2006). An analysis of Korean research on complementary and alternative therapy. *Thesis Collection, 41*, 529–539.

alternative therapies for use. The work of nurse scholars in South Korea described in Sidebar 29.1 illustrates this point.

Other outcomes are sought by healthcare consumers. That a therapy is shown to have beneficial health effects is not the only legitimate reason for its use. Immigrants tend to use complementary and alternative therapies first and then seek conventional medical help if these are not effective (Garcés et al., 2006). Such patterns and the use of complementary therapies as an alternative to conventional care may also be attributable, in part, to barriers to conventional care or a lack of insurance (Zhang, 2011). Certain therapies may also have cultural significance or be intricately tied with healing traditions, may lead to patients' peace of mind, or may meet patient and family expectations or lead to their increased satisfaction. For patients who have come to the United States from other countries, the cultural belief in alternative or complementary medicine is not changed. In considering the use of complementary therapies, the costs, risks, and value to recipients must be carefully weighed.

LONGITUDINAL STUDIES

Many studies have used small samples and examined the short-term effects of therapies. If we want to know the real risks and benefits of complementary and alternative therapies, we need longitudinal studies because we can determine the severity and occurrence of adverse events only when therapies are applied on a long-term basis. Recently, the first longitudinal analysis of predictive factors of new, continued, and discontinued use of complementary therapies was published (Scott et al., 2021). Data were collected over 20 years (three waves) and were able to report on trends over time on therapies such as massage therapy, meditation, and herbal products. This study is a start as foundational information on the use and discontinued use, although the authors acknowledge the ongoing need for confirmation of their findings and to explore these factors in subpopulations (Scott et al., 2021).

Although similar longitudinal studies using the same design are performed, different results may be obtained from people from different cultures. Therefore, it is important that we study complementary and alternative therapy using the same or similar designs in other countries and different cultures.

CURRENT STATE OF RESEARCH ON COMPLEMENTARY THERAPIES

As previously noted, the chapter authors have included the most recent research and have identified where more research is needed to provide knowledge to guide practice. Specific research challenges include the need for data-based decision support resources for combination therapies. Such resources would include data related to potential adverse interactions or the potentiating effects of therapies when given in combination. There is a need for research with special populations, including children, frail older adults, and the critically ill, as well as those from ethnically and culturally diverse populations. Research is needed to study the effects of complementary therapies in specific health conditions or disease states. Clearly, research lags behind the public's appetite for complementary therapies; knowledge of the putative mechanisms of action, the qualities of therapies, and the predictability of outcomes is uneven across therapies.

Insistence on the use of standard conventions of scientific inquiry has been helpful in increasing the amount of evidence systematically obtained to provide information for decision-making in complementary therapies. However, information is lacking on the appropriate dose and timing of interventions and on those for whom the interventions may have the most beneficial effects. A solid evidence base for complementary therapies would support decision-making in broad and complex patient situations. Complementary therapies may have different effects on people of diverse ethnic backgrounds and demographic characteristics. So, too, they may have potentially different indications and effects in people suffering from differing pathologies or medical conditions. The lack of such information is limiting to practitioners who rely on a more fully developed evidence base, and this may hinder the full integration of the use of complementary therapies in practice.

Often, studies have been done that have relatively small sample sizes and varying data collection tools; meta-analyses can be conducted to synthesize findings to estimate the "effect sizes" of therapies when examined across studies. These meta-analyses would greatly benefit from studies that consistently use the same instruments whenever possible. Also, large, multicenter studies may facilitate the recruitment of participants so that studies have overall larger sample sizes to enable the testing of hypotheses; such studies are important for scientifically testing the effects of alternative and complementary therapies (Singendonk et al., 2013). Synthesis and review articles would also contribute to the availability of well-organized, available information.

The NCCAM was established by Congress in 1998; in 2015, the center's name was changed to the National Center for Complementary and Integrative Health (NCCIH, 2019). The NCCIH's mission is "to define, through rigorous scientific investigation, the usefulness and safety of complementary and integrative interventions and their roles in improving health and healthcare" (NCCIH, 2019, para. 1). The NCCIH has a strategic plan that includes (a) advancing the fundamental science (such as determining the mechanism of action) and developing research methods; (b) focusing on research that advances the focus on the whole person and integration of findings; (c) fostering research on health promotion and restoration, resilience, disease prevention, and symptom management; (d) expanding the workforce of researchers in complementary health approaches; and (e) disseminating objective evidence-based to the public to promote informed decision-making by consumers (NCCIH, 2021h). The NCCIH website provides an authoritative up-to-date resource with summaries of a wide range of therapies (NCCIH, 2021g). The website also provides a listing of clinical trials that are alphabetized by the name of the therapies. The NCCIH has played a vital role in promoting the generation, organization, and dissemination of data for practice and research. It has fostered a standard language and is a source for arguably the most definitive information and funding. As part of its efforts to achieve its mission, the NCCIH has funded multidisciplinary research centers to foster more rapid development of the scientific knowledge base for the use of complementary and alternative therapies. These centers and their structure, functioning, and productivity have received intensive review, resulting in changes in the focus and mechanisms of funding over time (NCCIH, 2021a, 2021g). The work of the NCCIH promises to increase the scientific evidence base and improve the context and delivery of therapies in the years to come.

IMPLICATIONS FOR NURSING RESEARCH

There is a great need for nurses and scientists in other disciplines to develop ongoing programs of research related to specific complementary therapies, particularly from a holistic, whole-person perspective. As primary care providers, nurses are in an excellent position to address patients' need for complementary therapies. Nurses have a vested interest in generating information that can be used to build the knowledge database underlying the use of specific therapies that may benefit patients. They may also generate data that refute the use of therapies or reveal adverse risk/benefit ratios. Nurses have conducted research on a number of complementary therapies. Most nurse scientists are educated in both qualitative and quantitative designs. This gives them an understanding of multiple ways of constructing research studies to determine the effects of complementary therapies. The need for the expansion and dissemination of evidence and access to it has particular significance for the discipline of nursing and underlies recommendations for future directions in nursing research. As illustrated in the international sidebar and evidenced in the increasingly global contributions of health science researchers, we can draw on the diverse contributions and perspectives of international colleagues.

The need to generate information that can be used to build the evidence base for complementary therapies is compelling for nurse scientists. The specialized clinical expertise of nurse researchers can be used to select therapies to test and target outcomes of importance to their patient populations. Specialized clinical knowledge has the potential to enhance the identification of instruments that are sensitive enough to assess the potential effects of therapies (subjective, objective, or behavioral). Nurses play important roles in generating, disseminating, and using the evidence base for practice.

Interdisciplinary collaborations between nurse investigators and investigators from other disciplines who bring strengths from basic science, genetics, complementary therapies, or clinical practice may lead to a growth of the knowledge base and its breadth, depth, and relevance, which should ultimately improve the quality of care for patients. Collaborations between scientists who are capable of conducting research across disciplines may lead to new breakthroughs with regard to complementary therapies and integrative health approaches.

Broadening the frames of reference of nurse scientists to include global perspectives, genetic breakthroughs, new technologies, and information from around the world will ensure an appropriate and comprehensive view of the field. The WHO's global strategy for 2014 to 2023 will assist countries in blending complementary therapies with the respective countries' established system(s) of healthcare (WHO, 2013).

Such global initiatives and updated strategies on traditional and complementary therapies should serve as catalysts in making information available to practitioners worldwide and should advance the field of complementary and alternative medicine. Electronic means of posting new knowledge, warnings, or updated information on clinical trials speeds the availability of information and have the potential to bring a world of information to bear on practice—but only if used.

Electronic publishing speeds the transfer of research findings to practice settings. The mandate set forth by prominent medical publishers that requires investigators to enroll their studies in a registry of clinical trials for their results to be published in highly distinguished medical journals was a step in the right direction; there are worldwide listings of clinical trials (U.S. Department of Health and Human Services, 2015).

Clinical research is costly. Advanced research training may help hone nurse-investigators' grant-writing skills to pursue needed funds for investigative work to generate new knowledge in the field. Design skills that permit nurse investigators to rigorously test interventions and advance clinical knowledge about the use of complementary therapies are critical. However, studies conducted in non-clinical settings, including surveys of public use of complementary therapies, are also important. Nursing research is also needed to focus on the costs, relative cost-versus-benefits ratio, and ethical issues surrounding access to and delivery of therapies.

Nurses and other providers have responsibilities to provide the public with guidance in using complementary therapies, interpret and share scientific information, and contribute to the development of the knowledge base through investigation and research dissemination. Guidelines that are founded in the evidence base are clearly needed to set the standards for the appropriate use of complementary therapies. In addition, it is imperative that nursing consider and conduct research beyond patient populations to healthcare workers themselves. With the anticipated long-term mental health effects from the COVID-19 pandemic compounding the increasing burnout and compassion fatigue that was occurring pre-pandemic, nurses can play a vital role in accumulating evidence on how complementary therapies can assist colleagues in order to stem this crisis. This work directly relates to optimizing the care of patients since healthcare workers must be healthy and resilient to provide optimal care to the populations they serve.

Using available knowledge and methods to disseminate research electronically and making information available at the point of care is important. However, as noted in the concluding sections of the intervention chapters of this book, many questions remain to be answered for the application of therapies in general, as well as for populations and individuals with different cultures, ages, and comorbidities. More research is needed to answer the myriad questions that exist, and it is increasingly recognized that interdisciplinary, multicultural, and transglobal partnerships may be the most fruitful in answering these questions.

REFERENCES

AARP & National Center for Complementary and Alternative Medicine. (2011, April). *Complementary and alternative medicine: What people aged 50 and older discuss with their health care providers. AARP & NCCAM Survey Report.* https://nccih.nih.gov/sites/nccam.nih.gov/files/news/camstats/2010/NCCAM_aarp_survey.pdf

Agency for Healthcare Research and Quality. (2018). *Evidence-based decisionmaking.* https://www.ahrq.gov/professionals/prevention-chronic-care/decision/index.htm

Bauml, J. M., Chokshi, S., Schapira, M. M., Im, E-O., Li, S. Q., Langer, C. J., Ibrahim, S. A., & Mao, J. J. (2015). Do attitudes and beliefs regarding complementary and alternative medicine impact its use among patients with cancer? A cross-sectional survey. *Cancer, 121,* 2431–2438. https://doi.org/10.1002/cncr.29173

Black, L. I., Barnes, P. M., Clarke, T. C., Stussman, B. J., & Nahin, R. L. (2018). *Use of yoga, meditation, and chiropractors among U.S. children aged 4–17 year* (NCHS Data Brief, no. 324). National Center for Health Statistics.

Black, L. I., Clarke, T. C., Barnes, P. M., Stussman, B. J., & Nahin, R. L. (2015). Use of complementary health approaches among children aged 4–17 years in the United States: National Health Interview Survey, 2007–2012. *National Health Statistics Reports, 78*, 1–19. https://pubmed.ncbi.nlm.nih.gov/25671583/

Bothwell, L. E., Greene, J. A., Podolsky, S. H., & Jones, D. S. (2016). Assessing the gold standard—Lessons from the history of RCTs. *New England Journal of Medicine, 374*, 2175–2181. https://doi.org/10.1056/NEJMms1604593

Braithwaite, F. A., Walters, J. L., Moseley, G. L., Williams, M. T., & McEvoy, M. T. (2020). Towards more credible shams for physical interventions: A Delphi study. *Clinical Trials, 17*(3), 295–305. https://doi.org/10.1177/1740774520910365

Buchanan, D. R., White, J. D., O'Mara, A. M., Kelaghan, J. W., Smith, W. B., & Minasian, L. M. (2005). Research-design issues in cancer-symptom-management trials using complementary and alternative medicine: Lessons from the National Cancer Institute Community Clinical Oncology Program experience. *Journal of Clinical Oncology, 23*(27), 6682–6689. https://doi.org/10.1200/JCO.2005.10.728

Clarke, T. C., Barnes, P. M., Black, L. I., Stussman, B. I., & Nahin, R. L. (2018). *Use of yoga, meditation and chiropractors among U.S. adults aged 18 and older* (NCHS Data Brief, No. 325). National Center for Health Statistics.

Clarke, T. C., Black, L. I., Stussman, B. J., Barnes, P. B., & Nahin, R. L. (2015). Trends in the use of complementary health approaches among adults: United States, 2002–2012. *National Health Statistics Reports, 79*, 1–16. https://www.ncbi.nlm.nih.gov/pmc/articles/PMC4573565/#__ffn_sectitle

Dorn, S. D., Kaptchuk, T. J., Park, J. B., Nguyen, L. T., Canenguez, K., Nam, B. H., & Lembo, A. J. (2007). A meta-analysis of the placebo response in complementary and alternative medicine trials of irritable bowel syndrome. *Neurogastroenterology & Motility, 19*(8), 630–637. https://doi.org/10.1111/j.1365-2982.2007.00937.x

Frass, M., Strassl, R. P., Friehs, H., Mullner, M., Kundi, M., & Kaye, A. D. (2012). Use and acceptance of complementary and alternative medicine among the general population and medical personnel: A systematic review. *Ochsner Journal, 12*(1), 45–56. http://www.ochsnerjournal.org/content/12/1/45.abstract

Garcés, I. C., Scarinici, I. C., & Harrison, L. (2006). An examination of sociocultural factors associated with health and health care seeking among Latina immigrants. *Journal of Immigrant Health, 8*, 377–385. https://doi.org/10.1007/s10903-006-9008-8

Gross, D. (2005). On the merits of attention-control groups. *Research in Nursing & Health, 28*, 93–94. https://doi.org/10.1002/nur.20065

Gul, R. B., & Ali, P. A. (2010). Clinical trials: The challenge of recruitment and retention of participants. *Journal of Clinical Nursing, 19*, 227–233. https://doi.org/10.1111/j.1365-2702.2009.03041.x

Hopp, D. C. (2021). *NCCIH research blog. Finding answers to questions about drug-herb interactions.* National Center for Complementary and Integrative Health. https://www.nccih.nih.gov/research/blog/finding-answers-to-questions-about-drug-herb-interactions

Institute of Medicine & Committee on the Use of Complementary and Alternative Medicine by the American Public. (2005). *Complementary and alternative medicine in the United States.* National Academies Press. https://www.ncbi.nlm.nih.gov/books/NBK83799

Jazieh, A. R., Abuelgasim, K. A., Ardah, H. I., Alkaiyat, M., & Da'ar, O. B. (2021). The trends of complementary alternative medicine use among cancer patients. *BMC Complementary Medicine and Therapies, 21*, 167. https://doi.org/10.1186/s12906-021-03338-7

Jermini, M., Dubois, J., Rondondi, P-Y., Zaman, K., Buclin, T., Csajka, C., Orcurto, A., & Rothuizen, L. E. (2019). Complementary medicine use during cancer treatment and potential herb-drug interactions from a cross-sectional study in an academic centre. *Scientific Reports, 9*, 5078. https://doi.org/10.1038/s41598-019-41532-3

Latte-Naor, S. (2019). Managing patient expectations: Integrative, not alternative. *Cancer Journal, 25*(5), 307–310. https://doi.org/10.1097/PPO.0000000000000400

Lee, J. J., & Chu, C. T. (2012). Bayesian clinical trials in action. *Statistics in Medicine, 31*(25), 2955–2972. https://doi.org/10.1002/sim.5404

Leng, M., Zhao, Y., & Wang, Z. (2020). Comparative efficacy of non-pharmacological interventions on agitation in people with dementia: A systematic review and Bayesian network meta-analysis. *International Journal of Nursing Studies, 102,* 103489. https://doi.org/10.1016/j.ijnurstu.2019.103489

Lindquist, R., Tracy, M. F., & Savik, K. (2003). Personal use of complementary and alternative therapies by critical care nurses. *Critical Care Nursing Clinics of North America, 15*(3), 393–399. https://doi.org/10.1016/S0899-5885(02)00104-1

MacPherson, H. (2004). Pragmatic clinical trials. *Complementary Therapies in Medicine, 12*(2), 136–140. https://doi.org/10.1016/j.jchf.2021.04.016

Moonaz, S. H., Bingham, C. O., Wissow, L., & Bartlett, S. J. (2015). Yoga in sedentary adults with arthritis: Effects of a randomized controlled pragmatic trial. *Journal of Rheumatology, 42*(7), 1194–1202. https://doi.org/10.3899/jrheum.141129

National Cancer Institute. (2021). *Complementary and alternative medicine.* https://www.cancer.gov/about-cancer/treatment/cam

National Center for Complementary and Integrative Health. (2019). *The NIH Almanac: National Center for Complementary and Integrative Health.* https://www.nih.gov/about-nih/what-we-do/nih-almanac/national-center-complementary-integrative-health-nccih

National Center for Complementary and Integrative Health. (2020). *Placebo effect.* https://nccih.nih.gov/health/placebo

National Center for Complementary and Integrative Health. (2021a). *Clinical trials utilizing innovative study designs to assess complementary health approaches and their integration into health care.* https://nccih.nih.gov/about/strategic-plans/2016/Clinical-Trials-Utilizing-Innovative-Study-Designs

National Center for Complementary and Integrative Health. (2021b). *Herb-drug interactions: What the science says.* https://www.nccih.nih.gov/health/providers/digest/herb-drug-interactions-science#st-johns-wort

National Center for Complementary and Integrative Health. (2021c). *Home page.* https://nccih.nih.gov

National Center for Complementary and Integrative Health. (2021d). *Know the science.* https://www.nccih.nih.gov/health/know-science

National Center for Complementary and Integrative Health. (2021e). *NCCIH clinical digest for health professionals: Know the science of complementary health approaches.* https://www.nccih.nih.gov/health/providers/digest/know-the-science-of-complementary-health-approaches

National Center for Complementary and Integrative Health. (2021f). *Natural doesn't necessarily mean safer, or better.* https://www.nccih.nih.gov/health/know-science/natural-doesnt-mean-better

National Center for Complementary and Integrative Health. (2021g). *NCCIH clinical trial funding opportunity announcements.* https://nccih.nih.gov/grants/funding/clinicaltrials

National Center for Complementary and Integrative Health. (2021h). *NCCIH strategic plan FY 2021–2025: Mapping a pathway to research on whole person health.* https://www.nccih.nih.gov/about/nccih-strategic-plan-2021-2025

Ong, C. K., Bodeker, G., Grundy, C., Burford, G., & Shein, K. (2005). *WHO global atlas of traditional, complementary, and alternative medicine.* World Health Organization. http://apps.who.int/iris/bitstream/10665/43108/1/9241562862_map.pdf

Pew Research Center. (2017). *Vast majority of Americans say benefits of childhood vaccines outweigh risks.* https://www.pewresearch.org/science/2017/02/02/americans-health-care-behaviors-and-use-of-conventional-and-alternative-medicine/

Pradham, N., Gavali, J., & Waghmare, N. (2015). WHO (World Health Organization) guidelines for standardization of herbal drugs. *International Ayurvedic Medical Journal, 3*(8), 2238–2243.

Research Council for Complementary Medicine. (2016). *Evidence and best practice*. https://www.rccm.org.uk/

Scott, R., Nahin, R., & Weber, W. (2021). Longitudinal analysis of complementary health approaches in adults aged 25–74 years from the Midlife in the U.S. Survey (MIDUS) sample. *The Journal of Alternative and Complementary Medicine, 27*(7), 550–568. https://doi.org/10.1089/acm.2020.0414

Singendonk, M., Kaspers, G. J., Naafs-Wilstra, M., Meeteren, A. S., Loeffen, J., & Vlieger, A. (2013). High prevalence of complementary and alternative medicine use in the Dutch pediatric oncology population: A multicenter survey. *European Journal of Pediatrics, 172*(1), 31–37. https://doi.org/10.1007/s00431-012-1821-6

Therapeutic Research Center. (2017). *Natural medicines professional database*. https://naturalmedicines.therapeuticresearch.com/Login.aspx

Tracy, M. F., Lindquist, R., Savik, K., Watanuki, S., Sendelbach, S., Kreitzer, M. J., & Berman, B. (2005). Use of complementary and alternative therapies: A national survey of critical care nurses. *American Journal of Critical Care, 14*(5), 404–414.

U.S. Department of Health and Human Services. (2015). *Listing of clinical trial registries*. https://www.hhs.gov/ohrp/international/clinical-trial-registries/index.html

Ventola, C. L. (2010). Current issues regarding complementary and alternative medicine (CAM) in the United States: Part 2: Regulatory and safety concerns and proposed governmental policy changes with respect to dietary supplements. *Pharmacy and Therapeutics, 35*(9), 514. https://www.ncbi.nlm.nih.gov/pmc/articles/PMC2957745/#__ffn_sectitle

World Health Organization. (2013). *WHO traditional medicine strategy: 2014–2024*. http://who.int/medicines/publications/traditional/trm_strategy14_23/en

World Health Organization. (2019). *WHO global report on traditional and complementary medicine 2019*. World Health Organization. https://www.who.int/teams/integrated-health-services/traditional-complementary-and-integrative-medicine

Zhang, L. (2011). *Use of complementary and alternative medicine (CAM) in racial, ethnic and immigrant (REI) populations: Assessing the influence of cultural heritage and access to medical care* [Doctoral dissertation]. https://conservancy.umn.edu/handle/11299/104632

Zhang, Y., Peck, K., Spalding, M., Jones, B. G., & Cook, R. L. (2012). Discrepancy between patients' use of and health providers' familiarity with CAM. *Patient Education and Counseling, 89*(3), 399–404. https://doi.org/10.1016/j.pec.2012.02.014

30

Afterword

RUTH LINDQUIST, MARGO HALM, MARY FRAN TRACY,
AND MARIAH SNYDER

This book sought to bring its readers a firm foundation on complementary therapies and nurses' contemporary use of them. The chapters provide descriptive histories of the therapies as well as their current evidence base underlying applications for many different uses in a wide range of settings. In this new edition, closer attention was paid to the use of new technologies and new applications of old technologies in the delivery of the therapies, especially distant or online delivery—particularly salient in the peri-COVID era.

In the time since the start of the COVID pandemic, the use of therapies by some sources increased. During the pandemic, the world was struck with another epidemic: an "infodemic" (Kurcer et al., 2021)—the rapid and widespread generation of accurate and inaccurate information about COVID. Facts, rumors, and fears resulted from an inability to discern the truth about COVID.

Also observed as the pandemic unfolded was a dramatic rise in Google searches for *"immune boost"* and *"immune boosting"* (Wagner et al., 2020). Herbal and dietary supplement use was noted to be high across populations around the world, for example, in Saudi Arabia and Hong Kong (Alnajrany et al., 2021; Lam et al., 2021). Other therapies were increasingly utilized such as yoga in India (Zope et al., 2021). These are only a few examples. Although the precise cause of such adoption may not be known, increased use of complementary therapies may have been related to restrictions or fear of leaving home, limitations on healthcare to urgent/emergent needs, and the upswing of technology use to deliver health information and therapies. In the wake of the widespread interest and use of therapies, the National Institutes of Health cautioned there was "no scientific evidence any of these alternative remedies can prevent or cure COVID-19" (National Center for Complementary and Integrative Health [NCCIH], 2021a).

Using technologies for delivering interventions, or providing interventions from a distance is not new. However, contemporaneous access to information is unparalleled compared to the past. New research informs us, opening up new possibilities in ways to care for individuals and populations with ever greater precision. Online dissemination of cutting-edge research findings can be also accessed almost instantaneously. Technology helps us reach even the most geographically remote places (albeit access needs to be available). Nurses and other providers can readily explore and contemplate this evidence and its applicability to their practice, with the ultimate goal of translating it into practice in a timely manner. Likewise, laypersons around the world can also access, process, and apply knowledge related to these therapies.

In the peri-COVID pandemic era, headlines around the world swelled with stories of shortages of healthcare workers—especially nurses—as well as available staffed hospital beds. From the lack of effective treatments, worldwide mortality from the virus as it swept across the globe with surges of its variants; shortages of vaccines; the crippling of supply chains; the isolation of people from family members, friends, and community interactions; lockdowns of long-term care environments; and "sheltering in", intensified the experience of being and feeling alone for many. Essential workers often faced mandated work with shortages of protective equipment. Healthcare workers and first responders continued their work on the front lines of the pandemic. Nurses were among them.

And so, interest in using complementary therapies for self-care increased among nurses and nursing students as they faced the stress of long shifts, understaffing, and shortages of personal protective equipment. In a similar vein, Dr. Janice Post-White (2018) described the work of attendees at an annual meeting of the Oncology Nursing Society. While at the conference, nursing colleagues envisioned and created a healing therapies room at the conference—a model that still exists today—where colleagues can drop in and receive caring touch, healing energy, and respite from the task of always giving:

> We taught each other skills, gave each other permission, and learned compassion for each other and ourselves. It wasn't any one therapy that empowered us, as it isn't any one therapy that heals a particular patient. It was the spirit of caring and compassion that connected us. When we accept our own humanness and vulnerability, our patients come to accept theirs, opening the way toward healing. (Post-White, 2018, p. 524)

Endless opportunities exist to contribute to a future where complementary therapies are used for optimal benefits to the health and well-being of people around the world. The internet has become a highly relevant source of updated information, connecting people around the globe. We can learn much from international perspectives on successful complementary therapies, holding possibilities yet untapped in our communities, as they are adjusted to cultural nuances in local therapy implementation. Additionally, new or newly rediscovered therapies are being studied for their potential benefits, especially for stress and anxiety. Several interesting accessible and affordable examples that appear at face value to have benefits and appeal include sauna (Haseba et al., 2016; Laukkanen et al., 2018), forest bathing (Antonelli et al., 2021; Hansen & Tocchini, 2017; Mao et al., 2017; Qing et al., 2016), and wind therapy (University of Texas at Arlington, School of Social Work, 2021).

Throughout this text, the chapter authors highlighted the cultural applications and culturally sensitive delivery of the therapies. Included in their reflections were considerations of access to therapies, tailoring therapies to individuals and cultures, as well as the affordability and evidence base of complementary therapies. Care was taken to consider the integration of the therapies with cultural beliefs and other allopathic therapies received. As a "wrap-up," this chapter takes a 10,000-foot look at the "trends" across therapies.

VIEW ACROSS THERAPIES

We believe patient-centered care is better care. We live in a multi-cultural world comprised of indigenous and transplanted peoples. Many of the therapies presented in the text can be traced back thousands of years to cultural roots. Many definitions are derived from cultures and nations outside of their contemporary use. A number of therapies have lay definitions, as well as more official governmental definitions from regulation. Many have become part of contemporary healthcare as they have crossed time, space, and cultures. The enduring presence of the therapies testified to their utility and trust among people. Both the differing origins by nations, as well as adaptations of therapies in different cultures over time have resulted in varied interventional techniques. Massage, storytelling, meditation, and yoga are good examples of therapies that have had such cultural adaptations. Complementary therapies will endure as care honors the humanity of both patients and providers. The therapies build and strengthen trust in therapeutic relationships and foster the development of connecting bridges between human beings.

EVIDENCE CONSIDERATIONS

As described in the research chapter, it is difficult to generate good evidence to support the efficacy and, therefore, use of complementary therapies. Commonly accepted designs and the "gold standard" of randomized controlled studies may not be a good not fit for the study of all mind–body therapies. There may be problems pinpointing mind–body processes and "placebo effects." The general lack of research funding for the study of complementary therapies compounds the difficulty in establishing a solid evidence foundation. And yet a large increase in the number of studies and ongoing investigations related to complementary therapies is generating data for practice. It is noted, however, that more data do not translate into more insight. Strong information workers will be needed to translate evidence into meaningful knowledge that can be applied to care. Thus, nurses have a significant role to play with the interpretation and application to practice. The NCCIH Clearinghouse provides significant information on complementary and integrative health approaches (www.nccih.nih.gov/health/nccih -clearinghouse). Despite a solid evidence base across therapies, interest, demand, and the use of complementary therapies are growing among consumers as many therapies are generally recognized as safe.

PRACTICE IMPLICATIONS

New treatments and technologies do not themselves translate into more holistic care and greater satisfaction with care. Complementary therapies, as adjuncts to allopathic medicine, can enhance comfort, reduce pain, and help individuals adjust to illness, in addition to creating and maintaining well-being. Judging from their current popularity and extensive use by people around the world, complementary therapies will enjoy a prominent role in the future of healthcare. However, all therapies are not created equal. Appropriate consideration of indication and effects—including unintended and untoward effects—and therapeutic goals and recommendations by nurses are important to their success. From an array of therapies, practitioners can select useful, accessible, and affordable therapies for individual clients and monitor the effects of selected therapies over time.

As stated by more than one author, "natural doesn't mean safe," nor does it mean effective. As we continue to learn more about the safety and efficacy of therapies with certain populations and, more specifically, with individuals' responses to therapies, the evolving knowledge base will grow stronger for various complementary therapies. Nurses who are well prepared and educated about complementary therapies can offer clients advice and assist them in accessing credible sources of information. Consider, for example, a conversation neighbor to neighbor. Hearing of a newly prescribed drug, one neighbor extorted stopping that medication as soon as possible, sitting in the sun for at least 20 minutes a day unprotected without sunglasses, or eating a certain brand of butter. This neighbor did not know that her friend had a degenerative eye condition, a significant family history of melanoma, and a family history of heart disease. Furthermore, recently, it had been determined through annual bloodwork that her vitamin D level from vitamin D3 supplements was at a toxic level. This story illustrates first and foremost, armchair opinions should not outright take the place of advice from one's primary provider or another credible source. Nurses play a key role in assisting patients to deepen health literacy about complementary approaches for safe self-care. Students are also familiar with and prepared to recommend and refer a broad range of therapies and, as a result, will develop expertise to administer selected therapies. Moreover, they will be prepared to educate and refer patients and consumers to sources of credible information concerning complementary therapies. Furthermore, it is important to seek and utilize informed sources such as the National Institutes of Health or other credible sources.

We know there is not always rigorous evidence for traditional allopathic and nursing interventions. However, just as we would not always assume allopathic interventions have only positive results or are without unintended consequences, we must carefully review the evidence available with supporting rationale, surveillance, and safety-monitoring precautions in determining when complementary therapies are used—while continuing to gather more rigorous evidence. Health professionals have a role to play in reporting adverse events, as well as unique success in therapy application. Through remote monitoring and expert systems, clinical alerts can be in place, and practitioners who are practicing at the top of their license can better help people manage their health and disease conditions at home.

CONSUMER RECOMMENDATIONS

Complementary therapies may help people across the life span—including young people—to have a greater understanding of how their bodies work and what is needed to maintain and optimize their health and vital functions. As a number of chapter authors have stated, complementary therapies, as part of self-compassion and self-care, can be taught at an early age. Lifestyle problems, such as stress, addiction, diabetes, and obesity, will be reduced through not only allopathic medicine but also its integration with complementary therapies.

As one grows chronologically and biologically, it is beneficial to have regular routine laboratory tests. Bodies change, activities change, one's exercise and dietary needs change. Exposure from one's environment is impacted by changing elements and thus has various consequences on one's health. Habits started in one phase of life may be retained long beyond their usefulness. Far too often, a well-meaning neighbor, friend, or family member may prod and encourage others in their circle to "try this" or "try that," including supplements, dietary changes, or exercise. Testimonials such as this are possibly the most unreliable source of information, although possibly the most common. The downside is such recommendations may not be needed or have no benefits (and therefore have a zero cost–benefit ratio), or the practice/recommendation may even be detrimental to one's health. Thus, regular visits to one's provider can provide much-needed individualized information particularly since changes in one's body over time or inadvertent sequential layering of dietary changes (such as vitamins and fortified foods) may result in potentially more harm than good. Well-prepared providers understand the potential benefits and harms of a broad range of therapies and the specific risk of harm of such therapies to individual clients, as well as the need to monitor the changes in the effects of therapies over time.

Consumers need to be able to easily find credible practitioners and tap their expertise in using complementary therapies; these may be identified through one's primary care provider, community resources, or online listings offering providers' quality ratings. Finding the right primary care provider is an important first step to self-care. Selecting a provider needs to be based on one's ability to trust and communicate with them about complementary therapies. It is useful to review diet, laboratory values, and supplements frequently (or at least annually) with one's provider. Interested providers can both challenge and accept self-care and lifestyle choices and, therefore, plan healthcare treatments accordingly. Looking at the strengths and weaknesses, including the cost–benefit–harm ratio is extremely crucial. Additionally, it is vitally important to consider the source of information and avoid changes in health behaviors based on well-intended (although naïve) advice as previously described.

INTEGRATING COMPLEMENTARY THERAPIES AT THE HEALTHCARE-SYSTEM LEVEL

Precision medicine, personalized medicine, genotypes and genomics, and bionic organs and limbs promise to transform medical treatment options and open the door for new uses for therapies. Therapies addressing problems associated with aging and preventing and treating chronic illnesses will be in greater demand. It is well known that hard-to-manage symptoms such as pain, anxiety, and depression are common in many acute and chronic illnesses. The focus of care moves beyond the treatment of disease to managing the symptoms affecting function and health-related quality of life. Clinical studies testing these complementary therapies for symptom management will ensure appropriate use in clinical environments.

In the future, scientific evidence underlying the use of complementary therapies will be increasingly important, in keeping with the mega-trends of value-based models and data sharing (Weber, 2016). With an eye on aligning cost outcomes and quality, the role and place of complementary therapies in healthcare will be determined. Insurers will demand evidence to justify the costs of therapies, balanced with consumer demands, needs of patients, required therapy dosage and frequency amounts, known effects, and satisfaction with care ratings. Coverage/payment for evidence-based complementary therapies and integrative approaches would ensure greater access to therapies across subpopulations and sociodemographic circumstances.

The ideal use of complementary therapies involves tapping well-selected therapies intrinsically related to the body's natural healing powers, in harmony alongside the best therapies Western medicine can offer (Dean, 2018). Complementary therapies are important components of healthcare systems being embraced in countries and continents across the globe (Lin et al., 2021). The ability to routinely receive complementary therapies and allopathic treatments in one integrated healthcare system will result in more seamless care and greater consumer satisfaction. Providers with disparate expertise will work together within the same system and share information. In such systems, patients' needs will be fully assessed, with treatments selected from a menu of options and drawn together in a plan of care with the "right" blend of allopathic and complementary therapies. The plan of care will be crafted with precision to meet the needs and preferences of patients, thereby increasing their satisfaction with care. The result of the full integration of allopathic, complementary therapies, and integrative health approaches will be a "better blend" of therapies in the delivering true patient-centered care. Precision medicine, inclusive of complementary therapies, will take individual differences and characteristics into account in the plan of care/treatment to better match the needs of the individual. Needs can be met with a range of therapies that are culturally sensitive and tailored to patient preferences—appropriate for and aligned with consumers' needs and lifestyles. Such a system should result in consumers' greater health and well-being and satisfaction with care. The integration of complementary therapies into mainstream healthcare around the globe is viewed as a win–win situation in which the best of all worlds can be enjoyed.

CLOSING REMARKS

From editing the chapters and gathering and processing information published and presented over time, a bright future is envisioned. It is a future in which complementary therapies are increasingly offered that are accessible, affordable, safe, and evidenced-based.

A look into the future is informed by the NCCIH's strategic plan, which centers on the health of the "whole person." The mission of the NCCIH (2021b) is "to determine, through rigorous scientific investigation, the fundamental science, usefulness, and safety of complementary and integrative health approaches and their roles in improving health and health care" (p. 1). To accomplish this vision, the center has set forth a strategic plan available on the center's website (NCCIH, 2021b). The strategic plan and activities will go far in identifying evidence for best practices using complementary therapies and integrative health approaches. The NCCIH framework provides a great foundation for the future of complementary therapies and integrative health approaches. What is significant about the NCCIH's strategic plan is how these objectives work together to benefit all patients, with the potential to improve their health through safe, effective, and knowledgeable use of complementary therapies. The plan calls for more evidence and builds a knowledgeable public and provider workforce to effectively evaluate and use the evidence available in practice to improve the health and well-being of individuals and communities. Evidence is needed for practitioners to recommend or prescribe therapies and for insurers to pay for this integrated care. Meeting the objectives of the strategic plan will go far in ensuring the development of best practices and improving the quality of care delivered.

Transformative "leaps" into the future—based on desires, dreams, and actions—will successfully address the myriad of problems faced in our present day. For example, well-integrated complementary approaches will aid opioid and obesity epidemics and other present or future pandemics. We can welcome the positive changes that enhance our lives and work to counter those that have the potential to harm our health.

Imagine the future with a full and robust new culture of care. A culture that is open and offers a full menu of patient-centered care grounded in a well-established evidence base and inclusive of a well-honed set of complementary therapies alongside Western allopathic therapies. A future world in which care is viewed through the lens of the patient experience and integrates the best of Western medicine, as well as available nonallopathic remedies. Imagine care informed by the best knowledge from a global perspective—care that truly has the potential to be "the best in the world"—because what is available in the world is well known *and used*. A new world exploring therapeutic options including the consideration of allopathic and nonallopathic remedies by patients and their providers, followed by evaluation of outcomes of the selected therapies and revisions made, with doses and duration of therapy closely tailored to patient need, guided by research evidence.

With the exploding increase in the use of complementary therapies, there will be new and interesting therapies explored and adopted based on evidence supporting their efficacy. Imagination aside, new information regarding health practices of immigrant groups, increased global sharing of healing practices, and the globally expressed appetite for new ways to achieve better health, effect cures, or forestall aging—all guarantee the future use of complementary therapies by nurses, healthcare providers, and the public will always be fresh and interesting. We can envision the bright future . . . now, we just need to build it. In this work, nurses have a critical role.

It is a certainty technology will evolve and be an ever-present part of daily life. The future will expand today's technological advances such as online and group visits, team delivery, artificial intelligence, virtual reality, trackers, sensors and wearables, precision medicine/personalized healthcare, genome sequencing drug development, nanotechnology, and three-dimensional-printing robotics. The future will be increasingly portable, instantaneous, detailed, and digital. More information will be available "on demand," and real-time monitoring will be widely available. We can only imagine. These changes will transform the nature of the work we do. Much of what lies ahead will be nothing like we have seen before, so it is difficult to anticipate. Decisions and actions made now will have consequences rippling forward. Therefore, decisions made affecting healthcare and the environment must be made with careful foresight and subsequent actions need clear stakeholder accountability. A preferred future with foresight can be created by nurse leaders. It "will unfold if we activate and cultivate the future consciousness that is connected to our caring practices" (Pesut, 2018, p. 531).

New findings, methods, workforce strengths, and strategies spawned by the NCCIH's Strategic Plan for 2021–2025 can continue the work to transform healthcare as we know it, as well as promote our informed use of complementary therapies. This, in addition to staying true to goals of achieving "whole-person health," will require our attention to well-coordinated care and the thoughtful bringing together conventional and complementary approaches to the benefit of the whole person (NCCIH, 2021c).

WEBSITES

- Minnesota Board of Nursing (accountability for the use of complementary therapies in practice): https://mn.gov/boards/assets/Intgrtv_Therapies_Stmt _2017_7-19_tcm21-37140.pdf
- National Center for Complementary and Integrative Health (NCCIH): www .nccih.nih.gov
- World Health Organization (WHO): www.who.int/traditional-complementary -integrative-medicine/WhoGlobalReportOnTraditionalAndComplementary Medicine2019.pdf
- American Holistic Nurses Association (AHNA): www.ahna.org
- Earl E. Bakken Center for Spirituality and Healing (CSPH): www.csh.umn .edu/

REFERENCES

AlNajrany, S. M., Asiri, Y., Sales, I., & AlRuthia, Y. (2021). The commonly utilized natural products during the COVID-19 pandemic in Saudi Arabia: A cross-sectional online survey. *International Journal of Environmental Research and Public Health, 18*, 4688. https://doi .org/10.3390/ijerph18094688

Antonelli, M., Donelli, D., Carlone, L., Maggini, V., Firenzuoli, F., & Bedeschi, E. (2021). Effects of forest bathing (shinrin-yoku) on individual well-being: An umbrella review. *International Journal of Environmental Health Research*, 1–26. https://doi.org/10.1080/09603123.2021.1919293

Dean, P. J. (2018). Complementary therapies unmask the self-healing wisdom of the body (Sidebar 31.2). In R. Lindquist, M. F. Tracy, & M. Snyder (Eds.), *Complementary and alternative therapies in nursing* (8th ed., pp. 525–526). Springer Publishing Company.

Hansen, M. M., Jones, R., & Tocchini, K. (2017). Shinrin-yoku (forest bathing) and nature therapy: A state-of-the-art review. *International Journal of Environmental Research and Public Health, 14*(8), 851. https://doi.org/10.3390/ijerph14080851

Haseba, S., Sakakima, H., Kubozono, T., Nakao, S., & Ikeda, S. (2016). Combined effects of repeated sauna therapy and exercise training on cardiac function and physical activity in patients with chronic heart failure. *Disability and Rehabilitation, 38*(5), 409–415. https://doi .org/10.3109/09638288.2015.1044032

Kurcer, M. A., Erdogan, Z., & Kardes, V. C. (2021). The effect of COVID-19 pandemic on health anxiety and cyberchondria levels of university students. *Perspectives in Psychiatric Care*, 1–9. https://doi.org/10.1111/ppc.12850

Lam, C. S., Koon, H. K., Chung, V. C. H., & Cheung, Y. T. (2021). A public survey of traditional, complementary and integrative medicine use during the COVID-19 outbreak in Hong Kong. *PLOS ONE, 16*(7), e0253890. https://doi.org/10.1371/journal.pone.0253890

Laukkanen, J. A., Laukkanen, T., & Kunutsor, S. K. (2018). Cardiovascular and other health benefits of sauna bathing: A review of the evidence. *Mayo Clinic Proceedings, 93*(8), 1111–1121. https://doi.org/10.1016/j.mayocp.2018.04.008

Lin, L. W., Ananthakrishnan, A., & Teerawatananon, Y. (2021). Evaluating traditional and complementary medicines: Where do we go from here? *International Journal of Technology Assessment in Health Care, 37*, e45, 1–6. https://doi.org/10.1017/S0266462321000179

Mao, G., Cao, Y., Wang, B., Wang, S., Chen, Z., Wang, J., Xing, W., Ren, X., Lv, X., Dong, J., Chen, S., Chen, X., Wang, G., & Yan, J. (2017). The salutary influence of forest bathing on elderly patients with chronic heart failure. *International Journal of Environmental Research and Public Health, 14*(4), 368. https://doi.org/10.3390/ijerph14040368

National Center for Complementary and Integrative Health. (2021a). *In the news: COVID-19 and "alternative" treatments.* https://www.nccih.nih.gov/health/in-the-news-covid-19-and -alternative-treatments

National Center for Complementary and Integrative Health. (2021b). *Strategic plan: FY 2021–2025. Mapping a pathway to research on whole person health.* https://files.nccih.nih.gov/nccih-strategic-plan-2021-2025.pdf

National Center for Complementary and Integrative Health. (2021c). *Building our path to whole person health.* https://www.nccih.nih.gov/about/nccih-strategic-plan-2021-2025/introduction/building-a-path-to-whole-person-health

Pesut, D. J. (2018). Create the future with foresight (Sidebar 31.5). In R. Lindquist, M. F. Tracy, & M. Snyder (Eds.), *Complementary and alternative therapies in nursing* (8th ed., pp. 530–531). Springer Publishing Company.

Post-White, J. (2018). Future of complementary therapies in healthcare: Trends, trajectories, and visions (Sidebar 31.1). In R. Lindquist, M. F. Tracy, & M. Snyder (Eds.), *Complementary and alternative therapies in nursing* (8th ed., pp. 523–524). Springer Publishing Company.

Qing, L., Kobayashi, M., Kumeda, S., Ochiai, T., Miura, T., Kagawa, T., Imai, M., Wang, Z., Otsuka, T., & Kawada, T. (2016). Effects of forest bathing on cardiovascular and metabolic parameters in middle-aged males. *Evidence-Based Complementary and Alternative Medicine, 2016,* 1–7. https://doi.org/10.1155/2016/2587381

University of Texas at Arlington, School of Social Work. (2021). *Exploring the experience of wind therapy riders during the COVID-19 pandemic.* https://www.uta.edu/academics/schools-colleges/social-work/research/windtherapy

Wagner, D. N., Marcon, A. R., & Caulfield, T. (2020). "Immune boosting" in the time of COVID: Selling immunity on Instagram. *Allergy, Asthma & Clinical Immunology, 16*(1), 1–5. https://doi.org/10.1186/s13223-020-00474-6

Weber, M. (2016). Looking ahead: The future of healthcare delivery in 2017 and beyond. *HIT Leaders and News.* https://uk.hitleaders.news/press-releases/looking-ahead-the-future-of-healthcare-delivery-in-2017-and-beyond/

Zope, S. A., Zope, R. A., Biri, G. A., & Zope, C. S. (2021). Sudarshan Kriya Yoga: A breath of hope during COVID-19 pandemic. *International Journal of Yoga, 14*(1), 18–25. https://doi.org/10.4103/ijoy.IJOY_102_20

Index

Printed in the United States
by Baker & Taylor Publisher Services

Printed in the United States
by Baker & Taylor Publisher Services